ADVANCE PRAISE FOR THE SECOND EDITION OF
THE CHICKEN HEALTH HANDBOOK

"Twenty years ago, I got my first hen and turned to *The Chicken Health Handbook* for answers. Today, Damerow's work continues to provide sound counsel. This new edition — based in solid science, detailed and comprehensive — is an accessible and practical guide for anyone who has chickens."

— Terry Golson, **founder, HenCam.com**

"A wonderful reference book filled with practical advice that any new or experienced flock owner will find beneficial."

— Dr. Susan Watkins, **Professor of Poultry Science, University of Arkansas**

"A must-have book for all chicken lovers."

— Jeff Smith, **Cackle Hatchery**

"Accurate, valuable information that can be read with ease."

— Glenn Drowns, **author of *Storey's Guide to Raising Poultry***

"When it comes to questions on chicken health, this is the book I turn to for quick reference. We have one on every desk at Stromberg's and recommend it to everyone from beginners to longtime fanciers. The extensive pictures, illustrations, and explanations in the new edition should make it required reading for anyone interested in keeping a strong flock."

— Eric Stromberg, **Stromberg's Chicks and Game Birds Unlimited**

"Widely regarded as the Patron Saint of Poultry since her 1994 edition became the chicken keeper's bible, Gail Damerow has kept her finger on the pulse of chicken management innovations, advances, and trends, bringing us this completely recalibrated, modernized *Chicken Health Handbook*. More than a guide to chicken health, this book is a call to deliberate thought and informed decision-making, concisely providing the tools necessary in chapters that read like a novel."

— Kathy Shea Mormino, **The Chicken Chick®**

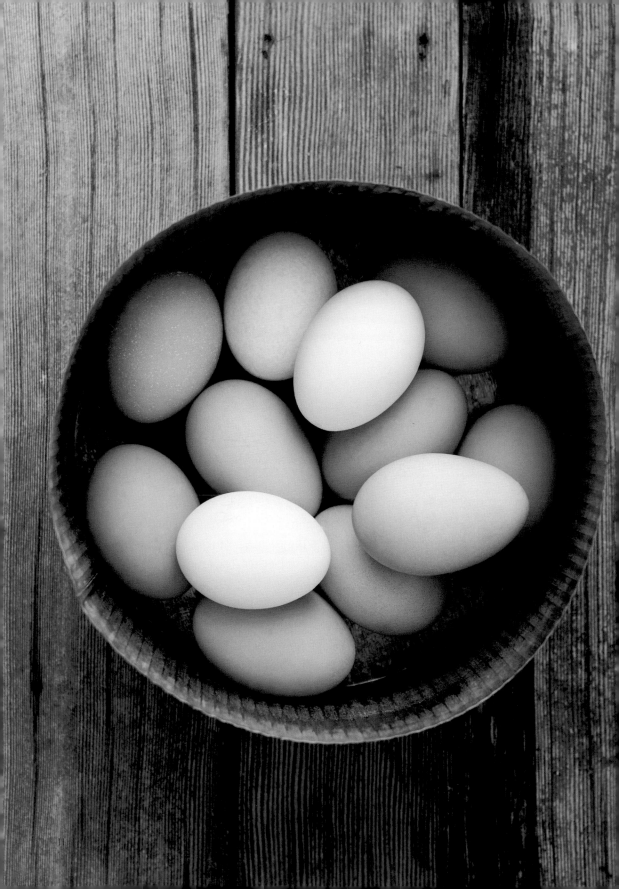

THE
CHICKEN
HEALTH
HANDBOOK
2ND EDITION

A Complete Guide to Maximizing Flock Health and Dealing with Disease

GAIL DAMEROW

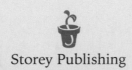

Storey Publishing

The mission of Storey Publishing is to serve our customers by publishing practical information that encourages personal independence in harmony with the environment.

EDITED BY Deb Burns
ART DIRECTION AND BOOK DESIGN BY Michaela Jebb
PRODUCTION DESIGN BY Liseann Karandisecky
INDEXED BY Samantha Miller

COVER PHOTOGRAPHY BY © Konstantin Petkov/iStockphoto.com
COVER ILLUSTRATIONS BY © Bethany Caskey

INTERIOR PHOTOGRAPHY BY © Elizabeth Cecil, ii, 412; © Elsbeth Upton, 333 (right); © Gail Damerow, 37, 40, 56, 83, 118, 124, 189, 295, 321, 333 (left and center); © Konstantin Petkov/iStockphoto.com, viii; © Krys Bailey/Alamy, 159
INTERIOR ILLUSTRATIONS BY © Bethany Caskey, except pages 5, 166, and 167 by © Elayne Sears

Storey Publishing
210 MASS MoCA Way
North Adams, MA 01247
www.storey.com

Printed in China by R.R. Donnelley
10 9 8 7 6 5

Library of Congress Cataloging-in-Publication

Names: Damerow, Gail, author.
Title: The chicken health handbook : a complete guide to maximizing flock health and dealing with disease / Gail Damerow.
Description: 2nd edition. | North Adams, MA : Storey Publishing, [2015] | Includes index.
Identifiers: LCCN 2015035875| ISBN 9781612120133 (pbk. : alk. paper) | ISBN 9781603428583 (ebook) | ISBN 9781612124797 (hardcover : alk. paper)
Subjects: LCSH: Chickens—Diseases. | Chickens—Health. | Chickens—Parasites.
Classification: LCC SF995 .D33 2015 | DDC 636.5/0896— dc23 LC record available at http://lccn.loc.gov/2015035875

Contents

Acknowledgments

Numerous knowledgeable specialists took time out of their busy schedules to help bring this edition up to date (any errors that remain are entirely my own). Thanks go to H. John Barnes, DVM, PhD, North Carolina State University (fungi); Paul Bukaveckas, PhD, Virginia Commonwealth University (algae); Gary Butcher, DVM, PhD, University of Florida (parasites); Ron Kean, poultry specialist, University of Wisconsin (small flock issues); G. Lynne Luna, DVM, Banfield Pet Hospital, Eugene, Oregon (diseases of backyard chickens); Larry L. McDougald, PhD, University of Georgia (parasites); Richard D. Miles, professor emeritus, University of Florida (nutrition); Eugene S. Morton, PhD, York University (technical guidance); Beth A. Valentine, DVM, PhD, Oregon State University (pathology); Susan E. Watkins, PhD, University of Arkansas (small flock issues). And, of course, to my wonderful husband, Allan Damerow, who patiently suffered through daily dialogs on the nature of chicken wellness.

Preface

A LOT HAS HAPPENED since the release of the first edition of this book. New technologies have changed the way we view the well-being of chickens, making us more certain of some things and less certain of others. The Internet has given us better access to academic research and to rapid communication with specialists.

More people than ever before raise chickens, providing unique insights due to their diverse educational and professional backgrounds. Online poultry forums have given us a clearer consensus on the issues of backyard flocks compared to problems of industrially produced chickens, or ailments induced and studied under laboratory conditions.

More small-animal veterinarians are accepting chickens as patients — indeed, many of them have chickens of their own — and today's chicken keepers are more inclined than in the past to seek veterinary care. And not least of all, I have had two decades of additional experience keeping my own chickens healthy.

So what started out as a simple update to the first edition has turned into a complete revision. As I reviewed where to start, I first decided to expand the chapter on incubation and brooding, which ended up becoming an entirely new and separate book, *Hatching & Brooding Your Own Chicks,* issued by Storey Publishing.

I then added a new chapter on metabolic disorders and split the old chapter on infectious diseases into three separate chapters, respectively, on bacterial diseases, fungi, and viruses. These changes provided more room to expand on emerging new diseases, our current understanding of old diseases, and how any disease gets a foothold in a backyard flock. By understanding how disease-causing organisms work, we have a much better chance to prevent them.

Critics of the first edition of this book took exception whenever I suggested that culling (euthanizing a hopelessly sick chicken) is sometimes the best option. I understand that urban and suburban flocks are smaller than rural flocks of the past, and that accordingly each chicken becomes a beloved family pet, resulting in the perspective that "culling is not an option." However, isn't allowing a chicken to suffer, or to spread an incurable disease to other chickens, a worse option?

To minimize the likelihood that you will ever reach that point, this edition focuses on a preventive approach and on methods of natural immunity enhancement. A chicken with a strong immune system is better able to keep itself healthy and less in need of being treated for one ailment after another.

Make no mistake, however: the longer you keep chickens, and the more chickens you have at one time, the more likely you are sooner or later to encounter problems. But you'll be less likely to find yourself dealing repeatedly with the same issues, *if* you learn how to manage or avoid each one the first time around.

This book is called *The Chicken Health Handbook* because its focus is on keeping your chickens healthy. By applying vigilance, knowledge, and common sense, you'll find it's not a difficult mission. Indeed, a few years ago the United States Department of Agriculture issued a report on small flock health and management that stated, "Owners of backyard flocks report very few health problems."

Here's to "very few health problems" in your own backyard flock!

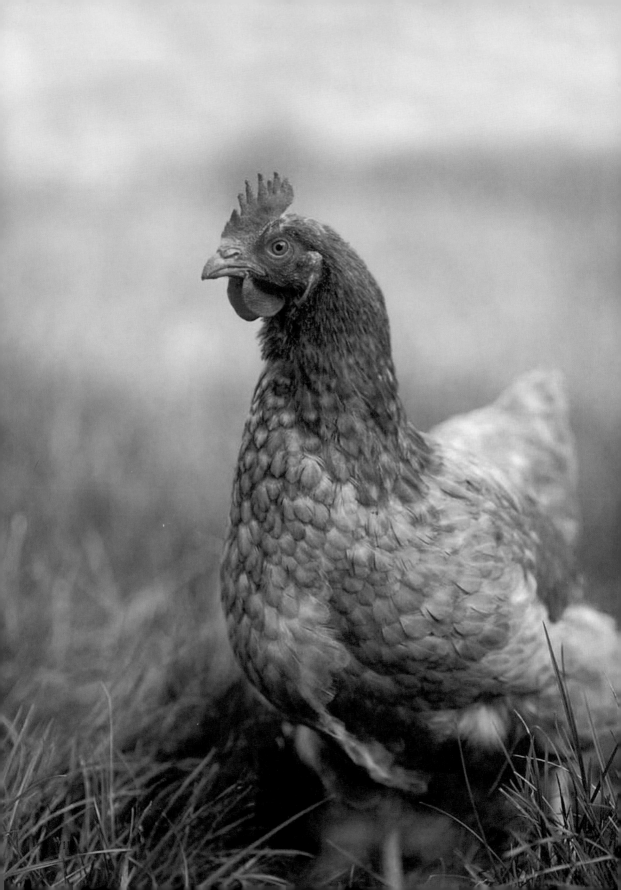

CHAPTER 1

Keeping Chickens Healthy

Healthy chickens are a joy to behold. They are bright-eyed, alert, curious, and lively as they chase butterflies or scratch in the soil and peck at a bug, a blade of grass, or a seed of grain — all the while vocalizing over their accomplishments. They regularly visit the feeder and drinker, take dust baths, groom their glossy feathers, stretch out to enjoy the warm sun, and take frequent catnaps. At dusk they flock inside to settle on the roost side by side for the night.

Even while a chick is growing within the egg, it has the beginnings of an active immune system that continues to develop after the chick hatches. Along with other natural defenses, the chicken's strong immune system helps it resist disease as long as the bird remains in a wholesome environment: one that is clean, free of hazards, and safe from predators; one that provides adequate space, light, ventilation, fresh water, and suitable feed; and one that protects the flock from unnecessary stress.

Speaking of Disease

biosecurity. Collective disease-prevention management practices

contagious. Readily transmitted from one individual or flock to another

fomite. Any inanimate object on which pathogens may be transported from one place to another

infectious. Capable of invading and multiplying in the living tissue of another organism, thus causing disease

opportunist. A pathogen that is noninfectious to a healthy individual but causes infection in one with reduced immunity

pathogen. A microorganism that causes infection, disease, or death by living on or in another organism as a parasite. Commonly called a germ

pathogenic. Capable of causing disease

primary pathogen. A pathogen that is capable of infecting an individual with a healthy immune system

The Nature of Disease

Disease is a departure from health, and it includes any condition that impairs normal body functions. Disease results from a combination of indirect causes that reduce resistance — in other words, stress in one form or another — and direct causes that produce the actual disease.

Direct causes of disease may be divided into two categories: infectious and noninfectious. Noninfectious diseases result from things other than an invading organism, such as nutritional problems (deficiency or excess), poisons, traumatic injury, or even excessive stress.

Infectious diseases result from invasion of the body by another living organism — bacteria, viruses, fungi, protozoa, and a variety of internal and external parasites. Some are always present but cause disease only under certain circumstances, such as when a chicken's resistance is weakened because of stress. Such microbes are called opportunists.

A few microbes produce disease wherever they occur. They are commonly known as germs, although technically they are pathogens and are described as being pathogenic. Variations in virulence among different strains of a specific pathogen can cause the same disease to appear in different degrees of severity or even in different forms altogether.

Reservoirs of Infection

Regardless of a disease's cause, before you can effectively control it, you need to know how the disease is introduced into a flock and how it spreads among the chickens. Diseases are introduced from reservoirs of infection, which can be any source or site where disease-causing organisms survive or multiply and from which they may be transferred to a susceptible host — in this case, a chicken. A reservoir of infection may or may not be another living being.

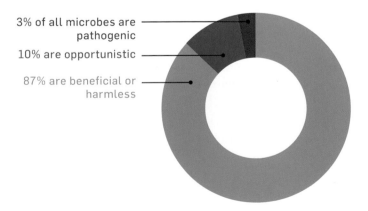

3% of all microbes are pathogenic

10% are opportunistic

87% are beneficial or harmless

A chicken can serve as its own reservoir of infection, as occurs when a disease is caused by a microbe that normally lives on or in a chicken's body without causing disease. Examples are streptococci and *Pasteurella* bacteria, both of which infect a chicken after its resistance has been weakened by some other cause. A sick chicken is, of course, a reservoir of infection, as is also an infected dead chicken that is pecked by other hens.

Some disease-causing organisms, such as the infectious bronchitis virus, are species specific to chickens, meaning they affect only chickens and no other type of animal. Other diseases may be shared by more than one species of poultry. Sometimes microbes that are harmless to one species can be devastating to chickens. One such microbe is the Marek's disease virus, which is common and harmless in turkeys but potentially deadly to chickens.

A reservoir of infectious microbes that affect chickens need not be some type of poultry. It might be a wild bird, or an exotic or cage bird kept as a household pet. Or it might not be a bird at all. Other pets, livestock, or rodents and other wild animals, even humans, can be reservoirs of an infectious disease that affects chickens. *Salmonella* bacteria is an example of a microbe that infects a wide variety of vertebrates, including humans. A few infectious organisms that parasitize chickens spend part of their life cycles living in arthropods — fleas, mites, ticks, lice, and mosquitoes — and can spread disease to chickens through those creatures' bites.

Inanimate reservoirs of infection are nonliving objects that harbor disease-causing microbes. Among them are accumulated droppings, litter, soil, dust, and feed or water in which an accumulation of pathogens survives or thrives.

When a chicken falls ill, knowing where the disease came from — the reservoir of infection — can help you control the disease and prevent future occurrences. You also need to know how the pathogen got from the reservoir of infection into the chicken.

CARRIERS

Carriers are major reservoirs of infection for many chicken diseases. A carrier is an individual that appears to be healthy even though its body harbors a pathogenic organism. A carrier may be a chicken that has recovered from a disease, or a chicken that never showed any signs of having been infected.

Either way, these stealth carriers are especially dangerous for backyard flocks, because they go around infecting other chickens without offering much indication that they might be the cause. A potential clue is that other chickens fall ill while the carrier remains apparently healthy.

The older a chicken is, the more exposure it has to disease-causing organisms in the environment, and the more likely it is to be a carrier of one disease or another. Since growing and adult chickens carry levels of microbes to which chicks and young birds have not yet developed resistance, mixing together chickens of various ages from various sources is always a hazardous practice.

Disease Happens

The vast majority of microbes are either harmless or actually beneficial. Beneficial microbes may live either on a chicken's skin or within its body, aiding digestion and/or enhancing the bird's immunity by fending off pathogenic microbes, a process known as competitive exclusion. (For more on this subject, see Probiotics and Prebiotics, page 378.)

Given the opportunity, however, some organisms that normally live on or in a healthy chicken can multiply to the point that they become harmful. Such an opportunity most commonly occurs in a chicken with an immune system that has been somehow weakened, perhaps by poor nutrition, a parasite overload, or excessive stress.

In contrast to these opportunistic organisms, other disease-causing organisms are primary pathogens. These organisms are not commonly found in the typical poultry environment, but when they arise from a reservoir of infection, they are capable of infecting a chicken with a perfectly healthy immune system.

Such an organism enters the chicken by being inhaled into the bird's respiratory system or taken into its digestive system with feed or water. Or the pathogen might be on or burrow into the chicken's skin, scales, or feathers, or invade the body through an open wound.

How Diseases Spread

Once introduced into an individual chicken, a disease may or may not be capable of spreading to other chickens. A disease that is caused by a primary pathogen is more likely to be contagious than one caused by an opportunistic organism. Brooder pneumonia, for example, is caused by opportunistic fungi and does not spread from chick to chick, while ringworm is caused by a primary pathogen and is contagious.

A contagious disease can spread either vertically or horizontally. Vertical transmission always involves direct contact between the infected chicken and the one that becomes infected. Horizontally transmitted diseases may be spread by either direct or indirect contact.

Diseases Spread by Carriers

DISEASE	CAUSE	PREVALENCE
Air sac disease	Bacteria	Common
Arizonosis	Bacteria	Rare
Avian influenza	Virus	Rare
Blackhead	Protozoa	Rare
Campylobacteriosis	Bacteria	Uncommon
Canker	Protozoa	Uncommon
Chlamydiosis	Bacteria	Rare
Chronic respiratory disease	Bacteria	Common
Erysipelas	Bacteria	Rare
Fowl cholera	Bacteria	Sporadic
Fowl typhoid	Bacteria	Rare
Infectious bronchitis	Virus	Common
Infectious coryza	Bacteria	Common
Infectious synovitis	Bacteria	Uncommon
Laryngotracheitis	Virus	Common
Listeriosis	Bacteria	Rare
Lymphoid leukosis	Virus	Common
Marek's disease	Virus	Common
Parasites	Worms	Common
Paratyphoid	Bacteria	Common
Pullorum	Bacteria	Rare
Ulcerative enteritis	Bacteria	Uncommon

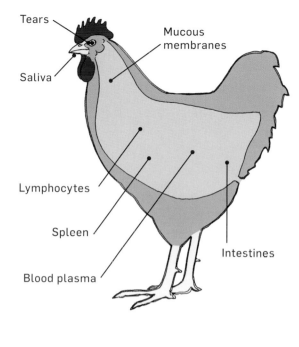

Tears
Mucous membranes
Saliva
Lymphocytes
Spleen
Intestines
Blood plasma

Where microbes are normally found on and in a healthy chicken

Vertical transmission is the spread of a disease from an infected hen to her eggs, and subsequently to chicks that hatch from the infected eggs. Some viruses can be vertically transmitted to chicks from an infected cock through the semen that fertilizes a healthy hen's eggs.

Horizontal transmission is the spread of a disease from one chicken to another by means other than from an infected breeder to offspring through eggs that hatch. Horizontally transmitted diseases don't necessarily require direct contact between a healthy chicken and a sick one.

DIRECT AND INDIRECT CONTACT

Direct contact occurs when an infected bird and a susceptible bird mate with, peck, or preen one another. Diseases that spread through contact with the skin of an infected bird include pox and influenza (caused by viruses) and staphylococcal and streptococcal infections (caused by opportunistic bacteria). Staph and strep infections also spread through mucus-to-mucus contact during mating.

Indirect contact occurs when pathogens are mechanically transported from a reservoir of infection to a chicken that becomes infected. As with reservoirs of infection, modes of transportation can be either animate or inanimate. However, here the animal or object doing the transporting is not itself the original source of infection but is merely giving the pathogen a ride from one place to another. Logically enough, an object that gives a pathogen a lift is called a vehicle.

VEHICLES OF TRANSMISSION

Animate vehicles of transmission are living beings, which might be wild birds, rodents, household pets, or other animals that transport pathogens on their feet, feathers, or fur (as distinct from diseased animals that are reservoirs of infection, spreading disease through their saliva or droppings). Flies and other arthropods can transport pathogens on their feet or bodies (as distinct from infected arthropods that spread disease by injecting contaminated saliva). Humans can transport pathogens on their clothing, shoes, hair, or hands when they visit each other's flocks, travel from flock to flock to inspect or vaccinate, make deliveries, or attend a poultry show.

Inanimate vehicles of transmission are nonliving objects on which pathogens are transported from one place to another. They include shed skin, feathers, droppings, broken eggs, and

Vertical Transmission

Infected cock or hen

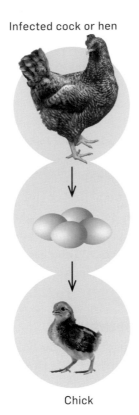

Chick

Horizontal Transmission

DIRECT CONTACT

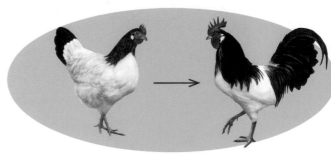

Infected cock or hen   Susceptible cock or hen

INDIRECT CONTACT

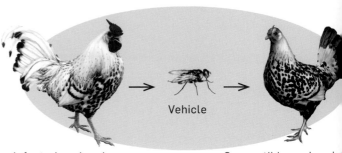

Vehicle

Infected cock or hen   Susceptible cock or h

other debris from infected birds. These bodily discharges can be transported to healthy chickens in contaminated feed or water. They might also be transported by air, which wafts dust, fluff, fine bits of dried droppings, and droplets of respiratory moisture expelled by breathing, sneezing, or coughing. Luckily, most airborne infections don't spread far.

A common vehicle is a single needle used for flockwide vaccination or blood sampling of both infected and susceptible birds. Reused items, such as egg cartons, feeders, drinkers, and tires (of a car, truck, tractor, mower, or wheelbarrow), are other objects to which body discharges containing pathogens may cling and be transported.

In veterinary jargon any inanimate object on which a pathogen hitches a ride is called a fomite, from the Latin word *fomes*, meaning tinder. A pathogen can travel on a fomite for hundreds of miles before setting off a new disease outbreak.

Biosecurity

Biosecurity encompasses all precautions you take to protect your flock from infectious diseases. The fewer precautions you take, the greater the risk that sooner or later a disease will affect your chickens.

On the other hand, no set of biosecurity measures, no matter how strict, is 100 percent foolproof in preventing disease. The best you can do to protect your flock is to follow a well-thought-out program of interrelated measures that are grounded in old-fashioned common sense. Your biosecurity program should include the following measures:

- Start with healthy chickens.

- Feed them a balanced ration (discussed in the next chapter, in Chicken Feed, page 37).

- Maintain a flock history.

- Provide a sound environment.

- Routinely clean their housing.

- Disinfect as necessary.

- Keep a closed flock, or quarantine newcomers.

- Exclude wild birds.

- Minimize stress.

- Medicate only as necessary.

Acquire Healthy Chickens

Maintaining a healthy flock is difficult unless you start out with healthy chickens. The best way to make sure new birds are healthy is to purchase locally, so you can see whether or not they come from a healthful environment. You can then ask the seller, eye to eye, about the birds' ages and health history, and you can see for yourself if any of the seller's birds show signs of diseases that might be carried by the birds you plan to buy.

You'll have the least chance of getting diseased birds if you start with newly hatched chicks. The older the bird, the more disease problems it has been exposed to. If you do purchase older chickens, take your time inspecting them. Make sure they have glossy plumage, look perky and active, and don't show any signs of stress behavior (see Stress Management, page 23).

Flocks and hatcheries enrolled in the National Poultry Improvement Plan are certified to be free of several serious infectious diseases (see NPIP, next page). Unfortunately, you may not find a member who has the kind of birds you want.

Don't buy any chicken unless you are completely satisfied with its background in terms of genetics, management, sanitation, and health history. Above all, avoid chicks or grown chickens from live-bird auctions, flea markets, wheeler-dealers, traders, uncertified hatcheries, and any other source where chickens are brought together from far-flung places.

The National Poultry Improvement Plan (NPIP) is a nationwide collaboration between state and federal departments of agriculture to certify member flocks as being free of the following diseases:

- **Avian influenza** — a potentially serious viral infection of chickens that can also infect humans

- **Chronic respiratory disease** — and other infections caused by pathogenic species of mycoplasma bacteria

- **Fowl typhoid** — an egg-transmitted bacterial disease that kills both baby chicks and mature chickens

- **Pullorum** — an egg-transmitted bacterial disease that kills baby chicks, as well as hatchlings of many other poultry species

- ***Salmonella enterica*** — an egg-transmitted bacterial disease of poultry that can affect humans who eat contaminated eggs

An online keyword search for NPIP will yield detailed information on the program, including a directory of certified hatcheries and flocks.

Keep a Flock History

A flock history is essentially a diary that documents anything and everything pertaining to your flock. Start it the moment you acquire your first chickens, noting the date (or date of hatch — if you purchase by mail, it will be on the shipping carton), source, strain (if known), anything the seller tells you about the birds and their history, and any health certificates that come with them.

Document your feed source(s), feeding and management practices, and any changes you make as you go along, including vaccinations you give and medications you use. Write things down as they occur, rather than trusting your memory to reconstruct events should you later need the information to help trace a health problem.

You don't need to make elaborate notes. In most cases, the date, along with a few key words, should be sufficient. The Flock History table on page 326 lists some of the information that would be vital should your chickens come down with an infectious disease.

A Sound Environment

The way you house your chickens can influence their continuing state of health. Most poultry housing falls into one of the following categories:

- Cage confinement — favored for show birds and pedigreed breeders

- Confinement housing — favored for fast-growing broilers, breeder flocks, and floor-managed layers

- Range confinement — favored for pasture-raised broilers and sometimes layers

- Free range — favored for laying flocks where sufficient forage is available

- Coop and yard — the most common method used for urban and suburban flocks, and others where space is limited

Chickens raised on an industrial scale are confined entirely indoors for several reasons, among them that lighting can be strictly controlled, air can be filtered, water systems can be easily medicated, and diseases that are spread by flying insects and wild birds can be more effectively excluded. If there is a major problem, the manager will remove all the chickens, clean and disinfect the facilities, and then bring in an entirely new flock.

While confined flocks are protected from some diseases, as a trade-off they incur other health issues due to lack of sunshine, fresh air, and activity. In addition, if a contagious disease does manage to get into their crowded environment, it spreads like wildfire.

Backyard chickens typically have more space to roam, as well as having access to fresh air and sunshine. They not only develop stronger immune systems, but pathogens that might wander in are more likely to get diluted by air and space.

By far the most common method of housing backyard chickens is in a coop constructed in a fixed location, with a fenced run attached. The challenge in keeping chickens healthy in such a situation is that microbe and parasite populations accumulate over years of constant use. Therefore, the single most important feature of any chicken facility is ease of cleaning. If cleanup is a hassle, you won't do it as often as you ought, and your chickens will suffer for it.

FLOORS

A coop's flooring influences its ease of cleaning. Several different types of flooring are common in backyard coops.

A dirt floor is simple and cheap, and it keeps birds cool in warm weather. Its disadvantages are that it's colder in winter, does not exclude burrowing rodents, and cannot be effectively sanitized.

A wood floor invariably has cracks that get packed with filth, and most are too close to the ground, providing a hiding place that invites invasion by rodents. (For more on rodents, see Rodent Control, page 291.)

Sheet linoleum covering a wood floor is a popular option in small and suburban coops because it's easier to clean than plain wood. The chief disadvantages are that it may not hold up under repeated cleanings, and bored chickens may take a notion to peck it to pieces. (For potential toxic issues, see Vinyl Flooring, page 312.)

A droppings pit fashioned from wooden slats or welded wire covering a boxlike pit may be set up directly beneath the nighttime roost, where most poop accumulates, or it can cover the entire coop floor. It has the advantage that poop will fall through, where chickens can't pick in it. The pit must be periodically cleaned out before the accumulated droppings reach the slats or wire.

A droppings board is a smooth shelflike surface suspended beneath nighttime roosts. The collection of overnight poop is then scraped off each morning. The disadvantage is that cleaning the board is a daily chore. The advantage is that you will become well acquainted with your chickens' droppings and can readily detect any changes in appearance or odor. For more information on examining droppings, see Intestinal Disorders, pages 331 to 335.

Concrete, when well finished, is the most expensive flooring, but it requires minimal repair and upkeep, is easy to clean, and discourages rodents and other burrowing predators.

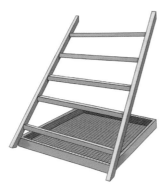

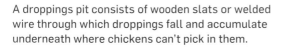

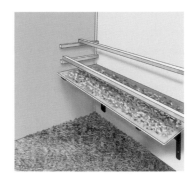

A droppings pit consists of wooden slats or welded wire through which droppings fall and accumulate underneath where chickens can't pick in them.

A droppings board is a smooth, wide shelf installed underneath nighttime roosts, where droppings accumulate and are scraped off each morning.

FLOOR SPACE

Crowded conditions get filthy fast, reduce the flow of fresh air, and cause stress — all inducements to disease. When building a new chicken coop, the trick is to figure out how much space is adequate for the number of chickens you want plus their feeders, drinkers, roosts, nest boxes, and doorways, all arranged to allow the chicken keeper access for easy maintenance. Despite all best intentions, most chicken coops end up being too small. One of the main reasons is that coop designers forget to allow sufficient floor space for all the necessary fixtures.

Feeders and drinkers. When planning a new coop, figure 1 square foot for each feeder and each drinker. If your climate turns hot in the summer, allow space for an extra drinker to make sure your chickens don't run out of water. If you have a big enough flock to accommodate more than one rooster, minimize territorial disputes by providing one feeder and one drinker for each rooster — spaced well apart — around which he can gather his harem of hens without conflict.

Nest boxes. Furnish one nest box per four to five hens and allow 1 square foot per nest box. If the nests are stacked in two rows, one on top of the other, allow 1 square foot (0.1 sq m) per lower row. For instance, for two nests stacked on top of two nests, allow a total of 2 square feet; for three on top of three, allow 3 square feet. Nests that are constructed on the outside of the coop do not require additional floor space.

Roosts. Allow at least 8 inches (20 cm) of roosting space per bird. If your roost is built on upright braces that rest on the floor, add 1 square foot (0.1 sq m) per brace that touches the floor. A smaller coop housing just a few chickens may manage with a roost that's attached to the walls and therefore doesn't require additional floor space.

Doors. For each people-size door that swings inward, allow 3 square feet (0.3 sq m). A door that swings outward does not require extra floor space, and neither does a pophole doorway.

Square footage per chicken. For each mature chicken allow the square footage indicated in the table on page 12. If your final calculation doesn't handily accommodate dimensional lumber, round upward — a slightly larger than needed coop is always better than one that's slightly too small.

LITTER MANAGEMENT

Litter covering the floor absorbs droppings and moisture expelled by the flock. For chicks, use 3 inches (75 mm) or more of clean litter that's absorbent, nontoxic, and free of mold, and has particles too large to be eaten. For adult birds, litter should be at least 8 inches (20 cm) deep.

A variety of different litter options is available. Dry pine shavings make excellent litter. Hardwood shavings, on the other hand, should be avoided because they tend to harbor molds that cause the respiratory disease aspergillosis. Cedar shavings, as well as pine that hasn't been thoroughly dried, release toxic phenol fumes that can cause respiratory distress and therefore should not be used in confined spaces such as nest boxes or brooders.

Whether you remove and replace the litter once a week, once a month, or once a year will depend on the type of litter you use, how many chickens you have, and how big the coop is relative to flock size. The important thing is to maintain the litter so it remains fluffy and absorbent, not damp, packed, or smelly. Frequently raking the surface and sprinkling a little fresh litter on top is often all that's needed for the bedding to keep doing its job.

Between thorough cleanings, remove and replace any litter that becomes packed or moist. Litter tends to pack at pophole openings and around feeders and can become damp at pophole openings (if rain can blow in) and around drinkers. Moist litter favors the growth of molds (such as those causing aspergillosis) and bacteria (that produce ammonia and other unpleasant gases), and aids the survival of viruses, protozoa (such as those causing coccidiosis), and nematodes (worms).

As necessary, but at least once a year, empty your coop, clean out and replace all the litter, and scrape droppings from the perches and walls (see Keep It Clean, page 16). Fall is the best time for this chore, since it gives your chickens fresh litter at the start of winter, when bad weather keeps them indoors much of the time. Compost the used litter, or spread it on soil where your chickens will not range for at least 1 year.

VENTILATION

Fresh air dilutes the population of microbes, especially those that cause airborne diseases. Good ventilation keeps air in motion without causing drafty conditions and removes suspended dust and moisture. Moisture tends to be particularly high in a chicken house because birds breathe rapidly, thereby using more air in proportion to their size than any other animal. Other important benefits of good ventilation are to prevent the buildup of ammonia fumes and to avoid frostbitten combs and wattles in winter.

Providing an adequate flow of fresh air may require a fan to move out stale air and bring in fresh air. Fans are sold according to how many cubic feet of air they move per minute (cfm). A good rule of thumb is to get a fan that provides 5 cfm per bird.

A fan designed for use in your home won't last long in the dust and humidity generated in the normal chicken shelter. To find a fan

Let's say you plan to have six Plymouth Rock hens. Rocks are midweight chickens, so allow 21 square feet (6 × 3.5) for the birds. You'll have one feeder (1 square foot), one drinker (1 square foot), and two nests, stacked one on top of the other (1 square foot). Your door will swing outward (no floor space). You need only 4 feet (120 cm) of roost, which therefore could be attached to the walls (no floor space). Your total required floor space is 24 square feet, so your coop could be, for instance, 6 feet by 4 feet.

As another example, you plan to have 18 Araucanas, a light breed. The chickens will need 54 square feet (18 × 3). You plan to have one large hanging feeder (1 square foot) and two drinkers (2 square feet). You'll need 12 feet of roosting space, which could consist of three 4-foot horizontals on two vertical braces (2 square feet), plus four stacked nest boxes (2 square feet) and a door that swings inward

(3 square feet). The total is 64 square feet, or a coop measuring 8 feet by 8 feet.

Use the same method to determine how many chickens can be comfortably housed in an existing building. Let's say the building is 75 square feet, the people door swings outward (no floor space required), and you plan to add nest boxes on the outside wall (no floor space required). You plan to have one feeder (1 square foot), two drinkers (2 square feet), and a roost with two upright braces (2 square feet) for a total of 5 square feet for fixtures. The floor space available for chickens is therefore 70 square feet (75 – 5). You want Rhode Island Reds, a midweight breed requiring 3.5 square feet per chicken, so the most chickens you should house in your retrofitted coop is 20 (70 ÷ 3.5).

Sizing a Chicken Coop
(PER FIXTURE)

FIXTURE	SPACE PER FIXTURE
Feeder	1 sq ft
Drinker	1 sq ft
Roost Brace	1 sq ft
Nest	1 sq ft
Door	3 sq ft

Metric conversion: 1 square foot = 930 square centimeters

Sizing a Chicken Coop
(PER CHICKEN)

BREED	SPACE PER BIRD
Heavy	4 sq ft
Midweight	3.5 sq ft
Light	3 sq ft
Bantam	2 sq ft

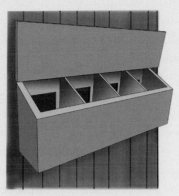

— no floor space —

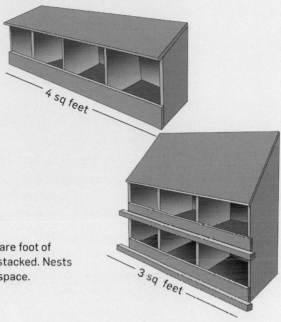

4 sq feet

3 sq feet

Allow one nest box per four to five hens, and 1 square foot of floor space per nest box; half that if the nests are stacked. Nests constructed outside the coop do not take up floor space.

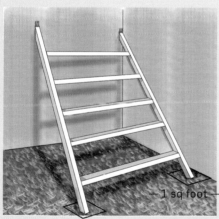

— 1 sq foot —

— 1 sq foot —

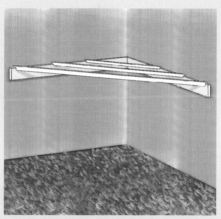

— no floor space —

Allow 8 inches (20 cm) of roost space per chicken, and 1 square foot of floor space for each vertical brace. A roost attached entirely to the wall does not take up floor space.

suitable for agricultural use, visit a farm store or rural-oriented builder's supply, or do an Internet keyword search for "barn fan" or "agricultural fan."

THE CHICKEN YARD

A fenced yard gives chickens a safe place to get the sunshine, fresh air, and exercise they need to remain healthy. A nice spacious area provides 8 to 10 square feet (0.75 to 1.0 sq m) per chicken. If your soil is neither sandy nor gravelly enough to provide good drainage, site your yard at the top of a hill or on a slope, where puddles won't accumulate when it rains. A south-facing slope, open to full sunlight, dries fastest after a rain.

As many advantages as a fenced yard offers, it has one big disadvantage — chickens can quickly destroy the vegetation by pecking at it, scratching it up, pulling it up, and covering it with droppings. The smaller the yard, the quicker it will turn to either hardpan or mud, depending on your climate.

Where space for a yard is truly limited, and you have only a few pet chickens, one way to avoid the problem is to level the yard area and cover it with several inches of clean sand. Go over the sand every day with a grass rake to smooth out dusting holes and remove droppings and other debris.

The larger your yard, the better chance you'll have of maintaining some vegetation in it. Since chickens are most active near their shelter, denuding will start around the entrance and work progressively outward. The best way to cope with this problem is to fence off part of the yard and let the chickens into only one section for several weeks or months before letting them into the next section. If you have enough space, you might establish two or more yards with a separate pophole door into each.

Keeping the chickens out of each yard long enough for vegetation to regrow reduces the concentration of pathogens and parasites. If this system is to work, the chickens must stay out of any resting yard(s), which means no flying over or ducking under fences. How often to rotate the flock from one yard to another depends on how fast the vegetation is destroyed and how long it takes to reestablish, which in turn depends on such things as the type of vegetation, your climate, the number of chickens, and the size of the yard.

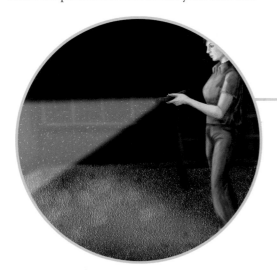

To tell if your coop would benefit from a fan, stir up dust by scuffing your foot in the litter. Wait 5 minutes for the dust to settle. Then look at a light beam coming through a window, or use the beam of a strong flashlight to check the air. If dust is still hanging in the air, the coop is not adequately ventilated.

AMMONIA CHECK

Ammonia is a pungent-smelling gas released by bacteria that decompose manure. It not only smells bad and can be a health hazard for chickens and their keeper, but it is also an indication that nitrogen is literally evaporating — not a good thing if you count on using composted litter to fertilize your garden.

High levels of ammonia in the coop's air can discourage chickens from eating, affecting the growth rate of young birds and the production of laying hens. Ammonia gas dissolves in fluid around the eyes, causing irritation, inflammation, and blindness. A chicken that can't see to find sufficient feed and water may die. Even if affected chickens don't die from ammonia blindness, they may contract (and die from) a respiratory infection caused by pathogenic bacteria entering through membranes in the upper respiratory tract that have been damaged by inhaled ammonia fumes.

Signs of ammonia-induced conjunctivitis are rubbing the eyes, reluctance to move, and staying away from sunlight. High levels of ammonia can also damage the mucous membranes of a bird's respiratory tract, allowing bacteria, dust, and viruses to travel farther down the tract to cause disease.

Before the ammonia level is concentrated enough to cause conjunctivitis or respiratory damage to chickens, it is concentrated enough to be detected by the human sense of smell. To check the ammonia level in your coop, squat or bend down until your head is 1 foot (30 cm) above the litter, or about the height of a chicken's head. Breathe normally for a moment or two. If your eyes, nose, or throat burn, the ammonia level is too high for your birds — refresh litter to decrease litter moisture, and improve ventilation. Once the condition is corrected, a chicken's cells that were damaged by ammonia fumes should repair themselves within a couple of weeks.

The time-honored practice of attempting to neutralize odors by sprinkling agricultural lime on a dirt floor during coop clean-out actually turns out to be counterproductive. Lime is alkaline, and the bacteria that produce ammonia thrive in an alkaline environment. By increasing the pH level, lime accelerates the release of ammonia. Better options for neutralizing ammonia, as well as reducing litter moisture, are diatomaceous earth (DE) and absorbent clay (bentonite or montmorillonite), sold as horse-stall conditioners. Some stall fresheners contain a combination of DE and clay.

Keep It Clean

After a period of continuous use, chicken housing becomes contaminated with pathogens that may eventually reach infectious levels. Regular cleanup (at least once a year) does not eliminate microbes, but it does keep them at bay. A thorough cleaning will remove an estimated 95 percent of contamination.

Dry cleaning is not nearly as effective as using water, and hot water cleans better than cold water. Detergent (or a 4 percent washing soda solution) added to the hot water reduces surface tension and helps the water penetrate and soften organic matter. In addition to this benefit, detergents are mildly germicidal.

During cleanup, wear a dust mask and avoid inhaling poultry dust, which can cause human respiratory problems. Methodically follow these steps:

1. Choose a warm day when the facility will dry quickly.

2. Suppress dust by lightly misting everything with water and a bit of detergent.

3. Remove all equipment that's portable, including feeders, drinkers, nests, and perches.

4. Remove all used litter; compost it or spread it on land where your chickens will not range for at least a year.

5. Use a broom, brush, or shop vac to remove dust and cobwebs from all surfaces, including the ceiling and walls.

6. Brush, blow, or vacuum dust from such fixtures as fans, vents, and heaters.

7. Use a hoe or other scraper to remove manure and dirt clinging to the floor, walls, and perches; as long as you can see manure or dirt, keep scraping.

8. Turn off electricity, and protect electrical equipment and outlets with watertight covers or duct tape.

9. Systematically apply hot water, mixed with detergent or washing soda, to the ceiling, walls, floor (other than dirt), and washable equipment with a long-handled brush or a fruit-tree sprayer that delivers a pressure of 400 pounds per square inch (psi) for good penetration.

10. Open doors and windows, and turn on the ventilation fan, to air out and dry the housing before letting the chickens back in.

11. Finish the job by removing any discarded equipment or other debris that may have accumulated in the yard since your last cleanup.

Disinfection

A thorough cleaning is usually all that's needed to effectively sanitize a chicken coop and related equipment. In this case, sanitizing is defined as reducing the number of microbes to a tolerable level. Soap or detergent used during cleaning does not function as a disinfectant, but once coop debris has been thoroughly removed, most remaining microbes can't survive long.

Following a disease outbreak, however, or prior to introducing used equipment into your chickens' environment, disinfection is essential. As distinct from sanitizing, disinfecting involves using some means to either inactivate or kill any microbes that might remain after a thorough cleaning.

Not all disinfectants work equally well against all pathogenic organisms. Following a disease outbreak, a veterinarian or poultry pathologist can help you select the appropriate disinfectant for your situation. Once you have a positive diagnosis, the published manufacturer/label information sheet for any given disinfectant will tell you if it is effective against that pathogen. Manufacturer/label information sheets are available online, usually in PDF format, from manufacturers, as well as from many disinfectant suppliers.

CHEMICAL DISINFECTANTS

A suitable disinfectant should be readily available, relatively inexpensive, and easy to use. Other characteristics of a good disinfectant include the following:

- It should be safe for use around your chickens and you.

- It should not be corrosive to the equipment it's used on.

- It should not have an unpleasant or lingering odor.

- It should be effective against a wide range of pathogens.

- It should remain effective for some time following application.

- It should be stable when diluted in water or exposed to air.

If you have hard water, an additional essential attribute is solubility in hard water. Here are some chemical disinfectants suitable for use in a poultry environment:

Bleach. One of the most readily available and inexpensive disinfectants is ordinary household bleach (such as Clorox and Purex), the active ingredient of which is sodium hypochlorite. The average strength of sodium hypochlorite in laundry bleach is approximately 5 percent, although strength varies from brand to brand and decreases with length of storage. Bleach works best when mixed in warm water but evaporates rapidly, so prepare a fresh solution before each use. For disinfecting purposes use ¼ cup bleach per gallon of hot water (15 mL/L).

The effectiveness of bleach as a disinfectant depends in part on how much bleach is added to water, but more so on the water's pH. The less alkaline the water, the better bleach works as a disinfectant against bacteria and many viruses.

The chief disadvantages to bleach are that it is irritating to the skin, eyes, and respiratory tract and is corrosive to metal. And if you're not careful, you can end up with bleached-out blotches all over your clothing.

Another type of bleach that makes a stronger disinfectant than sodium hypochlorite, but is safer for both birds and humans, is chlorine dioxide. Like sodium hypochlorite, chlorine dioxide is used to sanitize municipal drinking water. It is also used by manufacturers to bleach flour white. Oxine AH (animal health) is a brand sold for livestock use. It is more effective than sodium hypochlorite; has no odor; works against a broad range of bacteria, viruses, and fungi; and is relatively inexpensive because only low concentrations are needed. On the downside it degrades rather rapidly and therefore has no lasting effectiveness.

Vinegar. Vinegar contains acetic acid, which kills most bacteria and many fungi and viruses. It is biodegradable and deodorizing and at low strengths is nontoxic to humans and chickens. Most brands of vinegar — whether apple cider, raw, or distilled — contain about 5 percent acetic acid, making them relatively expensive because they must be used full strength to be effective. Heinz cleaning vinegar, at 6 percent acidity, is more effective as a disinfectant. Horticultural vinegar (such as Bradfield and Nature's

Survivability of Common Poultry Pathogens

DISEASE	PATHOGEN	SURVIVAL OF BIRDS
Avian influenza	Virus	Days to weeks
Avian pox	Virus	Months
Avian tuberculosis	Bacteria	Years
Chlamydiosis	Bacteria	Hours to days
Coccidiosis	Protozoa	Months
Erysipelas	Bacteria	Years
Fowl cholera	Bacteria	Weeks to months
Infectious bronchitis	Virus	Week or less
Infectious bursal disease	Virus	Months
Infectious coryza	Bacteria	Hours to days
Laryngotracheitis	Virus	Days
Marek's disease	Virus	Months to years
Newcastle disease	Virus	Days to week
Mycoplasmosis *Air sac disease* *Chronic respiratory disease* *Infectious synovitis*	Mycoplasma bacteria	Hours to days
Salmonellosis *Arizonosis* *Fowl typhoid* *Paratyphoid pullorum*	Salmonella bacteria	Weeks to months

Wisdom), marketed as a weed killer, is 20 percent acidity, making it highly corrosive to metal, and toxic if swallowed or inhaled. Further, concentrations of acetic acid greater than 11 percent are extremely caustic and can burn your skin on contact and cause permanent eye damage. For use as a disinfectant, horticultural vinegar should be diluted to 10 percent acidity by carefully mixing it half-and-half with water.

Citric acid. Citric acid alone does not have a broad spectrum of effectiveness unless it is combined with some other substance with disinfecting properties. The brand PureGreen24, for instance, is combined with ionic silver. Citric acid disinfectants are rapidly effective against bacteria, fungi, and viruses, nontoxic to humans and chickens, and need not be rinsed after application. They are effective deodorizers, noncaustic, and noncorrosive. They are, however, extremely expensive, especially since they are used full strength.

Iodine. Organic iodines (such as Betadine) are less toxic to humans and chickens than any other disinfectant used around poultry, but are not practical for routine use because they can leave yellow or brown stains, and because most products are used full strength, making them costly. They may, however, be prescribed for disinfection following a disease outbreak. They are effective against most bacteria and some fungi, protozoa, and viruses. Organic iodines consist of iodine combined with something that makes it readily soluble in water of any temperature, and in hard water, but they lose effectiveness in alkaline water.

Phenols. Phenol is another name for carbolic acid, a coal-tar derivative and the standard by which all other disinfectants are measured. Common brand names include Lysol and Tek-Trol. Phenol smells like pine tar and turns milky when diluted in water. Mixed according to directions on the label, phenols are effective against bacteria, fungi, and many viruses; work in hard water; don't leave stains; and have a long residual effect. Their chief disadvantages are that they are highly irritating to the skin,

eyes, and respiratory tract; are known to be carcinogenic; and are especially toxic to cats.

Quats. Quaternary ammonium compounds (referred to as quats or QACs) are widely available at drugstores, pet shops, feed stores, and poultry supply outlets, and vary in composition from brand to brand. Common brand names include Germex and Roccal-D. Quats have no strong odor and leave no stains, and are deodorizing, noncorrosive, nonirritating, and relatively nontoxic. They are effective over a wide pH range against bacteria and somewhat effective against fungi and viruses. They are relatively expensive, but a little goes a long way when diluted according to the directions on the label. However, when inhaled or ingested, these products are toxic to birds; following disinfection a thorough rinsing and drying is therefore advised.

FACTORS AFFECTING CHEMICAL DISINFECTANTS

Five main factors influence the effectiveness of a chemical disinfectant. They are as follows:

- **Concentration.** Too little disinfectant won't do the job; too much can be toxic.

- **Temperature.** Most, but not all, disinfectants work best at temperatures between 55°F and 110°F (13°C to 43°C).

- **pH.** Quaternary ammonium compounds are more active at a high pH; bleach, iodine, and phenols are more effective at a low pH.

- **Contact.** A disinfectant must have direct contact with microbes, which can't happen if the microbes are hidden by droppings or other debris.

- **Contact time.** Disinfectants take time to work; allow at least 20 minutes, unless a longer period is specified on the label.

USING CHEMICAL DISINFECTANTS

Most disinfectants don't penetrate beyond the surface of chicken coop debris, and in some cases poop and other organic matter actually deactivate a disinfectant, so follow the steps on page 16 for a thorough cleanup before applying any disinfectant. While you disinfect, keep the chickens out of the coop. Some disinfectants are toxic if consumed, can cause irritation on skin contact, and may be irritating to the eyes and respiratory system — especially if sprayed.

Don't be tempted to increase a disinfectant's effectiveness by combining it with detergent, washing soda, or any other cleaning product without first checking the label for compatibility. Mixing a disinfectant with another product may destroy the disinfectant's effectiveness — or worse: in some cases the resulting chemical reaction is highly toxic.

Store disinfectants in a cool place, ideally away from children, pets, livestock, food, and feeds. To avoid the possibility of a dangerous error through misuse, keep disinfectants in their original containers with the labels intact.

Always dilute a disinfectant according to either directions on the label or instructions provided by a vet or poultry pathologist. Disinfectants that don't work well in alkaline water may require the addition of an acidifier. Some disinfectants work best in hot water, while others evaporate quickly in warm or hot water.

When applying any disinfectant, avoid getting it on your skin or inhaling the fumes. Wear goggles to protect your eyes and a respirator to protect your respiratory tract. Work systematically, starting with the ceiling, then the walls, and finally the floor. Using a long-handled push broom to scrub in the disinfectant is safer than spraying, as it is less likely to get on your skin or be inhaled as droplets.

If the disinfectant changes color or looks dirty, it probably isn't working well anymore, so mix a fresh batch. When you're done inside the coop, don't forget to disinfect your shovel, broom, rake, hoe, and other cleanup tools, as well as your boots.

Wait at least 20 minutes to give the disinfectant time to do its job before rinsing housing, fixture, and tools with plain water. Some disinfectants must be left in contact longer than 20 minutes, while others need not be rinsed at all, so check the label for rinsing requirements.

To protect your chickens from skin injury, respiratory irritation, or a potential toxic reaction from consuming disinfectant, allow housing to dry thoroughly, and leave it empty for as long as possible before letting your chickens back in. The safe time between application and letting your chickens in varies from 4 hours to 2 days and should be specified on the label.

NONCHEMICAL DISINFECTANTS

Not all disinfectants are chemicals. Here's the rundown on readily available nonchemical disinfectants:

Hot water increases the effectiveness of some chemical disinfectants, and boiling water and live steam are both effective disinfectants in their own right.

Resting the coop by keeping chickens out for 2 to 4 weeks after cleanup further reduces the microbe population, since many microbes can't live long in the absence of chickens.

Freezing weather deactivates some microbes, but not most viruses. The longer empty housing is exposed to freezing temperatures, the fewer microbes will survive.

Drying for a period of time after cleanup also reduces the population of microbes, but killing a significant number by drying can take a long time.

Sunlight speeds up drying of portable equipment (such as feeders, drinkers, nests, and roosts) and the parts of housing that can be opened up to direct rays. Sunlight does not penetrate deeply but will destroy microbes on the surface. Sunlight and normal soil activity will effectively disinfect a yard or run once the accumulation of organic wastes has been removed from the surface.

Heat produced by composting will destroy most of the bacteria, viruses, coccidial oocysts, and worm eggs present in litter. Heap the litter into a pile (but not on a wood floor, where it could start a fire). If the litter is dry, dampen it a little to start fermentation. Let the pile heat up to at least 125°F (52°C), leave it for 24 hours, then turn it so the outside is on the inside. Let it heat for another 24 hours before spreading the litter back out. Composting litter to destroy microbes is always a good idea, even when the litter will be used to fertilize a garden or field.

Flame is an effective disinfectant, but a hazardous one, especially around wood structures. It is best reserved to disinfect concrete pads and to sear away feathers stuck to wire cages, but take care: if you hold a torch to wire long enough for the wire to get hot, the galvanizing will be damaged. In some extreme cases (such as a severe tick infestation), burning contaminated housing is the only way to eliminate the contamination.

Closed Flock

Each flock is exposed to its own combination of pathogens, causing each to develop its own combination of immunities. Chickens from two perfectly healthy flocks, when mixed together, can therefore give each other diseases for which the others have developed no defenses.

Once your flock is established, the best way to avoid diseases is to keep a closed flock. Keeping a closed flock means your chickens have no direct or indirect contact with other birds. Complete avoidance is not always possible, but knowing where the dangers lie can help you keep them to a minimum. Maintaining a closed flock means you never:

- mix chickens from various sources;

- introduce new chickens into your flock;

- return a chicken to your property once it's been elsewhere;

- visit other people's flocks;

- let owners of other flocks visit yours;

- borrow or lend equipment; or

- hatch eggs from outside sources.

Unfortunately for biosecurity, visiting other flocks is part of the fun of having chickens. If you do visit other flocks, wear rubber chore boots that you can scrub and disinfect afterward; keep a supply of inexpensive disposable overboot covers; or slip large plastic bags over your shoes and secure them with large rubber bands. When the visit is over, place the chore boots in a large plastic bag until you get them cleaned, or seal the overboot covers or plastic bags in a garbage bag for disposal. If other flock owners visit you, ask them to do the same, or have a supply of overboots or plastic bags for them to wear over their shoes. You may feel foolish and overly cautious, but you'll feel even more foolish if visiting spreads a disastrous disease from one flock to another.

Quarantine Incoming Chickens

Trading and showing your chickens are other fun activities that create a nightmare for biosecurity. Although diseases are more likely to be spread by trading than by showing, occasionally a highly contagious disease (often infectious laryngotracheitis) makes the show rounds.

To be on the safe side, isolate any returning show bird (or incoming new chicken) for a month, and feed it only after you've taken care of all your other chickens. As an added security measure, house two or three sacrificial chickens from your flock with the isolated chicken to serve as sentinels. If your old chickens remain healthy by the end of the month, chances are pretty good the incoming chicken is also healthy.

Exclude Wild Birds

Wild birds can transmit diseases to chickens either by mechanically carrying pathogens on their feet and feathers, or by becoming infected and shedding pathogens in their poop and saliva as they travel around in their daily activities. Wild birds are attracted to chicken yards where gaps in coop construction provide suitable nesting sites and feed is readily available.

Native North American birds are not as problematic as nonnative species, which are much more numerous and tend to congregate in large numbers. Further, native birds are seriously endangered because of deforestation, wetland draining, being preyed on by nonnative species, and other disturbances to their natural environment. Disrupting the nesting sites of native species is therefore a federal offense. To discourage birds from visiting your chicken yard, don't provide birdseed or nesting sites in or near your chicken yard; keep chicken feeders indoors, so spilled grain won't attract wild birds; and, where possible, cover the top of your chicken run with wire or plastic netting.

Three species of nonnative birds that spread diseases to chickens are particularly pesky and are not protected by federal law. House sparrows, European starlings, and rock pigeons (also called rock doves) are introduced species that have become invasive pests. European starlings and house sparrows steal the nests of native birds, evict the occupants, and destroy their eggs. Rock pigeons are prodigious poopers — each produces 25 pounds of pathogen-laden droppings per year — and they don't carry away the droppings of their nestlings like other birds do, so a pigeon nest eventually becomes a heavy mess of poop, unhatched eggs, and dead hatchlings. Besides spreading diseases to chickens, rock pigeons, as well as European starlings, can pose a health hazard for humans that inhale dust from their dried droppings (see Histoplasmosis, page 405).

Once any of these three nonnative birds discovers a good nesting area and comes back year after year, it can rapidly become numerous and problematic for chickens and humans alike. To discourage these birds from nesting, cover their preferred sites with 1-inch mesh wire, such as chicken wire or bird netting. If they remain persistent, trapping is a sure way to get rid of them. The Internet offers a variety of plans for homemade traps, as well as ready-made options, such as the reliable Troyer S&S (sparrow and starling) Controller. You can find out more about the habits of nonnative species, and learn to identify them through photographs and sound recordings, at the Cornell Lab of Ornithology website, www.allaboutbirds.org.

Chicken Diseases Spread by Wild Birds

DISEASE	CAUSE	PREVALENCE
Avian influenza	Virus	Sporadic
Avian pox	Virus	Common
Blackhead	Protozoa	Rare
Chlamydiosis	Bacteria	Rare
Chronic respiratory disease	Bacteria	Common
Cryptosporidiosis	Protozoa	Common
Fowl cholera	Bacteria	Sporadic
NEWCASTLE DISEASE		
Lentogenic	Virus	Common
Mesogenic/velogenic	Virus	Rare
SALMONELLOSIS		
Arizonosis	Bacteria	Rare
Fowl typhoid	Bacteria	Rare
Paratyphoid	Bacteria	Common
Pullorum	Bacteria	Rare

Stress Management

Like all living things, a chicken has a limited energy reserve with which to cope with day-to-day life and has just enough extra energy to adjust to minor unusual events or adapt to small changes. Stress occurs when events or changes are so intense or numerous that they rapidly use up the chicken's energy reserve, leaving too little for the bird's normal daily needs and reducing its resistance to disease. Although some microbes are so strong (or virulent) they readily overcome a bird's normal resistance, most cause no illness or only mild illness, except in birds with weakened immunity due to stress.

Disease itself is a stress factor. Even a disease that is not itself serious can reduce a bird's resistance to a more serious infection. Internal parasites (worms) are an example of a mild infection that can open the door to something more serious, or that can become serious when combined with other stress factors.

No matter how much natural resistance a chicken has, stress reduces its resistance to some extent. Stress cannot be avoided. It is normal in every chicken's life. Most chickens are able to adapt, even to times of peak stress, such as hatching out of an egg, reaching sexual maturity, and molting. Additional stresses are caused by the environment (such as chilling, heating, and excessive humidity) and by routine management procedures that involve handling individual chickens or herding the entire flock.

Stress management involves being a good steward to your chickens — providing adequate protection from the elements; clean, dry litter and range; good ventilation without draftiness; contamination-free feed and water; adequate feed and water space; proper nutrition; and freedom from crowding. Avoidance of crowding is especially important for chicks, since they grow fast and can rapidly outgrow their quarters. As birds grow, they develop immunities through exposure to disease-causing microbes. Stress due to crowding can result in disease instead of immunity.

Stress reduction also involves avoiding the indiscriminate or improper use of medications, as well as avoiding handling birds at critical times, such as when pullets are just starting to lay, when a flock has recently been moved or vaccinated, and when the weather is extremely hot or cold.

Gentle handling as a stress-reduction measure is more important to chicken health than fancy housing. Gently treated birds are calmer, are easier to handle, and experience less stress

Common Stressors in a Chicken's Life

USUALLY MINOR	MODERATE	SERIOUS	SEVERE
Too much time between hatching and first feed or water	Being chilled or overheated during first weeks of life	Overcrowding	Combining chickens of various ages
Nutritional deficiency in chicks due to inadequate breeder-flock diet	Extremely rapid growth	Extreme heat	Piling due to fright or cold
	Being transported	Nutritionally imbalanced feed	Inadequate feeder or drinker space
Cold damp floor	Being moved to different housing		Lengthy periods without feed
Rough handling	Being chilled or overheated during a move		Lengthy periods without water
Low-grade infection	Extreme changes in weather or temperature		Onset of any disease
Eating spoiled feed	Unsanitary feeders, drinkers, or litter		
Unusual or sudden loud noises	Internal or external parasites		
Unusual or sudden motions	Insufficient ventilation		
Extremely high egg production	Drafty conditions		
	Vaccination		
	Competition between sexes or individuals		
	Disruption to the pecking order		
	Medication (severity depends on drug used)		
	Injury (severity depends on degree of injury)		
	Exhibition (severity depends on travel and show conditions)		

Adapted from: Farm Flock Management Guide, *Floyd W. Hicks, Pennsylvania State University*

CHICKEN VETS

Because veterinarians willing to treat chickens remain few and far between, Metzer Farms of Gonzales, California, has compiled a list of avian vets throughout the United States and Canada. It may be found online at www.metzerfarms.com/Veterinarians.cfm.

during any procedure that requires handling. Compared to birds that are largely ignored or are treated roughly, chickens that are handled gently are more resistant to infections.

Conditioning is another stress-reduction technique. Whenever you make a management change, condition your birds by making the change gradually so that each step is relatively minor. For example, as chicks grow and require a larger feeder and drinker, leave the smaller feeder and drinker in place while the chicks get used to the new ones. If you plan to move or separate breeders, give them plenty of time to adjust to their new surroundings before you start collecting their eggs for hatching.

SHOWING AND STRESS

Showing causes stress by exposing a bird to unfamiliar and confusing surroundings, strange people, different-tasting water, and any number of new and potentially frightening experiences. Excessive showing can be so stressful that it affects the fertility and hatchability of eggs. Exhibited hens experience more stress than exhibited cocks.

If you show your chickens, condition them by coop-training them prior to the show so they'll get used to being caged alone and handled frequently. At show time bring along your own feed and water — if your chickens don't like the feed or water at the show, they won't eat or drink well, their stress level will go up, and they'll be more susceptible to diseases.

Some exhibitors add antibiotics or electrolytes to water during a show, but if a bird doesn't like the taste, it won't drink, and its stress level will go up. Skip the antibiotics altogether; offer electrolytes before and after, but not during, the show.

STRESS BEHAVIOR

By becoming familiar with the way your chickens normally act, you can readily notice changes caused by stress and can take appropriate action. You may be able to alleviate the stress behavior through a simple management change. Continuing stress that causes long-term behavioral changes seriously reduces a chicken's resistance to disease.

Sometimes the stress behavior itself is a first sign of disease. Stress behavior falls into three basic categories.

1. **Loose, watery droppings** become evident as a stress sign when you suddenly grab a chicken and it reacts by pooping on you. Loose droppings can also be a sign that something is wrong with the feed or water, or that your birds are suffering from a digestive disorder.

2. **Labored breathing** can be caused by crowding, panic, high temperatures, or respiratory distress. It may indicate that the coop is too dusty, ammonia fumes are too strong, or the chickens are coming down with a respiratory disease.

3. **Changes in normal behavior** or activity can be triggered by any number of factors, including boredom, fear, crowding, the introduction of new birds, frequent showing, insufficient or unpalatable water, uncomfortable temperatures, and disease. Veterinary ethologists, who study animal behavior and its relationship to health, organize the behavior of chickens into the following categories for observation purposes.

REFLEX BEHAVIOR involves any automatic reaction, such as flinching or shying away from sudden movement. A frightened chicken, for example, shakes its head from side to side. A sick chicken reacts more slowly than usual to perceived danger.

FEEDING BEHAVIOR includes both how often a chicken eats and drinks and how much it ingests. Under normal circumstances, a chicken visits feeders and drinkers often and eats or drinks a little at a time. Stress makes a bird eat and drink less, although some diseases increase thirst. Abnormal feeding behaviors that require management action include feather picking, cannibalism, drinking excessive amounts of water, eating litter or soil, and egg eating.

REST PATTERNS, including sleep, are easily disturbed during times of stress. The classic restlessness of chickens at roosting time, for example, is caused by fear of being bitten by the external parasites that feed on the birds at night. Predators, including rats, that routinely prowl beneath roosts can also make chickens nervous at bedtime.

EXPLORATORY BEHAVIOR involves investigating new things in the environment, including newly introduced chickens. But the sudden introduction of something a bird can't see or doesn't understand (such as a sudden loud noise or sudden rapid motion) can induce excessive stress, which leads to overreaction, often in the form of flightiness (the Chicken Little syndrome). Flightiness is relative, however, since some breeds naturally are more flighty than others. Loss of interest by a chicken in exploring its surroundings may be an early sign of disease.

BODY ACTIVITY relates to motion, including wing flapping and moving from place to place. A stressed-out chicken may pace up and down, indicating anxiety (in the case of a chicken that finds itself on the wrong side of a fence), frustration (as in the case of one cock being harassed by another), or boredom (in the case of a chicken that doesn't take well to close confinement).

GROOMING ACTIVITIES include head scratching, preening, mutual grooming, and dust bathing. If you're not familiar with dust-bath behavior, the first time you see your chickens laid out in the dirt, you might think they died a sudden death. A scruffy appearance, indicating loss of interest in grooming behavior, is a common early sign of disease.

SEXUAL BEHAVIOR on the part of a cock involves chasing hens, courtship (pecking the ground, dancing in circles, and wing fluttering), and crowing (to establish location and warn off competitors — a behavior that's territorial as well as sexual). Sexual behavior on the part of a hen largely involves crouching when a cock puts his foot on her back in preparation for mating. Hens that are low in the pecking order will crouch as a rooster nears and will be mated more often than other hens. You can readily identify these subordinate hens by the broken or missing feathers on their backs, and sometimes by wounds inflicted by the mounting cock. Such wounds may be serious enough to require isolating the hen and treating her injuries.

PARENTAL BEHAVIOR refers to the relationship between a hen and her chicks, since a cock develops no special relationship with his offspring. A hen protects her chicks, leads them to feed and water, and communicates with them (and they with her) through vocalizations. Abnormal parental behavior includes leaving the nest before the eggs hatch (perhaps because the hen was bothered by mites), attacking chicks when they hatch, or abandoning chicks after they hatch. Some breeds, particularly those best known for their laying abilities, have been selectively bred not to have parental instincts, because a hen stops laying when she starts incubating eggs in a nest.

TERRITORIALISM involves aggressive behavior that enables chickens to maintain personal and territorial space. Crowding increases aggression, which increases stress. Displacement activity is a common form of stress behavior in which a chicken suddenly shifts gears, as when two roosters are sparring and one suddenly starts preening or pecking the ground. Abnormal territorial behavior includes unprovoked attacks on intruders, other chickens, or humans and refusing (or being unable) to move out of fear.

SOCIAL RELATIONS basically involve the pecking order. Chickens that are low in the peck order get chased away from feeders, don't get enough to eat, and don't grow as well or lay as many eggs as others. The larger your flock, the more feeders and drinkers you need to provide, and the farther apart they should be so each social group within the flock has ready access. Stress goes up when the peck order is disrupted for any reason, including when chickens are removed from or added to the flock.

RELATIONSHIP TO HUMANS starts with imprinting, which occurs in chicks during their first day of life. By the time a chick is 3 days old it starts experiencing fear, which is why developing a friendly relationship with chicks hatched at your place is easier than developing a relationship with mail-order chicks or grown chickens. Whether or not your chickens are imprinted on you, to minimize stress, talk or sing softly when you move among them so they can keep track of where you are, and always move calmly and avoid abrupt broad gestures.

Medicate with Caution

Flock owners who routinely give antibiotics to new chickens, returning show birds, and newly hatched chicks aren't doing their chickens any favors. Such casual use of drugs only increases costs and eventually increases problems.

Instead, work out a disease-prevention program based on the issues prevalent in your area. Vaccinate only against serious diseases your flock is likely to be exposed to. Pay attention to your chickens, and know what to look for, so if a problem does occur you'll be prepared to treat it promptly and properly. And help your chickens resist potential diseases by managing for optimal immunity.

Sources of Immunity

Immunity is the ability to resist infection. Another word for immunity is resistance; the opposite of immunity is susceptibility.

A chick hatches with a certain amount of innate, or inherited, immunity and acquires new immunities as it grows. Since domestic chickens are confined to an unnatural environment, they often need help to develop immunities against diseases in their environment.

Inherited Immunity

Chickens are immune to some diseases because of inherited or genetically controlled factors.

When the entire species is resistant, immunity is complete. Chickens have complete immunity to a long list of diseases that infect other birds or animals but never infect chickens.

As a species, chickens are immune to some pathogens they commonly carry in their bodies but that make them sick if their resistance is broken down. The protozoan *Histomonas meleagridis* is an example. It commonly lives in the poultry environment, causing chickens to get blackhead only when their resistance is drastically reduced by a massive infestation. (Turkeys, on the other hand, are highly susceptible to blackhead and often get it from chickens that carry the protozoa without being infected.)

When only certain breeds, strains, or individuals are resistant to a disease, immunity is partial. Chickens have partial immunity to Marek's disease, since some strains never succumb to this common killer of other strains. In nearly every disease outbreak, some individuals do not become infected, thanks to inherited immunity. Those are the birds you'll want in your breeder flock if you wish to breed for resistance, as described on page 30.

Acquired Immunity

Acquired immunity is any resistance to disease that is not genetic but instead is conferred by antibodies. How a chicken acquires these antibodies determines whether the immunity is passive and short term or active and long term.

PASSIVE IMMUNITY

Passive acquired immunity is resistance conferred by antibodies produced by some source other than the chicken's own immune system. Passive immunity may be acquired naturally or artificially.

Natural passive immunity is acquired by a chick from a hen via the egg. The source of maternal antibodies is immaterial — they may result from a disease the hen once had or from a vaccine designed specifically to build up her antibodies so she can pass immunity along to her chicks. Unless a hen has been either exposed to a pathogen or vaccinated against it, she cannot pass along maternal immunity to it. Chicks that lack maternal immunity to a disease are more susceptible to that disease, and so are their future offspring.

Artificial passive immunity is acquired by a chicken when it gets an injection of an antiserum containing antibodies to counteract a specific pathogen, or an antitoxin to counteract toxins produced by bacteria, such those that cause botulism. Such antiserums and antitoxins consist of fluid taken from the blood of an animal that has been immunized against a disease and therefore has antibodies against that disease. Because an antiserum or antitoxin confers immediate immunity, it may be used to treat an existing disease.

The immunity is only temporary, however, since it is passively acquired. When antibodies are not produced within the chicken's own body, the resulting short-term immunity lasts only about 4 weeks. During this time, the passive immunity can interfere with the development of active immunity.

ACTIVE IMMUNITY

Active immunity differs from passive immunity in three important ways:

- It is caused by antibodies produced within a chicken's own body.

- It is not immediate but takes time, usually weeks, to develop.

- The immunity is longer lasting than passive immunity.

Although active immunity always lasts longer than passive immunity, it may be temporary (as in the case of a staphylococcal and streptococcal infection), it may be permanent (as in the case of fowl typhoid), or it may be permanent unless stress weakens the bird's resistance. As a general rule, active immunity against viruses is absolute and long lasting, while active immunity against bacteria is temporary and dependent on stress avoidance.

Like passive immunity, active immunity may be acquired naturally or artificially. Natural acquired active immunity occurs when a chicken's body produces antibodies to fight a particular disease (see Immune System, page 62). If the chicken recovers, its body continues to contain antibodies specific to that disease — they confer immunity only to that one disease. A bird can acquire active immunity as an embryo during incubation or at any point after it hatches.

Artificial active immunity is acquired from a vaccine that contains antigens that cause a chicken's body to produce antibodies against those particular antigens. Active immunity resulting from vaccination takes about 2 weeks to develop and, in some cases, must be renewed through one or more booster shots to keep the level of antibodies high enough to ward off the disease. The booster dose, which is usually smaller than the original vaccination dose, must be administered at a specified time following the original vaccination. For more information on vaccinations, see page 278.

Acquired Immunity

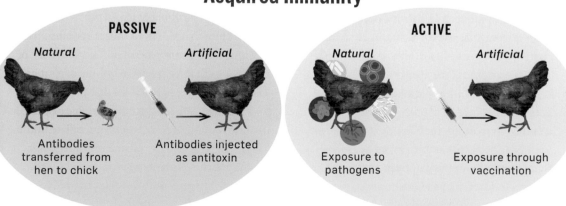

PASSIVE

Natural

Artificial

Antibodies transferred from hen to chick

Antibodies injected as antitoxin

Short-term immunity

ACTIVE

Natural

Artificial

Exposure to pathogens

Exposure through vaccination

Long-term immunity

A frequently repeated recommendation is to keep growing chicks healthy by raising them away from mature chickens. You have to wonder, then, how chicks brooded by a mother hen ever manage to survive. The answer is that the chicks start with maternal antibodies acquired from the egg during incubation and develop additional immunities through the process of trickle infection resulting from gradual exposure to the pathogens in their environment. Think of it as natural vaccination.

Chicks raised in a brooder don't enjoy the same benefit. Instead, they are kept in an unnatural environment apart from other chickens. If they are later brought into a mature flock, their immune systems may be overwhelmed by exposure to too many pathogens at once, resulting in disease.

A simple solution is to expose brooded chicks early to the pathogens they are likely to encounter later in life by giving them a little soil to scratch in while they are still in the brooder. The sooner chicks have an opportunity to peck and scratch in natural soil, the quicker they will develop immunities to the pathogens in their future environment.

Breeding for Resistance

Among the many consequences of industrialized chicken production is the development of various methods to control disease-causing pathogens. The National Poultry Improvement Plan focuses on complete eradication of the worst pathogens. Biosecurity measures emphasize preventing pathogens from entering a chicken's environment. The use of vaccines attempts to keep the pathogens a chicken does encounter from causing disease. Medications are used to control pathogens once disease occurs.

Little attention these days is paid to preventing diseases through the development of genetic resistance. A chicken that is resistant to a pathogen tolerates invasion by the pathogen with little or no physical damage. A chicken that is immune to the pathogen remains completely unaffected by it. One hundred percent resistance to a pathogen results in immunity to that specific pathogen.

If you raise a few backyard chickens for table eggs or as pets, their genetic resistance to diseases is out of your control. But if you selectively breed your chickens and hatch their eggs to perpetuate certain bloodlines, such as engaging in a conservation program or breeding for exhibition excellence, genetic resistance is an important trait to encourage.

Constitutional Vigor

Old poultry books make frequent reference to constitutional vigor. The concept is quite simple: In every flock some individuals are less affected by diseases than others. Susceptible birds get sick or die when exposed to a disease. Resistant birds (those with constitutional vigor) get mildly ill and recover quickly or don't get sick at all.

Developing genetic resistance in your flock means breeding only those birds that are less affected by disease, so their offspring will be as vigorous as they are. Any birds that don't measure up should be removed from the breeding flock.

A legendary example of genetic resistance is the Hellevad hen, developed by Denmark's Wolf family by crossing New Hampshire and White Leghorn bloodlines to get a productive layer of brown-shell eggs. For generations the Wolfs used no medications (other than Newcastle vaccine, required by Danish law), while removing from their breeder flock any chicken that did not appear to be perfectly healthy. Researchers are now studying the Hellevad to determine what, exactly, makes the breed so robust compared to other industrial layers.

The trouble with most selective breeding programs is that they emphasize traits other than resistance to diseases. Industrial egg-laying breeds are selected in favor of high egg production on low feed input. Industrial meat-producing breeds are selected in favor of rapid growth on low feed input. Exhibition breeds are selected in favor of size, shape, and color.

When chickens are artificially bred for traits other than disease resistance, vigor declines in succeeding generations. Chickens bred for extreme egg production or rapid meat production, for example, use their energy elsewhere than for immune response. Conversely, chickens that are deliberately bred for disease resistance tend to be somewhat less productive.

Indeed, Hellevad hens are not as productive as other industrial layers, but their greater vigor makes them much healthier and therefore more economical. Breeds available in North America that have superior disease resistance include Fayoumi, Kraienköppe, and Naked Neck. Because of either deliberate selection or chance, some strains within any breed have a higher level of resistance than other strains.

Breeding Guidelines

Breeding in favor of disease resistance is not difficult. Resistance may be improved in just a few generations by inbreeding gradually, using only healthy breeder cocks and hens that are free of skeletal defects and other deformities, exposing chicks to the environment inhabited by their parents, and continuing to breed only the healthiest and defect-free offspring. Here are a few additional guidelines on breeding for disease resistance:

- Keep a minimum breeding flock of about 50 birds, so you'll have the leeway to cull vigorously and still maintain genetic diversity in your flock.

- Chickens that remain healthy despite never having been vaccinated or medicated are the best candidates for your breeding flock.

- Use breeders that are at least 2 years old, which opposes the conventional wisdom that the older the bird, the more diseases it has been exposed to and the less healthy it is likely to be. Chicks hatched from survivors of exposure to pathogens are particularly hearty and may carry maternal antibodies that give them further immunity. (Be sure, of course, that your hens are not infected by a pathogen that is egg-transmitted from survivor-carriers to their chicks.)

- Progeny-test, meaning evaluate your breeders based on the health of their offspring. Progeny testing requires pedigreeing your birds; in other words, you must know exactly which cock and hen produced each chick. If the majority of offspring from a particular mating live and remain healthy for 1½ years, keep the parents in your breeder flock; if the majority of offspring don't survive that long, or fail to remain healthy, cull the parents and any remaining progeny.

- Learn about indicators known to relate to susceptibility or resistance to the diseases prevalent in your area. Some indicators may be identified through blood typing, a potentially impractical, expensive, and time-consuming practice. Other indicators are more accessible, such as associations between resistance to some infections and higher than normal body temperatures.

- Give your flock a head start by selecting a breed, or a strain within your chosen breed, that already has some natural resistance to the diseases and parasites they will encounter in your area.

Breeding for genetic resistance does have a downside — resistance to a pathogen cannot occur where that particular pathogen is not present. Therefore your birds can develop resistance only to diseases present in your yard. If a new disease is introduced, your chickens may have no defenses against it. Since no flock can be exposed to all possible diseases, no flock can be immune to all possible diseases. Even while you breed for genetic resistance to diseases prevalent in your chickens' environment, take care not to introduce new diseases.

Another aspect to breeding for resistance is that disease-causing organisms can evolve right along with the development of resistance in your strain of birds. These evolving new forms of pathogens make breeding for resistance a never-ending process.

ABILITY TO RESIST DISEASE

Whether a chicken succumbs to a particular infection, recovers from it, resists infection, or is completely immune to the disease depends on a combination of factors, which include the following:

- The presence or absence of the pathogen in the chicken's environment

- The concentration of pathogens in the chicken's environment

- The virulence (severity) of the pathogen

- Immunity conferred by vaccination

- Immunity resulting from previous exposure to the pathogen

- Maternal immunity conferred by a mother hen to her chicks

- The chicken's age in relation to its ability to develop immunity

- The chicken's condition, affecting normal immune response

- The chicken's genetic resistance to developing signs of infection

- The chicken's genetic resistance to being infected by the pathogen

CHAPTER 2

Good Nutrition Means
Healthy Chickens

AN OBSERVANT READER of my several poultry books and magazine articles once asked about an apparent contradiction she had detected. She quoted me as saying in one place that chickens are not vegetarians and in another place that I don't feed my chickens commercial rations containing protein from animal sources. How could both statements be true?

Simple. My chickens free-range and therefore get their animal protein from nature in the form of bugs, worms, and the occasional mouse or toad unfortunate enough to attempt a shortcut through the chicken yard.

My chickens get additional animal protein from surplus Nubian goat milk. Whenever I clean out the goats' hay manager, I save the fines — those bits of leaves and seeds that accumulate at the bottom of the manager. When I have extra milk, I mix in a handful of fines and let the milk ferment overnight. By morning it has turned to a soft cheeselike consistency with a divinely herbal odor. As tempting as it smells, I've never tasted it, but my chickens mob me when they see the milk bucket coming.

So you see, my chickens get plenty of animal protein. Just not from commercial rations.

The Nature of Nutrition

Nutrition and health interact in many ways, making proper nutrition an essential part of keeping chickens healthy. Disease isn't always caused by bacteria, viruses, or other parasites. Disease may result from a nutritional deficiency, which can inhibit the body's immune response, opening the way for infection.

Conversely, an infection can reduce a bird's appetite or inhibit the absorption of nutrients from its digestive system. Interference with the absorption of nutrients, or malabsorption, can be caused not only by disease but also by parasite loads such as worms or coccidiosis, as well as by medications and environmental stresses such as extremes in temperature or humidity. Any of these conditions can make even the most perfectly formulated rations insufficient to prevent a deficiency. The result may either delay recovery from an infection or further reduce the bird's resistance, increasing its susceptibility to additional infections.

Besides reducing resistance to disease, an improperly balanced diet can result in poorly growing chicks, poorly laying hens, low fertility in roosters, and low hatchability of eggs. To complicate things, a chicken's nutritional requirements change with age, season, and breeding status.

Too much of any nutrient, or a lack of balance among the nutrients, can be just as devastating as a deficiency. Well-meaning flock owners can easily cause nutritional problems by feeding their chickens too many treats or pumping them full of unnecessary nutritional supplements.

More than 36 nutrients have been identified as being essential to chickens. Since no single feed ingredient contains all the necessary nutrients, the best diet includes a combination of ingredients that together satisfy all of a chicken's dietary needs. The most essential nutrient in any healthy chicken diet is water, which is needed to carry all other nutrients in solution.

Drinking Water

Water makes up 50 percent of a chicken's body weight and 65 percent of an egg's total weight. Among its many important functions are helping transport other nutrients throughout the body, removing the waste products of metabolism, and keeping the body cool through evaporation.

An old saying points out the perversity of chickens: "A flock's water supply is no better than the poorest drinking water available." You can bring your flock the purest, freshest water, yet given the chance your birds will persist in drinking from filthy puddles. Good yard drainage prevents stagnant puddles where disease-causing microbes and parasite-carrying insects thrive. If your soil is neither sandy nor gravelly, enhance drainage by locating your coop on a slight slope. Many microbes and parasites can't survive long in the absence of moisture.

Minimum Water Needs

AGE	WATER PER DOZEN BIRDS	
1 day–1 week	1 quart	1 liter
1–4 weeks	2 quarts	2 liters
4–12 weeks	1 gallon	4 liters
12 weeks and up	1½ gallons	6 liters

Provide your flock with water from a clean, reliable source. Avoid surface tanks, ponds, or streams, all of which are easily contaminated, especially if the chickens can walk in them. Chickens prefer to drink water with a temperature of about 55°F (13°C) and will drink less if their water is much above or below that temperature.

How Much a Chicken Drinks

A chicken doesn't drink much at a time, so it needs to drink frequently throughout the day. An average chicken drinks between 1 and 2 cups (240 to 475 mL) of water per day, depending on numerous factors, including its size, the ambient temperature, water palatability, feed intake, feed composition, condition of health, and whether or not the bird is laying.

The average layer drinks twice as much as the average nonlayer. Some disease conditions cause chickens to drink more, as do rations that are high in protein or salt. Chickens drink less if the water contains a medication or an excessive amount of dissolved minerals they find unpalatable. Chickens that don't drink enough because the water tastes bad, is dirty or too warm, or frequently runs dry can suffer kidney failure.

Under normal conditions, a chicken will drink approximately twice as much as it eats, by weight. A layer, for example, may eat ½ pound (225 g) of feed and drink 2 cups (475 mL), or 1 pound (450 g), of water per day. As the temperature goes up, the ratio of water to feed also goes up, since high temperatures cause a chicken to eat less and drink more.

Effect of Environmental Temperature on Water Use

TEMPERATURE	PINTS OF WATER/POUND OF FEED
60°F (16°C)	1.8
70°F (21°C)	2.0
80°F (27°C)	2.8
90°F (32°C)	4.9
100°F (38°C)	8.4

The Danger of Dehydration

A chicken can survive longer without feed than without water. Insufficient water slows growth in chicks, reduces egg production in hens, and increases the potential for heat stress during warm weather.

Water deprivation and resulting dehydration can occur at any age and for a variety of reasons. Water may be available to chicks, but perhaps they are too small to reach the drinker level. Chickens of any age will go without water if the quality is poor or they simply don't like the taste of it. Diarrhea causes dehydration by passing water through the body too quickly to be absorbed. In warm weather, water deprivation occurs when a flock's water needs go up but the supply remains the same, causing drinkers to periodically run dry. Hens may have plenty of water in winter, but if the water freezes, egg production will drop.

Water is essential for the laying of eggs. If a hen goes without water for as little as 24 hours, she may take 24 hours to recover. If she goes without water for 36 hours, she may take 2 or 3 weeks to recover. If she goes without water for 2 days, she may go into a molt, followed by a lengthy period of poor laying from which she may not recover.

Brooded chicks will start to die on the fourth day without water. As they reach the point of death, they stop peeping. Otherwise, the signs of water deprivation in chicks are similar to those for older chickens.

Signs of Water Deprivation

BODY PART	SIGN
Comb and wattles	Shrunken and bluish
Tendons on backs of legs	Prominent
Droppings	Loose and off-color
Weight	Rapid loss
Breast muscle	Dark and dry
Activity level	Lethargic

Suitable Drinkers

A proper drinker encourages adequate water consumption. A good drinker has these features:

- It doesn't leak, drip, or tip over easily.

- It's easy to clean; one that's hard to clean won't be sanitized as often as it should be.

- It's designed so chickens can't roost over or step into the water.

- It may be adjusted so the water level is at the height of the birds' backs.

- It holds enough water that it won't run out before you can conveniently refill it.

Automatic watering is, of course, ideal, provided someone is available to check it daily to make sure the system continues to function properly. Nipples are a particularly popular type of automatic drinker. Properly installed, they are virtually trouble-free. They don't leak or spill over and dampen the bedding, they keep bedding and poop out of the water, and they don't need to be scrubbed daily. You do have to check them daily to ensure they aren't leaking or clogged (just tap with a finger to make sure water comes out). The one downside to nipples is that chickens tend to drink less, making it wise to offer additional sources of water during hot weather.

Numerous bacteria, protozoa, and viruses can be spread by means of drinking water contaminated with droppings or mucus from infected birds. No less often than once a week, scrub drinkers with soap and water. Then sanitize them with either vinegar or a solution of chlorine bleach — one part bleach to nine parts water.

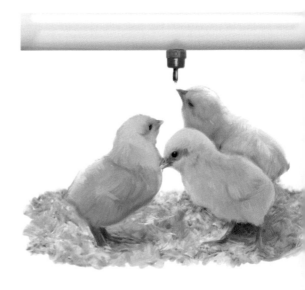

When used correctly, water nipples are extremely sanitary and virtually trouble-free.

In winter, coils or a heating pan will keep water from freezing. In summer place drinkers in a shady place where the water won't be warmed by the sun. A gravel or sand bed beneath the waterer, covered by a platform topped with slats or hardware cloth, will keep chickens from drinking spills and picking in the moist, poopy soil that invariably develops around a waterer.

Depending on the type of drinkers you use and the source of your water supply, biofilm may reduce the quality of your flock's drinking water. See Controlling Biofilm on page 303.

Chicken Feed

Your chickens' rations might be commercially prepared, homegrown, or a combination of both. They must be nutritionally balanced to meet the chickens' needs based on the season, the temperature, and each bird's age, size, weight, and expected rate of lay. For most chicken keepers, using a commercial ration is the easiest way to provide the basics on which to build a balanced diet.

Commercial rations are formulated according to stage of maturity and include chick starter, grower, developer, and layer rations. Layer ration may be available with different levels of protein, the higher levels used during hot weather when hens tend to eat less and also to improve the hatchability of eggs intended for incubation. Broilers have their own formulations for starter/grower and finisher rations intended to induce rapid growth.

Rations designed for mature chickens are usually in the form of pellets, which consist of ground-up ingredients that are mixed together, then compressed. Each pellet has an identical nutritional value so chickens can't pick out only what they like. Crumbles start out as pellets that are then crushed to make them small enough for chicks to swallow. Rations for mature chickens are sometimes crushed into crumbles to make eating take longer, which makes the chickens less likely to get bored and start picking on each other.

The variety of choices you have in commercially prepared rations will depend on where you live. In some areas developer, finisher, and breeder rations are not available, and lay ration comes in only one protein level. You'll have more choices if you live in an area where chickens are especially numerous.

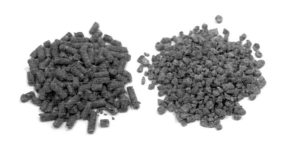

Pellets (left) contain ground-up and crushed ingredients. Crumbles (right) are crushed pellets.

Despite the inclusion of antioxidants to slow the deterioration of bagged rations, nutrients are gradually destroyed by heat, sunlight, oxygen, and a variety of spoilage organisms. Even the best ration loses nutritional value during prolonged storage at a warehouse or on your back porch.

A good rule of thumb is to buy only as much feed as you can use within 6 weeks of manufacture. Store the feed in such a way that it won't go rancid, moldy, or stale. Nutritional content holds up best in feed stored in a cool, dry place, away from direct sunlight. Once you open a bag, transfer the feed to a sealed container that keeps out insects and rodents.

Typical Schedule for Prepared Rations

FLOCK TYPE	AGE	FEED*
Broilers	1 day–5 weeks	Starter
	5–7 weeks	Finisher
	or 1 day–7 weeks	Starter/grower
Roasters	7 weeks–slaughter	Finisher + corn
Layers and breeders	1 day–6 weeks	Starter
	6–13 weeks	Grower
	13–20 weeks	Pullet developer
	or 1 day–20 weeks	Starter/grower
	20+ weeks	Lay ration + calcium supplement

In many areas, the only feeds readily available for small flocks are starter/grower and layer ration. Gradually make any feed change by adding progressively more of the new ration and less of the old until the changeover is complete.

Feeding Breeders

Nutritional research has largely focused on broiler chicks and laying hens, because that's where the money is. More is therefore known about the requirements for rapid early growth in heavy breeds and the maintenance needs of lightweight high-production hens than about requirements of the breeds commonly found in backyard flocks.

Furthermore, commercially prepared layer rations are formulated to ensure hens lay well but don't always provide sufficient nutrition for the eggs to hatch into strong, viable chicks. Some farm stores carry a breeder ration. The next best thing is a game bird ration. Since adding grain dilutes protein, vitamins, and minerals, eliminate grain during hatching season. Also add a vitamin/mineral supplement to the drinking water. Vitamins A and E are particularly important for males; a deficiency in either vitamin reduces fertility.

Introduce your flock to a breeder diet at least 1 month before you plan to start collecting eggs for hatching, and continue it throughout the breeding season. By improving your flock's level of nutrition, you should see at least a 10 percent improvement in the hatchability of their eggs.

Home-Mixed Rations

With chicken keeping such a popular backyard pastime, a lot of people are deciding not to feed their chickens commercially prepared rations. Here are a few of their many reasons:

- To avoid the ever-rising cost of commercially prepared rations

- To steer clear of genetically engineered feedstuffs

- To improve the nutritional value of chicken meat and eggs

- To avoid feeds to which the chicken keeper may be allergic

- To improve the chickens' health and longevity

Formulating your own rations is a complex undertaking. It involves a thorough understanding of the nutritional needs of chickens (about which entire books have been written), as well as the nutritive value of available feedstuffs capable of providing those needs.

If you decide to mix your own, you might purchase all the separate ingredients or grow some of them yourself. If your intent is to save money, you may be in for a surprise — buying first-quality ingredients separately will likely cost more than purchasing ready-mixed rations.

When you mix your own feed, you can either crush or grind the feedstuffs or feed them whole. Grinding lets you mix things together so each chicken can't pick out its favorite ingredient. To keep things fresh and avoid nutritional deficiencies, crack or grind the ingredients within about a week of feeding them.

The advantage to feeding whole grains is that they keep their nutritional value longer than cracked grains. When converting a flock from a commercial pellet or crumble to whole grains, do it gradually to give the chickens' gizzard muscles time to handle the extra workout. Whether you feed grains whole or cracked, use a combination of ingredients that furnish an appropriate balance of energy, protein, vitamins, and minerals.

Avoiding GMOs

One of the reasons people cite for mixing their own chicken feed is to avoid genetically modified ingredients. Most bagged chicken feed includes corn for energy and soybeans for protein; 88 percent of the corn and 94 percent of the soybeans grown in the United States are genetically modified.

A genetically modified organism (GMO) is a living thing into which genetic material from an unrelated organism has been artificially inserted. Unlike hybrids, which have been selectively bred from similar organisms, genetic modification involves altering the genetic structure of an organism in a way that would not occur in nature.

The purpose of most GM crops is to make the plants resistant to insects or to herbicides, or both.

Insect resistance is derived from the common soil-dwelling bacterium *Bacillus thuringiensis* (Bt), which is used as a natural insecticidal spray in both chemical-based and organic farming. It kills insects by binding to receptors in an insect's gut, causing the insect to stop feeding and die. Bt corn is engineered to kill insects without being sprayed; instead, the corn plants produce their own Bt, which kills any Bt-susceptible insect that chomps down on a corn plant. Different strains of Bt affect different types of corn pests.

Sprayed-on Bt is degraded by sunlight and therefore ceases to be effective in less than a week — 24 hours for some strains. Sprayed-on Bt also is rinsed off the crop by rain or overhead irrigation. In contrast, Bt in genetically engineered (GE) corn occurs in every cell of the plant, including the harvested corn. It is more concentrated than sprayed-on Bt and doesn't degrade or rinse

GRIT FOR THE GIZZARD

Grit is little more than a collection of coarse sand, pebbles, and similar small, hard objects that are eaten by a chicken. The grit lodges in the bird's gizzard, where the gizzard's muscular action grinds it together with tough feeds to break them down for digestion. Over time each piece of grit gets ground up, along with the feed, so the gizzard's grit supply needs to be constantly replenished.

Whether or not chickens require supplemental grit is a matter of some debate. Chickens that eat only commercially processed feeds — such as chick crumbles or layer pellets — don't need supplemental grit because saliva alone is sufficient to soften these feeds. Chickens that are fed whole grains can learn to manage without grit, provided the grains are introduced gradually to give the chickens' gizzard muscles time to strengthen.

On the other hand, chickens that have an opportunity to forage ordinarily pick up grit from the environment to help them digest fibrous plant material, making grit a regular part of natural digestion. To ensure that a flock has access to adequate amounts of grit, many chicken keepers offer it as a free-choice option.

Commercially available grit is available in two forms:

Mineral grit serves as a time-release source of minerals, most notably calcium carbonate (needed by laying hens to produce strong eggshells), and therefore is commonly called calcium grit. Oyster shell is a mineral grit that erodes less readily than other sources of calcium carbonate, so it serves double duty as a source of both calcium and grit for the gizzard.

Calcium grit is available in a variety of screened sizes, one of which is called chick grit or starter grit. But supplemental calcium should not be fed to birds that are not nearing the age of lay, as excess calcium can interfere with bone development and also cause kidney damage. Similarly, any chicken that does not need extra calcium (such as a cock or a poorly laying hen) can overdose if it eats mineral grit because it doesn't have access to inert grit.

Inert grit is a hard form of grit, such as granite grit or washed river sand, that is not readily ground up by the gizzard. Grit fed to young chickens, and to mature cocks, should be inert, to avoid calcium overdose. Laying hens that have access to both inert grit and mineral grit will choose one or the other based on whether or not they need more calcium.

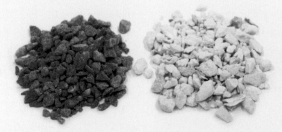

Inert grit (granite) Mineral grit (oyster shell)

off the plant. When a chicken (or a human) eats Bt corn, it gets an undesirable dose of insecticide.

Herbicide tolerance (HT) is another feat of genetic engineering. Roundup is a broad-spectrum systemic herbicide produced by Monsanto. Its main active ingredient is glyphosate. When sprayed on a plant, glyphosate is absorbed through the leaves and into the shoots and roots, disrupting the plant's ability to grow and causing the plant to die. Roundup is widely used by farmers to control weeds that compete with their commercial crops.

The problem with Roundup is that it kills crops as readily as it kills weeds. So starting with soybeans, Monsanto has engineered various crops to be resistant to the effect of glyphosate. This technology, called Roundup Ready, involves the insertion of an enzyme from the soil bacterium *Agrobacterium tumefaciens,* which is resistant to glyphosate. Plants sprayed with Roundup absorb the herbicide, but unlike weeds, modified HT crops don't die. As with Bt in crops, if we or our chickens ingest these crops, we also get the Roundup.

In a study published in 2013 in the journal *Current Biology,* glyphosate was tested against the gut bacteria normally found in chickens. Most of the pathogenic bacteria (*Salmonella* Enteritidis, *S. Gallinarum, S. Typhimurium, Clostridium perfringens,* and *C. botulinum*) were highly resistant to glyphosate, while most of the beneficial/probiotic bacteria (*Enterococcus faecalis, E. faecium, Bacillus badius, Bifidobacterium adolescentis,* and *Lactobacillus* spp.) were moderately to highly susceptible. Since the gut's good bacteria are responsible for keeping the bad bacteria under control, feeding chickens rations containing glyphosate has the potential for increasing

diseases caused by salmonella and campylobacter, as well as their related illnesses in people who eat contaminated meat or eggs.

Roundup Ready is not the only HT technology. There's also Libertylink corn and soy, which are resistant to the herbicide glufosinate, and the Enlist Weed Control System, which makes corn and soybeans resistant to the weed killer 2,4-D. And then there's stacking, where more than one GM trait is combined in a single plant. SmartStax, for instance, combines eight traits: six for insect resistance and two for tolerance to different herbicides.

So far no one has produced definitive proof that GMOs are or are not safe, yet modified corn, soy, and other crops have permeated the feed system to the point that you can pretty much assume anything derived from corn or soy (as well as from alfalfa, canola, cottonseed, or sugar beets) is GM unless it's labeled "non-GMO," "GMO-free," or "organic." By law farmers and processors of organic products must show they do not use GMOs and they make an effort to protect their crops and products from contact with GMOs. The Non-GMO Project and the Non-GMO Sourcebook are among websites that list GMO-free resources.

Basic Ration Formulas

The exact nutritional analysis of each ingredient varies with its source, the time of year it was grown, the place where it was grown, and the methods by which it was grown and harvested. Purchased feedstuffs may be labeled with some nutritional information. Average values are suggested in *Nutrient Requirements of Poultry* (periodically updated by the National Academy Press) and similar source books.

Feeding your chickens GM rations does not automatically make them, or their meat or eggs, genetically modified. Chickens that are genetically engineered, or transgenic, are created by inserting genetic material from some other organism into a developing chicken embryo that then hatches into a transgenic chicken. Some engineered traits are heritable, meaning they are passed on to the chickens' offspring; others aren't. Engineered chickens, which outwardly look like any other chicken, have been or are being developed for several different purposes.

Food-use chickens may at some point be engineered to grow faster and develop larger breast muscles. Such chickens may have a trademark string of DNA inserted as a sort of copyright tag to prevent unlicensed breeding. To date, consumer resistance has prevented transgenic chickens from being commercially grown for food.

Biopharm chickens are hatched from eggs into which human DNA has been inserted. They are used to produce substances for pharmaceutical use. Some biopharm lines produce insulin; others produce various antibodies that are made into vaccines; still others produce cancer-treating drugs. These biopharmaceuticals are collected from eggs, rather than from the chickens' blood, as is done with other animals engineered for drug production. Chickens with human DNA may be used, as well, to study the progression of human diseases and disorders. In a document about transgenic animals, the Food and Drug Administration (FDA) has stated, "In general, we do not anticipate that biopharm animals will be used for food."

Disease-resistant transgenic chickens may be used for either food or biopharm applications. One such line is engineered to be resistant to the avian leukosis virus (Marek's disease). Another line is engineered to prevent the spread of bird flu. These chickens still can be infected by a bird flu virus, but they can't transmit it to other chickens, transgenic or not, a trait that would prevent the virus from mutating into a more highly pathogenic form. To date, no disease-resistant transgenic chickens are available to the public.

A good, comprehensive resource for ration formulation is *Feeding Poultry* by G. F. Heuser (reprinted from the original 1955 publication). Although it includes some nutrient tables, its greater value is in its extensive discussions of nutrient sources and feeding methods, as well as its numerous recipes for complete starter/grower rations, layer rations, and breeder rations.

The table on page 44 offers an easy way to formulate your own well-balanced rations. It lists a variety of feedstuffs from which you can choose to mix 100 pounds (45 kg) of starter, grower, or layer ration. For the most nutritious blend, select a combination of ingredients from each category that adds up to the total weight for that line.

Although you needn't limit yourself to the specific ingredients listed, substitute only ingredients of similar nutritional value. As an example, instead of alfalfa meal you may use alfalfa pellets or alfalfa hay fines (the bits of vegetation that collect at the bottom of a livestock hay feeder) or provide pasture where your chickens can forage for fresh tender greens.

If you have a goat or a cow that produces more milk than your household uses, you may substitute fresh milk for the milk powder. Two pounds (0.9 kg) of milk powder is equivalent to about 20 pounds (9 kg) of liquid milk, needed for every 100 pounds (45 kg) of feed consumed. Since mixing milk into dry ration invites spoilage, offer the milk in a separate container. One time-honored way to feed chickens liquid milk is to fill drinkers with milk instead of water for half of each day.

Whatever you have available that's suitable for feeding chickens, determine where it fits in the table and substitute like amounts. If the feedstuff doesn't come with a nutritional label, you can determine approximate nutritional equivalents by consulting *Nutrient Requirements of Poultry* or a similar source that offers page after page of tables listing the average nutritional contents of various feedstuffs.

Nutritional Energy

Like a chicken's water use, its energy needs vary with temperature. Where the annual temperature range is extreme, adjust nutritional energy seasonally — upward during cold months, downward during warm months. You reduce energy by adding wheat bran (but not too much, which would affect laying) and increase it by increasing either protein or carbohydrates.

NUTRITION AND WEIGHT GAIN

Prevent Starvation

Starvation occurs when newly hatched chicks do not learn to eat early enough, causing them to rapidly lose energy until they can no longer actively seek food. In older birds, starvation occurs when rations are too high in fiber (such as might occur in discount feeds). Starvation may also be related to climate: during cold weather, chickens may not get enough to eat to keep warm; during hot weather, chickens eat less and therefore consume fewer nutrients; during extremely dry weather, chickens that rely on pasture may not find adequate vegetation. These issues may be overcome by adjusting the feed's nutritional content.

Avoid Obesity

Obesity is most likely to occur in inactive chickens kept as pets and fed more energy-rich feed than they need. Some breeds — especially New Hampshire, Plymouth Rock, and other dual-purpose breeds — have a tendency to put on fat. Fat hens do not lay well and are more subject to heatstroke and reproductive problems. Signs of obesity include poor laying, poor shell quality, laying eggs at night, frequent multiple yolks, and prolapse. To determine if a chicken is overweight, check the area below the vent — if it bulges and looks dimply, the hen is too fat.

Home-Mixed Formulas

INGREDIENT*	Imperial			Metric		
	STARTER	GROWER	LAYER	STARTER	GROWER	LAYER
Coarsely ground grain (corn, milo, oats, wheat, rice, etc.)	46 lb	50 lb	53.5 lb	20.5 kg	22.5 kg	24 kg
Wheat bran, rice bran, etc.	10 lb	18 lb	17 lb	4.5 kg	8 kg	7.5 kg
Soybean meal, peanut meal, cottonseed meal (low gossypol), safflower meal, sunflower meal, sesame meal, etc.	29.5 lb	16.5 lb	15 lb	13 kg	7 kg	6.7 kg
Meat meal, fish meal, soybean meal	5 lb	5 lb	3 lb	2.3 kg	2.3 kg	1.3 kg
Alfalfa meal (not needed for pastured birds)	4 lb	4 lb	4 lb	1.8 kg	1.8 kg	1.8 kg
Bone meal, rock phosphate	2 lb	2 lb	2 lb	1 kg	1 kg	1 kg
Vitamin supplement** (with 200,000 IU vitamin A, 80,000 IU vitamin D_3, 100 mg riboflavin)	+	+	+	+	+	+
Yeast, milk powder (not needed if vitamin supplement is balanced)	2 lb	2 lb	2 lb	1 kg	1 kg	1 kg
Ground limestone, marble, oyster shell, aragonite	1 lb	2 lb	3 lb	0.5 kg	1 kg	1.3 kg
Trace mineral salt or iodized salt** (supplemented with 0.5 ounce manganese sulfate and 0.5 ounce zinc oxide)	0.5 lb	0.5 lb	0.5 lb	200 g	200 g	200 g
Total	100 lb	100 lb	100 lb	45 kg	45 kg	45 kg

*Ideally, use a combination of ingredients in each category.

**Instead of a vitamin supplement and trace mineral salt, you can use a complete commercial vitamin/mineral premix per directions on the label (usually 3 lb/100 lb).

Adapted from "Feeding Chickens," Suburban Rancher, Leaflet #2919, University of California

A chicken's energy needs also change with its level of activity. A bird that spends a lot of time foraging requires more energy than one that gets its entire daily ration from a trough. Chickens that are fed a lot of kitchen scraps and garden waste may get insufficient energy, and protein, for good growth and egg laying.

Although protein contains a certain amount of energy, a more concentrated form of energy is the carbohydrates found in grain. Because grains are the most caloric form of energy, they must be used judiciously. If the ration is too high in carbohydrates, chickens get fat; if too low, they become underweight. Both situations affect laying and increase the birds' susceptibility to disease.

Grain Caution

⚠ When feeding grain to your chickens, make sure the grain is mold-free. Molds produce mycotoxins, which can be detrimental or even deadly to chickens, as described on page 247.

Corn is the grain most commonly fed to chickens because it is the easiest for them to digest. Other sources of energy include cereal grains and oilseeds, most of which have two major disadvantages as chicken feed: they contain antinutrients of one sort or another, and they are not as easily digested as corn.

An antinutrient is a natural compound that interferes with the absorption of vitamins, minerals, or other nutrients, resulting in diarrhea or pasting and, in chicks, slow growth. A diet that is heavy in one feedstuff can result in a deficiency of the nutrients that are bound by the antinutrients in that particular ingredient. Combine a variety of feedstuffs to help prevent deficiencies, since not all feedstuffs contain the same antinutrients. Commercial rations are fortified to compensate for antinutrients.

Feeding grains with low digestibility can result in sticky droppings. Among cereal grains, the worst offenders are barley, oats, rye, and wheat; among the offending oilseed meals are rape, soy, and sunflower.

When large amounts of these feeds go undigested, they become thick and sticky in the intestinal tract, resulting in loose, gelatinous droppings that stick to skin, feathers, feet, and eggs. Sticky droppings moisten litter, promoting an ideal environment for pathogens and increasing respiratory stress due to ammonia fumes. If your chickens consistently produce sticky droppings, take a good look at what you are feeding them.

Speaking of Feed Ingredients

amino acids. The basic constituents of proteins

antinutrient. A natural compound in a feedstuff that interferes with the absorption of nutrients

antioxidants. Organic chemicals of plant origin that destroy free radicals and reduce, prevent, or help repair the damage they do

free radicals. Unstable oxygen molecules that damage body cells and contribute to the development of such unhealthful conditions as impaired immunity, heart disease, and tumors

GMO. Genetically modified organism; a living thing into which genetic material from an unrelated organism has been unnaturally inserted; also called genetically engineered or transgenic

Protein and Amino Acids

Providing protein is the most expensive part of feeding chickens. Protein is furnished by any feedstuff that is high in amino acids, which are nutrients the body uses to make and maintain such things as muscles, ligaments, cartilage, skin, feathers, blood cells, hormones, and enzymes.

A chicken's body needs 22 amino acids, some of which (the essential amino acids) must be furnished by diet, while others (the nonessential amino acids) can be synthesized within the chicken's body. However, even the nonessential amino acids must be furnished in some amounts to prevent a shortage that causes essential amino acids to be converted into nonessential amino acids.

Sources of protein are classified as being either complete or incomplete. Complete protein, sometimes called high-quality protein, furnishes a good balance of all the essential amino acids. Complete protein comes from animal sources such as meat, fish, dairy products, and eggs. The tiny grain quinoa, although low in protein, also contains all the essential amino acids and therefore is considered to be a complete protein.

Incomplete protein is a source that is low in one or more of the essential amino acids. Incomplete protein comes from plant sources, including oilseed meals (such as peanut, safflower, and sunflower) and grain legumes (alfalfa, beans, and field peas). Grain sorghum, wheat, and similar cereal grains are often fed to backyard chickens as a source of protein, but along with corn they are particularly low in the essential amino acid lycine.

The most common source of protein in commercial rations is soybean meal, which is the residue remaining after the beans have been processed with solvents to remove the oil. Although soy is commonly considered to be a complete protein, it is deficient in the essential amino acid methionine, which is so important it has been called the queen of amino acids.

Not incidentally, while soybeans and other legumes contain more protein than any other plant-derived feedstuff, raw legumes also contain antinutrients that make them particularly undigestible. Roasting or steaming them improves their digestibility by destroying the antinutrients, but overheating reduces their nutritional value. Sprouting raw legumes is an easy alternative.

Incomplete proteins may be made complete by combining readily digestible protein-rich ingredients that have complementary amino acid profiles. Complementary proteins might consist of a combination of plant and animal sources, such as a legume or cereal grain plus a dairy product; for example, whey derived from cheesemaking.

Combining only plant sources, such as legumes plus either cereal grains or oil seeds, also works, although given the opportunity (or the need), chickens will opt for some animal protein in the form of such things as bugs and worms, or sometimes feathers and even each other.

Producers of commercial rations maximize profits by using sources of lesser-quality protein fortified with synthetic amino acids. If you prefer to mix your own, you can provide your flock with better-quality protein by judiciously choosing a variety of ingredients that, combined, equal the total protein values listed in the table on page 48.

FAT FACTS

Chickens need some amount of fat for health and growth. A chicken's body uses fat to store energy and fat-soluble vitamins, insulate body tissues, and cushion internal organs. In general an older chicken accumulates more fat than a younger chicken, and a hen has more than a cock of the same breed and age. Too much fat, however, can result in reduced health, laying, and fertility.

Fat consists of a group of compounds called fatty acids, which are divided into two main types: saturated and unsaturated. The latter is further subdivided into two types: monounsaturated and polyunsaturated. Polyunsaturated fatty acids are divided into two main groups: omega-3 and omega-6.

A chicken's body can metabolize nearly all the fatty acids it needs from normal daily rations. The single exception is the omega-6 fatty acid known as linoleic acid, which is required for both growth and egg production.

Linoleic acid comes from nuts, seeds, vegetable oils, and animal products. Animal sources include pork lard, beef tallow, and milk. An excellent nonanimal source is sunflower seeds. Linoleic acid is concentrated in polyunsaturated oils, such as safflower oil, sunflower oil, and corn oil.

The problem with polyunsaturated oils is that they can get rancid pretty quickly, especially when exposed to air, heat, and light. Rancid oils are unstable and create free radicals (see Antioxidants and Free Radicals, page 57). Refined oils have been exposed to air, heat, and light during processing and therefore get rancid more quickly than the whole seeds they came from. Oils used in home-formulated rations should be stored in a cool, dark place and mixed into the ration just before feeding.

PROTEIN AND HEALTH

If a chicken is deficient in a single amino acid, that amino acid is said to be limiting, because it restricts or limits growth, reproduction, and overall health. For optimal health at any given stage in a chicken's life, the bird needs a specific combination of amino acids, with none limiting or in excess. The best combination of amino acids for each stage of life is called ideal protein.

If you define "ideal" as being perfect, and you recognize that nothing is perfect, then ideal protein is not so readily attainable. For one thing, the amino acid content and digestibility of any particular feed ingredient varies with such factors as genetics and growing conditions. For another, despite all the research that has been done over the decades, we still don't know with 100 percent certainty exactly what a chicken's nutritional requirements are at each stage of its life.

Then throw in the nutritional effects of stress or ill health. A chicken's body needs complete protein to produce antibodies that fight disease. During infection a bird rapidly loses its protein stores, causing its protein requirement to go up. If the bird cannot obtain additional protein, its resistance drops. An adequate amount of complete protein is especially important for stressful periods experienced by chicks that are growing, hens that are laying, roosters that are expected to fertilize eggs, chickens displayed at exhibitions, and any chicken going through a molt.

Deficiencies in specific amino acids are linked to specific conditions, most of which are not common in backyard chickens, especially those that have some opportunity to forage outdoors. Marginal amino acid deficiencies, particularly in growing birds, can result in an increase in appetite, a decrease in lean muscle growth, and an excess of body fat.

Interestingly, general signs of overall protein deficiency are similar to general signs of infection: decreased appetite, slow growth in chicks or weight loss in mature birds, decreased laying, and smaller egg size. At the other extreme, excess protein in a chicken's diet is converted to uric acid and deposited as crystals in joints, causing gout.

Protein Needs

Chickens of different ages and levels of production need different levels of overall protein. Whenever the protein in a flock's diet is adjusted by more than 2 percent, make the change gradually to avoid intestinal upset and diarrhea.

TYPE	AGE	PROTEIN*
Broiler	0–3 weeks	20–24%
	3 weeks–butcher	16–20%
Layer	0–6 weeks	18–20%
	6–14 weeks	16–18%
	14–20 weeks	14–16%
	20+ weeks	15–17%
Cock	Maintenance	10–12%
Breeder	20+ weeks	18–20%

*As a percentage of total daily ration

UPPING PROTEIN

Since feathers are 85 percent protein, a little supplemental animal protein will help your chickens through a molt and improve the plumage of show birds. Compared to the protein in grains, animal protein is rich in the amino acids a chicken needs during a molt. Some good sources of animal protein include the following:

- High-quality cat food (not dog food, most of which derives protein from grains)

- Raw meat from a reliable source (not chicken; feeding an animal the meat of its own species can perpetuate diseases)

- Fish (but don't feed fish to a chicken you plan to eat anytime soon or the meat may taste fishy)

- Molting food, sold by pet stores for caged songbirds (it's expensive but lets you circumvent such issues as potentially toxic pet foods and bacteria-laden meats)

- Scrambled or mashed hard-boiled eggs

- Sprouted grains and seeds, particularly alfalfa and sesame seeds (sprouting improves protein quantity and quality)

- Mealworms and red worms (which are about 50 percent and 80 percent protein, respectively)

A hard molt — when feathers fall rapidly but grow back slowly — may indicate a deficiency in animal protein. Another indicator is feathers that become brittle and break easily. If the deficiency is unlikely to be caused by a dietary problem, look for a disease (recent or current) that may be inhibiting protein absorption.

ADJUSTING PROTEIN

Using a method called Pearson's square, you can easily determine how much of each protein ingredient you must combine to get the protein level you want. Begin by drawing a square on a piece of paper. In the upper left corner, write the percentage of protein in the first ingredient. In the lower left corner, write the percentage of protein contained in the second ingredient. At the center of the square, write the percentage of protein you want to end up with.

Moving from the upper left toward the lower right (following the arrow in the illustration), subtract the smaller number from the larger number. Write the answer in the lower right corner. Moving from the lower left toward the upper right (again following the arrow), subtract the smaller number from the larger number. Write the answer in the upper right corner. The number in the upper right corner tells you how many

pounds of the first ingredient and the number in the lower right corner tells you how many pounds of the second ingredient you need to mix together to achieve the desired level of protein.

The illustration on this page shows two typical examples. In the first case 16 percent lay ration is combined with 8 percent scratch to create a 10 percent cock maintenance diet. Note that since we want to reduce the protein content, the number in the lower left corner must be less than the number in the upper left corner. Pearson's square shows that to get a 10 percent cock maintenance ration we need to combine 2 parts of lay ration with 6 parts of scratch, or 1 part (pound or kilogram) lay ration to 3 parts (pounds or kilograms) scratch.

In the second example, 16 percent layer ration is combined with 31 percent cat kibble to create a breeder-flock ration containing 19 percent protein. Since we now want to

Pearson's Square

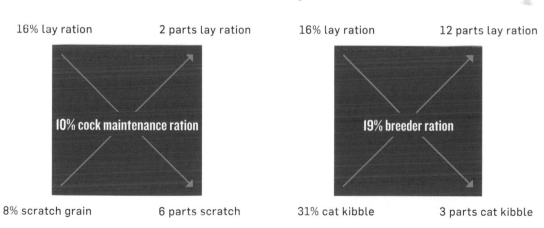

16% lay ration   2 parts lay ration

10% cock maintenance ration

8% scratch grain   6 parts scratch

16% lay ration   12 parts lay ration

19% breeder ration

31% cat kibble   3 parts cat kibble

Using Pearson's square, you can determine how much ration and how much supplement to combine together to get the desired protein content.

increase the protein content, the number in the lower left corner is greater than the number in the upper left corner. Pearson's square shows that to get a 19 percent breeder ration we should mix 12 parts of layer ration with 3 parts of kibble, or 4 parts (pounds or kilograms) of layer ration to 1 part (pounds or kilograms) of kibble.

Different feedstuffs have different weights, so you won't get an accurate mix if you measure by volume (bucketfuls) instead of by weight (pounds or kilograms). If you don't have a spring scale for weighing feed, weigh yourself on a bathroom scale holding an empty bucket. Add feed to the bucket until you increase the total weight by the amount you need.

In combining feedstuffs use rations of similar consistency. If, for example, you use soybean meal to boost the protein in pelleted ration, the meal will filter out and fall to the bottom of the trough. You'd do better to combine soybean meal with crumbles, perhaps moistening the result at feeding time to keep the meal from sifting out.

Whenever you adjust the protein in your flock's diet by more than a percentage point or two, make the change gradually. Too rapid a change can cause intestinal upset and diarrhea.

Vitamins

Derived from plant or animal sources, vitamins are needed in small quantities for normal growth and activity. Chickens need every known vitamin in some amount, and — unlike their needs for energy and protein — their vitamin requirements remain fairly steady year-round. However, a flock's vitamin requirements are interrelated with and must be balanced against other nutritional components — protein, minerals, and energy — whose sources

also contain some vitamins. Vitamins are either fat-soluble or water-soluble.

FAT-SOLUBLE VITAMINS

Vitamins A, D, E, and K, the fat-soluble vitamins, are stored in body fat to be used as they are needed. Because these vitamins are stockpiled in the fat, a diet that is too high in fat-soluble vitamins can result in toxicity, a condition known as hypervitaminosis. A deficiency in any of these vitamins, called hypovitaminosis or avitaminosis, can result from depressed appetite due to illness, hot weather, or other extreme stress. Because these vitamins are stored gradually and used gradually, signs of excess or deficiency can take a long time to appear.

Vitamin A is a group of related nutrients required for vision, growth, and bone development. It is called the anti-infection vitamin because it helps sustain the immune system. It aids disease resistance as an antioxidant (see Antioxidants and Free Radicals, page 57) and also by playing a role in maintaining mucus production in the linings of the digestive, reproductive, and respiratory tracts.

Vitamin A deficiency can occur in chickens that are fed stale commercial rations or an improperly balanced home-mixed ration without having access to green forage. It may also be caused by any health condition that interferes with nutrient absorption, such as coccidiosis or worms. A vitamin A deficiency, in turn, increases a chicken's susceptibility to coccidia and other internal parasites.

If a chicken consistently misses the mark while pecking, suspect poor eyesight due to a deficiency of vitamin A. Deficiency can also cause laying hens to take more time off between clutches, as well as reducing the hatchability of their eggs; chicks that hatch from such eggs will themselves be vitamin A deficient. An increase in blood spots in eggs is another sign, since the amount of vitamin A needed to minimize blood spots is higher than the amount needed to keep a hen healthy enough to lay.

Vitamin A deficiency interferes with the proper functioning of mucus-producing glands and can cause the upper digestive tract to develop blisters resembling those of fowl pox. The damage caused to linings of the upper digestive and respiratory tracts may open the way for a bacterial or viral invasion. Deficiency can cause a condition known as nutritional roup, which mimics a respiratory infection — characterized by runny eyes and nose, eyelids stuck together, ruffled feathers, weakness, and emaciation — and can increase the severity of any existing respiratory infection.

Green forage is an excellent source of vitamin A. For confined chickens cod liver oil mixed into the ration at the rate of 2 tablespoons per 5 pounds (65 mL per 5 kg) is another good source, used in moderation — too much can make eggs taste fishy. An excellent source is a vitamin AD&E supplement, used as directed on the label.

Take care not to go overboard with vitamin A supplements. Too much vitamin A is toxic to chickens. Ironically, the signs of vitamin A excess are similar to the signs of deficiency.

Vitamin D is a steroidlike compound necessary for the absorption of calcium to make strong bones, beaks, claws, and eggshells. A bird's body synthesizes vitamin D from sunshine, making deficiency more likely in confined chickens than in those having access to the outdoors.

In young chickens a vitamin D deficiency can cause rickets. Signs include bent or malformed beaks, bowed legs, and deformities of the ribs and spine. Where growing chicks cannot be provided access to unfiltered sunlight, full-spectrum fluorescent lighting for part of the day is the next best thing.

A typical sign of vitamin D deficiency in hens is a continuing cycle of normal egg production, followed by the appearance of thin- and soft-shelled eggs, followed by a drop in production, followed by a return to normal production. A deficient hen may have weak legs just before she lays an egg, causing her to squat in a penguinlike stance. If the deficiency is not corrected, her beak, claws, and keel will become soft, and her eggs will be small with reduced hatchability. Deficiency can be corrected easily with access to sunlight, or by adding cod liver oil to feed at the rate of 2 tablespoons per 5 pounds (65 mL per 5 kg) or using a vitamin AD&E supplement as directed on the label.

A chicken's need for vitamin D is intimately tied with its needs for the minerals calcium and phosphorus. A deficiency in any of these three nutrients can cause egg eating, as well as osteoporosis in older birds.

An excess of vitamin D can cause an excess of calcium in the blood, a condition called hypercalcemia. Excess calcium affects the heart and other organs, is toxic to the liver, and can cause the kidneys to calcify, which in mature chickens leads to gout. One sign of too much vitamin D in a hen's diet is the appearance of calcium pimples on eggshells, which, if scraped off, leave little holes in the shell.

Vitamin E is an antioxidant (see Antioxidants and Free Radicals, page 57) and a necessary nutrient for the normal functioning of the immune and reproductive systems. Vitamin E is concentrated in polyunsaturated fats, such as those found in fresh cod liver oil, corn oil, soybean oil, and wheat germ oil. Dietary deficiency most often results from feeding oil-rich rations that have gone rancid, which can occur rapidly when the temperature and humidity are high.

In mature chickens, deficiency produces no visible signs, but it can result in reduced fertility in cocks and the early death of embryos in incubated eggs laid by deficient hens. Deficiency in chicks can result in a potentially lethal nervous disorder (encephalomalacia) that, left untreated, destroys the brain. When started early, an effective treatment is a vitamin AD&E supplement, used as directed on the label and continued until signs disappear.

Vitamin E and the trace mineral selenium are closely linked. A deficiency of either nutrient can result in a readily treatable condition in which fluid accumulates under the skin (exudative diathesis). An adequate amount of vitamin E in the diet ensures the metabolism of sufficient selenium to prevent this deficiency.

Vitamin K is necessary for normal blood clotting. Signs of deficiency are profuse bleeding from slight wounds and internal bleeding (into the body cavity, or under the skin and appearing as a bruise). A deficiency of vitamin K in the breeder diet causes late, and bloody, embryo deaths during incubation. Alfalfa and leafy dark greens are good sources of vitamin K.

WATER-SOLUBLE VITAMINS

B and C, the water-soluble vitamins, are not stored by the body, which uses only what it immediately needs and expels any excess in droppings. Water-soluble vitamins must therefore be replenished more often than fat-soluble vitamins.

Vitamin B is actually a group of unrelated substances that often appear together in the same feed sources and therefore were once considered to be a single vitamin. After they were determined to be several different nutrients, they were given individual numbers and names. Today 8 of the 22 originally numbered B vitamins are identified as part of the B complex. The rest are no longer considered to be vitamins and therefore have been removed from the B

Fat-Soluble Vitamins

VITAMIN	ROLE	DEFICIENCY SIGN	SOURCE
A	Vision, growth, strong bones, immunity, antioxidant	Weakness, slow growth or emaciation, poor vision, reduced laying, low hatchability, blood spots in eggs, respiratory distress	Green forage, cod liver oil
D	Enable calcium absorption	Rickets, thin- and soft-shell eggs with low hatchability, leg weakness	Sunshine, cod liver oil
E	Antioxidant, immunity, reproduction	Encephalomalacia, reduced fertility in cocks, low hatchability of eggs	Cod liver oil, corn oil, soybean oil, wheat germ
K	Blood clotting	Easy bruising and bleeding	Alfalfa, leafy dark greens

list, which accounts for gaps in the numbering system: B_4, B_8, B_{10}, and B_{11} are missing.

All the B_1 vitamins aid in converting carbohydrates into energy-producing glucose, as well as helping metabolize protein and fats. The B complex is also important for the proper functioning of the brain and the rest of the nervous system, and for healthy skin, feathers, beaks, claws, eyes, and liver.

Most B vitamins come from plant sources. Vitamin B_{12} is unique among nutrients in being found almost exclusively in animal products. A vitamin B_{12} deficiency can occur in chickens confined indoors, especially if they are fed soymeal as the main or sole source of protein. Chickens raised on built-up floor litter get enough vitamin B_{12} by picking in the litter. Chickens pastured with other livestock get plenty of B_{12} by picking through cow patties and horse apples.

A deficiency of vitamin B_2 is notable because it can cause curled-toe paralysis in chicks that hatch from the eggs of penned breeder hens fed an unsupplemented layer ration. Greens, including young grass, are good sources of B_2. Milk, whey, and other dairy products are also good sources, but too much can cause diarrhea.

A deficiency is not always caused by the lack of a vitamin in the diet. For instance, the coccidiostat amprolium has a similar chemical structure to vitamin B_1. It therefore metabolically competes with vitamin B_1, so the prolonged use of amprolium can lead to a B_1 deficiency.

Choline was once called vitamin B_4. Although it is no longer considered to be a vitamin, it is an essential nutrient that is still grouped with the B vitamins. Among other things, choline aids in the maintenance of properly functioning nerves. Mature chickens synthesize choline, but chicks are susceptible to choline deficiency, which can result in poor growth. Choline is notable for being one of the nutrients that, when deficient in a chick's diet, can cause the potentially fatal condition slipped tendon (see Slipped Tendon on page 119). Good sources of choline are soybean meal and wheat bran.

Vitamin C helps prevent diseases both as an antioxidant (see Antioxidants and Free Radicals, page 57) and by reducing the harmful effects of stress. Chickens make their own vitamin C and do not need a supplement, except when the absorption of vitamin C and other nutrients is inhibited by stress, such as might occur because of hot weather, overcrowding, or the presence of a disease. Such periods of stress can reduce immunity by rapidly using up the body's stores of vitamin C.

Supplementing your flock's summer diet with a source of vitamin C can help them overcome heat stress, but be careful with a vitamin C supplement (ascorbic acid), as too much can upset digestion and cause diarrhea. A better choice is treating your chickens to some fresh produce. Among the best sources of vitamin C are uncooked pumpkins and other winter squash, sweet potatoes, and leafy dark greens.

Minerals

Minerals are soluble nutrients derived from the weathering of chemical elements in the earth's crust. They give bones rigidity and strength, and they interact with other nutrients to keep the body healthy. Like a chicken's need for vitamins, its mineral requirements do not fluctuate with the season. Unlike vitamins, minerals don't go stale.

Vitamin B Complex

B VITAMIN	ROLE	DEFICIENCY SIGN	SOURCE
B₁ Thiamin Thiamine	Healthy nerve cells	(Rare) Failure to eat; inflamed nerves; death	Legumes, sesame seeds, sunflower seeds, wheat bran
B₂ Riboflavin Vitamin G	Antioxidant; growth; red blood cell production; metabolize vitamin B₆	Emaciation while eating well; diarrhea; leg paralysis; curled-toe paralysis; death	Soybeans, sesame seeds, wheat germ, whole grains, milk products
B₃ Niacin Nicotinic acid	Metabolize carbohydrates, fats, and protein; hormone production; blood circulation	Swollen hocks; bowed legs	Fish meal, sunflower seeds
B₅ Pantothenic acid	Red blood cell production; healthy digestive tract; body fat	Sores on feet and face; rough, broken feathers; death	Corn, legumes, sunflower seeds, sweet potatoes, wheat bran, whey
B₆ Pyridoxine	Healthy nerve cells; brain function; hormone production; red blood cell production	Muscle weakness; death	Legumes, milk, sunflower seeds, wheat germ
B₇ Biotin Vitamin H	Metabolize carbohydrates, fats, amino acids; strengthen feathers, beaks, and claws	(Rare) Sores on feet and face; slipped tendon	Brewer's yeast, legumes, oats, wheat germ, manufactured in the intestine
B₉ Folate Folic acid Folacin	Brain function; DNA and RNA production; red blood cell production; growth	Slow growth; poor feathering; anemia	Leafy dark greens, legumes, milk, root vegetables, wheat germ, whole grains
B₁₂ Cobalamin	Healthy nerve cells; DNA and RNA production; red blood cell production; metabolize carbohydrates and fats	Slow growth; small eggs with low hatchability; death	Milk, fish meal, livestock manure

Ingredients for home-mixed rations should be chosen with their mineral content in mind, or a commercially prepared mineral premix (such as Fertrell Nutri-Balancer) must be included. Most commercial feeds contain adequate amounts of minerals, with the possible exception of calcium.

CALCIUM AND PHOSPHORUS

Calcium is the most prevalent mineral in a chicken's body and phosphorus the second most prevalent. Calcium and phosphorus are interrelated — each is needed for metabolism of the other — and both require the presence of vitamin D to be metabolized. A deficiency in vitamin D can cause a deficiency of calcium and/or phosphorus.

Calcium is needed for bone and eggshell development, as well as for blood clotting, muscle contractions, nerve impulses, heartbeat, enzyme activation, and hormone secretion. Phosphorus, too, is needed for bone and shell development, as well as for muscle formation and the metabolism of carbohydrates, fats, and protein.

Chicks that receive insufficient calcium and phosphorus for normal skeletal growth develop rickets. On the other hand, feeding chicks a ration that is too high in calcium for their age (feeding them a layer ration, for example) can cause kidney disease, visceral gout, and death.

The amount of calcium and phosphorus a hen needs to make strong eggshells varies with her age, diet, rate of lay, and state of health. Older hens, for instance, need more calcium than younger hens, because laying has depleted their bones. Chickens on pasture obtain some calcium and phosphorus by eating beetles and other hard-shelled bugs, but they may not get enough. Ironically, a deficiency of calcium and phosphorus increases a chicken's susceptibility to parasitic infection, and beetles can be a source of parasites.

In warm weather, when all chickens eat less, the calcium in a hen's ration may not be enough to meet her needs. A hen that gets too little calcium lays thin-shell eggs that break easily, and because she draws calcium from her own bones, she becomes susceptible to osteoporosis. Rough eggshells are a sign a hen is getting too much calcium, which can cause a phosphorus deficiency.

Since most grains are deficient in calcium, a source of calcium must be included in the ration. Although most grains contain a lot of phosphorus, they also have an antinutrient that makes the phosphorus unavailable.

Commercial rations therefore include sources for both minerals, although they may not furnish enough calcium for the best layers.

Eggshells consist primarily of calcium carbonate, the same mineral found in aragonite, limestone, and oyster shell. All laying hens should have access to a supplement of ground aragonite, crushed oyster shells, or chipped limestone (*not* dolomitic limestone, which can inhibit egg production). The calcium supplement should be offered separately and free choice, rather than mixed into the ration, to allow for differences in the needs of individual hens, so those needing less calcium don't get too much, which can cause kidney damage.

Calcium and Phosphorus Sources

SOURCE	% CALCIUM*	% PHOSPHORUS*
Aragonite	97	Variable
Bone meal	30	17
Dicalcium phosphate	22	18
Eggshells	39	0.3
Limestone (calcium carbonate)	40	0
Oyster shell	38	0
Soft rock phosphate	20	20

Average; actual percentage varies with origin.

To balance the calcium supplement, offer phosphorus in the form of bone meal, dicalcium phosphate, or soft rock phosphate in a separate free-choice hopper. When both supplements are offered separately and free choice, the hens will consume the proper balance.

POTASSIUM

Potassium is the third most prevalent mineral in a chicken's body. It is needed for membrane maintenance and cellular fluid balance, as well as for normal heart function. A potassium deficiency can occur during times of heat or other stress, resulting in decreased egg production, thin shells, and general muscle weakness.

Unlike grains, which contain little potassium, legumes and other protein sources are potassium rich. Additional sources include leafy dark greens, sweet potatoes, and cooked white potatoes.

SALT

Salt, in the form of sodium and chloride, is an important part of blood and other body fluids but is needed only in tiny amounts. Commercially prepared rations contain all the salt a flock needs. Pastured chickens that survive primarily on plants and grain may need a salt supplement.

Pastured chickens should always have loose salt (not rock salt) available in a separate hopper. Iodized salt is suitable, although either a trace-mineral salt mix or kelp will supply your chickens with many other necessary minerals in addition to salt.

Salt-deficient chicks grow slowly and have soft bones. An ongoing deficiency results in a general shutdown of body functions, eventually leading to shock and death. Salt-deficient hens experience a drastic drop in egg production, lay smaller eggs, lose weight, and may become cannibalistic.

Poisoning from getting too much salt is more likely than a salt deficiency. For details see Salt Poisoning on page 314.

MANGANESE

Manganese is needed for normal bone and skin development, wound healing, nutrient absorption, and eggshell quality. It is also a potent antioxidant (see Antioxidants and Free Radicals, facing page).

With the exception of corn, most things a chicken eats are manganese rich, but many of the same feedstuffs contain antinutrients that inhibit manganese absorption. Certain other minerals — including calcium, phosphorus, and iron — limit the retention of manganese when fed in excess. Coccidiosis also interferes with the metabolism of manganese.

Commercial rations are intended to provide a balance of manganese and other minerals. Chickens fed a home-mixed ration that includes a mineral salt supplement get plenty of manganese.

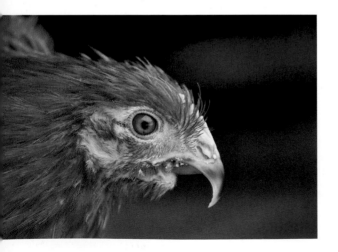

Parrot beak is one sign of manganese deficiency.

Hens that are manganese deficient lay poorly and produce thin-shell eggs with low hatchability. Chicks that do hatch from such eggs may have skeletal deformities such as thickened, shortened legs and wings (chondrodystrophy, or slipped tendon). Additional signs in hatchlings include parrot beak, in which the bottom half of the beak is too short, causing the top half to curl over it, and stargazing, or bending back of the neck so the head is above the back (or sometimes down, between the legs).

Although skeletal deformities are permanent, poor egg quality and hatchability may be corrected with a manganese supplement such as manganese sulfate, also known as Epsom salt, at the rate of 1 teaspoon per 50 pounds of ration (5 g/23 kg). Excess manganese is excreted, making it among the least toxic minerals and, when used with common sense, unlikely to result in overdose.

SELENIUM

Selenium is an interesting dietary mineral in that it was first identified, in 1818, as a toxin. Not until the 1950s was its role as a trace mineral essential for life and good health discovered. Because of its history as a toxin, the addition of selenium supplements to poultry rations and other livestock feed falls under the control of the Food and Drug Administration.

Selenium is now known to be an important antioxidant that, working together with vitamin E, helps maintain the immune system, as well as being essential for the proper development of muscles and the circulatory system. Fish meal and dried brewer's yeast are good sources of selenium, as are crops grown in the naturally selenium-rich soils of the United States and Canadian plains.

ANTIOXIDANTS AND FREE RADICALS

The metabolic production of energy from oxygen produces free radicals, unstable fragments of oxygen molecules that are missing an electron. Free radicals damage body cells and contribute to the development of such unhealthful conditions as impaired immunity, heart disease, arthritis, and tumors. Ironically, free radicals can also strengthen muscles and help the immune system fend off infection and tumors. So some free radicals are beneficial, but too many are harmful.

Antioxidants are organic chemicals that neutralize free radicals by replacing the missing electron, thus reducing or preventing damage by free radicals and also helping repair any damaged cells.

Plants produce antioxidants to protect themselves from pathogens, pollution, and harmful ultraviolet sunlight. The best-known antioxidants are selenium and vitamins A, C, and E. However, regular use of these antioxidants in the form of concentrated dietary supplements can lead to toxicity. On the other hand, treating your chickens to feeds that are naturally rich in antioxidants will help them live a long and healthy life.

Vitamin and Mineral Supplements

Trying to furnish your chickens each of the vitamins and minerals individually is impractical and so is attempting to identify signs of a deficiency in any specific vitamin or mineral. (See Signs of Deficiency, next page.) If you suspect your chickens are suffering from a vitamin or mineral deficiency, the best approach is to provide a complete supplement, of which many different brands are available specifically designed for poultry.

Giving your chickens a vitamin-mineral supplement will boost their immunity during times of stress, such as when their bodies are battling a disease, when the weather is unpleasant, during a move, before and after a poultry show, and during breeding season. To counteract any potential deficiencies in the breeder flock diet, chicks get off to a better start when given a supplement during their first 3 weeks of life.

Keep in mind, though, that some vitamins interact synergistically with each other or regulate the metabolism of certain minerals, and some minerals require the presence of other minerals to be effective. An excess of some minerals can interfere with the absorption of other minerals, and an excess of some vitamins can interact detrimentally with minerals or can themselves be toxic. Instead of making chickens healthier, the unnecessary use of packaged vitamin and mineral supplements can have the opposite of the desired effect. Never use a supplement, including electrolytes, for more than 10 days.

If you are formulating your own rations, the best way to guard against vitamin and mineral deficiencies is to include a mineral premix (for example, Fertrell Nutri-Balancer). Premixes are available in both standard and organic formulations. Since too much can be as detrimental as too little, carefully follow the directions on the label to avoid overdosing your chickens.

Feeders

Feeder design can affect health if it discourages eating; for example, because the chickens can't get their heads into the hopper, or the hopper rubs against the birds' combs. Such situations usually indicate that young chickens have outgrown their feeder.

A poor design might affect health by allowing droppings to accumulate in the feed. Droppings can be excluded by hanging a feeder from the ceiling or by fitting it with an antiroosting device that rotates and dumps any bird trying to perch on top.

Feeder design can affect health also by allowing feed to be scattered on the ground, where it not only attracts rodents but combines with manure and moisture to provide a good environment for disease-causing organisms. Beaking out — the bad habit chickens have of using their beaks to toss feed out of a trough — can be prevented by using a feeder with an inwardly rolled lip and by positioning the feeder so the hopper is approximately the height of the birds' backs. Here again, a hanging feeder is ideal because its height can be adjusted easily as the birds grow.

FEEDING STATIONS

Provide enough feeders so at least one-third of your chickens can eat at the same time. As a general rule, allow each mature chicken at least 1½ inches (40 mm) of space around a tube feeder or 1 inch (25 mm) of space along a trough feeder. If the trough is accessible from both sides, count both sides in your calculation; for example, an 18-inch (50 cm) trough with access from both sides has 36 inches (100 cm) of feeder space.

Even if one feeder would be enough for your flock, a good idea is to furnish at least two to ensure the weaker birds don't get chased away by the bullies. If you have more than one rooster, provide at least one feeding station per rooster. Each cock will gather his hens around a feeder, and fighting will be reduced.

Placing feeders inside the shelter keeps feed from getting wet but encourages chickens to spend more time indoors. Placing feeders under a covered outdoor area keeps feed out of the sun and rain and encourages the flock to spend more time in fresh air. But outdoor feeders attract wild birds, especially flocks of sparrows or starlings, and leaving a full feeder in the open overnight invites pilfering by opossums and other wildlife.

Feeder Space

AGE	SPACE PER BIRD
Layer breeds	
0–6 weeks	1.0" (25 mm)
7–18 weeks	2.0" (50 mm)
19 weeks and up	3.0" (75 mm)
Broiler breeds	
1 day–1 week	1.0" (25 mm)
1–4 weeks	2.0" (50 mm)
4–8 weeks	2.5" (60 mm)
8–20 weeks	4.0" (100 mm)
21 weeks and up	5.0" (125 mm)

SIGNS OF DEFICIENCY

In practical terms, identifying any single nutrient as the cause of a particular deficiency is difficult because most nutrients have multiple functions, many nutrients interact with one another in complex ways, and most signs of a deficiency apply to more than one nutrient.

Further, a deficiency may not result from a lack of nutrients in the diet, but from a bird's inability to metabolize existing nutrients; for example, because an intestinal disease is inhibiting nutrient absorption. Or a deficiency, especially in salt or vitamin B_1, may cause such a complete loss of interest in eating that the result is deficiency in all nutrients.

Except when a specific nutritional deficiency is induced for research purposes, most signs of deficiency appear as a gradual progression. By the time specific signs appear that might be associated with a specific deficiency, it's too late to correct the deficiency by improving the diet. The three main stages of this progression may be identified as follows:

- **Borderline:** Lack of energy, loss of appetite, poor or rough feathering, reduced weight gain in chicks, loss of weight in mature chickens, decreased laying, a reduction in egg hatchability

- **Serious:** Birds become crippled, hens stop laying

- **Extreme:** Chickens die

HOW MUCH A CHICKEN EATS

How much chickens eat varies with the ration's palatability, texture, and energy and protein content, as well as with the chickens' age, breed and strain, degree of activity, and condition of health. How much a chicken eats also varies with environmental temperature. In cold weather chickens eat more than they do during the heat of summer.

Because chickens eat less in hot weather, the ration's nutritional value must be increased to meet the bird's needs. Some chicken keepers feed their hens a higher-protein ration during summer. Others feed a high-protein ration year-round but add scratch grains during the winter to increase the energy level.

Under most conditions, chickens should be fed free choice, meaning the ration is available to them any time they feel like eating. Restricted feeding, or withholding rations for part of the day, is sometimes done to prevent lameness in broilers that grow too fast, to delay the onset of lay while breeder pullets mature, or to prevent older hens from getting fat and lazy. A less stressful plan is to adjust the nutritional content of the ration; for instance, by introducing low-energy high-fiber feeds.

How Much a Chicken Eats
(Basic Guidelines)

BREED	IMPERIAL	METRIC	TIME PERIOD
Bantam	0.5 lb	0.25 kg	Week
Light Breed	2 lb	1 kg	Week
Dual-Purpose	3 lb	1.5 kg	Week
Heavy Breed	4 lb	2 kg	Week
Broiler	10 lb	4.5 kg	Lifetime

WHEN CHICKENS WON'T EAT

Chicks that don't eat enough won't grow well, and hens that don't eat enough won't lay well. Circumstances that can cause chickens to eat too little include the following:

- The feeder is positioned where the chickens can't reach the feed.

- The amount of feeder space is inadequate for the number of chickens, causing some not to get their share.

- Chickens that are abruptly switched to unfamiliar feed, or are fed moldy or rancid rations, may stop eating.

- Chickens eat to meet their energy needs. High-energy feeds cause chickens to stop eating before they meet their needs for protein, vitamins, and minerals.

- A ration that is deficient in vitamins or minerals can suppress a flock's appetite. Chicks that are severely deficient in either salt or vitamin B_1 simply stop eating.

- Chickens that don't get as much water as they want will eat less, getting fewer nutrients than their bodies need.

- Uncomfortably high temperatures cause chickens to eat less than usual.

- The first sign of many diseases is loss of appetite; watch for other signs.

CHAPTER 3

The Inner Chicken

When you see a chicken off by itself, hunkered down and looking miserable, you know it's not feeling well. That part is easy. Unfortunately, the bird can't tell you where it hurts. More often than not, to determine what's ailing the bird you have to figure out what's going on inside its body. Different conditions affect different parts of a chicken's body in different ways, so knowing what part of the body is having a problem is a big step toward identifying the problem.

If several chickens in the same flock continue to contract diseases that always affect the same body system, some management change may be in order. Frequent bouts with digestive disorders, for example, may signal a need for improved sanitation, while repeated respiratory problems may require an improvement in ventilation.

Speaking of Anatomy

atrophy. To shrivel up or waste away

cilia. Short, tiny hair-like structures that vibrate to keep the trachea clear of debris

diverticulum. A finger-shaped blind pouch

microbe. A microorganism, especially one that causes disease

microflora. Beneficial microorganisms living in the gut of a healthy chicken

microorganism. A microscopic organism, especially a bacterium, virus, or fungus

mucosa. Membranes that secrete mucus and that line the body cavity and the tubular passages of the digestive and respiratory systems

myopathy. Any disease of the muscles

pathogen. Any disease-causing organism

stem cell. A cell that is capable of producing an unlimited number of like cells with the potential to develop into many other kinds of cells with differing functions

Immune System

The functions of a chicken's immune system are to defend the body against disease-causing microorganisms, or pathogens, and to minimize the harm done by any pathogens that do manage to invade the body. A chicken's immune system has these three basic lines of defense:

1. Feathers, skin, and mucous membranes that hinder the penetration of pathogens into the body

2. Cells and chemicals circulated from the blood to any organs affected by invading pathogens, resulting in inflammation and other responses, as described on page 327

3. Enhanced immunity, as discussed in depth in chapter 14

Protective Feathers

Six to 8 percent of a chicken's weight is feathers. A chicken's feathers protect the skin from injury and sunburn, conserve the bird's body heat, and furnish some degree of waterproofing.

Like most birds, chickens lose and replace their feathers at approximately 1-year intervals. The process, called molting, usually occurs over a period of weeks, so most chickens don't go completely naked — although occasionally one comes close. A chicken normally molts gradually over a period of 14 to 16 weeks during the late summer or early fall. Finding lots of feathers in the yard is a sign that your chickens are molting and will soon develop healthy coats of fresh new feathers. This annual loss and renewal of feathers is perfectly normal and is not an indication of disease.

A chicken's feathers do not cover the entire body, but grow from follicles arranged in 10 symmetrical tracts located on the head, neck, shoulder, wings, breast, back, abdomen, rump, thigh, and legs. The feathers' follicles are linked by a network of tiny muscles that allow the chicken to raise and lower its feathers; for instance, to trap warm air by puffing out the feathers in cold weather.

The feather tracts (technically, pterylae) are separated by featherless areas (apteria) that may contain some down. These bare areas facilitate cooling when a chicken holds out its wings in hot weather and pants, attempting to stay cool by exposing bare skin and by losing internal body heat via the respiratory system (as described later in this chapter).

Feather Tracts

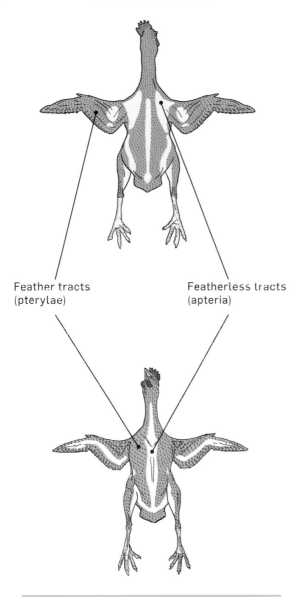

Feather tracts
(pterylae)

Featherless tracts
(apteria)

Feathers are arranged in symmetrical tracts
(pterylae) separated by featherless areas (apteria).

Skin and Mucosa

The chicken's skin is its largest organ — making up another 8 percent of the bird's total weight — and the main organ by which it comes into contact with its environment. A chicken's skin is thinner and more delicate than that of humans and other mammals. The color of the skin varies depending on the bird's breed, diet, age, rate of egg production, and state of health. A yellow-skin breed that isn't feeling well or for some other reason isn't eating well has paler skin than its flock mates. A young chicken with little fat may have bluish-looking skin.

The majority of disease-causing organisms enter a chicken's body either through the skin protecting the outside of its body or through the mucous membranes (mucosa) lining the openings on the inside of its body. On the skin live certain beneficial microbes that, through competitive exclusion, keep harmful microbes away. If the skin is broken, the good microbes themselves may get into the body and cause disease.

The mucosa, too, host beneficial microorganisms, or microflora, that fend off invaders through the process of competitive exclusion. These microbes are assisted by moving fluids (mucus and tears) and by enzymes that rush to destroy any invaders.

Lymphatic System

Many pathogens can't penetrate uninjured skin or mucosa. A nutritional deficiency (such as biotin deficiency), however, or an infectious disease may weaken the body coverings, allowing pathogens to penetrate.

Unlike humans, chickens don't have sweat glands. The only skin gland is the pea-size uropygial gland at the base of the tail. Also called the preen gland or oil gland, it consists of two symmetrical lobes that come together into a small nipple at the center, with a tiny tuft of feathers in the middle of the nipple. This gland secretes oil the chicken uses to condition and waterproof its feathers. During preening, the chicken releases oil by rubbing the gland's nipple with its beak, then distributes the oil by rubbing its beak against its feathers.

When pathogens manage to break through the defenses of the skin or mucosa, the bird's lymphatic system takes up the battle. All body tissues are lubricated by lymph, a watery fluid derived from the blood that accumulates in the spaces between the body's tissue cells. Lymph contains specialized white blood cells that are technically called lymphocytes but popularly known as killer cells. These killer cells neutralize or destroy invading microbes, which they recognize as antigens. An antigen is any protein that differs from the proteins naturally occurring within a chicken's body.

When lymphocytes detect an antigen, they respond by producing substances to fight off the invader. These substances are antibodies, or immunoglobulins. The antibodies attach to the antigens, breaking down the antigens' defenses to make the killer cells' job easier.

Unlike humans, chickens do not have a system of organized lymph nodes but instead have several lymphoid organs — the term "lymphoid" referring to any body tissue that produces lymphocytes and antibodies. This tissue occurs primarily in the spleen, thymus, and cloacal bursa, but is dispersed elsewhere in the body, including in the bone marrow, intestines (GALT), respiratory system (BALT), and head (HALT) as described on page 66.

Vital Statistics

Average life span	5–8 years
Maximum life span	18–22 years
Maximum productive life	12–15 years
Body temperature* (average)	
Adult	103°F (39.4°C)
Adult, deep body	107°F (41.7°C)
Chick	106.7°F (41.5°C)
Respiration rate (at rest)	
Cock	12–21 breaths per minute
Hen	31–37 breaths per minute
Heart rate* (average)	
Adult, large breed	250 beats per minute
Adult, small breed	350 beats per minute
Chick	300 beats per minute

*A chicken's temperature is too variable and its heart rate too fast to count, making this information difficult to determine in real life, and therefore not much use in diagnosing an illness.

SPLEEN

The spleen is a dark red, round organ normally about ¾ inch in diameter. The view through a microscope reveals that it is made up of red pulp and white pulp. The red pulp destroys worn-out red blood cells. The white pulp forms white blood cells, or leukocytes, colorless cells that circulate in blood and body fluids and help counteract pathogens and other foreign invaders. Both the red pulp and white pulp produce antibodies.

Many diseases affect the spleen, causing it to swell (paratyphoid), turn mushy (histoplasmosis), or atrophy (infectious anemia). The spleen is not a vital organ, however, and if it ceases to function, other organs take over its job.

THYMUS

A chicken's thymus is made up of several paired, flattened, pale-pink lobes of irregular shape strung out along the jugular vein on both sides of the neck and running down nearly the entire length of the neck. The number of pairs in a given chicken may be anywhere from five to eight. As a bird ages, the thymus naturally shrinks. Disease can also cause this organ to atrophy.

The thymus and cloacal bursa are the chicken's primary lymphoid organs. Both organs produce functional immune cells that are stockpiled by other (secondary) lymphoid organs.

CLOACAL BURSA

A pale-colored, grape-shaped organ above the cloaca is largely responsible for controlling immunity and activating antibody production in chicks. It is called the cloacal bursa, or the bursa of Fabricius after Italian anatomy professor Hieronymus Fabricius, who first described the organ in 1621. The inside of this organ consists of about two dozen parallel folds bearing some 10,000 follicles that provide an ideal environment for the development of antibodies.

The cloacal bursa of a young bird reflexively takes in fluids, a phenomenon known as cloacal drinking, as a way to inoculate the bird against pathogens in the environment. The bursa continues to grow, reaching its maximum size in chicks between 6 and 12 weeks old. It then begins to shrink until it nearly disappears and is no longer functional by the time a bird

T CELLS AND B CELLS

Small lymphocytes produced in the thymus are called T cells, while the somewhat larger lymphocytes produced in the cloacal bursa are called B cells (some B cells are also produced elsewhere in the body). Each type of cell has a specific role in a chicken's immune response.

T cells put up a defense on the cellular level, so their work is called cell-mediated immunity. B cells produce antibodies that defend body fluids, so their job is called noncellular, or humoral, immunity, from the Latin word *humor*, meaning moisture.

T cells and B cells both begin as stem cells produced during incubation in the embryo's yolk sac, liver, and bone marrow. The circulatory system delivers these cells to the chick's thymus and cloacal bursa, where they mature to perform their distinctive functions.

is sexually mature at 4 to 5 months. Certain diseases and nutritional conditions can cause early atrophy of the cloacal bursa, permanently compromising the bird's immune system.

Conditions Causing Atrophy of the Cloacal Bursa

CONDITION	CAUSE
Aging	Normal
Avian influenza	Virus
Cryptosporidiosis	Protozoa
Colibacillosis	Bacteria
Infectious bronchitis	Virus
Infectious bursal disease	Virus
Marek's disease	Virus
Mycotoxins in feed	Fungi
Newcastle disease virus (velogenic)	Virus
Vitamin A deficiency	Nutritional
Water deprivation	Dehydration

GALT, BALT, AND HALT

Clusters of organized lymphoid nodules occur along a chicken's digestive tract, particularly in parts of the small intestine, where they are called Peyer's patches (after the seventeenth-century Swiss anatomist Johann Conrad Peyer, who first described them in 1677); at the base of the ceca, where they are called cecal tonsils; and in the Meckel's diverticulum (described on page 81). Collectively, this tissue is known as gut-associated lymphoid tissue, or GALT. Its function is to protect the chicken against intestinal diseases.

As a chick matures, the accumulations of GALT increase, reaching a maximum by the time the bird reaches 16 weeks of age. Along with the thymus and cloacal bursa, GALT then begins to regress until, by the time the bird reaches 1 year of age, most of the tissue clusters are gone.

Similarly to GALT, the respiratory tract develops lymphoid tissues, referred to as bronchial-associated lymphoid tissue, or BALT, in the trachea and bronchi to help protect the chicken against inhaled pathogens. Like GALT, it gradually develops as a chick grows, becoming well developed by the time the bird reaches 8 weeks of age.

Head-associated lymphoid tissue, or HALT, includes the nasal glands, tear glands, mucous membranes of the eyes, and a relatively large Harderian gland behind each eyeball (named after physician Johann Jacob Harder, who discovered the glands in 1694). HALT protects the eyes, nasal cavity, and upper airways.

Muscular System

Muscles are the most familiar part of a chicken's body system for most people, especially for those of us who enjoy eating chicken meat in various recipes — muscles are the meat. Muscle is made up of bundles of fibrous tissue with the ability to contract, thus allowing the chicken to walk, run, fly, and otherwise move around and to maintain its position when standing still or perching. Like other animals, a chicken has these three kinds of muscle:

Cardiac muscle, which controls movements of the heart;

MEMORY CELLS

When T cells or B cells are exposed to a new antigen, they develop both antibodies targeted against that specific antigen and memory cells that store information about the particular antigen. If the same type of antigen again enters the chicken's body in the future, the memory cells spring into action to produce antibodies that attack the antigen. As a chick grows to maturity, the pathogens it encounters in its environment stimulate its immune system to develop a wide range of antigen-specific memory cells.

Once the chicken matures and various of its lymphoid organs atrophy, the antigen-specific memory cells take over much of the responsibility for maintaining the chicken's immunity. Should the chicken be exposed to pathogens not encountered during its youth, the immune system has no information in its memory bank, and the chicken therefore has no immune defense against it. Chickens that are raised in different places, then brought together into one flock, therefore may not all be immune to the same diseases, and indeed may share diseases to which others in the flock have developed no immunity.

Smooth muscle, which is controlled by the autonomic, or involuntary, nervous system, the part of the nervous system that is responsible for body functions the chicken does not have conscious control over, such as respiration and digestion; *and*

Skeletal muscle, which is responsible for voluntary movement; for the chicken's shape, which varies with breed; and for providing us with delicious meat on our dinner plates.

Skeletal muscle develops from different kinds of fibers, making some muscles dark (dark meat) and some light (white meat). Dark muscle generally occurs in legs and thighs, which are heavily used, while light muscle occurs in the breast and wings, which get less exercise. A bird uses breast muscles for flying and leg muscles for walking, but chickens do more walking than flying. Active muscles need oxygen, and oxygen is carried in blood cells.

The more active the muscles, the more blood they require, and the more blood they require, the darker the muscle.

Dark muscle is denser than light muscle. The older the chicken, the greater the difference between the density of the active leg muscles and the less active breast muscles.

Because muscles get their energy from fat stored within the muscle cells, the more the muscles are exercised, the more energy they need and the more fat they store. Consequently, the leg muscles contain more fat than the breast muscles.

Muscles allow movement by alternately contracting and relaxing, using a system of levers created by the chicken's joints and skeletal system. Many of the chicken's bones have ridges, bumps, and other irregularities to which the muscles can readily attach.

The word "muscle" derives from the Latin word *musculus*, meaning "little mouse," because the appearance and movement of a bulging muscle can resemble a mouse under the skin. In Greek the word *mys* means both "mouse" and "muscle," giving rise to the prefix "myo-," referring to muscles, as in myoglobin and myopathy.

Myoglobin is a red protein that carries and stores oxygen in the muscle cells. It is responsible for the dark color of a chicken's more active skeletal muscles.

Myopathy is any muscle disease, *pathos* being the Greek word for suffering. Two muscle diseases a chicken may suffer from are white muscle disease, or nutritional myopathy, and green muscle disease, or deep pectoral myopathy (the latter is discussed in detail on page 122).

Skeletal System

The skeletal system of a chicken has these functions:

- To provide a framework for muscles, allowing movement

- To support the body

- To protect the internal organs

- To store and release calcium

- To aid in respiration

Skeletal problems may be caused by insufficient calcium, either because the diet is deficient or because a disease or other condition keeps calcium from being properly metabolized. By far the most common skeletal problem is weak legs, which may be related to genetics, nutrition, infection, or some combination thereof. In hens the problem is usually the result of mineral imbalance.

Skeletal Issues

Leg weakness is more likely to occur in heavy breeds than in light breeds. Guard against it by keeping young birds off slippery surfaces, by feeding a balanced diet, and by not breeding lame or deformed birds. Be aware that lameness is not always a skeletal disorder but may result from nerve or muscle damage.

Another common skeletal problem is inflammation of the joints and synovial membranes, thin membranes lining joint cavities and tendon sheaths. The synovial membranes secrete synovia, a fluid resembling thin egg white that lubricates joints. Inflammation of the synovial membranes, called synovitis, causes excess synovia to be secreted, making the joint swell and become warm and painful. The most likely joint affected is the hock. Noninfectious synovitis may be caused by injury or nutritional problems. Infectious synovitis may be caused by bacteria, staphylococci, or viruses.

Skeletal System of a Chicken

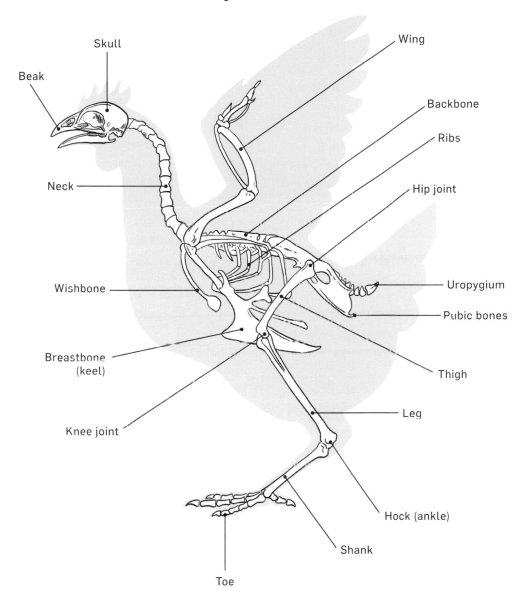

Skull

Beak

Wing

Backbone

Ribs

Neck

Hip joint

Wishbone

Uropygium

Pubic bones

Breastbone
(keel)

Thigh

Knee joint

Leg

Hock (ankle)

Shank

Toe

Near the joints, at places where a tendon or muscle crosses a bone or muscle, are small fluid-filled sacs, called bursa, that cushion pressure points. Inflammation of the bursa (bursitis) may be caused by pressure, friction, or injury to the membrane surrounding the joint. If the injury does not become infected or the bird is not reinjured, after a time the excess fluid is resorbed by the bloodstream.

The most common form of bursitis is keel bursitis, popularly known as breast blister. Breast blister is caused by pressure against the keel, usually in a bird with weak legs (so it cannot keep its weight off the keel while resting) or poor feathering (offering little protection to the keel).

Medullary Bone

A chicken's skeleton includes some bones that contain marrow and a fluctuating substance called medullary bone, from the Latin word *medulla* (derived from *medius*, meaning "middle" or "central"). Medullary bone lies inside the structural bone, both lining the structural bone and extending as numerous tiny needle-like projections into the marrow. This feature is unique to female birds.

As a pullet approaches sexual maturity and estrogen kicks in, about 2 weeks before she lays her first egg, her system switches from developing structural bone to packing some of the structural bones with medullary bone. From that point on, as long as the hen continues laying, specialized cells within her bones resorb both medullary bone and, to some extent, structural bone to provide calcium for the development of eggshells.

A really good laying hen that produces an egg nearly every day can't absorb calcium from her diet fast enough to put a sturdy shell around each egg. Instead she uses up a considerable amount of skeletal calcium to form each eggshell. Throughout a hen's productive life, she gradually loses structural bone, which is characteristic of osteoporosis, a condition in which the bones become brittle and fragile and fracture more easily.

Along with osteoporosis, highly productive hens housed in cages (as has been widely practiced in industrial egg production) may develop cage fatigue, a form of paralysis that can end in death because of the hen's inability to get to food and water. Interestingly, if the cage is fitted with a solid bottom, or the hen is removed from the cage, she may recover in a matter of days.

Along with genetics and environment, a hen's bone loss is influenced by nutrition. If a hen's diet is deficient in calcium, she will rapidly deplete her body of calcium. As a result, her eggs will have thinner shells and she will gradually lay fewer eggs until she stops laying. When an otherwise healthy hen stops laying, her body reduces the production of estrogen and resumes the formation of structural bone, restoring the strength of her skeletal structure.

Pneumatic Bones

Another type of bone in a chicken's skeleton, which occurs in both genders, contains blind tubes, or diverticula, extending from air sacs that are part of the respiratory system. Being hollow, these bones reduce the bird's weight for flight and, being filled with circulating air, they both increase the flow of oxygen for metabolism and serve as a chicken's cooling system.

Called pneumatic bones — from the Latin word *pneumaticus*, meaning "belonging to the air" — these bones directly connect a chicken's skeletal system with its respiratory system. A chicken that fractures a pneumatic bone may have difficulty breathing and is subject to air sac infection.

Medullary and Pneumatic Bones

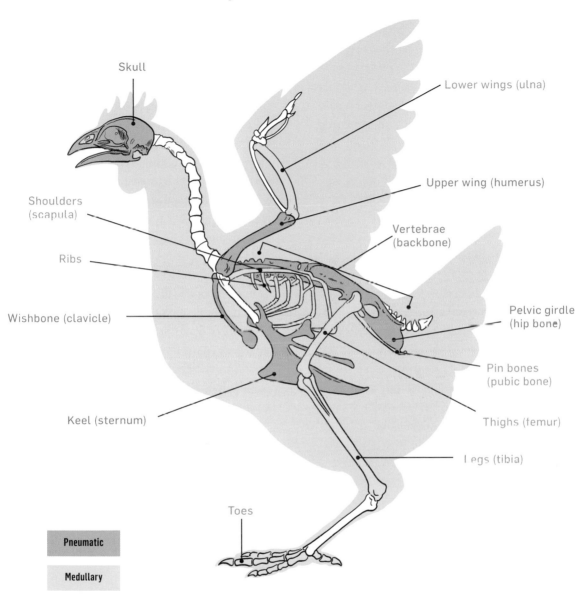

Skull

Lower wings (ulna)

Upper wing (humerus)

Shoulders (scapula)

Vertebrae (backbone)

Ribs

Wishbone (clavicle)

Pelvic girdle (hip bone)

Pin bones (pubic bone)

Keel (sternum)

Thighs (femur)

Legs (tibia)

Toes

Pneumatic

Medullary

The hard outer covers of a mature cock's spurs grow like a human's fingernails and are made of the same material, keratin. Some spurs grow so long they interfere with walking; may curl back toward the leg and pierce the shank, causing lameness; or may accidentally stab the cock's own body, leading to infection and death. Long spurs can slice into a hen's back when the cock treads during mating. And a spur can cause serious damage to the cock's handlers. For all these reasons, you may need to trim the spurs of a mature cock by blunting the spur or removing the entire outer shell.

The ends of spurs may be blunted with a Dremel cutting wheel, wire cutters, or a pair of quality toenail or canine clippers, and the edges smoothed with a file. Cutting off too much of a spur will damage the quick, or soft tissue underneath, causing pain and bleeding. Depending on the rooster's breed, age, and time since last spur trim, the quick will be between one-third and two-thirds the length of the outer spur, so cutting off no more than one-third of the spur from the tip should be a safe bet.

You may remove the hard outer cover of each spur entirely, revealing the quick, which in 2 to 4 weeks will harden into a new spur. Grasp the spur with a pair of pliers and twist it back and forth until the hard cover pops off. A spur that doesn't easily twist off may be softened by sticking it into a hot baked potato — taking care to avoid burning the shank with the potato — for about a minute. Remove the potato, and wiggle the spur back and forth until it slips free. Reheat the potato for the second spur. (Some roosters will hold still for this procedure; others must be held by a helper or confined, as in a towel. Usually, if the bird is turned on its back it will not struggle.)

A spur without the hard outer cover remains sensitive for a week or two, during which time the cock should be isolated from other chickens to avoid damage to the soft spur tissue. Keeping the cock in a separate, clean pen within the same area as the other chickens will minimize fighting when he returns to the flock.

If the freshly uncovered spur bleeds, stop the bleeding by applying a wound powder such as Wonder Dust or styptic powder or an astringent such as witch hazel, or hasten clotting with a little flour, cornstarch, or table sugar. The new spur will gradually harden and begin to grow long and eventually will need to be removed again.

Respiratory System

Because chickens are particularly subject to respiratory diseases, and because their respiratory system is much different from a human's, understanding how their system works is an important step toward maintaining a healthy environment for your flock.

The respiratory system includes the nasal cavity, sinuses, larynx, trachea (windpipe), syrinx, bronchi, lungs, and air sacs. A chicken's respiratory system serves several functions, including the following:

- It circulates oxygen throughout the body.

- It removes carbon dioxide from the body.

- It aids in temperature regulation.

- It allows the chicken to cackle, crow, and make other sounds.

Air Sacs

Like other birds, chickens are peculiar among animals in having an extensive system of air sacs, or thin-wall bubblelike pockets that circulate fresh air into various parts of the body. The system of air sacs extends around the internal organs, filling nearly all of the rest of the body cavity that's not occupied by other organs, and into the pneumatic bones.

The air sacs are organized into two sets, one toward the front of the body (the anterior, or cranial, air sacs) and the other toward the rear (the posterior, or caudal, air sacs). Soon after a chick hatches, the forward air sacs expand into the vertebrae of the neck. As the chick grows, the rear air sacs expand into the vertebrae toward the pelvis. By the time a chicken is mature, air sacs have spread throughout the vertebrae.

THE CHICKEN'S VOICE BOX

In humans the voice box consists of vocal cords within the larynx at the top of the windpipe. In chickens, the voice box has no vocal cords and consists of the syrinx at the bottom of the windpipe, where the trachea splits at an upside-down Y-shape junction to create the bronchi that go into the two lungs. The function of a chicken's larynx is solely to make sure food doesn't get sent down the windpipe when the chicken swallows.

All the sounds a chicken makes, including the cock's crow, require a cooperative effort among the tracheal muscles, syrinx, air sacs, and respiratory muscles. Some muscles contract to force air from the air sacs into the syrinx, while other muscles exert tension to alter the syrinx's shape to create different sounds. Because the syrinx is located at a critical juncture between the windpipe and the bronchi, it cannot be surgically removed to prevent a rooster from crowing.

Syrinx and Air Sac System

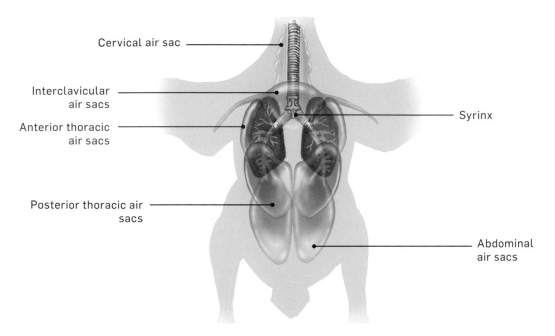

Cervical air sac

Interclavicular air sacs

Anterior thoracic air sacs

Posterior thoracic air sacs

Syrinx

Abdominal air sacs

Of the chicken's nine air sacs, all but one come in pairs. The largest pair is in the abdomen, surrounding the intestine. The air sacs fill with and release air based on the size of the body cavity, which is controlled by muscle movement. When a chicken is resting, the abdominal muscles control its breathing. When a chicken is active, the greater amount of muscle movement causes its body cavity to expand and contract, increasing airflow into the air sacs.

If a chicken needs still more oxygen, it flaps its wings to generate a greater airflow, expanding the air sacs even farther and drawing more air into its pneumatic bones. A rooster flaps its wings prior to crowing to fill its air sacs so it can let out a mighty "Cock-a-doodle-do!"

While the air sacs are flexible, the lungs are rigid, being solidly attached between the ribs and therefore unable to expand. Instead of the lungs expanding and contracting with each breath, the air sacs expand and contract. Incoming air goes directly from the trachea into the rear air sacs but passes through the lungs before going into the forward air sacs. Outgoing air goes out directly from the forward air sacs but passes through the lungs before going out of the rear air sacs. Air thus always passes through the lungs in the same direction, and since oxygen is captured by the lungs, the bird obtains oxygen both when it breathes in and when it breathes out. This steady flow gives the chicken sufficient oxygen to maintain its high rate of metabolism.

Air Sacs

NUMBER	NAME	LOCATION
Forward Air Sacs		
1	Cervical	Neck, above esophagus
2	Interclavicular	Shoulder, between wishbones
2	Thoracic, anterior	Below lungs
Rear Air Sacs		
2	Thoracic, posterior	Behind lungs
2	Abdominal	Surrounding intestine

Airflow

Inhaling

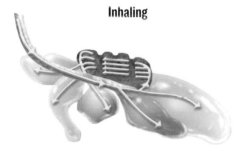

Exhaling

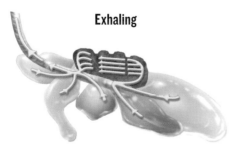

Please Don't Squeeze

⚠ A chicken's breathing is controlled by muscle movements of the breast and ribs, which in turn control the size of the bird's body cavity to allow its air sacs to expand and contract. Holding a chicken tightly enough to restrict movement of its breast and ribs can inhibit breathing and cause the bird to suffocate, which occurs especially when a child gets a too-tight grip on a baby chick. If a chicken appears to have trouble breathing, sometimes lifting its wings or letting the bird drop down a short distance so it reflexively flaps its wings will generate enough airflow to get it breathing again.

Respiratory Defenses

The chicken's trachea is lined with short, tiny hairlike structures called cilia that, by vibrating, whisk pathogens and dust particles back up toward the beak to keep them away from the lower respiratory system. Excessive amounts of dust in a chicken's environment can overload the cilia and cause them to become ineffective.

The chicken's trachea produces mucus to help the cilia trap inhaled particles. A poorly ventilated chicken coop or one that is crowded and accumulates manure too rapidly, resulting in a high level of ammonia in the air, can cause the trachea to produce thicker than normal mucus. Mucus that is too thick inhibits the movement of cilia.

The lungs host scavenger cells that seek out and destroy pathogens and dust particles that get past the cilia, in an attempt to prevent them from spreading into the air sacs. Excessive ammonia levels can reduce the effectiveness of these scavenger cells, allowing pathogens to gain a foothold in the respiratory system.

An environment that is excessively dusty and laden with ammonia can cause dust particles and thick mucus to accumulate at the

Respiratory System

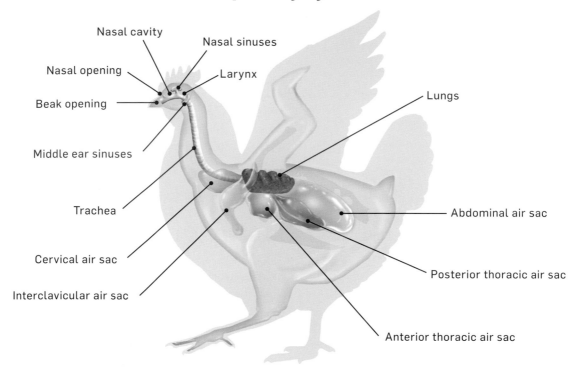

Nasal cavity
Nasal sinuses
Nasal opening
Larynx
Beak opening
Lungs
Middle ear sinuses
Trachea
Abdominal air sac
Cervical air sac
Posterior thoracic air sac
Interclavicular air sac
Anterior thoracic air sac

bottom of the trachea, where it divides into two narrower bronchi. This accumulation of sludge can eventually clog up the bronchi with solid plugs that block air from getting into the lungs and air sacs, causing the chicken to suffocate.

Airsacculitis

Inflammation of the air sacs, or airsacculitis, is a condition that is usually caused by a bacterial infection. Air sac disease generally affects young chickens, especially intensively raised broilers. Signs include failure to eat, rapid weight loss, stunting, and a high death rate. Since air sacs contain few blood vessels, and since most antimicrobial medications are delivered through the bloodstream, infected air sacs are difficult to treat.

Ruptured Air Sac

A chicken of any age can puncture or tear a delicate air sac membrane from being handled roughly, too much roughhousing in the coop, or a crash landing off a high perch. Considered a form of airsacculitis, a ruptured air sac allows air to leak into the chicken's body, causing the skin to puff up as if the bird has been inflated.

For this reason it is also called windpuff or, more technically, subcutaneous emphysema — subcutaneous meaning "under the skin," and emphysema deriving from the Greek word *emphusan*, meaning "to puff up." The skin in front of the neck might swell, looking as though the chicken has swallowed a small balloon. A bubble might develop under a wing, causing the wing to stick out at an unnatural angle. Or the air pocket may appear elsewhere on the chicken's body.

Often the ruptured air sac will heal on its own. If the chicken has trouble getting around, and especially if the poultry yard does not offer a tranquil environment, isolating the affected bird may help the air sac heal more quickly.

If the chicken is obviously in pain, or it can't move or breathe normally, the air pocket may be deflated with a sterile needle and syringe. Deflation may need to be done more than once and runs the risk of introducing pathogens into the respiratory system, so it should be undertaken only if the bird is suffering.

An air sac that has been seriously torn may not heal at all. In such a case the bird — usually a chick — will eventually die.

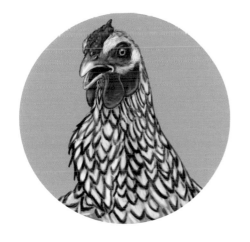

A ruptured air sac can cause the front of a chicken's neck to swell, as if the bird swallowed a small balloon.

Conditions Affecting Respiration

CONDITION	CAUSE
Common Conditions	
Air sac disease	Bacteria
Avian influenza (low path)	Virus
Brooder pneumonia	Fungus
Chronic respiratory disease	Bacteria
Infectious bronchitis	Virus
Infectious coryza	Bacteria
Laryngotracheitis	Virus
Marek's disease	Virus
Newcastle (lentogenic)	Virus
Uncommon Conditions	
Canker	Protozoa
Cryptosporidiosis (respiratory)	Protozoa
Fowl cholera (chronic)	Bacteria
Gapeworms	Parasite
Infectious synovitis	Bacteria
Ornithobacteriosis	Bacteria
Pox (wet)	Virus
Rare Conditions	
Aspergillosis (chronic)	Fungus
Avian influenza (high path)	Virus
Chlamydiosis	Bacteria
Newcastle (mesogenic)	Virus
Newcastle (velogenic)	Virus
Pseudomonas	Bacteria
Roup (nutritional)	Metabolic
Ruptured air sac	Injury

Respiratory Diseases

Respiratory diseases have always been a problem in poultry and today remain the most common cause of death (aside from predation). At one time all respiratory diseases were lumped together as a cold or roup. Today they are recognized as several separate, sometimes unrelated, infections with common characteristics similar to a human cold: labored breathing, sniffling, gasping, coughing, sneezing, runny eyes and nose.

Respiratory diseases may be classified according to their cause, whether nutritional, parasitic, bacterial, fungal, viral, or environmental. Most serious respiratory diseases are caused by viruses, which spread easily in moist air, expelled by a sick bird that coughs, sneezes, or simply breathes. Respiratory distress can also be a reaction to vaccination, especially for Newcastle disease or infectious bronchitis.

Respiratory diseases often occur in combination, so a flock cured of one disease may continue to have signs produced by a second disease. The best defense against respiratory illness is to develop your flock's genetic resistance. The best management practices are to provide good ventilation and avoid introducing carriers into your flock.

General Signs of Respiratory Disease

Labored breathing	Sneezing
Sniffling	Wheezing
Gasping	Runny nose
Coughing	Watery/foamy eyes

Digestive System

A chicken has no teeth. When it finds something tasty to eat that's too big to swallow, the chicken attempts to tear it apart by tidbitting, repeatedly picking up and dropping it to break it into smaller pieces. Once the chicken pecks a piece that's small enough, its tongue pushes the item toward the back of its throat.

Occasionally a chicken will pick up a string or a long, thin blade of grass that partially goes down its throat while the remainder hangs out the beak. You may be able to pull out the string or grass with a gentle tug. If you can't easily get it out, cut off the part that's hanging out to prevent strangulation.

Saliva contains enzymes that start breaking down feed as soon as it enters the bird's mouth, and moisture from the saliva helps dry feed move along more easily. The feed slides down the esophagus, a tube leading to the crop, where the feed is softened while being temporarily stored.

As prey animals, chickens are designed to be able to eat quite a bit at once, then rest in a protected place while they digest what they've eaten. The crop, being a stretchy storage sack, allows them to do that. You can readily see, and feel, a bulging crop at the base of a bird's neck. When it's full, a normal crop is about the same shape and size as a golf ball.

The crop releases feed a little at a time. Exactly how long the crop takes to empty depends on how full it is, the hardness and consistency of its contents, and the amount of moisture that's included. A crop full of grain may take as long as 24 hours to empty; commercial pellets or crumbles pass through considerably faster.

Crop Binding

The crop can become jammed full of feed, a condition called crop impaction or crop binding. Impaction may occur when feed is withheld prior to deworming, causing chickens to gobble down too much afterward. Offering a moistened ration 1 hour after deworming will prevent hard, dry feed from jamming up in the crop.

A crop may become packed with bedding if appropriate rations are not available, causing the bird to be hungry enough to eat inappropriate matter. A crop may also become packed when a bird free-ranges where little is available to eat other than tough, fibrous vegetation. The swollen crop will prevent nutrition from getting through, starving the bird to death, or can cut off the windpipe, suffocating the bird. Mow pasture often enough to keep plants tender and succulent.

A chicken that is losing weight, yet has a full crop that feels hard when you press it with your fingers, and perhaps is not pooping, likely is suffering from crop impaction. To verify that the crop is indeed impacted, isolate the chicken from feed overnight; in the morning a normal (not impacted) crop should be empty or nearly so.

Once you ascertain that the crop is impacted, you can sometimes relieve the congestion by putting a few drops of vegetable oil down the chicken's throat using an oral syringe, then gently massaging the crop to get the contents moving. If that doesn't work, a vet can surgically clean out the crop.

If no avian vet is available and the chicken is in danger of dying, here's how to relieve an impaction:

1. Disinfect the skin over the crop.

2. Use a sharp blade (such as a fresh razor or box cutter) to make a small slit just through the skin.

3. Pull the skin to one side and make a small slit through the crop (the two slits should *not* line up with each other when the skin is in normal position).

4. Gently remove the crop's contents, and rinse out the crop with saline-solution wound wash in a clean oral syringe.

5. Isolate the bird, and keep the wound clean until it heals (see Wound Washes, page 396).

Pendulous Crop

Sometimes a crop becomes so fully distended that the muscles get stretched beyond their ability to bounce back. The more the chicken eats and drinks, the more the crop bulges, until it hangs down and swings back and forth like a pendulum. Unlike an impacted crop, which feels round and hard, a pendulous crop feels baggy and squishy.

Why a crop becomes pendulous in the first place is something of a mystery. Since backyard chicken owners today tend to keep their birds as pets, resulting in lives longer than most farmyard chickens had in the past, a pendulous crop may be due to a loss of muscle tone as a chicken ages. This possibility is suggested by the fact that pendulous crop is not as uncommon as it once was. Irregular access to feed and water (or unpalatable feed or water) may play a role, causing a chicken to stuff itself when it does get something to eat and drink. Genetic predisposition also may be involved.

Various treatments have been suggested for resolving a pendulous crop, although in most cases the crop muscles are so severely stretched they never return to normal. Some birds get along quite well despite having a distended crop. Since the crop can never fully empty, however, the accumulating contents may ferment, eventually leading to the bird's death (see Sour Crop on page 255).

Tale of Two Stomachs

From the crop, feed trickles down to the proventriculus, or true stomach, where acid and enzymes begin the process of digestion. Feed is then passed along to the gizzard, the ventriculus or mechanical stomach, which grinds things up and is therefore sometimes referred to as the chicken's teeth. Feed particles that are not digested well enough to suit the gizzard may be sent back to the proventriculus.

The gizzard has strong muscles — their strength being influenced by the chicken's diet — a tough lining, and usually a collection of small stones or grit to help grind up grains and plant fibers. Acquiring fresh grit is a continuing process, because each particle eventually becomes eroded by acids and is ground up and digested, providing the chicken with mineral nutrients.

Chickens fed only commercially prepared mash or pellets do not need grit; digestive juices are sufficient to soften and digest the feed. Digestive efficiency may be impaired, however, if a chicken eats grains without having access to grit to help grind them up. (See Grit for the Gizzard, page 40.)

Hardware Disease

Because chickens naturally eat small pebbles and bits of sand, they may also eat small, sharp objects such as snips of wire or shards of glass. Such a sharp object is likely to lodge in the chicken's gizzard and, because of the strong grinding motion of the gizzard muscles, may eventually punch a hole in the gizzard wall and invite infection.

This condition is technically known as traumatic ventriculitis, from the Greek word *trauma*, meaning "wound," the Latin word *ventriculus*, meaning "stomach," plus the suffix *itis*, referring to an inflammation. The condition is more commonly known as hardware disease. An affected bird will waste away and eventually die — reason enough to keep your chicken yard free of hazardous bits and pieces.

LIVER COLOR AND AGE

A chicken's liver changes in color and consistency as the bird ages. The liver of a baby chick is soft and pale, because it contains a lot of fat. By the time the chick reaches 1 week of age, its liver becomes firm and is a normal brownish-red. Barring illness, it remains that way while the chicken matures.

When a hen starts laying, fat again begins accumulating in the liver, making it soft and giving it a paler, yellowish color compared to the liver of a cock the same age. Although these changes are normal, a high-producing hen fed an imbalanced diet that is too high in grains, with little exercise opportunity to burn off the excess calories, can develop a potentially fatal condition known as fatty liver syndrome.

The Intestines

The gizzard passes feed, a little bit at a time, into the intestine for nutrient absorption. The small intestine has three main parts, the duodenum, the jejunum, and the ileum. Along the small intestine where the jejunum transitions into the ileum is a tiny blind pouch (open only at one end), the Meckel's diverticulum, and between the small intestine and the large intestine are two large blind pouches, the ceca.

The duodenum, or upper portion of the small intestine, forms a loop. Within the duodenal loop is the pancreas, which secretes enzymes to aid digestion, bicarbonate to neutralize acids, and hormones to regulate blood sugar. Sharing a common duct with the duodenum is the liver, located at the end of the duodenal loop. The liver secretes green bile (or gall) to aid in the absorption of fats. Attached to the liver is a transparent pouch, the gallbladder, where bile is stored until it is needed. The duodenum uses enzymes to break down feed for digestion and also regulates the rate of digestion.

The jejunum is in the middle of the small intestine and is the first part of the lower small intestine. It specializes in absorbing fully digested carbohydrates and proteins.

The Meckel's diverticulum is a small blind pouch, roughly in the shape of a comma, protruding from the lower small intestine along the area where the jejunum gradually transitions into the ileum. It is a permanent vestige of the yolk stalk that connected the yolk sac to the developing embryo during incubation and through which the yolk sac was absorbed soon after the bird hatched. During necropsy the Meckel's diverticulum is helpful in identifying conditions that affect the jejunum but not the ileum, and the ileum but not the jejunum.

Conditions Affecting Intestines

CONDITION	CAUSE
Common	
Coccidiosis (cecal)	Protozoa
Coccidiosis (intestinal)	Protozoa
Cryptosporidiosis (intestinal)	Protozoa
Newcastle disease (lentogenic)	Virus
Paratyphoid	Bacteria
Pasting	Environmental
Uncommon	
Blackhead	Protozoa
Canker	Protozoa
Ulcerative enteritis	Bacteria
Rare	
Arizonosis	Bacteria
Chlamydiosis	Bacteria
Fowl typhoid	Bacteria
Necrotic enteritis	Bacteria
Newcastle disease (velogenic)	Virus
Pullorum	Bacteria

The ileum is not nearly as long as the jejunum but functions much like the jejunum in absorbing nutrients, primarily vitamin B_{12} and other substances the jejunum does not absorb. The ileum also absorbs moisture, causing digestive contents to grow progressively thicker as they move through.

The ceca branch off as a pair of blind pouches where the small intestine joins the large intestine. The ceca gather in fluids, materials dissolved in the fluids, and extremely fine digestive particles to maintain a reservoir of microflora for the proper fermentation of digestive

JOURNEY THROUGH THE DIGESTIVE SYSTEM

A chicken's diet greatly influences how rapidly feed passes through its digestive system. In a healthy chicken, feed generally passes through in 3 to 4 hours, but may take as little as 2 hours or as long as 24. Feed moves fastest through young chickens, which require a lot of nutrients for growth, and through laying hens, which need a steady supply of nutrients for egg production. The consistency of feed changes dramatically as it moves through the digestive system.

- **Crop:** whole grains, lengths of grass, and so on, mixed with saliva
- **Stomach:** mucoid and creamy with some pieces of feed still intact
- **Gizzard:** small pebbles mixed with ground-up fibers and crushed grains
- **Duodenum:** watery and tan to yellow
- **Far side of bile ducts:** greenish
- **Jejunum and ileum:** progressively thicker
- **Ceca:** dark, pasty fermented matter
- **Colon:** drier than in small intestine
- **Cloaca:** normal feces mixed with urates

Digestive System

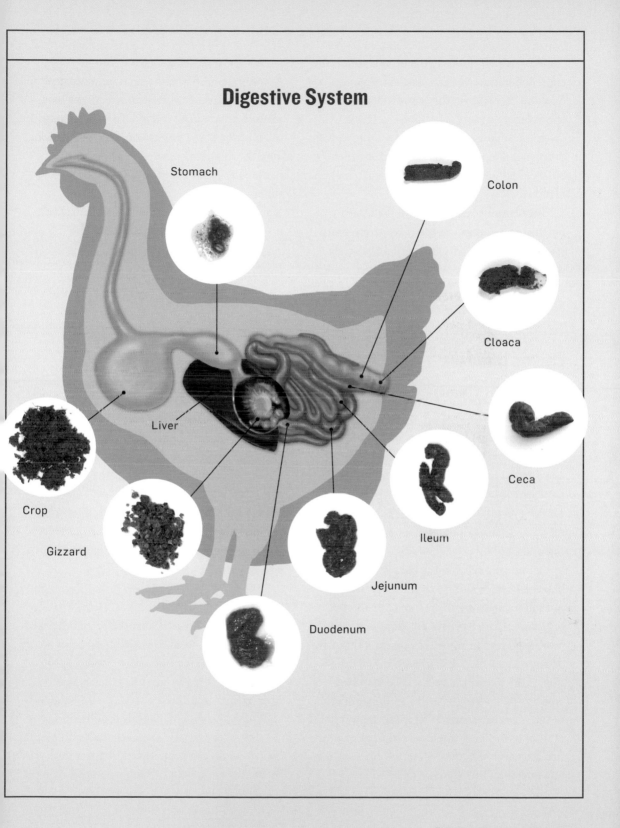

Stomach

Colon

Cloaca

Liver

Ceca

Crop

Gizzard

Ileum

Jejunum

Duodenum

contents, which results in the production of all eight B vitamins. The ceca also absorb moisture and digest fiber. They empty their contents approximately twice a day, producing soft droppings that may smell stronger than regular droppings. Depending on the chicken's diet, cecal droppings might be mustard yellow, chocolate brown, or greenish brown.

The colon, or large intestine, is the last portion of the intestine and is relatively short. It absorbs moisture from digested feedstuffs, which accumulate in the fecal chamber at the end of the colon until passed as droppings. A healthy chicken produces normal gray-brown droppings 12 to 16 times each day.

Enteric Diseases

The word "enteric" refers to the intestines, deriving from the Greek word *enterikos*, meaning "intestinal." Both the small and large intestine are normally populated by beneficial microbes, referred to as microflora (from the Greek word *mikros*, meaning "small," plus the Latin word *Flora*, the goddess of flowers). Microflora aid digestion and enhance immunity by guarding their territory against invading microbes.

An intestinal disease occurs when the balance of microflora is upset or the normal microflora are overrun by too many foreign organisms, which are usually ingested in contaminated feed or water. The result is enteritis, or any disease characterized by an inflammation of the intestine. (Technically speaking, enteritis refers specifically to an inflammation of the small intestine, while colitis is an inflammation of the large intestine, although in practice the word "enteritis" is commonly used for any intestinal inflammation.)

Enteric diseases tend to be complex. Combinations of and interactions among various organisms — worms, bacteria, protozoa, viruses, and natural microflora — determine the severity of the disease. Successfully treating enteritis requires knowing what organisms, or combination of organisms, are causing the illness.

General Signs of Enteritis

Diarrhea	Loss of appetite
Increased thirst	Weakness
Dehydration	Weight loss or slow growth

The Cloaca: Where It All Comes Together

The large intestine ends at the cloaca, from the Latin word *cloaca*, meaning "drain" (and a Latin euphemism for sewer). The digestive, reproductive, and urinary tracts all meet at the cloaca, which is bell shaped and loosely divided into three chambers or compartments that are partially separated by sphincterlike muscular ridges.

The fecal chamber at the end of the colon is the first and largest compartment, where a final bit of moisture is absorbed from digested materials until fecal pressure causes the chamber to stretch and evert, expelling the droppings. This chamber has the ability to hold great amounts of poop, as witnessed by the infamous and enormous broody poop, held by a setting hen until she makes her brief daily trip off the nest. The ability to retain feces allows the hen to keep her eggs warm for long periods without having to relieve herself and prevents contamination of the eggs with droppings. Feces retention can also be detrimental, as might occur when a chicken is deprived of water — because the water runs out, has frozen, is too hot, or tastes bad. In such a case the fecal chamber may become packed with feces that are too dry, resulting in constipation.

The middle and smallest compartment is the urogenital chamber, where both the urinary tract and reproductive systems end. From the urinary tract come urine salts, which appear as a white cap on droppings. The reproductive system of a rooster deposits semen into this chamber; a hen's reproductive system deposits eggs. How eggs avoid being contaminated with feces and urine salts is described later in this chapter; see Reproductive System, page 87.

The final cloacal chamber is the discharge chamber, which is the shortest and ends at the vent. The cloacal bursa opens into the upper wall of this chamber. A young bird's cloacal bursa can therefore readily sample the outside environment through the vent by means of cloacal drinking, described earlier in this chapter; see Cloacal Bursa, page 65.

Cloacitis

Since all of these body systems empty their contents into the cloaca, it is subject to any disease organism related to any of the systems, resulting in inflammation or cloacitis, which is often called vent gleet, from the Latin *glitem*, meaning "sticky soil." A typical sign of cloacitis is smelly slime oozing from the vent and sticking to the feathers. Cloacitis is not a specific disease but a condition that can be caused by many things — bacteria, fungi, yeast, protozoa, and parasites, to name a few. Successful treatment therefore depends on identifying the cause of the infection.

Cloacitis can start simply as the result of a chicken experiencing a highly stressful situation (as described on page 23). A chicken under

Cloaca

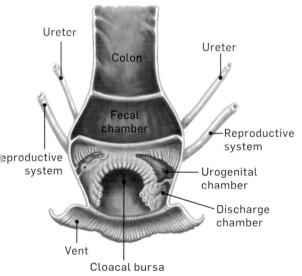

Ureter

Colon

Ureter

Fecal chamber

Reproductive system

Reproductive system

Urogenital chamber

Discharge chamber

Vent

Cloacal bursa

Signs of Cloacitis

EARLY	ADVANCED
Loose, watery droppings	Slimy (sometimes bloody) droppings
Soiled feathers below vent	Straining
Soft, bloated abdomen	Bad odor
Gas	Hard, solid abdomen
Reduced egg production	Red, swollen (sometimes bloody) vent
Eating normally	No longer eating

stress tends to expel loose, watery droppings, an indication that the cloaca is not functioning as it should; a poorly functioning cloaca becomes susceptible to infection. Cloacitis may also result from an infection in the intestines or, in the case of a hen, an infection in the uterus.

TAKING ACTION

At the first sign, clean the vent feathers with warm, soapy water. Using an oral syringe, gently squirt saline-solution wound wash into the vent, and massage the area around the cloaca. If the chicken is constipated, you should be able to work out an accumulation of hard feces. Once the cloaca is clean, follow up with an iodine-based antiseptic such as Betadine. To encourage beneficial bacteria, add vinegar to the drinking water at the rate of 1 tablespoon per gallon (15 mL per 4 L) — double the vinegar dose if the water is alkaline.

Continue this treatment for 3 to 4 days, isolating the chicken if it is in distress or being picked on by others in the flock. If the chicken does not get better, take a fecal sample to the vet for culturing, to find out what type of pathogen is causing the infection. (If the chicken is valuable, you might want to get a fecal culture at the start.)

An advanced case of cloacitis becomes more difficult to treat, and the infection can spread into the colon or uterus. Cloacal infection typically doesn't spread from bird to bird, but when the entire flock experiences the same stressful condition, all the birds become equally susceptible to infection. The appearance of cloacitis in more than one bird during the summer could be the result of heat stress; in fall or winter it could be an indication of parasites, nutritional deficiency, contaminated feed, or contaminated water. At any time of year, droppings that stick to vent feathers can result from feedstuffs chickens have a hard time digesting, as described in Grain Caution, page 45.

Urinary System

The urinary system consists basically of the kidneys (lying along the chicken's backbone) connected to the cloaca's urogenital chamber by means of tubes called ureters. The kidneys are responsible for maintaining an appropriate balance of electrolytes and for filtering water and removing wastes from the blood. In humans these waste products are expelled in urine. A healthy chicken does not excrete much liquid urine but expels blood wastes in the form of semisolid uric acid, called urine salts or urates, that appear as white, pasty caps on fecal droppings.

Urates may be improperly metabolized because of water deprivation, excess dietary protein or calcium, or certain diseases. Droppings may then contain more than the usual amount

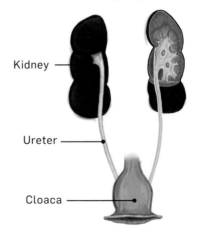

Urinary System

Kidney

Ureter

Cloaca

of urates (as occurs in spirochetosis), or urates may accumulate as pasty deposits in the joints (as happens in articular gout) or collect as crystals that block the ureters (as in the case of infectious bronchitis). A chicken that is frightened or otherwise under stress, especially heat stress, may pass liquid urine.

Reproductive System

One of the main reasons most people keep chickens is to get delicious fresh eggs. Not all eggs are eaten, of course. Some are incubated to make more chickens. Understanding how a rooster's or a hen's reproductive system works will help you recognize any issues that may come up relative to egg laying and fertility.

The Rooster

The rooster has only a rudimentary penis. In place of a single penis, each semen duct ends in a small nipplelike bump, or papilla; this pair of papillae serve as the rooster's mating organs.

Male Reproductive System

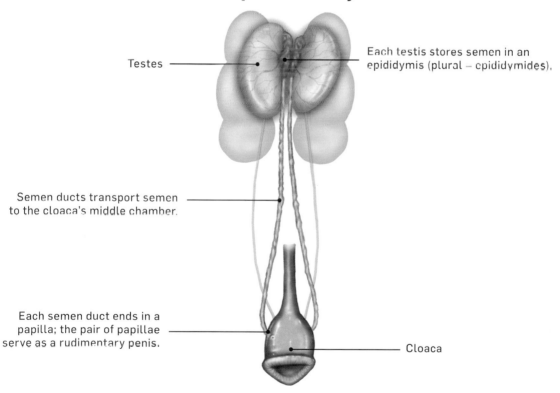

Testes

Each testis stores semen in an epididymis (plural – epididymides),

Semen ducts transport semen to the cloaca's middle chamber.

Each semen duct ends in a papilla; the pair of papillae serve as a rudimentary penis.

Cloaca

The sperm-producing testes are yellowish white, shaped like large kidney beans, and lie along the backbone just below the upper end of the kidneys.

He injects sperm into a hen by pressing his cloaca against hers in a process called the cloacal kiss. To ensure that the two cloacas come together for the transfer of semen, the hen squats, the cock does a balancing act on her back, and when the timing is right she lifts her tail up and to one side while he bends his tail downward for the cloacal kiss.

While the cock is attempting to keep his balance, his claws slide against the hen's back, side, and wing feathers in a process called treading. A hen that's mated often will eventually lose feathers, and the unprotected areas of skin then may become wounded by the cock's claws and spurs. To prevent such injuries, a hen that loses feathers from treading may be fitted with a protective mating saddle until her feathers grow back.

FERTILITY

The inability of a cock to produce sperm or a hen to produce eggs can have many different causes. Determining the reason for infertility therefore can be difficult. Health-related causes of infertility include:

- Stress
- Temperature extremes
- Nutritional deficiency
- Obesity
- Poor condition (too thin)
- Reaction to a medication, pesticide, or toxin, especially aflatoxicosis
- Parasites (internal or external)
- Disease

MATING SADDLE

Mating saddles are worn by hens that have been defeathered by overzealous roosters. Saddles are available ready-made or may be homemade, in a variety of sizes that must properly fit the specific chicken. A saddle that is too tight will chafe, rub off breast feathers, injure the wings, or strangle the bird. A too-loose saddle, or one constructed of droopy material, will flop to one side and be useless.

To prevent skin wounds, apply a saddle as soon as you notice a hen's feathers start to disappear. At first the hen will try to back out of the saddle but will soon get used to it. A saddle is not intended as permanent clothing but should be worn until the hen is well protected by a full set of feathers.

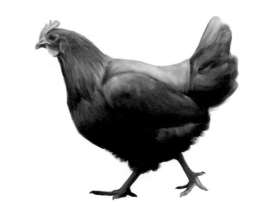

A well-fitted mating saddle protects a hen's back from being defeathered by an amorous rooster.

Roosters past the age of 2 years may lack fertility, or experience significantly reduced fertility, as a result of stones accumulating in the epididymis region, a condition known as epididymal lithiasis. This term derives from the Greek words *epi*, meaning "upon," *didumos*, meaning "testicle," and *lithos*, meaning "stone." Such stones are similar to those commonly occurring in a human's kidney or bladder (and, in fact, roosters and male humans are the only animals known to get stones in their reproductive tracts). As a result of epididymal stones, a rooster's testes atrophy.

No one knows exactly why such stones develop. Theories include hormone imbalance, infection, and heredity. The facts that male chickens are the only birds known to develop this condition, that it is more common in industrial flocks (approaching 100 percent) than in backyard flocks (about 50 percent), and that an affected industrial rooster typically develops more stones than an affected backyard rooster support the theory that epididymal lithiasis results from centuries of genetic selection in favor of efficient calcium mobilization for rapid growth and high egg production.

Season also affects fertility, which tends to be lowest during the heat of summer and at those times of year when daylight hours total fewer than 14. At such times hens may stop laying and a cock's testes temporarily shrivel.

The Hen

A hen's reproductive system consists of one ovary and a multicompartmented passageway or oviduct that's slightly more than 2 feet (60 cm) long. A female chick embryo actually starts out with a pair of reproductive organs. Typically only the left ovary and oviduct continue to develop and become functional, while the right side remains undeveloped. One possible reason is to protect a hen from the stress of potentially producing two eggs at the same time.

Occasionally, often following illness from infectious bronchitis, the right oviduct fills with fluid and becomes cystic. A cyst that remains small may have no effect, but if it grows large it may eventually press against other internal organs and cause the hen's death. Signs are not usually visible until the cyst grows large enough to press against, and cause damage to, internal organs. The chief sign is a bloated abdomen. A veterinarian examining such a hen can determine if a cyst is involved and, if so, provide relief by draining the fluid.

THE YOLK'S JOURNEY

A properly functioning left ovary consists of a clump of undeveloped yolks or ova (a single one is an ovum) located just below the hen's backbone, approximately halfway between the neck and tail in the vicinity of the upper end of the kidneys. As each ovum develops and matures, it is released into the oviduct, usually about an hour after the previous egg was laid. Double-yolked eggs, laid most often by pullets and by heavy-breed hens, occur when two yolks are released within a short time of each other.

During a yolk's journey through the oviduct, it is fertilized (if sperm are present), encased in

Female Reproductive System

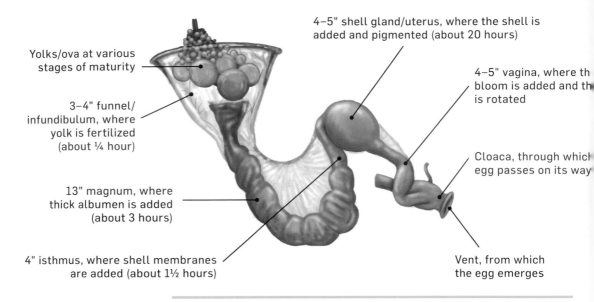

Yolks/ova at various stages of maturity

4–5" shell gland/uterus, where the shell is added and pigmented (about 20 hours)

3–4" funnel/infundibulum, where yolk is fertilized (about ¼ hour)

4–5" vagina, where the bloom is added and the is rotated

13" magnum, where thick albumen is added (about 3 hours)

Cloaca, through which egg passes on its way

4" isthmus, where shell membranes are added (about 1½ hours)

Vent, from which the egg emerges

A hen's oviduct is about 25 inches long, and an egg takes about 25 hours to travel through, from start to finish.

albumen, wrapped in a couple of membranes, sealed in a shell, and given a thin protective coating called the cuticle or bloom. The whole process takes about 25 hours, causing the typical hen to lay each day's egg a little later. Since a healthy hen doesn't lay in the evening, as her cycle progresses and her laying time approaches 3:00 in the afternoon, she'll skip a day and start a new cycle the following morning. A group of eggs laid within one cycle is a clutch.

A typical clutch size for a backyard hen is five eggs. A hen with a longer cycle (say, 28 hours) lays fewer eggs per clutch than a hen with a shorter cycle.

Any interruption in normal cycling (such as a predator attack or being moved) can result in abnormal shell patterns. Abnormal patterns also

occur when yolks are released less than 25 hours apart, causing two developing eggs to move through the oviduct close to each other. The second egg may have a thin, wrinkled shell that's flattened toward the pointy end. If it bumps against the first egg, the shell may crack and sometimes is mended with a new layer of shell covering the crack. The occasional appearance of abnormal shells is nothing to worry about.

Egg shape is inherited, so you can expect to see family similarities. Occasional variations are normal, and so are seasonal variations. Shells will be thicker and stronger in winter but will get thinner in warm weather due to a reduction in calcium mobilization. Soft-shelled eggs are common when production peaks in spring.

A hen that stops laying, hunkers down in the nest, and puffs up her feathers and hisses or growls when she's disturbed is not sick. She's broody, meaning she has motherhood on her mind. The instinct to brood, or to sit on eggs until they hatch, is generally triggered by increasing day length in the springtime. When a hen goes broody, her pituitary gland releases the hormone prolactin, which causes her to stop laying so she won't continue to deposit fresh eggs among the partially incubated eggs in her nest.

PULLET MATURITY AND DAY LENGTH

Pullets are normally hatched in spring and reach maturity during the season of decreasing day length. If you raise pullets between August and March, the increasing day length that normally triggers reproduction will speed up their maturity, the more so as they approach laying age. Pullets that start laying before their bodies are ready will lay smaller eggs with thinner shells, and fewer of them, and are more likely to suffer reproductive issues such as prolapse.

To prevent premature egg laying in pullets raised out of season, consult an almanac to determine how long the sun will be up on days occurring 24 weeks from the date the pullets hatch. Add 6 hours to that day length, and start your pullet chicks under that amount of light (daylight and electric combined). Reduce the total lighting by 15 minutes each week, bringing your pullets to a 14-hour day by the time they start laying. When they reach 24 weeks of age, add 30 minutes per week for 2 weeks to increase total day length to 15 hours.

Since spring is the natural season for chicks to hatch, pullets hatched from April through July and raised in natural light will mature at the normal rate, making them less likely to experience reproductive issues.

Lightweight breeds generally start laying at 18 to 22 weeks of age. Larger-bodied hens usually begin laying at 24 to 26 weeks of age. About 2 weeks before you expect your pullets to start laying, gradually change them over from grower ration to layer ration, which contains more calcium, needed for sound eggshells. Do not feed layer ration to pullets before they reach the age of lay, as the high calcium content can cause serious kidney damage.

REPRODUCTIVE DISORDERS OF THE HEN

A hen lays best during her first and second year. Thereafter, as long as she is healthy, she may continue to lay, but not efficiently enough for commercial production. (See Effect of a Hen's Age on Laying on page 319.) Regardless of a hen's age, the number of eggs she lays, their size, shape, and internal quality, and shell color, texture, and strength can be affected by many things, including environmental stress, improper nutrition, medications, vaccinations, parasites, and disease.

Soft-shelled, thin-shelled, or misshapen eggs, ruptured yolks within eggs, reduced production, and prolapse may be the result of either poor nutrition or infection. A coccidiostat in a hen's rations may alter egg size, color, and shell texture. Watery whites and weak or misshapen shells with altered texture and strength can be caused by a viral respiratory disease, such as infectious bronchitis or Newcastle, or sometimes by vaccination. For more information on disorders that affect eggs and their numbers, see Conditions Affecting Egg Production on page 343.

EGG BINDING

An egg is shaped in the uterus pointed end first. As it moves through the vagina into the cloaca, it is turned end for end so it will be laid large end first. Sometimes an egg gets stuck, in which case the hen is egg bound or suffering from oviduct impaction. Some of the reasons for egg binding include the following:

- The egg may be too large, for example, if a pullet starts laying too young or a hen lays a double yolker.

- The hen is too fat, putting too much pressure on the muscles responsible for egg laying.

- Extremely cold weather can make a hen's egg-laying muscles stiff and therefore unable to contract properly to push the egg out.

- Calcium, needed for the muscle contractions that push the egg out, may be deficient, especially in a better layer or an older hen with depleted calcium reserves.

- A disease may cause the oviduct to swell or its muscles to lose tone.

When a hen becomes egg bound, unlaid eggs accumulate behind it, distending the hen's abdomen. Unless you can get things moving again, the hen will go into shock and die.

Signs of Egg Binding

Sluggishness	Swollen vent
Straining	Pasting
Bloated abdomen	Sudden onset

First make sure the hen is truly egg bound; similar-appearing conditions include ascites, cystic right oviduct, infected uterus, internal laying, and egg peritonitis. One way to find out for certain that a hen is egg bound is to have the hen X-rayed. A vet who ascertains the hen is indeed egg bound can treat her on the spot, including prescribing an antibiotic in the event the cloaca has been damaged or the oviduct has become contaminated with backed-up feces.

You know a hen is egg bound if she strains to release an egg and you can see the egg protruding from the vent. If the egg is not visible, lubricate a finger with K-Y Jelly or other water-based lubricant, and gently insert it into the vent until you feel the hard shell with the end of your finger. Do not attempt to stretch the vent, which could tear delicate tissue.

TAKING ACTION

Once you have ascertained the hen is egg bound, lubricate the vent and egg with K-Y Jelly and/or gently squirt in warm (not hot) saline-solution wound wash or warm soapy water. Sometimes at this point the egg will emerge on its own. Otherwise, gently insert your lubricated finger to help maneuver the egg, while with your other hand you push gently against the abdomen and try to work the egg out. Be careful not to break the egg, which can cause internal injury.

When an egg won't slide out easily, warming the vent area may relax the muscles enough to release the egg. Moisten an old towel, warm it in the microwave (make sure it's not hot enough to burn), and apply it to the hen's bottom. Reheat the towel as needed to keep it warm, or use two towels and warm them alternately, to maintain moist heat. If you don't have a microwave oven handy, put warm, not hot, water in a bucket or basin, and stand the hen in it with the water reaching just above her vent. After warming the pullet's bottom for about 15 minutes, give her a rest, and if she doesn't soon release the egg, try again.

If all else fails, you may need to collapse the shell to remove the egg. This maneuver is tricky and, unless you work slowly and carefully, can injure the hen and result in infection and death. On the other hand, if the egg doesn't come out, the bird won't make it anyway; you may want to solicit the help of a veterinarian.

To attempt removing the egg yourself, first suck out the contents of the egg by piercing the shell with a needle at the end of a syringe. Use a large-bore needle, 18 or lower gauge; otherwise, emptying the shell will take forever.

Once the shell is empty of its contents, try to collapse it while keeping the shards together. This part is the trickiest, as you must take great care to avoid injuring the hen with a sharp shard. For this reason, don't squeeze the abdomen to crush the egg, but rather work gently with your fingers directly on the shell, or at least one or two fingers on the inside and the other hand gently pressing from the outside.

Using lots of warm saline or soapy water as a lubricant, carefully remove as much of the shell as possible, then rinse away remaining pieces with squirts of saline gentle enough not to wash the shell bits deeper. Don't worry about getting the last tiny bits; once the egg is out, the hen is better off left to rest, and any bits left

behind should come out on their own. If tissue protrudes outside the vent, treat the pullet as you would for prolapse.

PROLAPSE

Prolapsed oviduct, also called eversion, is a natural process by which eggs are laid. The word "prolapse" derives from the Latin word *prolapsus*, meaning "to slip forward"; eversion derives from the Latin word *evertere*, meaning "turn out."

A hen's vagina grips a completed egg and pushes it through the cloaca by prolapsing, or turning itself inside out, to deposit the egg outside the vent, then withdraws back inside the hen. If an egg is too big, a hen is too fat or is

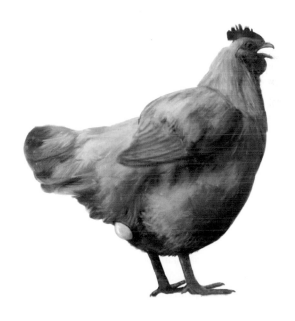

Prolapse is the normal process by which an egg moves through the vagina, but it becomes a serious problem if the protruding tissue does not immediately retract after the egg is laid.

calcium deficient, or a pullet is immature when laying begins, the vagina may be weakened and unable to retract back inside. Uterine tissue that protrudes outside the vent and remains prolapsed is a serious condition called blowout.

Caught in time, the prolapse can sometimes be reversed by cleaning the protruding tissue, applying an anti-inflammatory cream (such as hydrocortisone), and gently pushing the tissue back inside the hen — repeating the treatment as needed. Isolate the hen until she improves. Otherwise the other chickens will be attracted to pick at the protruding tissue, eventually pulling out her insides and causing the hen to die from hemorrhage and shock, a condition known as pickout.

Discouraging the hen from laying will help her heal more quickly. Arrange her recovery unit in a place where she gets no more than 8 hours per day of light, which may be accomplished by letting her outdoors for 8 hours, then bringing her into a darkened area for the rest of the day.

INTERNAL LAYER

An egg does not always develop and get laid in a nest according to schedule but instead ends up inside the hen's body cavity. Internal laying is also known as ectopic eggs, from the Greek word *ektopos*, meaning "out of place." When an affected hen visits the nest regularly without laying, she's called a false layer. Several different conditions can cause internal laying.

Oviduct malfunction. A malfunctioning oviduct may fail to accept mature yolks. An injury can cause such a malfunction. A chickhood infection, particularly infectious bronchitis virus, can prevent the oviduct from developing properly. Or a bacterial infection such as *Escherichia coli* or *Mycoplasma gallisepticum*

can cause a blockage that prevents the oviduct from accepting mature yolks.

Instead, the yolks drop into the hen's abdominal cavity and are partially resorbed by the hen's body. Such a hen fails to lay eggs but otherwise appears normal, unless yolk material gets into the air sacs and from there into the lungs, resulting in pneumonia. A postmortem examination will typically reveal large quantities of orange fat in the abdominal cavity.

Reverse peristalsis. A developing egg is moved through the oviduct by means of a rhythmic, wavelike motion known as peristalsis. Reverse peristalsis can move a fully or partially developed egg in the opposite direction, up and out of the oviduct and into the hen's body cavity. Reverse peristalsis can occur in a hen that is overly fat or can be caused by tumors resulting from lymphoid leukosis. The hen may lay irregularly, and her eggs may be oddly shaped. A postmortem examination may reveal the presence of shell membranes in the hen's abdomen.

Oviduct impaction. An impacted oviduct can cause internal laying. When a fully formed egg gets stuck and cannot emerge, subsequent eggs will back up behind the stuck egg. If the condition is not corrected, and the hen lives long enough, eventually some of the backed-up eggs may get pushed into the body cavity.

Egg peritonitis. Egg material that accumulates in the abdomen without being resorbed eventually becomes infected with bacteria. Sometimes a bacterial infection of the oviduct initiates the egg accumulation. If more than one hen is affected, an infectious bacterial disease may be involved.

OVARIAN ATROPHY

A hen's ovary may atrophy from either disease or severe stress. Infectious diseases that can lead to ovarian atrophy include avian influenza, exotic Newcastle, fowl cholera, and pullorum. Stress conditions typically result from a lack of feed or water, as might occur if the hens are overcrowded, an insufficient number of feeders is provided, or the hens are kept on restricted rations. If a hen is not getting enough nutrients to maintain her body weight, she certainly has insufficient nutrients to maintain a healthy ovary.

As the ovary atrophies, some yolks may drop into the abdomen (see Internal Layer, facing page). Signs of atrophy include emaciation and dehydration accompanied by a neck or body molt. Once the ovary has atrophied, the hen stops laying.

TUMORS

Tumors occur in the reproductive organs of hens more often than in any other animal and are a common cause of poor laying. Some tumors have known causes, notably lymphoid leukosis and Marek's disease; others do not. Slow-growing tumors that occur in older hens are understood least of all, since only young hens are kept in commercial flocks that sponsor most of the research.

SEX CHANGE

Spontaneous sex change is a phenomenon whereby a hen develops the characteristics of a cock. When a hen's left ovary atrophies, the latent reproductive organ on the right side may develop into a combination ovary-testicle. While the dysfunctional left ovary reduces estrogen output, the testicular component of the right ovary releases testosterone. A tumor in the left ovary, or elsewhere, may also result in the production of testosterone.

As a result, the hen's comb grows larger, she may molt into male plumage, she may crow, and she may mount other hens. She may even produce viable sperm to fertilize eggs that hatch into chicks. Spontaneous sex change is more common in an older hen reaching the end of her productive life.

In a younger hen hormonal change may result from an infection. If the infection is successfully treated, the "cock" will revert back to a hen at the next molt. If the infection is cured before the next molt, the apparent "cock" will lay eggs. This phenomenon was once considered witchcraft, the most famous case being a "cock" named Basel that was burned at the stake in 1474 for laying eggs.

Nervous System

The nervous system is a complex network that coordinates all the other systems to control all body functions. It consists of the central nervous system, which includes primarily the brain and the spinal cord, and the peripheral nervous system, a network of nerves connecting the organs and other body parts to the brain and spinal cord.

Whenever anything stimulates the peripheral nervous system, it sends a signal to the central nervous system for an interpretation. Based on this interpretation, the peripheral nervous system reacts through one of the following two groups of nerves:

Somatic nerves, which use the skeletal muscles to control voluntary movements such as running, eating, and feather ruffling

Autonomic nerves, which are responsible for involuntary body functions such as breathing, heartbeat, and digestion

The nervous system may be disrupted by any number of things, including poisoning, a virus, a tumor, or a hereditary defect. Typical signs of a nervous disorder are incoordination, trembling, twitching, staggering, circling, neck twisting, convulsions, and paralysis of a wing, leg, or the entire body.

General Signs of a Nervous Disorder

Incoordination	Circling
Trembling	Neck twisting
Twitching	Convulsions
Staggering	Paralysis

Eyes

The eyes are part of the central nervous system. When the eye detects an image, a network of nerves in the retina at the back of the eyeball sends a signal to the brain for interpretation, which then tells the chicken how to react. Like most other birds (and other prey animals), a chicken's eyes are on the sides of its head, giving it a larger range of peripheral vision but a smaller range of binocular vision, compared to other creatures (including humans) with eyes positioned toward the front so both can focus on an object at the same time.

A chicken, by contrast, has a right-eye system and a left-eye system, each with different and complementary capabilities. The right-eye system works best for activities requiring recognition, such as identifying items of food close by on the ground. The left-eye system works best for activities involving depth perception, such as warily watching an approaching hawk.

Compared to most other animals, birds have large eyes in relation to the size of their heads, giving them keen eyesight that is 10 times sharper than a human's to help them guard against predators. Chickens have better color vision than most animals, including humans, because their retinas are organized primarily for seeing in the daytime, when chickens spend most of their time looking for things to eat. The trade-off of having superior day vision is that they don't see well at night.

EYE STRUCTURE

The protective covering of a chicken's eye consists of three eyelids. The upper and lower eyelids are much like those of a human, except that a chicken's lower eyelid moves more freely than the upper. The third eyelid, called the nictitating membrane (from the Latin word *nictare*, meaning "to blink"), lies between the eye and the other two eyelids and has its own lubricating duct, similar to a human's tear duct. The nictitating membrane moves horizontally across the eye from front to rear and is transparent, so the chicken can see even with this eyelid closed. The chicken draws this third eyelid across its eye to clean and moisten the eye and sometimes for protection, such as when a hen's chick tries to peck her eye.

Environmental conditions that can cause eye irritation include ammonia fumes from accumulated droppings, any strong chemical fumes, and excessive dust. Eyes may be scratched or otherwise injured from altercations between chickens or from dust, dirt, or bits of bedding getting into the eye. Numerous diseases can affect a chicken's eyes, causing them either to swell or to sink, get foamy, stick shut, become cloudy, or go completely blind. Disorders that affect a chicken's eyes are listed under Conditions Affecting Eyes on page 341.

Congenital loco, also known as stargazing, is a nervous condition that causes a chick's neck to bend so far back that its head touches its back and its beak points toward the sky. The epileptic-like muscle spasms that pull the head back typically cause the bird to tip over. After a few days of flopping around, the chick dies from lack of food and water.

Chicks exhibiting this condition are discarded by commercial hatcheries and dedicated backyard breeders. Because they are rarely kept for study, no one is certain how common the condition is or exactly what causes it. The fact that it occurs only occasionally in chicks at the time of hatch indicates that it may be a recessive genetic trait. The few studies that have been done revealed a possible defect in the ear structure.

A similar condition appears several days after hatch, occurs sporadically, lasts a few days, then disappears as mysteriously as it came. Although the condition looks identical to congenital loco, the fact that it does not occur at the time of hatch, and is not lethal, indicates that it may be a separate condition with a different cause. To make this distinction the term "congenital loco" might best be used to refer to the condition when it occurs at the time of hatch and "stargazing" for transient occurrence in older chicks.

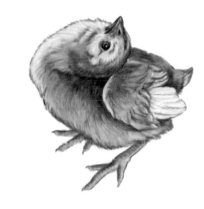

Typical posture of congenital loco and stargazing

HOW TO TELL IF A CHICKEN IS BLIND

A blind eye usually takes on a smoky, gray look, and the pupil becomes irregular in shape. When only one eye is blind, the pupils are usually of unequal size.

If you slowly move a finger toward the affected eye, a blind chicken won't blink or dodge your hand, as would a bird that can see. Don't wave your hand, though, because the chicken may feel the stirred air and blink or move its head even if it can't see.

A chicken can usually do relatively well despite being blind, provided feed and water are readily available, the chicken has companion chickens, and the blind bird is confined to a limited area where it won't lose its way or be vulnerable to predation. Even when a partially or fully blind chicken seems to be doing well, keep a close watch to make sure the bird is getting enough to eat to maintain its normal weight.

Ears

The ears are also part of the nervous system. They consist of small openings on each side of the chicken's head, below and behind the eyes. Unlike a dog, cat, or human, a chicken has no external ear part, so its ears more rightly might be considered ear holes. Instead of an external ear, each ear is covered by a clump of tiny, stiff feathers that protect the ear opening and also direct sounds into the ear.

The chicken's ear consists of three chambers: outer, middle, and inner. The outer and middle ears are filled with air and are separated by the eardrum. Even though the chicken's middle ear structure is not as complex as that of a human, the bird hears pretty well, because the middle ear includes a well-developed sound-conducting structure.

The inner ear is more complex than the other two chambers and is filled with fluid. Similarly to a human's ear, the chicken's inner ear is responsible for the bird's sense of balance. Whenever the chicken moves its head, sensitive hairs in the inner ear are moved by flowing fluid, transmitting information to the brain via auditory nerves that keep the brain notified as to exactly where the chicken's head is at any given time. If this signal gets disrupted, the chicken loses coordination.

Problems involving a chicken's ears are not common but do occasionally occur. Such issues include the following:

Infection of the outer ear, typically caused by bacteria or fungi, which may result in itching, swelling, fluid leakage around the ear opening, and waxy/cheesy material in the ear

EYE TREATMENT

To treat a chicken's eye, confine the bird under your arm and hold its head with one hand while working on the scratched or crusted-over eye with the other hand. Working without a helper can be an exercise in frustration if the chicken won't hold its head still. A simple trick is to hypnotize the chicken (as described on page 398), which will keep it calm long enough to treat the eye.

Use a cotton swab to gently clean the eye of any debris that can be removed easily. If debris is crusted in, soften it by gently laying a gauze pad or cloth dampened with warm water against the eye. Gently rinse the cleaned eye with saline wound wash (see Make a Saline Wound Wash, page 397) or quality eyedrops such as Systane, then apply an eye-safe antimicrobial such as colloidal silver or Vetericyn ophthalmic gel. Repeat as necessary until the eye heals.

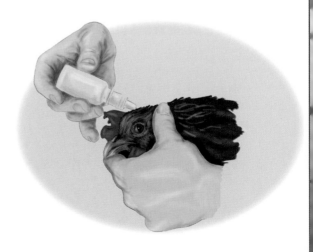

A rapid, jerky movement of the head from side to side is not necessarily a sign of ear infection. Such head shaking, particularly by roosters, is often a sign of nervousness or fear. This behavior pattern may be distinguished from head shaking caused by ear discomfort in two ways:

- The chicken will keep an eye on the feared object (or person) while moving away from it.

- Behavioral head shaking is not accompanied by head scratching or rubbing.

Infection of the middle ear, typically from a chronic bacterial infection, resulting in swelling

Infection of the inner ear, typically resulting from a virus, causing loss of coordination and twisting of the neck (torticollis), similar to the stargazing posture described on page 97

A tumor in or pressing against the ear, resulting in signs similar to those of a chronic infection

An infection in the outer ear is relatively easy to treat by cleaning out the ear, applying an antimicrobial, and repeating as necessary. Infections of the middle and inner ear involve identifying and treating the underlying cause. A tumor may be identified by eliminating the possibility of a chronic infection or by obtaining an X-ray, and is not treatable.

Circulatory System

The circulatory system consists primarily of the heart, spleen, blood, and blood vessels. Blood makes up approximately 6 percent of a chicken's body weight. The blood serves these important functions:

- It transports oxygen, hormones, and nutrients throughout the body.

- It carries away carbon dioxide and other waste products.

- It forms blood clots to minimize bleeding from wounds.

- It carries antibodies and infection-fighting cells.

- It helps regulate body temperature.

A chicken may have one of 12 blood types, each with its own set of antigens. Blood type therefore influences a chicken's resistance to disease, a hen's egg production and vigor, and the hatchability of her eggs. Some breeds and strains therefore are more vigorous and less susceptible to disease than others.

The heart is a four-chambered pump that keeps blood circulating through the vessels. The spleen's function is to clean the blood of microorganisms, unhealthy blood cells, and other debris. The blood is susceptible to invasion by bacteria, viruses, fungi, protozoa, and other parasites that get into the blood through mucous membranes or through the skin, introduced by wounds or insect bites. Some species of parasitic worms temporarily travel through the bloodstream on their way to the organ or tissue in which they will grow to maturity.

Septicemia

When any infectious organism enters the bloodstream and becomes generalized, or systemic, by invading the whole body, septicemia occurs. Typical signs that a disease has gone septicemic are weakness, listlessness, lack of appetite, chills, fever, and prostration. In acute septicemia chickens that are in good condition and appear healthy die suddenly. Sudden death with a full crop is a typical indication of acute septicemia, since most other conditions cause loss of appetite.

Signs of Septicemia

GENERAL	ACUTE
Weakness	Sudden death in an apparently healthy bird in good flesh with a full crop
Listlessness	
Lack of appetite	
Prostration	

Anemia

Anemia, or going light, is a condition in which the blood is deficient in quantity (blood loss) or quality (low red blood cell count). Red blood cells, or erythrocytes, are the most numerous kind of blood cells. They are responsible for transporting oxygen throughout the body and removing carbon dioxide and other waste gases. Hemoglobin is an iron-rich protein within red blood cells that carries oxygen and carbon dioxide. It is bright red, giving red blood cells their color.

Red blood cells rapidly become worn out and die, but under normal conditions they are replaced by fresh red cells. Anemia occurs when a disease or other abnormality causes these cells to die out faster than usual or fail to regenerate at a normal rate.

Anemia may be caused by dietary copper or iron deficiency, blood-sucking parasites (mites and lice), aflatoxins, some infectious diseases, or an internal tumor. It may also result from an inability to absorb nutrients, such as might occur because of a worm load or coccidiosis.

Signs of anemia include pale skin and mucous membranes, loss of energy, loss of weight, and death. Anemia from iron deficiency also causes faded plumage in red-feathered breeds.

Aside from the viral disease infectious anemia, which does not typically afflict backyard flocks, anemia itself is not a disease. Rather, it occurs as a result of some other unhealthful condition. Treating a chicken for anemia is therefore futile unless the underlying condition is successfully treated.

With appropriate treatment of the underlying disease, combined with proper nutrition, a chicken will recover from anemia. If the chicken appears to need a nutritional boost, the vitamin/mineral Red Cell supplement (formulated for horses) can provide small amounts of a large number of necessary nutrients when added to drinking water at the rate of 1 teaspoon per gallon.

CHAPTER 4

Mysteries of
Metabolism

METABOLISM, A WORD deriving from the Greek *metabole*, meaning "change," encompasses the collective life-maintaining changes that take place within the body. It occurs when food is digested, absorbed, and converted into either the acids that become the building blocks that make up the physical body or sugars that provide energy to run the body.

Metabolic processes — which include breathing, blood circulation, body temperature control, the maintenance of brain and nerve function, muscle contraction, and cell growth — are of two distinct types.

Constructive metabolism involves the step-by-step synthesis of complex substances from simpler ones to store energy and to produce the carbohydrates, fats, and proteins that form body tissue. Another word for this process is anabolism, from the Greek word *anabole*, meaning "to build up."

Destructive metabolism involves the breaking down of complex substances into simpler ones to release the energy needed for constructive metabolism. Another word for destructive metabolism is catabolism, from the Greek word *katabole*, meaning "to tear down." Destructive metabolism produces waste matter in the form of urine and feces expelled as poop, and carbon dioxide released during breathing.

As a chemical activity occurring within cells, metabolism stores energy, releases energy from nutrients, and uses energy to create bodily substances. Metabolism is therefore measured in terms of energy use: in other words, calories.

Speaking of Metabolism

basal metabolism. The amount of energy (fuel) needed to keep a chicken alive and healthy but not engaged in activity, growth, or egg production

core temperature. The temperature of internal organs; also called deep body temperature

critical high temperature. The air temperature at which a chicken starts suffering heat stress

critical low temperature. The air temperature at which a chicken starts suffering cold stress

metabolism. The collective life-maintaining processes creating physical and chemical changes that produce, maintain, or destroy substances forming the physical body, as well as chemical changes that provide energy for the body to run on

thermoregulation. The ability to maintain core temperature within certain limits despite changes in air temperature

Metabolic Rate

A chicken's basal, or base, metabolic rate is the amount of energy, or number of calories, the bird needs to keep its body functioning at rest in a temperate environment. A chicken that doesn't get enough feed and water to furnish its basic energy needs for survival becomes emaciated and dies.

A chicken's metabolic rate is the actual amount of energy, or number of calories, it uses within a specific amount of time. The heavier the chicken, the higher its metabolic rate tends to be, even at rest. Other things that increase the metabolic rate include activity, stress, fear, fever, disease, and temperature extremes.

Birds, in general, have a high metabolism because they're always on the go, and because they have a high internal temperature compared to other animals. A chicken's deep body (or core) temperature ranges between 105°F and 107°F (40.6°C and 41.7°C) compared to a human's average core temperature of about 99.5°F (37.5°C).

One reason chickens, and other birds, operate at a high temperature is that they can eat a lot at one time and digest it rather rapidly. This feature evolved to help chickens in the wild stay ahead of predators by eating fast, then moving to a safe place to digest what they've eaten. In a healthy chicken, feed passes through the entire digestive system within 3 to 4 hours.

Another reason healthy birds have a high body temperature is that they naturally have high blood sugar — about twice that of a human. High blood sugar gives chickens the energy to spend most of their daylight hours on the move.

Normal activity accounts for 20 to 25 percent of the calories a chicken burns each day. Its basal metabolic rate accounts for the remaining 60 to 75 percent, some 10 percent of which is used for digestion.

A metabolic disorder is any condition occurring because of a disruption in normal metabolism. Such disruptions may — rarely — result from a genetic defect. More often they result from faulty nutrition, which might be caused by insufficient rations, an inappropriate diet, or a disease that leads to the failure of an organ and thus impairs the body's ability to use nutrients the chicken consumes. Bottom line: a metabolic disorder results when a chicken's body does not get enough energy to remain healthy.

Thermoregulation

A chicken's body operates most efficiently at an effective air temperature between 70°F and 75°F (21°C and 24°C), which is the ideal temperature range for good health and productivity. Somewhat above and below this range, chickens remain comfortable by modifying their behavior, which allows them to maintain a satisfactory body temperature without expending a lot of energy.

The warmest temperature that defines this comfort zone is the critical high temperature, above which chickens suffer heat stress. The lowest temperature is the critical low, below which chickens suffer cold stress. The degree of heat stress or cold stress a chicken suffers depends on how fast the temperature changes and how long the extreme temperature lasts. Chickens that are gradually exposed to high or low temperatures become acclimated, causing their critical high temperature to move upward in a warm climate and their critical low temperature to move downward in a cold climate.

So the exact temperature range that defines the comfort zone depends, in part, on how well acclimated the chickens are to temperature extremes. Other factors that define the comfort zone include the chickens' age, weight, diet, and state of health. Environmental factors that influence the comfort zone's temperature range include degree of air movement and ambient relative humidity.

Heat Stress

When hot weather or a fever increases a chicken's core temperature, its enzymes speed up their activity, which increases the chicken's metabolic rate. If the chicken gets hot enough for its enzymes to lose stability, they stop functioning altogether, and the chicken dies.

The problem is that the temperature at which a chicken's enzymes lose stability is not much higher than the bird's normal internal body temperature. So when a chicken starts feeling too warm, it looks for ways to cool off. Luckily, although a chicken's relatively large body surface absorbs heat rather quickly, given suitable conditions its body can release heat nearly as fast.

KEEPING COOL

Since a chicken has no sweat glands, it needs other ways to stay cool. One evolutionary adaptation that is common in chickens from hot climates — such as the Leghorn and other Mediterranean breeds, as well as the Fayoumi,

UNHAPPY ENZYMES

The entire process of metabolism relies on enzymes. These complex proteins are produced by living cells and function as biological catalysts for every aspect of metabolism. But unhappy enzymes don't function at all well.

Among the many things that adversely affect a chicken's enzymes are dehydration, pH imbalance, excessive salt, chemical toxins, extreme cold, and extreme heat. The most common cause of enzyme malfunction in chickens is extreme heat.

Temperature Zones

Fatal: The chicken's core temperature becomes too high.

Heat stress: Chickens pant, gular flutter, drink more, hens stop laying.

Warm: Chickens move away from each other, lift their wings, eat less.

Ideal: Optimal temperature for good health.

Cool: Chickens huddle together, ruffle feathers, eat more.

Cold stress: Chickens shiver, cover legs, hens stop laying.

Fatal: The chicken's core temperature drops too low.

115°F
110°F (43°C)
105°F
100°F
95°F (35°C) Critical High
90°F
85°F
80°F
75°F (24°C)
70°F (21°C)
65°F
60°F (16°C) Critical Low
55°F
50°F
45°F
40°F
35°F
30°F
25°F (4°C)
20°F
15°F
10°F
5°F
0°F
-5°F
-10°F

Comfort zone: Chickens do not use much energy to maintain a comfortable core temperature.

Temperature zones vary depending on breed, age, weight, diet, state of health, how well acclimated the chickens are, and how well they are protected from the elements.

Fatal Core Temperatures

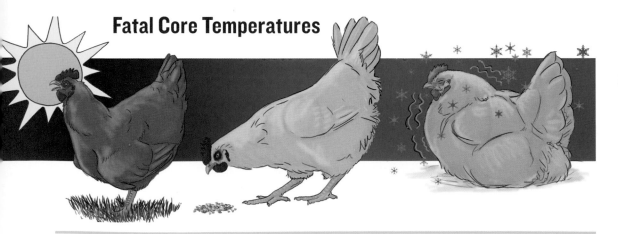

A typical chicken's average deep body temperature is 106°F (41°C). Any condition that causes the deep body temperature to rise above 115°F (46°C) or drop below 25°F (4°C) is fatal.

which originated in Egypt — is a large comb and wattles, through which blood circulation increases in hot weather to more rapidly dissipate body heat. Since feathers trap heat close to the body, another warm-climate adaptation is sparse feathering on the body and no feathers on the legs and feet.

Still, when the temperature soars, such adaptations go only so far. The first thing any overheated chicken does is move to a place that's cooler than its body, which allows heat to radiate from the bird into the environment. On hot summer afternoons chickens hang out in shady places, and to help reduce their metabolic rate, they take a break from their normal busyness.

A breeze will move heat away from the too-hot chicken by replacing warm air close to its body with cooler air. To enhance this effect, chickens lift their feathers to let heat escape from their skin and spread their wings so the breeze can blow across the sparsely feathered areas underneath. But a breeze can cool a chicken only as long as the air is cooler than the bird's body.

Transferring body heat to cool objects is another way chickens keep cool. Holes for dust bathing in cool soil or fresh litter can be significant cooling devices. Standing in cool water helps dissipate heat through the legs. As with the comb and wattles, blood flow to the legs increases when a chicken feels hot. Furnishing a wading pool filled with cool water for the chickens to stand in helps dissipate heat from their legs more rapidly.

AVOIDING HEAT STRESS

When the temperature exceeds a chicken's comfort zone, external cooling mechanisms become insufficient, and the chicken must increase the loss of internal body heat through excretion and evaporation. Excretory heat transfer is accomplished by drinking lots of cool water. The chicken's body warms the water, then eliminates the water in droppings. At high temperatures chickens increase the rate of excretory heat loss by drinking much more than usual, which causes their droppings to become loose

VARIABLE BODY TEMPERATURE

The core, or deep body, temperature of chickens normally ranges between 105°F and 107°F (40.6°C and 41.7°C). In each of the following pairs, the first chicken typically has a higher core temperature:

- Active chicken versus sleeping chicken
- Mature chicken versus hatchling
- Cock versus hen
- Small breed versus large breed

Temperature/Humidity Heat Stress Index for Chickens

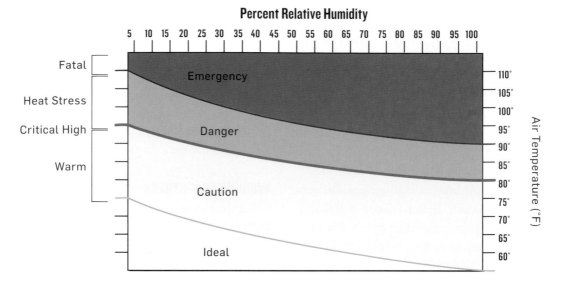

The heat stress index combines air temperature with the relative humidity to determine how increasing humidity affects the comfort zone. Note, for example, that the typical critical high temperature of 95°F (35°C) drops to about 85°F (29°C) at 45 percent relative humidity and to about 80°F (27°C) at 90 percent relative humidity.

and watery. Off-color droppings during the heat of summer may be a sign your birds aren't getting enough to drink.

Evaporation is accomplished through respiratory heat transfer, which occurs when a bird inhales air that's cooler than its internal body temperature and exhales moisture-laden warm air. The bird's extensive respiratory system — which includes not only the lungs but also the air sacs among its organs and the air spaces within some of its bones — is an important mechanism for removing internal body heat.

The rate of heat loss increases when a chicken pants. Panting is an efficient way to lose heat, because (unlike in humans) air passes through a chicken's lungs in one direction, so outgoing warm air doesn't mix with incoming cooler air. Not only does this feature increase

the chicken's cooling capacity, but it also increases oxygen levels to accommodate the higher metabolic rate.

When panting isn't enough to keep its body temperature from rising, the chicken increases the rate of evaporation by rapidly vibrating its throat muscles. This technique is known as the gular flutter, from the Latin word *gula*, meaning "throat." Gular flutter increases the rate of evaporation from the moist lining of the chicken's throat and mouth, accounting for as much as 35 percent of the total heat dissipation.

When the environmental temperature approaches the chicken's body temperature, as happens in the southern U.S. nearly every summer, evaporation can help remove excess body heat through liquid vaporizing on the body's surface. Each 17°F (9.5°C) increase in air temperature doubles the air's capacity to carry moisture, up to a point — air at any temperature can accept only so much moisture, and if the air is already saturated with humidity, it just can't hold any more. Although the critical high air temperature is generally considered to be 95°F (35°C), an air temperature of 82°F (28°C) can be just as uncomfortable if the humidity is above 65 percent.

COOLING STRATEGIES

But when the humidity is low, you can take advantage of evaporation to cool your chickens by frequently hosing down the coop's outside walls and roof and occasionally misting adult chickens. Use these cooling techniques when the following conditions prevail:

- Air temperature is above 95°F (35°C)
- Air humidity is below 75 percent
- Air circulation/ventilation is good

In hot weather chickens attempt to reduce their metabolic rate by eating less. The consequence is that young birds don't grow well, and hens lay fewer and smaller eggs of lesser quality. Since fat requires less energy to metabolize than corn and other carbohydrates, feeding some calories as fat in place of carbohydrates during hot weather helps keep up the chickens' energy level while minimizing an increase in body heat caused by digestion.

As a further measure to maintain adequate energy when heat causes chickens to lose appetite, encourage them to eat while temperatures are cooler than they are at midday. Feed them early in the morning and late in the afternoon.

If necessary, turn on lights inside the coop before dawn and after dusk so they can eat and digest their feed before the daytime temperature rises and after it cools down.

The shells of eggs laid by hens suffering heat stress get thinner, because the increased respiratory rate caused by panting decreases the carbon dioxide level in their blood, which causes the blood's pH to rise, which in turn reduces the amount of ionized calcium in the blood. Since hens need this calcium to make eggshells, the eggs they lay in hot weather tend to have thinner than normal shells. Adding ¼ cup of sodium bicarbonate (common baking soda) to each gallon of drinking water, or offering an electrolyte supplement, can reduce the effects of heat stress by helping restore the chicken's acid/base balance. (For more on electrolytes, see Electrolytes on page 385. See also When *Not* to Use Vinegar on page 384.)

Where hot weather is common, insulating the coop roof helps reduce radiant heat from the sun. Chickens that get relief from the heat by roosting in a cool coop during the night are better able to cope with heat during the day.

A chicken that is unable to maintain a core temperature below about 115°F (46°C) dies. How likely a chicken is to die because of heat stress depends on many factors, including the bird's age and size, the degree to which it has acclimated to hot weather, how rapidly the temperature rises, how high it goes, how long it stays high, and how humid the air is. Factors that help chickens survive a hot spell include the birds' ability to get out of the sun, the presence of air circulation (if no breeze, then from a fan), and access to plenty of cool drinking water.

Cold Stress

One of the reasons a chicken's body temperature is naturally high is so the bird can remain active during cold weather. When the temperature drops, the chicken's body speeds up metabolism to keep the bird warm. As a result, chickens generally suffer less in cold weather than in hot weather and are less apt to die from cold stress, as long as they have adequate nutrition and drinking water, and their housing is neither damp nor drafty.

COLD WEATHER STRATEGIES

Adaptations that help chickens cope in cold climates include dense body feathers, as well as additional feathering on normally exposed body parts — such as on the legs and feet, surrounding the beak (beards and muffs), or on top of the head (crests) — and combs and wattles of minimal size.

Just as chickens increase the blood flow to their legs during summer, they decrease the flow during winter to minimize the escape of body heat from their bare legs. The overlapping scales on their legs and feet also help conserve heat to some extent, but when a chicken feels really cold, it will try to keep its legs and feet warm by sitting on them or tucking them under its breast. Similarly, heat also escapes from the beak, and a cold chicken will warm its head during the day by tucking it under a wing.

Developing fat reserves is another cold-climate adaption, as a chicken with some body fat suffers less in cold weather than a thin chicken does. The cold-hardy American breeds are notorious for how easily they accumulate body fat, to the detriment of egg production.

Cold chickens also ruffle up their feathers, creating an air space near their skin that traps body heat. And unlike too-hot chickens that tend to move apart, cold chickens tend to congregate and huddle together to conserve their collective body heat. On a cold winter morning, notice how chickens linger longer cuddled among their companions on the roost.

When huddling and feather ruffling aren't enough to keep chickens warm, they start to shiver. Shivering increases the metabolic rate, generating more body heat, but also requires more calories. Chickens therefore eat more in winter and suffer if the feeder goes empty. A chicken that doesn't eat for just 1 day drops about 2.5°F (1.4°C) in body temperature, and one that doesn't eat for a second day drops another degree or so. A chicken that goes hungry in cold weather won't last long.

Aside from keeping the feeder full, offer your chickens a little scratch grain just before they go to roost to give them the extra calories they need to stay warm during the night. For additional calories give them a suet block to peck at during cold weather.

AVOIDING COLD STRESS

In the same way that heat stress is influenced by a combination of air temperature and relative humidity, cold stress is influenced by a combination of air temperature and wind chill. A well-feathered bird may be perfectly comfortable at an air temperature of 50°F (10°C) in still air and sunshine, while the same chicken out in the wind and rain will be miserable at 68°F (20°C).

Environmental conditions therefore play a major role in how well a chicken can avoid the lethal core temperature of 73°F (23°C). Important considerations are how rapidly the temperature drops, how cold it gets, how long it stays cold, and whether the chicken can stay dry and out of the wind.

TAKING ACTION

Reduce drafts. To keep warm a chicken needs protection from drafts that carry away warm air trapped in its ruffled feathers. If you suspect that your coop is too drafty, hold out a strip of survey tape or tissue paper in the roosting area. If the tape or paper moves while you are holding it still, the coop is too drafty.

Reduce humidity. One of the most important environmental factors inside the coop in cold weather is humidity. Although relative humidity tends to be low in winter months, the air inside a chicken coop is typically high in humidity from breathing and pooping. When the air trapped under a chicken's feathers is damp, the chicken's body needs to generate more heat energy to warm it. Otherwise the chicken will feel a chill.

Temperatures low enough to freeze moisture in the air can also freeze combs, wattles, and toes. Frostbite is therefore more likely to occur in damp housing than in dry housing. (For more information, see Frostbite, page 299.)

Good ventilation helps reduce a coop's humidity. Ventilation involves a steady air exchange whereby stale air goes out and fresh air comes in. If moisture accumulates on coop windows, ventilation is inadequate. But unlike a draft, good ventilation doesn't necessarily stir up a breeze. One way to ensure good ventilation without draftiness is to place windows and air vents higher than the chickens' roost.

Another way to help reduce coop humidity during winter is to avoid keeping chickens confined during the day, but let them go outside. As long as they can get back in when they want to, and provided it's not windy out, they just may prefer to be outdoors, despite the cold. They might even find a sunny nook where they can enjoy the sun's warming rays.

Avoid heaters. If humidity is controlled inside the coop, installing a heater is not the best idea, unless the temperature drops so far so fast that your chickens didn't have time to acclimate. The routine use of a heater interferes with the chickens' ability to acclimate to the cold. And many heaters used in chicken coops pose a serious fire hazard. The safest type of heater to use in a cold-weather emergency is a flat-panel radiant space heater, an infrared panel heater designed specifically for pets, which may be hung from the ceiling or affixed to the wall.

The only heat source your coop might benefit from is one that keeps the drinking water from freezing. An alternative is to fill drinkers with warm water several times a day to ensure your chickens get their fill. As long as your chickens get enough to drink, they will generally eat enough to stay warm in cold weather.

Heart Failure

Metabolic processes create the tissues that make up the circulatory organs — heart, blood vessels, and blood — and these organs, in turn, are collectively responsible for delivering oxygen and digested nutrients needed for the metabolic processes of all body cells.

The chicken's high metabolic rate places great stress on its heart. The chicken's heart rate can be as high as 400 beats per minute, compared to a human's heart rate of 60 to 100 beats per minute. To handle the greater stress, the size of a chicken's heart relative to its body mass is about 0.8 percent, compared to a human's heart size to body mass of about 0.6 percent.

The heart operates two distinct blood flow patterns — pulmonary circulation, which gathers oxygen from the lungs, and systemic circulation, which delivers the oxygen throughout the chicken's body. The left side of the heart is responsible for pumping oxygen-rich blood into the body. The right side of the heart receives the returning oxygen-emptied blood and pumps it into the lung's blood vessels, where it gathers more oxygen. The oxygen-rich blood from the lungs goes back to the left side of the heart to be carried back into the body.

Ascites

Also known as waterbelly or dropsy, ascites is not itself a disease but a sign of heart failure, resulting in an accumulation of fluid in the chicken's body cavity. An excessive amount of fluid causes the abdomen to bloat, which is where the condition gets its name. The word "ascites" (pronounced as-EYE-tease) derives from the Greek word *askos*, meaning "sac," a word used by scientists to denote a cavity enclosed by a membrane and containing, in this case, a liquid.

ASCITIC BROILERS

Although ascites occurs in older laying hens, it is commonly considered to be primarily a problem in fast-growing broilers. Such a broiler — bred for rapid growth and efficient feed conversion — has an especially high rate of metabolism, which requires so much oxygen that its immature heart and lungs can barely provide enough to sustain its body. If the need for oxygen exceeds the abilities of the normally functioning heart and lungs, the heart attempts to supply the body with more oxygen by pumping more than the usual amount of blood into the lungs.

The result is an increase in blood pressure between the heart and lungs. Since this condition is related to the lungs (pulmonary) and involves abnormally high blood pressure (hypertension), it is technically known as pulmonary hypertension syndrome.

Compared to expandable human lungs, a bird's lungs are more rigid, and they can't handle the increased pressure, which makes the heart work even harder to overcome the increased resistance. All that exercise makes the heart muscle enlarge and thicken, until the right heart valve can no longer close, causing blood to back up into the liver. As a result of the increased pressure to the liver, liquid leaks from the liver into the body cavity. This protein-rich liquid, called ascitic fluid, consists of a combination of blood plasma — the colorless fluid part of blood — and lymph fluid. It may be a clear waterlike liquid or yellowish and jellylike.

All that fluid filling the abdomen restricts the abdominal air sacs, causing the bird to pant, even at temperatures too cool to trigger heat stress, and sometimes make gurgling sounds. Because the chicken is not getting enough oxygen, its skin turns bluish, especially around the comb and wattles. Eventually, the heart fails entirely and the bird dies — sometimes suddenly, without showing any signs.

Ascites in broilers may be prevented by slowing their growth rate. One way to slow the growth rate is to reduce the energy and protein levels of the ration. Another way is to limit the amount of total ration fed each day.

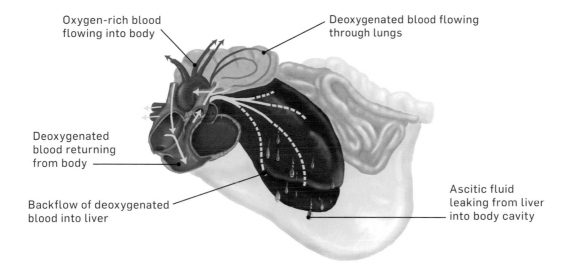

Oxygen-rich blood flowing into body

Deoxygenated blood flowing through lungs

Deoxygenated blood returning from body

Backflow of deoxygenated blood into liver

Ascitic fluid leaking from liver into body cavity

Ascites occurs when a chicken's need for oxygen exceeds the ability of its heart to pump enough blood through its lungs, causing deoxygenated blood to back flow into the liver, where the increased pressure causes ascitic fluid to leak into the body cavity.

ASCITIC LAYERS

Ascites in broilers is known to result from their too-rapid rate of growth, but the causes in laying hens have not been as thoroughly researched. In older chickens, as in older people, heart failure can have many different causes. Either tumors or internal laying can cause breathing difficulty, thus restricting oxygen intake and causing the heart to work harder. Sometimes it's not just one big thing, but an accumulation of lesser things over the years. Factors that can contribute to pulmonary hypertension in layers include these:

- Genetic predisposition

- Obesity, causing clogged arteries

- Excessive stress, which increases oxygen demand

- Poor ventilation, which limits available oxygen

- Ammonia fumes, which irritate the lungs and inhibit oxygen intake

- Respirable dust, which inhibits oxygen intake

- Aspergillosis or other lung condition affecting lung capacity

- Cold or hot temperatures, which increase blood flow through the lungs

- Moldy feed or other toxin causing liver damage

- Infections that cause liver damage

- High-energy feed, which increases the metabolic rate

- Altitudes above 3,000 feet (915 m), where the oxygen level is low

- Salt poisoning due to excessive sodium in feed or drinking water

Avoiding ascites in layers basically involves providing the same wholesome environment that minimizes any unhealthful condition. For today's pampered backyard hens, guarding against obesity is a major step in the right direction.

Sudden Death Syndrome

Sometimes a chicken with pulmonary hypertension dies suddenly before reaching the ascites stage. Such a death is difficult to distinguish from sudden death syndrome (SDS), which is caused by acute heart failure. A distinguishing feature of SDS is that although a dead chicken is occasionally found lying on its side or breast, more often it flips over onto its back with one or both legs raised or extended. A graphic name for this dire condition is "flip-over disease," and chickens that die in this way are "flippers."

SDS is a serious problem in fast-growing industrial broilers, which can die as young as 3 days of age. Large birds, usually cockerels, are the most likely to be affected. Laying hens can also die of acute heart failure, sometimes while laying an egg.

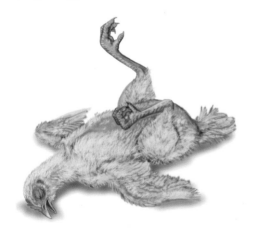

A chick stricken by sudden death syndrome typically dies on its back with one or both legs in the air.

Chickens that die of acute heart failure don't show any sign of illness. The only warning sign is convulsions that occur just moments before death.

The exact cause of sudden death syndrome hasn't been determined. Genetic and environmental factors may be involved, but nutrition is a major contributor. Excessive carbohydrates, along with possible vitamin or mineral deficiencies, are usually involved.

SDS may be avoided in broilers by reducing their rate of growth during their first 3 weeks of life and in layers by ensuring adequate dietary potassium and phosphorus and by preventing obesity. A more likely cause of sudden death in obese backyard laying hens is liver rupture.

Ruptured Liver

The most common noninfectious cause of sudden death in backyard layers is a ruptured liver. The condition is known as fatty liver syndrome, or fatty liver hemorrhagic syndrome, because dead hens often have yellow, mushy, fat-filled livers. However, about half the time the ruptured liver has little or no fat, in which case the condition is more appropriately called hemorrhagic liver syndrome.

Although in nearly all cases the dead hens are extremely fat, the exact reason their livers rupture hasn't been determined. One explanation involves a hormone imbalance: egg laying is influenced by estrogen, which also triggers fat accumulation in the liver. Another explanation — since this condition commonly occurs during the summer, when a hen's need for dietary energy decreases — is that it may be related to a diet that is too high in energy relative to protein. Supplementing a layer's diet with brewer's yeast or fish meal helps prevent this syndrome.

Dysfunctional Kidneys

Instead of excreting urine, a chicken normally expels blood wastes in the form of white, semi-solid urates. A kidney dysfunction can cause urates to be retained by the chicken's body instead of being expelled along with the poop.

The urates may solidify into kidney stones that block the ureters, or they may appear as chalky deposits in soft tissues around the joints or in various organs. Technically called urate deposition, the latter condition is more commonly known as gout.

Chickens are subject to two different forms of gout: articular, from the Latin word *articularis*, meaning "pertaining to joints"; and visceral, from the Latin word *viscera*, meaning "internal organ." Note that neither kidney stones nor gout is a disease but a sign of whatever has caused the kidneys to malfunction.

Articular Gout

Articular gout is likely due to a genetic defect that causes the kidneys to function improperly but may also be triggered by a diet that is too high in protein. It is more common in cocks than in hens, generally doesn't appear in birds until they are at least 4 months old, and usually affects individuals rather than an entire flock.

The usual sign is swollen joints of the feet and toes, resulting in lameness and shifting of the weight from leg to leg to relieve discomfort. Because of the swelling the bird is unable to bend its toes. The feet may redden and blister, and the blisters may develop into sores. Because walking is painful, the bird may spend a lot of time sitting in one place and grooming to the point of pulling out its own feathers. In a severe case the comb and wattles may also become swollen.

Because articular gout is so uncommon, the foot swelling and sores are often mistaken for bumblefoot, described on page 221. The swelling and deformity resulting from articular gout also could be confused with a severe case of scaly leg mite, described on page 129. Unlike bumblefoot and scaly leg, though, articular gout has no cure. But you can take measures to make an affected bird more comfortable.

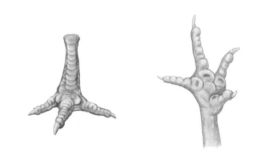

Articular gout always causes swelling of the joints in the feet and toes, which *may* also be a sign of visceral gout. The swelling and deformity (left) may be mistaken for scaly leg mites. Sores developing beneath swollen toe joints (right) may be mistaken for bumblefoot.

TAKING ACTION

Because articular gout is a form of arthritis that makes walking and perching uncomfortable, install wide roosts and keep the bird's toenails clipped to help reduce discomfort. A chicken that doesn't want to walk may need to be encouraged to spend time outdoors in the sunshine and fresh air.

Increased moisture intake helps flush the system, thus increasing the amount of urates expelled and reducing the amount retained in the body. Encourage an affected bird to increase its moisture intake by changing water frequently, by offering cool water in summer and warm water in winter, and by feeding moisture-laden fruit and vegetable treats, such as fresh sprouts, bits of apple, or slices of watermelon. Reducing dietary protein may help keep articular gout from getting worse.

Visceral Gout

Visceral gout is more common than articular gout and affects both hens and cocks. It has many causes, including water deprivation; excess dietary protein; electrolyte excess or deficiency; moldy feed; diseases affecting the kidneys, such as infectious bronchitis and intestinal cryptosporidiosis; excessive exposure to toxic chemicals, including insecticides and disinfectants; overuse of antibiotics, particularly gentamicin and related aminoglycosides, and sulfa drugs; or any combination of these factors. Either tumors or kidney stones can obstruct the ureters, causing urates to accumulate in the kidneys and other organs.

Typical signs of visceral gout include increased thirst, decreased appetite, and emaciation accompanied by lethargy, dull plumage, white pasty droppings, and reduced laying. Swelling of the feet and toes may occasionally occur, in which case visceral gout can be difficult to distinguish from articular gout. However, unlike articular gout, visceral gout eventually progresses into kidney failure and death.

Because it happens so gradually, signs may not become readily apparent until the situation reaches the acute stage and chickens start to die. By that time, ascertaining the original cause can be decidedly difficult. Further, chickens, like humans, tend to naturally lose some kidney function as they age, so combining the natural loss of function with kidney degeneration from other causes can create a critical situation for the older chicken.

TAKING ACTION

As with articular gout, no cure is known for visceral gout. Once a diagnosis has been made, the best treatment is to increase water intake using the same methods described for articular gout.

Kidney Stones

Kidney stones are urates that harden into irregular white stonelike objects that can be large enough to block a ureter. Kidney stones are technically called uroliths — from the Greek words *ouron*, meaning "urine," and *lithos*, meaning "stone" — and the condition of having kidney stones is urolithiasis. This degenerative condition affects primarily laying pullets and hens and may eventually progress into visceral gout.

When kidney stones block a ureter, the associated portion of the kidney atrophies. Unaffected lobes may then enlarge in an attempt to continue normal kidney function.

Causes of kidney stones include water deprivation, insufficient dietary phosphorus, excess dietary calcium (feeding high-calcium layer ration to pullets before they are ready to lay), and excess sodium bicarbonate (prolonged addition of baking soda to drinking water to relieve heat stress). Kidney stones have also been associated with infectious bronchitis and improper vaccination for infectious bronchitis.

Affected birds may become lethargic, emaciated, and dehydrated; develop pale combs; and lay less well. Or they may appear perfectly fine and die of kidney failure without any warning.

Kidney Dysfunctions

	ARTICULAR GOUT	KIDNEY STONES	VISCERAL GOUT
Prevalence	Sporadic	Common	Common
Earliest age	4–5 months	4–5 months	1 day
Gender	Mostly male	Female	Both
Progression	Usually chronic	Chronic	Usually acute, sometimes chronic
Most common sign	Swollen, deformed feet	Lethargy, weight loss	Sudden death
Percent affected	Individual birds	Up to 100%	Up to 100%
Mortality	None	Up to 50%	Up to 100%
Postmortem (see chapter 13, What's Going on Inside)			
Kidneys	Usually normal unless bird was dehydrated	Atrophy of portion blocked by stones, enlargement of unaffected portion	Abnormal size, covered with white, chalky deposits
Other organs involved	Rare	If progressed to visceral gout	Common
Joints involved	Always, especially feet	If progressed to advanced visceral gout	Sometimes
Possible causes	Genetic defect; excess dietary protein; kidney damage	Water deprivation; excess dietary calcium	Kidney failure due to dehydration; toxins; antibiotics; injury; infection; tumors; vitamin A deficiency; kidney stones

TAKING ACTION

Adding vinegar to the drinking water may help prevent kidney stones. Because chickens like the taste of vinegar, it encourages them to drink more and therefore expel more urates rather than retain them in the body. Add vinegar to drinking water at a rate of 1 tablespoon per gallon (15 mL per 4 L); double the dose if your water is alkaline.

A veterinarian may recommend a urine acidifier, such as ammonium chloride (commonly used to prevent urinary stones in male goats) or DL-methionine (a common ingredient in commercially prepared nonorganic poultry feeds). Natural sources of the amino acid methionine include fish meal and oilseed meal, such as safflower, sesame, or sunflower meal.

Kidney Failure

The kidney is subdivided into six lobes. As long as two of the lobes are functional, a hen can survive and continue to lay eggs. Unless at least two lobes remain functional, the kidney can no longer keep up with normal metabolism, and urates flood the bloodstream, resulting in the chicken's death. This condition is technically known as hyperuricemia — from the Greek words *hyper*, meaning "excess"; *ouron*, meaning "urine"; and *hamia*, meaning "blood."

The most common cause of kidney failure is water deprivation, which can affect newly hatched chicks that are held in the incubator too long, are in transit too long when shipped, or are unable to access drinkers in the brooder. In older birds kidney failure from dehydration can occur when drinkers frequently run dry, such as may happen in hot weather, or the chickens don't like the taste of the water and therefore won't drink it.

A common cause of kidney failure in growing birds is being fed a high-calcium layer ration instead of an appropriate chick starter or grower. Identifying water deprivation or excessive calcium as the cause of kidney failure is not difficult, and neither is preventing kidney failure resulting from either of these causes. However, in older chickens, if visceral gout progresses into kidney failure, determining the original cause may be impossible.

The Calcium Connection

To encase an egg in shell, a hen's shell gland draws calcium from her blood. This withdrawal of calcium sets off a chain reaction: the medullary bone releases calcium into the bloodstream, the kidneys conserve calcium by excreting less of it, the intestines absorb more calcium from digesting matter, and the ovaries release a spurt of estrogen, which signals the body to create more medullary bone.

Causes of Low Calcium

The rapid cycling of calcium through the hen's body mobilizes ready calcium for eggshells, but any disruption in her body's response to the initial decrease in blood calcium is potentially life-threatening. The condition of low blood calcium is called hypocalcemia, from the Greek words *hypo*, meaning "under," and *khalix*, meaning "small pebble" (from which we get the word "calcium").

The results of hypocalcemia are muscle weakness, paralysis, and death. Since calcium is needed for muscle contractions, weakened uterine muscles that can't contract and push the egg out result in an egg-bound hen. (For more on egg binding, see Egg Binding, page 92.) Chronic low blood calcium can lead to brittle bones that easily fracture (osteoporosis), especially in older hens. Possible causes of hypocalcemia include these:

- **An electrolyte imbalance.** The body's electrolyte balance is maintained by both the intestinal tract, which is responsible for absorption of calcium into the body and excretion of dietary excess, and the kidneys, which are responsible for calcium retention and excretion of metabolized excess. Any condition or disease affecting either the intestines or the kidneys can interfere with electrolyte balance, as can the hen's diet. A dietary imbalance between calcium and phosphorus, for example, can interfere with the metabolism of calcium. (For more on electrolytes, see Electrolytes on page 385.)

- **Alkalosis.** An increase in blood pH, or alkalosis, occurs when blood calcium changes from an active (ionized) form to an inactive (protein-bound) form and therefore becomes unavailable. Alkalosis can be caused by an electrolyte imbalance, a metabolic disturbance, or heat stress. Low levels of the electrolyte chloride, for instance, affect the body's acid-base balance, increasing blood pH. Due to a metabolic malfunction, the kidneys may retain sodium, which causes a rise in blood pH. Panting as a result of heat stress increases the release of carbon dioxide through respiration, which causes a loss of bicarbonate from the blood, increasing the blood's pH.

- **Reduced calcium absorption.** Calcium in the bloodstream is absorbed by the intestines from digesting food. The faster digesting matter moves through the intestines, the less time the intestines have to absorb calcium. Feed moves more quickly through the intestines if it is highly fluid (moistened mash, for instance, compared to dry pellets), the chicken drinks a lot of water (such as during hot weather), or the chicken has a condition causing diarrhea. Intestines that have been damaged by a previous illness, such as a bout with coccidiosis, are also less absorptive.

- **Calcium supplement particle size.** The larger the particle size of the calcium supplement, the longer it takes to move through the digestive system, and the more of it will be absorbed. Oyster shell or limestone granules remain in the gizzard longer than the more powdery calcium supplements and therefore release more calcium into the bloodstream.

Classically, hypocalcemia affects pullets that are just starting to lay, but it can occur in a hen of any age, particularly during hot weather. Since most eggs are laid early in the day, signs of hypocalcemia most commonly appear in the morning. Often a hen dies in the nest while trying to lay an egg.

A hen that is experiencing muscle weakness because of low blood calcium is less able to get away from amorous roosters and therefore may lose a lot of back feathers to treading. However, loss of back feathers is not necessarily a sign of hypocalcemia; the lower a hen is in the peck order, the more readily she will submit to mating and the more likely she is to have feathers rubbed off her back, regardless of her state of health.

Preventing Low Calcium

Hypocalcemia is easily prevented with good pullet and hen management. For starters, don't feed layer ration to pullets until they are ready to start laying and their bodies have matured enough to mobilize calcium. Feeding excess calcium too soon can damage the kidneys, making them less efficient at metabolizing calcium. When in doubt, wait until your pullets lay their first eggs before starting the gradual switch to layer ration.

After pullets start laying, offer a large-particle calcium supplement in the form of oyster shell or limestone granules. Compared to powdery supplements, a large particle size acts as a time-release calcium tablet, extending the period of calcium absorption, minimizing the loss of medullary bone, ensuring replacement of depleted medullary bone, and overall improving shell quality.

Avoid heat stress in layers of all ages. Make sure they have access to good airflow and plenty of fresh drinking water to help them better cope with changes in blood pH.

An additional measure that helps control blood pH during hot weather and other times of stress is to add ¼ cup of sodium bicarbonate (common baking soda) to each gallon of drinking water. It will restore lost blood bicarbonate and help hens maintain their natural buffering system. Alternatively, a complete water-soluble electrolyte supplement that includes both sodium and bicarbonate, as well as chloride and potassium, will help hens maintain their electrolyte balance.

Pasting

Pasting — also known as pasty butt, paste up, or sticky bottoms — is a common condition in newly hatched chicks. Soft droppings that stick to the vent harden and seal the vent shut, eventually leading to death.

Although pasting may be caused by disease — typically in chicks older than 1 week — during a chick's first week of life it is more likely to be caused by chilling, overheating, or improper feed. If only one or a few chicks in the brood paste up, they were likely chilled or otherwise stressed. If most of the chicks are pasting up, the issue likely relates to something they are eating or drinking.

Shipped chicks that get chilled in transit may paste, as may dehydrated chicks that get too-cold water as their first drink. Pasting is less apt to occur if the first drink is brooder temperature and the chicks are drinking well before they start eating.

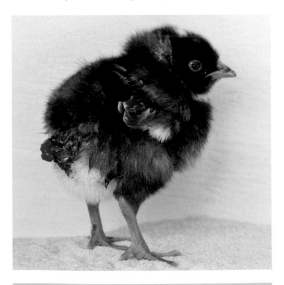

Sticky droppings clinging to a chick's vent eventually dry up, sealing the vent shut unless cleaned off.

Pasting can occur if too much sugar is added to the first water as an energy booster. Some types of feedstuffs, particularly soybeans, can also trigger pasting.

TAKING ACTION

Where the problem is ration related, it usually can be alleviated by feeding only chick scratch, or starter combined with chick scratch, for the first day or two, while the chicks are still deriving nutrients from residual yolk. If your farm store doesn't carry chick scratch, run regular chicken scratch through the blender, or crush uncooked oatmeal and combine it with an equal amount of cornmeal, or feed the chicks mashed scrambled egg. A better solution is to change to a higher-quality starter ration.

Meanwhile, poop clinging to a chick's vent must be cleaned off before it hardens and plugs up the works. Run a light stream of warm tap water over the chick's bottom, then take your time gently picking off the mess with your fingers, being careful not to rip out down or tear tender skin.

Depending on how thick and hardened the poop is, you may have to repeatedly pick off a little at a time, then apply more warm water. When all the droppings have been cleaned off, dry the chick's bottom by gently dabbing it with a paper towel. Apply a little hydrogen wound ointment or petroleum jelly (Vaseline) to protect the affected area and prevent fresh poop from sticking.

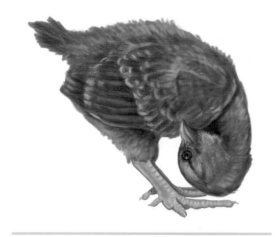

A sign of crazy chick disease is a downward bending of the neck with the head between the legs.

Crazy Chick Disease

A rare condition caused by vitamin E deficiency, crazy chick disease is technically known as encephalomalacia, from the Greek words *enkephalos,* meaning "brain," and *malakos,* meaning "soft." Encephalomalacia is a softening of the brain tissue that, if not treated early, results in permanent brain damage.

Although the primary cause of this disease is a deficiency in vitamin E, the vitamin may actually be present in the diet but unavailable for metabolism. For instance, when vitamin E is furnished in the form of polyunsaturated fats — such as cod liver oil, corn oil, soybean oil, or wheat germ oil— that have become rancid, the vitamin oxidizes and is no longer available for absorption. Since vitamin E's powerful antioxidant property is responsible for preventing crazy chick disease, the condition is even more likely to occur if the ration is also low or deficient in other antioxidants (see Antioxidants and Free Radicals, page 57).

Eggs laid by vitamin E–deficient hens don't hatch well, and chicks that do hatch show signs of crazy chick disease within their first week of life. Chicks that develop this condition because their starter ration lacks sufficient metabolizable vitamin E show signs within 2 weeks of being fed a deficient diet.

Vitamin E–deficient hens do not exhibit any visible signs, but in chicks the signs are pretty dramatic. The first sign is usually muscle weakness and loss of coordination. A classic indication is a downward bending of the neck with the head between the legs, sometimes with the head turned or twisted to one side. This position puts the chick so far out of balance that if it tries to walk it tumbles over. Eventually the brain deteriorates to the extent that the chick can no longer function, whereupon it lies down and dies.

TAKING ACTION

If treated early enough to prevent serious damage to the brain, hefty doses of vitamin E can reverse the condition. Vitamin E is not particularly toxic for chickens, making overdose highly unlikely.

Foot and Leg Deformities in Chicks

Common deformities in chicks involve their legs and feet. While such deformities can be metabolic, they are more often caused by injury. Since metabolic deformities tend to be confused with environmental injuries, both types of deformity are discussed here to help you distinguish between them.

Slipped Tendon

Slipped tendon is a metabolic condition in which the legs' long bones are shorter than normal, the hock joint becomes swollen and flattened, the hock rotates, and the leg can no longer support the bird's weight. As the condition progresses, the Achilles tendon slips away from the back of the joint, causing the foot and shank to extend diagonally toward the back. When both legs are affected, the bird can't stand up and eventually dies for lack of food and water.

An old term for slipped tendon is perosis, from the Greek words *peros*, meaning "deformity," and *osis*, meaning "condition." The word "perosis" is still more often used than the current term, which is a mouthful — chondrodystrophy, from the Greek words *chondros*, meaning "cartilage," *dys*, meaning "bad," and *trophe*, meaning "nourishment."

The cause of slipped tendon, as you might guess, is a nutritional deficiency. It can result from a lack of any one of several different nutrients. At one time manganese deficiency was blamed, but today the finger more often points to inadequate vitamin B_7 (biotin) or other B vitamins, as well as the vitamin choline, any of which is more likely than manganese to be inadequate in starter ration.

Slipped tendon usually appears in chicks that are less than 6 weeks old. Chickens with mature bones do not develop this deformity, but hens suffering from the same nutritional deficiencies lay fewer eggs, with thin shells that break easily, and if the eggs are incubated, they don't hatch well. Developing embryos from such eggs usually die late in incubation with short, thick legs, short wings, and parrot beaks. The few chicks that do hatch have short legs and develop the same deformity as would an otherwise healthy chick on a deficient diet.

TAKING ACTION

Prevention starts by adequately feeding breeders prior to collecting their eggs for hatching. Once the chicks hatch, add a vitamin/mineral supplement containing manganese, choline, vitamin B_7 (biotin), and other B vitamins to their drinking water, and feed them a balanced starter diet.

Slipped Tendon versus Splayed Leg

Slipped tendon looks similar to splayed leg in chicks, except slipped tendon typically involves one leg extended diagonally backward and doesn't appear in newly hatched chicks; splayed leg is much more common, usually involves both legs that extend to the sides, and appears

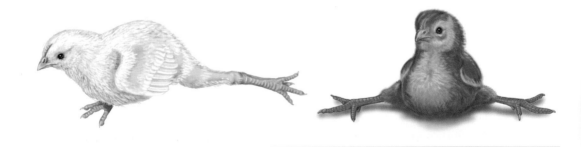

Slipped tendon (left) is a relatively uncommon deformity resulting from a nutritionally inadequate breeder flock ration or starter ration. Splayed leg (right) is a common injury experienced by newly hatched chicks when their feet slide on slick flooring. Note the differences between these two leg positions and that of Marek's disease on page 263.

at or shortly after hatch. Splayed leg is an injury that can occur during incubation, during the hatch, or after hatch. It may be caused by a too-high incubation or hatching temperature, which affects the development of bones, muscles, and tendons and results in legs that are not strong enough for the hatchling to stand on. Lack of sufficient strength may also be the result of an inadequate breeder-flock diet.

A common cause of splayed leg during or shortly after the hatch is footing that's too smooth to provide good traction, so the chicks' legs slide out to the side. As a result, the leg muscles don't get sufficient exercise to develop properly; the bird can't walk; and, if the condition is not corrected, the chick will die. Lining a smooth-bottom hatcher or brooder floor with paper toweling or rubber shelf liner helps keep little legs from splaying.

Curled-Toe Paralysis

Curled toe paralysis in chicks is a metabolic condition caused by a deficiency of vitamin B_2 (riboflavin), which is needed for proper functioning of the nerves. Deficiency leads to degeneration of the sciatic nerve, which runs down the back of the leg to the foot. As a result, the toes curl under, giving the foot the appearance of a fist. Since the chick can't walk on its feet, it attempts to move around on its hocks. While some affected chicks survive, others become so deformed they can't get around to eat and drink and eventually starve to death.

Riboflavin deficiency in hatching eggs may occur when the breeder diet consists solely of layer ration without vitamin supplementation or access to green forage. The hens lay fewer eggs that don't hatch well, if at all. Chicks that do hatch have clubbed down, a condition in which

the sheaths surrounding the down fail to rupture, which bends each bit of fluff so it bulges at the shaft base. The combination of clubbed down and curled toes in chicks is a clear sign of riboflavin deficiency in the breeder flock diet.

Because riboflavin-deficient eggs tend not to hatch, this deficiency is more likely to result from a poor-grade starter ration, in which case the condition appears around 2 weeks after the hatch. The chicks' growth rate slows; the chicks become thin and weak even though they eat well; and after about a week they may develop diarrhea.

As the chicks get weaker and their toes curl into their feet, they become increasingly more reluctant to move. When they do move, they tend to use drooping wings to help with locomotion. Eventually the legs atrophy and one or both may extend out from underneath the chick's body. Unless treated early with a correct diet or a water-soluble vitamin supplement, an affected chick will die from starvation.

Curled Toes versus Crooked Toes

Curled-toe paralysis is sometimes confused with crooked toes, in which a chick's toes bend to the side rather than curling under the foot. Crooked toes appear at an earlier age than curled toes and may occur because of inappropriate conditions during incubation, during the hatch, or after the hatch. They may result from high temperature early in incubation, low temperature throughout incubation or during the hatch, or excessive activity too soon after hatching. Brooder conditions associated with crooked toes are overcrowding and a too-smooth floor. Other potential causes include nutritional deficiency, injury, and heredity.

If treated early, crooked toes may be corrected with splints. Crooked toes don't affect

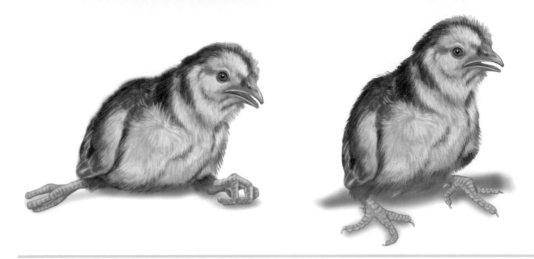

In curled-toe paralysis (left), which appears in chicks around 2 weeks of age, the toes curl under the foot and the chick can't walk. Crooked toes (right) that curve to one side are much more common, appear at or shortly after hatch, and don't affect the chick's ability to get around.

a chicken's ability to get around and therefore are mainly cosmetic. However, if you can't determine the cause, don't include birds with crooked toes in your breeder flock; if the condition is genetic, you will have more crooked-toe chicks in future generations.

Green Muscle Disease

A disorder that affects heavy-breasted broilers — cockerels more often than pullets — green muscle disease is not evident until the broiler is slaughtered and its tenders are found to be discolored, which can be disconcerting for anyone who raises chickens to put meat on the table. The tender is the part of the breast, or pectoral, muscle that lies deep within the breast, closest to the breastbone. When the breast is removed from the bone, the tender is the strip that has a tendon running through it and that readily separates from the main part of the breast. Because the tender is the inner, or deep, pectoral muscle, green muscle disease is technically known as deep pectoral myopathy.

This condition is a direct result of industrial-strength broilers having been bred for excessively large breast muscles, which can be as much as 25 percent of a bird's total body weight. Further, heavy broilers do little more than sit around eating, so their muscles don't get enough exercise to allow for a well-developed system of blood flow.

The deep pectoral is the muscle used to raise the wing. It is surrounded by a tough, inflexible sheath. When a broiler flaps its wings, blood flow increases to the muscle, causing the muscle to expand until it becomes restricted by the sheath, at which point the blood flow stops. If the wing flapping continues, the muscle is deprived of oxygen. As a result, the tenders bruise, atrophy, and die. They may look bloody or yellowish or be an unappetizing green color, depending on how long before the broiler was slaughtered the incidence of wing flapping occurred.

Green muscle disease is more likely to affect broilers that are raised to heavier weights, such as for roasting, and broilers raised in cooler weather, since they grow faster than those raised in the warmer months. It also can be a bigger issue for pastured broilers than confined broilers, because chickens kept outdoors are subject to a greater variety of scary experiences — such as prowling predators, large birds flying overhead, or sudden loud noises from passing vehicles.

Since green muscle disease produces no outwardly visible signs, no treatment is possible. Prevention involves taking measures to ensure heavy-breast broilers are not startled into excessive wing flapping. Keep small children and household pets from chasing broilers. Do not catch or carry them by their wings or legs. Do not provide perches, from which they would fly down while flapping their wings.

Lactose Intolerance

Chickens raised on homesteads and family dairy farms have long enjoyed the benefits of surplus milk as a source of calcium and animal protein, yet today we frequently see warnings that chickens are lactose intolerant and therefore should never be given milk or milk products. What's the deal?

Lactose, otherwise known as milk sugar, is a type of sugar found only in dairy products. Lactose is a disaccharide — from the Greek *di*, meaning "two," and the Latin *saccharum*, meaning "sugar." For lactose to be digested, it must be broken down into its two constituent simple sugars, or monosaccharides (*mono* being Greek for "single"). The two readily digestible single sugars are glucose (from the Greek *glukus*, meaning "sweet") and galactose (from the Greek *galakt*, meaning "milk").

Lactose and Lactase

Baby mammals, including humans, are born with the enzyme lactase, which breaks down the lactose in mother's milk so it can be digested as glucose and galactose. As some mammals mature and move on to other foods besides milk, their bodies produce fewer lactase enzymes, and they become less able to digest milk. The result is a genetically determined condition known as either lactase deficiency or lactose intolerance. One of the signs of lactose intolerance is diarrhea.

Chickens, of course, are not mammals, and in their natural environment they would not normally encounter mammalian milk or products derived from it. Oddly, however, their bodies still produce some lactase. So technically they are not entirely lactose intolerant — defined as an inability to fully digest lactose — since they can tolerate small amounts.

Some dairy products are naturally low in lactose. Cottage cheese, for instance, is particularly low in lactose. And some of the lactose in a live-culture dairy product such as yogurt gets predigested by the culturing microbes. At the opposite extreme, dried dairy products such as milk powder and buttermilk powder are high in lactose.

TAKING ACTION

If you feed milk to your chickens, avoid the temptation to include Lactaid or any similar product to overcome their lactase deficiency. Such products work by breaking down lactose into glucose and galactose, and a large amount of galactose is toxic to chickens. Giving your chickens a lactase substitute so you can increase the amount of dairy products you feed them is therefore a bad idea. On the other hand, if you drink lactose-free milk and want to share it with your chickens, that's okay. A little galactose can actually be beneficial.

Researchers at the University of Illinois found that feeding galactose to broilers at the rate of 2 to 4 percent of their total diet improved their growth rate, while feeding galactose at the rate of 10 percent or more resulted in deaths. From the table below you know that fluid milk is approximately 5 percent lactose. Figuring half of that is galactose, and assuming all of it is digested (which is unlikely), a broiler that eats or drinks nothing but milk would have a diet consisting of 2.5 percent galactose — well within the safe and beneficial range.

However, a diet consisting solely of milk will not provide chickens with complete nutrition, and anything you add to improve the nutritional profile reduces the overall percentage of lactose and therefore galactose. So feeding fluid milk to chickens is a pretty safe bet.

Percentage of Lactose in Dairy Products
(approximate)

DAIRY PRODUCT	LACTOSE
Milk, fluid	5%
Milk powder, whole	38%
Milk powder, nonfat	51%
Yogurt, kefir	4%
Sour cream	4%
Buttermilk	4%
Buttermilk powder	48%
Whey (liquid)	5%
Cottage cheese	0.4%
Cottage cheese (2% fat)	3.6%
Cottage cheese (1% fat)	2.7%

Benefits of Milk

Milk is 87 percent water. The remainder is loaded with protein, carbohydrate, fat, vitamins, and minerals. When fermented into live-culture yogurt, milk makes a good probiotic for chickens, as described on page 379. Because too much lactose causes diarrhea, some farmers use milk powder as a flush, described on page 392.

As for routinely feeding surplus milk to chickens, one rule of thumb is to feed hens no more than 10 pounds (5 quarts) of milk per 50 pounds of ration they consume. A routine practiced by old-time farmers — which works well and doesn't require weighing or calculating — is to fill drinkers with milk instead of water for half the day, then clean them and fill them with plain fresh water the other half day.

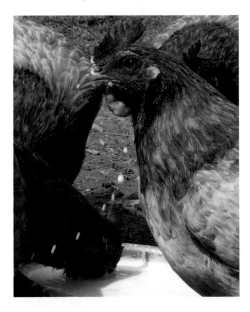

Chickens love milk and can benefit from its animal protein and other nutrients.

CHAPTER 5

What's Bugging Your Birds

A PARASITE IS A LIVING organism that invades the body of another living organism, relying on its host for survival without providing benefit in return, and in fact sometimes causing harm. Any living thing that invades a chicken's body and produces an infection is, by definition, a parasite. Compared to bacteria and viruses, however, the organisms commonly called parasites may be seen without a microscope.

Parasites are divided into two groups: internal parasites that invade the internal organs — including worms and protozoa, discussed in the next two chapters — and external parasites, which generally stay on the outside of a chicken's body.

External parasites, in turn, are divided into two groups: insects (bugs, fleas, flies, lice) and mites (chiggers, mites, ticks). Most external parasites produce similar results: weight loss or slow growth, reduced egg production, and aesthetic damage to show birds and meat birds. A serious infestation may cause death, particularly to a young chicken. Some parasites carry diseases from one bird to another. A show bird with external parasites will likely be disqualified and required to be removed from the showroom.

Mites and Ticks

Mites are by far the most common external parasite of chickens. They are spiderlike creatures with single-segmented bodies, exterior skeletons, and four pairs of jointed legs.

Mites are quite small, usually under $\frac{1}{25}$ inch (1 mm) in length; some are microscopic. All have mouths designed for piercing or chewing. Depending on the species, they live on blood, tissue cells, or feathers.

Some mites spend a lot of time off the bird and are spread by contaminated equipment, shoes, or clothing. They are also spread by infested birds, including wild ones.

Other mites remain on a chicken's body at all times. They may live on the skin, hide in feather parts, burrow under the skin, or make their way deep within the body to live in the lungs, liver, or other organs. Mite infestation (technically called acariasis) causes irritation, low energy, feather damage, and increased appetite accompanied by low egg production, reduced fertility, retarded growth in young birds, and sometimes anemia and death.

Red Mites

Also called chicken mite, poultry mite, or roost mite, the red mite (*Dermanyssus gallinae*) is the most common mite found in warm climates. It is a bigger problem in summer than in winter, becoming inactive when the temperature drops.

Red mites are so small they can barely be seen without magnification. They are gray until they get a blood meal and turn red. They live and lay their eggs in cracks near roosts or nests, crawling onto chickens to feed at night. They survive for a month off chickens, so housing may remain infested long after chickens have been removed.

Mites and Ticks That Affect Chickens

COMMON NAME	SPECIES	WHERE FOUND	SEASON	LIFE CYCLE	SURVIVAL OFF CHICKENS
Red mite, chicken mite, poultry mite, roost mite	*Dermanyssus gallinae**	At night on birds; during day in nests and cracks	Summer	7–10 days	1 month
Northern fowl mite	*Ornithonyssus sylviarum**	On vent, tail, back, and neck	Cooler seasons (northern states)	7–14 days	3–4 weeks
Tropical fowl mite, bird mite, starling mite	*Ornithonyssus bursa*	Fluffy vent feathers	Spring and early summer (southern states)	7 days	10 days
Scaly leg mite, scaly face mite	*Knemidocoptes mutans**	On unfeathered shanks (sometimes face)	Year-round	10–14 days	4–6 weeks
Depluming mite, itch mite	*Knemidocoptes gallinae*	Feather follicles on back, wings, breast, thighs, vent	Spring and summer	10 14 days	Limited
Air-sac mite	*Cytodites nudus*	In respiratory system	Year-round	Unknown	Unknown
Chigger mite, berry bug, harvest mite, jigger, red bug	*Trombicula* spp.	Vent, thighs, breast, underside of wings	Late spring through fall (South, Southeast, Midwest)	50–55 days	1 year (larva feed on chickens once for up to 2 weeks)
Fowl tick, argas tick, blue bug	*Argas* spp.*	Under wings at night; during day in wood litter, cracks	Warm, dry weather	1 month	1 year
Lone star tick	*Amblyomma americanum*	Head area	Spring and summer (eastern states)	1–3 years	14 months
Gulf Coast tick	*Amblyomma maculatum*	Neck area	Winter in warm climate; late spring and summer in cool climate (southern states)	Unknown	Unknown

Most common

The red mite completes its life cycle in 7 to 10 days, and one female lays as many as 120,000 eggs, resulting in a rapid population increase in hot weather. In a heavy infestation some mites may stay on birds during the day and can cause a drop in laying, as well as causing the death of chicks and setting hens. In a particularly severe infestation, red mites invade the roof of a bird's mouth, causing serious anemia. Red mites, when abundant, will also attack humans.

TAKING ACTION

Check birds at night, when red mites are on the prowl. Look for tiny specks crawling on the roost or on the birds themselves. Since red mites leave the chicken during the day, they may be controlled solely by cleaning up the coop — no need to treat individual birds. Clean facilities thoroughly (especially remove all bedding, which may be infested) and apply a pesticide approved for poultry (see Parasite Control, page 146), with particular attention to all cracks and crevices. Treat again in 5 to 7 days.

REPEAT TREATMENT

Few methods of pest control destroy unhatched parasite eggs. To avoid a reinfestation by freshly hatched parasites, coordinate repeat treatments with the life cycle of the parasites involved.

Fowl Mites

The northern fowl mite (*Ornithonyssus sylviarum*) is the most serious external parasite of chickens and the most common one found in cooler climates. Female mites lay their eggs on a chicken's feathers. Young mites hatch and develop without leaving the chicken, completing their entire life cycle in approximately 7 to 14 days, so an infestation rapidly gets worse.

In contrast to red mites, northern fowl mites increase more rapidly in cool weather. This mite differs from the red mite in another way: it survives no more than 2 to 3 weeks off the bird. It feeds on blood and lives its entire life on the bird and therefore does more damage than the red mite.

The irritation causes chickens to scratch, and loss of blood can cause anemia, with a resulting drop in laying among hens and reduced fertility in cocks. Other evidence that northern fowl mites are present includes mites crawling on eggs in nests and large numbers of mites on the skin of birds — especially around the vent, tail, back, and legs — during the day. These dark red to black mites are so tiny they may be hard to see without a magnifying glass, so look for darkened vent feathers and blackened, scabby skin, especially around the vent. Wounds caused by mites around the vent can result in eggs being streaked with blood.

Northern fowl mites move quickly and will crawl up your arms when you handle your chickens. Control involves treating individual birds as described under Parasite Control, page 146. Repeat treatment in 5 to 7 days.

The tropical fowl mite (*Ornithonyssus bursa*) resembles the northern fowl mite but is more common in the warm southern states. In contrast to the northern fowl mite, the tropical mite may lay its eggs in nests as well as on chickens, where it prefers soft, downy feathers surrounding the vent. Also called bird mite or starling mite, it is spread by starlings and other wild birds nesting in the eaves of a chicken coop. When the wild birds leave the nest, the mites move into the coop. If they can't find a bird to bite, these mites will happily feed on people. Control involves treating nests as well as individual birds.

Leg Mites

A tiny pale, gray, round creature, the scaly leg mite (*Knemidocoptes mutans*) is only about $\frac{1}{100}$ inch (0.25 mm) in diameter. It is more likely to attack older birds but also affects young birds kept with old birds. It burrows under the scales on a chicken's shanks and feet, raising the scales by generating debris that accumulates beneath them. As a result, the shanks thicken and crust over and eventually become deformed.

TAKING ACTION

Scaly leg mites spread slowly by traveling from bird to bird along the roost. Their spread therefore may be controlled by brushing perches once a month with a mixture of one part kerosene to two parts linseed oil (not motor oil), or twice a month with an old-time natural poultry product called VetRx Veterinary Remedy, which has a corn oil base.

Once scaly leg mites settle in, they burrow deeply under the leg scales and spend their entire lives on the chicken, so you'll have a hard time getting rid of them. Every poultry keeper, it seems, has a favorite method. One such method is to use the drug ivermectin, as described on page 157.

Other methods involve physically smothering the mites by dipping affected legs in vegetable oil, linseed oil, or VetRx. In a pot or can 5 to 6 inches (13 to 15 cm) deep, place about 4 inches (10 cm) of vegetable oil. Dip each affected leg until it is well coated with oil up to the feathered part; repeat every 3 days for a mild infection, daily for a severe infestation. Continue until the old scales pop off and the shanks appear normal, indicating the legs are completely free of mites, although don't expect severely damaged scales to return to normal.

Less messy than using drippy oil is liberally coating the shanks and feet with petroleum jelly (brand name Vaseline), which stays on longer than oil and therefore needs to be repeated only about once a week. No matter which method you prefer, the easiest way to handle individual chickens is to pick each chicken off the roost at night and treat them.

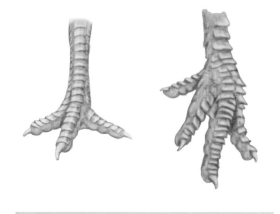

Scaly leg mites burrow under the scales on a chicken's shanks and feet (left). If left untreated (right), accumulating debris causes the legs to thicken and crust over, eventually crippling the bird.

Feather Mites

Feather mites live on and eat plumage, ruining feathers by chewing stripes across them or by damaging the feather base. In North America the most common feather mite is the depluming mite (*Knemidocoptes gallinae*), which is related to and resembles the scaly leg mite but is even tinier and barely visible to the naked eye.

The depluming mite is especially active in warm weather, burrowing into the skin at the base of feathers and causing the chicken to try to reduce the irritation by scratching and pulling at feathers. A sign of infestation is numerous broken or missing feathers, or the appearance of molting out of season. Broken skin where feathers have been pulled out can lead to infection or cannibalism. Depluming mites are controlled by the same methods as fowl mites.

Respiratory Mites

The air-sac mite (*Cytodites nudus*) invades a chicken's respiratory system (and sometimes other internal organs), where it seems to do little damage unless it becomes abundant, usually in older chickens. The result of a severe infestation is pneumonia.

Signs are similar to those of any serious respiratory disease: gasping, sneezing, coughing, head shaking, and lethargy. If a chicken can't get sufficient oxygen, its comb turns dark blue, and death soon follows.

No one knows how common these mites are, and little is known about their life cycle. What is known is that, unlike other mites — which lay eggs — female air-sac mites give birth to larvae that spend their entire lives in the windpipe, air sacs, lungs, and bone cavities of chickens and other birds.

The only way to diagnose the presence of air-sac mites is through a postmortem examination (as described in chapter 13). Look for tiny (0.4 by 0.5 mm) slow-moving white dots inside the air sacs and other respiratory organs. If one bird in a flock has air-sac mites, it's a pretty good bet others do, too, since these mites easily spread from bird to bird in respiratory mucus coughed up or sneezed by infected chickens.

No effective treatment has been discovered, other than culling affected birds. One of the few possible treatments, ivermectin, apparently requires a large enough dose to be toxic to chickens as well as to the mites.

Chigger Mites

The larvae of chigger mites (*Trombicula* spp.) — also called berry bugs, harvest mites, jiggers, or red bugs — leave welts on the skin of birds, humans, and other animals. Chiggers are prevalent primarily in hot and humid areas of the South, Southeast, and Midwest. In the southernmost states they go through four generations per year; farther north, they go through only two or three generations.

Mature chiggers feed on plants or small insects, including mosquito eggs. They are about ⅕ inch (1 mm) long, bright red, and hairy — giving them a velvety appearance. The body has somewhat of a figure-eight shape but is larger at the back than at the front. Females produce up to 400 eggs, laying them in clusters when the spring soil temperature reaches 60°F (16°C).

The larvae may be yellowish, pinkish, or bright red and are about ¹⁄₁₅₀ inch (0.18 mm) long — so small they can barely be seen without magnification. They are a little less hairy than adults and have three pairs of legs instead of the usual four of mature chiggers and other mites.

Chigger larvae remain close to where they hatch, climbing up grass stems and the tips of weeds to await a suitable host on which to feed. They are most active on warm afternoons, becoming inactive when soil temperatures are below 60°F (16°C) or above 99°F (37°C).

They prefer birds to humans and are fond of attacking where the skin is thinnest around a chicken's vent and on the thighs, breast, and underside of wings. A chigger pierces the skin with its mouth and injects an enzyme that liquefies the skin. The surrounding tissue hardens to create a feeding tube through which the chigger continues to gorge for up to 2 weeks. The longer the chigger feeds on its once-in-a-lifetime meal of liquefied skin, the deeper the tube penetrates into the skin until the chigger drops off.

Meanwhile the bite gets red and swollen, and the resulting scab itches intensely for days. Chickens scratching chigger scabs can develop a bacterial skin infection. Heavily infested young birds become lethargic, lose interest in eating and drinking, and may die.

TAKING ACTION

Chiggers tend to congregate in transition areas between pasture and woodland, posing a problem for free-range chickens. Keeping such areas mowed or keeping chickens away from these areas during chigger season helps prevent infestation. Dusting or spraying with sulfur repels chiggers from hot spots near the coop.

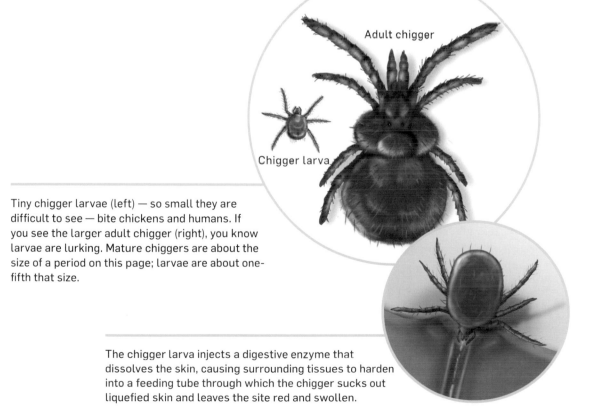

Adult chigger

Chigger larva

Tiny chigger larvae (left) — so small they are difficult to see — bite chickens and humans. If you see the larger adult chigger (right), you know larvae are lurking. Mature chiggers are about the size of a period on this page; larvae are about one-fifth that size.

The chigger larva injects a digestive enzyme that dissolves the skin, causing surrounding tissues to harden into a feeding tube through which the chigger sucks out liquefied skin and leaves the site red and swollen.

Individual chickens may be treated by bathing them in warm water with a mild dish soap (such as Ivory liquid) or flea and tick shampoo for household pets. Itching may be relieved by adding a generous amount of Epsom salt to the wash water.

Ticks

Ticks are nothing more than big mites. They are divided into three families, one of which is found only in southern Africa. The remaining two are Argasidae, or soft ticks, and Ixodidae, or hard ticks.

Of the several species of soft ticks, *Argas persicus* is the most prevalent in the United States and the most likely to attach to chickens. Two kinds of hard ticks affect chickens in North America — the lone star tick and the Gulf Coast tick.

FOWL TICK

The soft tick *Argas persicus* is variously known as the adobe tick, argas tick, blue bug, chicken tick, or fowl tick. It likes warm climates and therefore is found primarily throughout the southern and southwestern states.

Fowl ticks are oval, leathery, flattish, and up to ⅓ inch (8.5 mm) long. They feed only on blood and can survive a year or more between feedings. They are tan or reddish brown until they feed; then they turn bluish.

A female tick lays as many as seven batches of eggs containing up to 500 eggs each. She deposits her eggs under tree bark and in cracks and crevices in coop walls. In warm weather the eggs hatch in about 10 days; in cool weather they take up to 3 months. Tick larvae search until they find a host, attach themselves, and feed for about a week. They leave the bird to molt, then return for another blood meal, repeating the procedure until they reach maturity, which can take as long as 11 years.

Ticks are particularly active during dry, warm weather. They hide during the day and come out at night to feed. Feeding takes 15 to 30 minutes and leaves red spots on the bird's skin, typically under the wings. Chickens that anticipate being bitten grow restless at roosting time.

Other signs of infestation are ruffled feathers, paleness, weakness, depressed appetite, weight loss, and a drop in laying. Bite wounds may become infected with bacteria. In a growing or mature hen, toxins released from the ticks' saliva can cause transient paralysis that is sometimes mistaken for botulism or Marek's disease. Soft ticks also spread a number of diseases, including spirochetosis, also known as tick fever (described on page 238). A large infestation of ticks causes anemia, emaciation, and (rarely) death.

LONE STAR TICK

The lone star tick (*Amblyomma americanum*) occurs in the eastern part of the United States as far west as Texas and as far north as Maine. It is found in densely wooded and brushy areas and attaches to chickens foraging on the forest floor.

This tick gets its common name not from the state of Texas but from the single white spot on the female's back. The male tick has several small white spots on the lower part of its back, which sometimes join to create the appearance of a pair of horseshoes. The markings on both genders stand out against the chestnut-brown color of the tick's roundish body.

The adult male lone star tick dies soon after mating with one or more females. The female dies soon after laying thousands of eggs in forest-floor litter. The eggs take about 32 days to hatch into straw-colored six-legged larva, or seed ticks, that crawl around in bunches looking for their first meal. This swarming activity makes them more visible than would be a single tiny seed tick, which is only about the size of a poppy seed. After a blood meal the seed tick molts and develops into an eight-legged tan nymph, which is smaller than an adult tick and lacks the distinctive markings.

The life cycle of the lone star tick takes 1 to 3 years, during which it feeds three times on three different hosts. Seed ticks and nymphs are the most likely stage to feed on chickens. Depending on the climate, seed ticks tend to be most active from June through August, while nymphs are active in spring (March through May) and again in late summer (July and August).

Free-range chickens scratching and pecking in woodland debris can pick up a lone star tick, which becomes highly visible if it attaches on the head or a wattle. The lone star tick has longer mouthparts than most other ticks and raises an awful-looking lump that does not necessarily indicate a serious infection.

GULF COAST TICK

The Gulf Coast tick (*Amblyomma maculatum*) is chestnut-brown with a colorful pattern on its back. The female has a white shield-shape marking on its upper back, near the head, while the male's back is marked with a black-and-white netlike pattern.

This tick occurs along the Atlantic Coast from Virginia southward into Florida, westward along the Gulf Coast into Texas, and northward into Oklahoma and Kansas, decreasing in numbers as it moves farther from the coast. Although it attacks chickens, it prefers

humans, dogs, and other large animals. Larvae usually attach themselves to the neck area and feed in groups.

As with the lone star tick, the seed tick and nymph stages of the Gulf Coast tick are most likely to attach to chickens. In warmer climates their peak activity tends to occur during winter, while in cooler inland climates they are usually most active in late spring and summer.

Hard Ticks

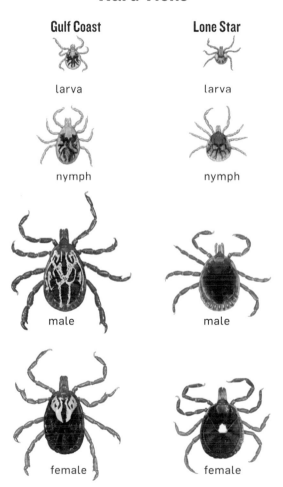

Gulf Coast

larva

nymph

male

female

Lone Star

larva

nymph

male

female

TICK REMOVAL

A tick's mouth is made up of a backward-barbed feeding tube (the hypostome), a pair of fanglike devices (chelicerae) that protect the tube when the tick isn't feeding, and a pair of jointed feelers (palps) that flank the fangs. To feed, it uses the fangs to pierce the skin, inserts the feeding tube into the incision, and spreads the feelers on the skin's surface, which provides stability and also prevents the tick's main body from entering the skin. Saliva released into the incision cements the tick in place, keeps the accumulating blood from clotting, and suppresses pain so the tick won't get scratched off before it's had its fill.

The feeding tube's barbs are what make a tick so difficult to remove. The trick is to remove the tick without squeezing or tearing it, for which pointy tweezers work better than blunt tweezers. Grasp the tick firmly as close as possible to where it enters the skin, and pull straight out without jerking or twisting the tweezers. Don't worry about any mouthparts that stay behind.

If you don't have tweezers handy, scratching the tick off with a fingernail is better than leaving it in. Protect your finger with a tissue, plastic bag, or disposable glove, and wash your hands afterward. After the tick has been removed, rub the site with alcohol or other antiseptic to prevent infection.

TICK CONTROL

Because ticks spend most of their time off the chicken, their control involves treating housing, as described under Parasite Control, page 146. However, once they get a foothold, controlling them is especially hard because they have such a long lifespan, they are able to survive for long periods without a blood meal, and their secure hiding places are difficult to reach with pesticides.

A tick feeds by using its fangs to pierce the skin, inserting its feeding tube into the incision, and spreading its feelers for stability.

Feeler (palp)

Feeding tube (hypostome)

Fang (chelicera)

Using pointy tweezers, firmly grasp the tick close to the chicken's skin, and pull straight out without jerking or twisting.

To rid a coop of ticks, start with a thorough cleaning, including the use of a high-pressure sprayer or a steam cleaner (see Steam 'Em on page 164) to get deeply into nooks and crannies, then follow up with an appropriate pesticide, as described under Parasite Control. Since ticks molt several times before reaching maturity, and the entire process can take several weeks, treat housing every week for at least 8 weeks to destroy all stages in the life cycle, then treat once a month thereafter.

Where ticks can be a significant issue, preventive measures include keeping grass and weeds mowed around the coop to eliminate tick hiding places; removing any nearby trees where ticks can hide and where chickens may acquire ticks by roosting; installing suspended roosts that ticks can't easily climb onto; and constructing housing to eliminate as many hiding places as possible. Moving infested chickens to fresh housing will only transfer the problem, unless each bird is first individually treated to destroy larval ticks.

Insects That Bug Chickens

Bugs, fleas, flies, and lice all belong to the class Insecta. They all have three-part bodies — a head, a thorax, and an abdomen — and three pairs of legs attached to the thorax, or middle part. They develop to maturity in stages, and young insects do not look like mature ones.

Most insects spend at least part of their lives off the bird's body, making it possible to control them by eliminating their favorite hiding places and breeding grounds — inside buildings and in junk piles on the outside.

Bedbugs

Bugs are flat-bodied, oval-shaped insects with sucking, beaklike mouths. The most likely bug to affect chickens is the common bedbug (*Cimex lectularius* in temperate areas, *C. hemipterus* in Florida and other warm, humid areas). Bedbugs feed on blood, and in biting to get a meal, they inject saliva that causes a small, hard welt that swells and itches like the dickens.

Mature bedbugs are reddish brown, about ¼ inch (6 mm) long, and look something like little cockroaches. Immature bedbugs look like miniature adults, except they are lighter brown or yellowish in color. Bedbugs don't fly but scuttle along walls, ceilings, and floors. They spread by hitchhiking on the shoes or clothing of people and on cages or other equipment transported from an infested coop.

The female bug finds secluded places in which to lay an egg or two each day until she has produced anywhere from 70 to 200 eggs. Each egg is no bigger than about the size of a speck of dust and is sticky enough to cling to the surface where it was laid.

Depending on the temperature, eggs hatch in 1 to 2 weeks. Within 1 to 3 months, again depending on temperature, young bedbugs shed their skin (molt) five times before reaching maturity and beginning to reproduce. Each stage requires a blood meal, as does the laying of eggs.

Bedbugs can produce three or more generations a year. They hide in protected places such as the corners of nest boxes, in housing, and in litter, where they can survive for as long as a year without a blood meal. They usually feed in the early morning, for about 10 minutes, while chickens are still on the roost, then leave, so they are rarely seen on birds during the day.

Evidence of bedbug infestation includes irritated vents, unusual feather loss, sores on breasts and legs, and black bug poop deposited in congregating areas and on eggs. Blood loss from an extreme infestation can cause chickens to become anemic, resulting in increased feed consumption and reduced laying.

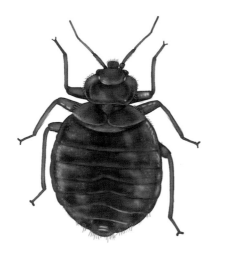

Bedbug (*Cimex lectularius*)

MORE BEDBUGS

Resembling the common bedbug is the poultry bug (*Haematosiphon inodora*), also called adobe bug, curuco, or Mexican chicken bug. It occurs mainly in the arid Southwest and favors chickens but will bite people.

Also resembling the common bedbug is the swallow bug (*Oeciacus vicarius*), which can be spread to chickens by barn swallows. It has a fierce bite and, like the poultry bug, may bite humans.

The conenose bug (*Triatoma sanguisuga*) is not closely related to the common bedbug, although it is variously called the big bedbug or the Mexican bedbug. It's also called the kissing bug, because its preferred site for biting people while they sleep is on the mouth. The blood-feeding bite is usually not much, but if this bug bites in self-defense, you'll know it, so handle with care.

Unlike the common bedbug, the conenose bug has wings and can fly but not well, especially after having a blood meal. It is about ¾ inch (2 cm) long and has a dark body with six distinctive bright orange stripes on each side. It has a long cone-shaped head ending in a long beak through which it sucks blood.

Like common bedbugs, conenoses like to hide in cracks and crevices and lay eggs after having a blood meal. They favor rodent nests, which offer both a hiding place and a source of blood meals. They feed at night, when their victims are asleep, and are known to feed on roosting chickens, taking about 20 minutes to tank up on blood.

The conenose has a long life cycle, requiring 2 years or more to reach maturity. Since chickens relish this bug, young conenoses in a chicken coop often don't live long enough to become a serious problem.

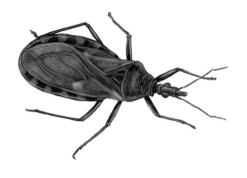

Conenose bug (*Triatoma sanguisuga*)

CONTROLLING BUGS

Once bedbugs get a foothold, they are difficult to eliminate, especially since they are becoming resistant to the usual line of defense, synthetic pyrethroids. Effective chemical alternatives require a licensed exterminator and are as toxic to chickens as they are to bugs. Natural pyrethrins work, although they deteriorate rather quickly and therefore must be frequently reapplied.

In a dry environment, diatomaceous earth (described on page 155) will provide long-term control when liberally applied to all potential bug hiding places.

If all else fails, remove the chickens — thus eliminating them as potential blood meals — thoroughly clean out the coop, and leave it empty until the bugs starve or leave.

Fleas

Fleas are insects with an enlarged third pair of legs that allow them to jump. They spend most of their lives off their host, usually in bedding or grass. They live for weeks off the host but survive for up to a year after temporarily visiting for a blood meal. Female fleas lay several eggs per day, which hatch in bedding, litter, or grass.

Most fleas are brown and large enough to see without magnification. They are particularly abundant in temperate and warm climates, where they attack not only chickens but also rodents and humans. Of the six species that attack poultry, three are important in North America.

CHICK FLEA AND HEN FLEA

The European chick flea (*Ceratophyllus gallinae*), also called the European chicken flea or nest flea, occurs throughout the United States. Mature fleas stay on birds, or people, only long enough for a blood meal. The larvae live in nests and litter, feeding on organic matter and undigested blood secreted by mature fleas. The larvae spin cocoons, where they overwinter, to emerge when spring brings warmer temperatures.

The Western hen flea (*C. niger*), also called the Western chicken flea or black hen flea, is common along the Pacific coast and northward into Alberta. It is similar to the European chick flea but occurs in a different geographical area. It breeds in poultry droppings and only occasionally returns to birds for feeding.

STICKTIGHT FLEAS

The sticktight flea (*Echidnophaga gallinacea*), also called southern chicken flea, tropical hen flea, or stickfast flea, is quite common all across the southern United States and as far north as New York. It is particularly prevalent in sandy areas and becomes most active in late spring and early summer.

These tiny, reddish-brown fleas attack humans and other mammals as well as chickens. Rather than jumping, like other fleas, they burrow in clusters of a hundred or more into the skin of a chicken's head (or sometimes vent), where they remain for life, feeding on the chicken's blood. The resulting blood loss may lead to death, especially in young birds. Numerous fleas congregating around an eye can cause infected sores that lead to blindness.

Sticktight fleas look like small brown dots clinging to the skin. They are easy to control on birds by coating them with a common household pet flea spray or poultry-safe insecticide, applied with a cotton swab. A follow-up with petroleum jelly will smother any stragglers. Dead fleas remain attached, so they must be removed with tweezers.

Unfortunately, sticktight fleas are less easy to remove from housing because of the female's habit of forcefully ejecting eggs so they will land and hatch in sand or litter. The eggs take about 4 days to hatch into wormlike larvae that feed on organic matter in the litter. After a couple of weeks and several molts, they burrow into the litter and spin cocoons, from which they emerge in another couple of weeks, work their way to the litter's surface, and look for a warm body to feed on. The entire life cycle can take as little as 4 weeks or as long as 8 months, depending on the temperature.

Controlling sticktight fleas involves removing infested litter and heavily dusting the floor with diatomaceous earth or a chicken-safe insecticide. Repeat the insecticide application two or three times at 10- to 14-day intervals to kill larvae that hatch between times.

Life Cycle of a Sticktight Flea

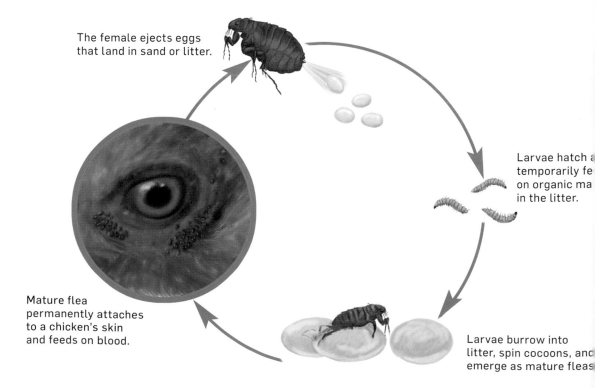

The female ejects eggs that land in sand or litter.

Larvae hatch a temporarily fe on organic ma in the litter.

Larvae burrow into litter, spin cocoons, and emerge as mature fleas

Mature flea permanently attaches to a chicken's skin and feeds on blood.

Flies

Flies are insects of the order Diptera, meaning two-winged. One pair of wings is for flying, the other for balance. Flies that bother chickens fall into two categories: biting flies and filth flies. Both kinds spread diseases and parasitic infections.

BITING FLIES

Biting flies are found primarily around bodies of water. The two main kinds that bother chickens are blackflies and biting gnats.

Blackflies (*Simulium* spp.) are approximately the same size as mosquitoes but are stouter and have rounded or humped backs. Also called buffalo gnats (because of their humped backs) or turkey gnats (because they favor free-range turkeys), they reproduce at the edge of flowing water, although they may migrate many miles in search of a blood meal. Sometimes, usually after a heavy rain that produces a lot of runoff, they attack chickens in swarms large enough to cause anemia and death.

Blackflies go through two to four generations in a year. Each female lays several hundred eggs, but before laying can commence, the females must have a blood meal. They feed in the daytime during late spring and early summer. On sunny days the worst attacks are in the evening, just before dusk, but they will also attack in midmorning. On overcast days they feed at any time of day, becoming worse as a storm approaches.

Since blackflies are difficult to control, the best plan is to manage your chickens to avoid attacks during peak blackfly season. And since blackflies tend not to enter buildings, bringing chickens into a darkened coop during late afternoon helps protect them from an attack.

Biting midges (*Culicoides* spp.) are variously known as no-see-ums (because you can feel their stinging bite without seeing the tiny insect that causes it), punkies (possibly from the Algonquian word *ponk*, meaning "a speck of dust"), five-Os (for their preferred mealtime), pinyon gnats (because they lay eggs in the bark of pinyon pines in the Southwest), and (incorrectly) sand flies. In addition to annoying people, midges irritate chickens, causing them to become restless.

Midges reproduce in moist soil that is high in organic matter, such as swampy areas, marshes, and bogs. In a dry climate they seek out moisture-collecting tree holes and saturated rotting wood. Unlike blackflies, they do not travel far from their breeding ground. They produce several generations in a year, and the females need a blood meal to lay eggs.

Depending on climate, the midge season runs from June through August. The peak biting time occurs around dusk, but midges also bite at dawn. If attracted by light they will enter a coop and bite at night. And they will bite at any time on cloudy, windless days.

Like blackflies, they are extremely difficult to control. A good start is to eliminate sources of stagnant water, as midge eggs cannot survive drying, and the larvae also need moisture to survive. Avoidance techniques during peak season include letting the chickens out late in the morning and closing them in late in the afternoon. Midges can get through ordinary window screening, but they are weak fliers and therefore are sensitive to air movement, so installing fans in the coop helps deter indoor attacks.

Homemade Fly Trap

Fly traps are easy to make from items commonly found around the home. For each trap, all you need is a 2-liter soda bottle, a piece of string, and some fly bait. How many traps you need depends on how big your chicken coop is and how bad the fly problem is.

1. Cut off the top of the bottle below the neck, creating a cup and a funnel. Use an X-Acto or utility knife to start the cut, then finish up with a pair of heavy scissors. Invert the funnel into the cup and wedge it in.

2. Use a hole punch or the tip of the scissors to make a hole through both pieces, then make a second hole on the opposite side. Thread a 2-foot (60 cm) piece of string through the holes and knot it to create a loop to hang the trap from.

3. Slide the funnel up the string and drop fly bait into the bottom (or, if the funnel is wedged in good and tight, pour in the bait through the funnel), taking care to leave about a ½-inch (13 mm) gap between the top of the bait and the bottom of the funnel for flies to get in.

4. Hang the trap close to the ceiling. Once a week, or whenever the trap gets full of flies, replace it with a fresh one.

Supplies

- X-acto or utility knife
- 2-liter soda bottle
- Heavy scissors
- Hole punch
- 2-foot (60 cm) length of string
- Fly bait

Fly Bait

For bait you can use commercial fly bait; a bit of raw hamburger covered with water; or a homemade solution. Combine 3 cups water (700 mL) with ¼ cup white vinegar (60 mL), ¼ cup table sugar (50 g), and a few drops of dish soap. Drop in a bit of ripe fruit, such as a slice of orange, a chunk of watermelon or banana, or a piece of banana peel.

The sugar and fruit attract the flies. The vinegar discourages honeybees. The soap serves as an insecticide and is optional because the flies can't get back out of the trap anyway (they tend to climb up the outer wall and then hit a dead end) and will eventually drown.

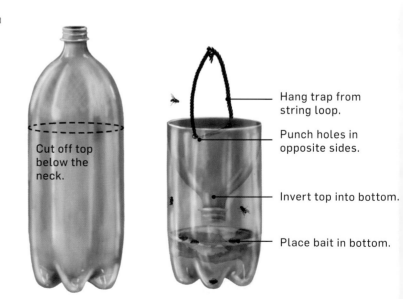

Cut off top below the neck.

Hang trap from string loop.

Punch holes in opposite sides.

Invert top into bottom.

Place bait in bottom.

FILTH FLIES

Fly problems result from keeping chickens in an unnatural environment that lacks proper management. Moist droppings provide an ideal environment for flies to lay eggs and for the eggs to develop into larvae (maggots). Droppings won't dry out sufficiently to discourage flies where ventilation is poor, drinkers leak, or rainwater runoff seeps into the coop.

The common housefly (*Musca domestica*) and other filth-breeding flies don't bite, but they irritate birds, transmit tapeworm (by ingesting tapeworm eggs that infect a chicken when the bird eats the fly), transmit roundworm (by worm eggs clinging to the feet of flies, which then infect a chicken that eats the flies), and spread bacterial and viral diseases. Flies also leave annoying specks on eggs, and they bother neighbors, sometimes leading to nuisance-abatement lawsuits.

TAKING ACTION

To control flies, minimize fly breeding sites. The following simple measures make a good start.

- Maintain dry bedding. Avoid such moisture sources as a leaky drinker, a leaky roof, and runoff seepage from an improperly graded yard.

FLY PREDATORS AND PARASITOIDS

A number of biological pest controls can help suppress fly populations. Given favorable conditions, they will usually populate a chicken coop on their own.

The hister beetle (*Carcinops pumilio*) is commonly found in poultry manure. It is a member of the Histeridae family, from which it gets its name. It is a small black oval beetle, about ⅛ inch (3 mm) long, that feeds on fly eggs and developing maggots.

Fuscuropoda vegetans is a predaceous mite that does not attack chickens but instead forages in manure for developing fly maggots. A healthy population of these mites can help minimize flies in the coop.

Parasitic wasps, or parasitoids, are tiny wasps (1–2 mm long) that attack filth flies, but not chickens or humans. Different wasp species prefer different fly species. Mature wasps feed on, thereby killing, fly pupae. The female wasp deposits eggs in the killed pupae, providing a food source for wasp larvae to feed on until they mature and emerge 2 to 3 weeks later. You can find out if your coop has fly parasites by collecting a few fly pupae, putting them in a jar, and waiting to see whether flies or wasps emerge.

Although parasitic wasps appear on their own when conditions are prime, they may also be purchased from biological pest control suppliers. The advantage to releasing them in your coop early in the spring is that they will start reproducing before flies have a chance to get out of control. Most suppliers provide information on what kind of wasps you should get, how many you need, and when you should release them.

Insecticides do not discriminate between beneficial and harmful insects. To encourage biological pest controls, minimize your use of pesticides.

- Likewise, avoid damp breeding sites in the yard. Keep a weedy yard well mowed, and eliminate low spots that accumulate runoff.

- Install a ceiling fan to improve ventilation and help dry out droppings and litter. Since flies don't like moving air, a ceiling fan also keeps them from bothering the chickens.

- Remove manure accumulations and soiled bedding periodically, but leave enough behind to ensure the survival of biological controls. Dispose of used litter where it won't attract more flies — compost it, bury it, or spread it on a field or fallow garden.

Even if flies get out of hand, avoid using insecticides. They affect biological controls more than they affect flies, because the latter have developed some degree of resistance to many commonly used products. Limit fly-control measures to those that attract flies without coming into contact with manure, such as fly sticky tape or fly traps.

Mosquitoes

The occasional mosquito does not seriously bother a chicken, but a mass attack lowers egg production and can cause death. Several mosquito species (*Aedes, Culex,* and *Psorophora* spp.) feed on chicken blood and can transmit pox and other poultry diseases. Mosquito attacks are most likely to occur in late summer and early fall, on cool nights when a chicken coop's warmth and lights attract large populations of mosquitoes.

Most female mosquitoes require a blood meal before they can lay eggs but usually don't travel far from their breeding site to obtain it. Each female lays up to 300 eggs at a time and may produce up to 3,000 offspring within her lifetime. The eggs are laid in water or moist soil, where they hatch into larvae that remain in the water until they emerge as adult mosquitoes. The entire process takes 1 week or less. Only the females feed on blood; the males feed on plants.

Since most female mosquitoes feed at night, fitting windows with screens helps keep them out of the coop. And since their life cycle requires water, they may be effectively controlled by eliminating their principal breeding grounds: stagnant water in persistent puddles, old tires or buckets, and swampy areas. Where mosquitoes are particularly dense in a pox-prone area, you may need to vaccinate your chickens against pox. (For more on pox, see page 265.)

Lice

Lice come in two varieties: blood-sucking and biting. Blood-sucking lice attack only mammals. Biting lice attack both mammals and birds. Several species infest chickens — more, in fact, than affect any other bird — and a chicken may host more than one species at a time.

How badly chickens become louse infested depends in part on their strain; some strains are more resistant than others. Debeaked birds, because they can't groom properly, are more likely to become seriously infested than chickens with their beaks intact.

An infested bird can be so irritated from being chewed on that it won't eat or sleep well. Egg production may drop by as much as 15 percent, and fertility may also drop. Chickens become restless, scratching and pecking their own bodies. In the process, feathers are damaged — not a good thing when birds are raised for show. In a serious infestation, especially in chicks, birds die.

Louse infection — technically called pediculosis — often accompanies poor management and is associated with such problems as malnourishment, internal parasites, and a variety of other infections. Whether louse infestation causes these problems, or these other problems make chickens more susceptible to lice, is arguable but entirely academic: poor nutrition, infection, worms, and lice are all undesirable.

LOUSE SPECIES

Louse species vary in shape and size, ranging in length from ⅟₂₅ to ¼ inch (1 to 6 mm). Most lice are yellow or straw colored, making them difficult to see on white chickens but easier to spot on dark-feathered varieties.

Interestingly, northern fowl mites are not compatible with lice, because lice will either eat the mites or starve them by outcompeting them. A chicken with lice is therefore not likely to have mites, which is a good thing because lice are easier to get rid of than mites.

All species of lice are wingless and spend their entire lives on the chicken, quickly dying otherwise. Young lice look like mature lice, only smaller and lighter in color. All species attach their eggs to feathers. Each female louse lays 50 or more eggs, and the life cycle from egg to egg-laying louse is about a month, so you can see how quickly a chicken can become overrun with lice.

Each louse species has a preference for feeding on certain parts of a chicken's body, resulting in descriptive common names such as wing louse, head louse, and fluff louse. Most lice eat feathers, dried skin, and other organic matter on the skin.

The head louse (*Cuclotogaster heterographus*) is the most serious louse pest of young birds, particularly in such heavily feathered

breeds as Polish and Cochin. Mature lice are oblong, gray, and rather large. Females lay one egg at a time, gluing it to down or a feather on the top or back of the head, under the beak, and sometimes on the neck. Head lice spread from a hen to her chicks, causing the little guys to become droopy and weak. Seriously infested chicks may die.

The body louse (*Menacanthus stramineus*), sometimes called the chicken body louse or yellow body louse, is the most common louse that bothers mature chickens. It is flat, straw colored, and one of the largest of lice. It lives on the skin of less densely feathered areas of the body, such as below the vent and under the wings. In a heavy infestation some lice may move onto the breast, head, or other parts of the chicken's body. Signs include numerous scabs on the bird's skin and pearl-colored egg masses at the base of small feathers. In mature chickens egg clusters are typically attached to feathers around the vent; in chicks they might be found on the throat or head. Body lice move fast — when you part a bird's feathers, take a quick look before the lice scurry into hiding.

The shaft louse (*Menapon gallinae*), also called the feather louse, looks like the body louse, only about half the size and paler in color, and spends its time on feather shafts rather than on skin. It does not bother chicks until they are fully feathered. It punctures soft quill feathers near the base to feed on blood, and leaves strings of light-colored eggs on feathers. It likes to rest on feather shafts but scurries toward the bird's skin when the feathers are parted.

The fluff louse (*Goniocotes gallinae*) stays mainly on fluff at the bases of feathers on the chicken's back and vent. It has a pale yellow, nearly circular body and is among the smallest louse that affects chickens. It usually does not occur in large enough numbers to cause a serious problem, although a massive infestation results in feather damage, anemia, restlessness, and reduced laying.

The brown chicken louse (*Goniodes dissimilis*) is a large, reddish-brown louse that favors a temperate climate. A similar species, the large chicken louse (*Goniodes gigas*), occurs in more tropical climates. These lice live on both skin and body feathers and can irritate chickens to the point that they injure themselves with incessant scratching and feather pulling. Young chickens in particular may get too restless to eat, causing them to become thin and weak and eventually die.

The wing louse (*Lipeurus caponis*) favors the undersides of the large feathers on a chicken's wings and tail. It is a slender (longer than it is wide), gray louse that moves rather slowly when disturbed. Aside from prompting the usual restlessness caused by all lice, the wing louse is not a serious threat to chickens that are otherwise in good health.

LIFE CYCLE

A louse lives for several months, going through its entire life cycle on a bird's body. It can survive less than a week off the body. The female louse lays her eggs, called nits, on a chicken's feathers and makes sure they stay there by sticking them down with glue.

Nits hatch in 4 to 7 days. Young lice, called nymphs, are unlike other insects in that they look like adults, only they're smaller and nearly transparent. They go through several molts and develop color as they grow.

When a louse matures, it mates on the bird and starts laying nits. One female may lay as many as 300 nits in her lifetime. Since lice go through one generation in about 3 weeks, in just a few months one pair explodes into thousands.

Lice usually travel to chickens by way of wild birds or used equipment. They spread by crawling from bird to bird or through contact with infested feathers, especially during a molt.

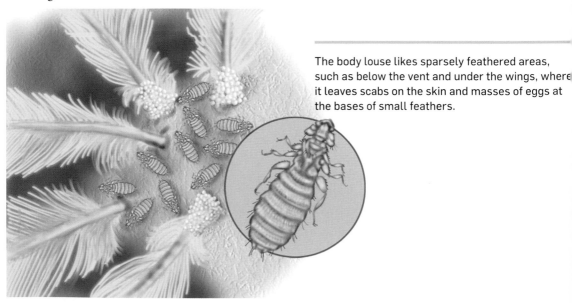

The body louse likes sparsely feathered areas, such as below the vent and under the wings, where it leaves scabs on the skin and masses of eggs at the bases of small feathers.

Lice

COMMON NAME Female/Male	SCIENTIFIC NAME	WHERE FOUND	APPEARANCE OF LOUSE	APPEARANCE OF EGG	OTHER NATURAL HOSTS
Brown chicken louse	*Goniodes dissimilis*	Skin and body feathers	Reddish brown, 3 mm	In clusters near feather base	None
Chicken body louse, yellow body louse	*Menacanthus stramineus**	Close to skin in sparsely feathered areas of vent, breast, head, under wings	Straw color, 3.5 mm, moves fast	In clusters near base of small feathers	Guinea, pea-fowl, pheasant, turkey
Fluff louse	*Goniocotes gallinae*	Body feather fluff on back and vent	Round, yellow, 1.5 mm, moves slowly	In clusters near feather base	None
Head louse	*Cuclotogaster heterographus*^	Base of feathers on head and neck	Oblong, gray-ish, 2.5 mm	White, attached singly to down or feather base	Many
Large chicken louse	*Goniodes gigas*	Skin and body feathers	Brown, 3.5 mm	In clusters near feather base	None
Shaft louse, feather louse	*Menopon gallinae**	In groups on shafts of new quill feathers on thighs and breast	Pale yellow, 2 mm, moves fast	In strings on feathers	Duck, turkey
Wing louse	*Lipeurus caponis*	Skin and under-sides of large wing and tail feathers	Thin, gray, 2.2 mm, moves slowly	In clusters near feather base	None

*Most common

TAKING ACTION

Lousiness is usually worse in fall and winter. Suspect lice if your chickens are restless and constantly scratch and pick themselves. Look for moving lice on feathers and skin, and for white or grayish egg clusters at the base of feathers. If you see lice on one bird, chances are good the whole flock has them, or soon will.

Inspect your birds at least once a month, especially during fall and winter when the concentration of lice is greatest. As soon as you spot lice, treat the entire flock as described under Parasite Control, below. For head lice, insecticidal powder may be combined with Vaseline and rubbed onto each bird's head and neck. Repeat any treatment twice at 7-day intervals.

Avoiding lice largely involves preventing their introduction. Discourage wild birds from nesting in the coop. Treat newly purchased infested chickens before putting them in with an existing flock. When acquiring used feeders, carriers, or other equipment, thoroughly disinfect them to make sure they are not harboring lice.

Parasite Control

Many external parasites may be effectively controlled through good management, including providing proper nutrition and a healthful environment, and giving the coop a periodic thorough cleaning. Once parasites get a foothold, however, stronger measures are needed.

Apply treatment either to infected birds individually or to the coop environment. Parasites that remain on chickens can be eliminated only by treating each bird. Parasites that spend part of the time away from chickens may be controlled by repeatedly treating the environment until they are eliminated. In a heavy infestation, control may require treating both individual chickens and the coop.

Many products are used against poultry pests, most of which are not labeled as being approved for use on or around chickens, and please note: approval for treating housing does not imply approval for use directly on birds. Many of the products described below fall into the nonapproved category, even though they are commonly used by owners of backyard chickens. They are included here not to imply endorsement but to provide accurate information so you can make informed decisions about which measures you feel comfortable using on your own flock.

Insecticide Formulations

A formulation is a combination of ingredients prepared for a specific purpose. Each insecticide formulation contains some percentage of an active ingredient — the one that immobilizes or kills parasites — along with an inactive or inert carrier. The carrier might be a powder that helps evenly spread the active ingredient as a dust. It might be an emulsifier that allows mixing of the active ingredient with water to create a spray. It might be something tasty that encourages parasites to eat the insecticide. Or it might be something that makes the active ingredient more potent. Unfortunately, manufacturers are required to identify only ingredients that are active but not those considered to be inert.

Many insecticides come in more than one formulation with varying percentages of active ingredient, so the dosage to be applied or the amount mixed with water to create a spray will vary. Read labels carefully to make sure you are getting the correct formulation for your purpose, targeted to the specific parasite you wish to control and designed to be used in the way you intend to use it.

DARKLING BEETLES

The darkling beetle (*Alphatobius diaperinus*) and its larva the lesser mealworm are not, strictly speaking, parasites of chickens, but are often found in and around poultry houses, especially where deep litter bedding is used. Also called black poultry beetle or litter beetle, it can spread a variety of bacterial and viral diseases, as well as parasitic worms and coccidiosis.

The wormlike larvae are yellowish-brown and up to ⅜ inch (9.5 mm) long. The mature beetle is about ¼ inch (6 mm) long and has a shiny black or dark brown shell with parallel ridges and grooves along the back. The darkling beetle's life cycle takes from 42 to 97 days, depending on the temperature.

Although this beetle can fly well, it prefers to crawl, usually at night. During the day it likes to hide in corners and under feeders. Each female beetle produces hundreds of eggs during her lifetime, which can be a year or more. These beetles survive by eating such delicacies as damp or moldy spilled feed, chicken poop, and each other.

Darkling beetles are difficult to control without the use of highly toxic insecticides. Diatomaceous earth (described on page 155) sprinkled near walls and other areas where beetles tend to travel, as well as in feed and on the litter, helps control both beetles and larvae but also affects fly predators and other beneficial insects.

Life Cycle of the Darkling Beetle (*Alphatobius diaperinus*)

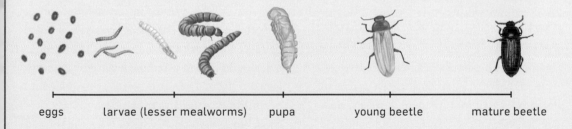

| eggs | larvae (lesser mealworms) | pupa | young beetle | mature beetle |

The National Pesticide Information Center offers comprehensive information on all types of pesticides at npic.orst.edu, including a link to each state's regulatory agency at npic.orst .edu/reg/state_agencies.html. The Extension Toxicology Network (EXTOXNET) maintains a database of pesticide profiles at pmep.cce .cornell.edu/profiles/extoxnet. The Organic Materials Review Institute maintains a database of insecticides acceptable for certified organic production under the USDA National Organic Program at omri.org.

Parasite Resistance

When an insecticide is used on a pest population, some pests may survive. The offspring of these survivors may then become better able to withstand exposure to that insecticide. In other words, they are resistant to it. The more you use that particular insecticide, the larger becomes the resistant population.

Resistance may occur in a number of different ways. The surviving parasites may have uncommon enzymes that allow them to render the insecticide ineffective, or they may have behavioral habits that let them avoid contact with the insecticide. In either case, they pass these survival mechanisms along to their offspring. Alternatively, the population may gradually mutate in a way that confers immunity to the insecticide.

A second problem related to the overuse of pesticides is that most of them don't discriminate between chicken parasites and biological pest controls. The combination of a loss of biological controls and increasing resistance of parasitic pests makes the latter even more difficult to control.

Once a population of parasites becomes resistant to a once successful insecticide, that insecticide will no longer be effective, and a different one must be found that is not in the same class as the original. Occasionally using an alternative insecticide helps delay the development of resistance, but routinely alternating two different insecticides can rapidly lead to resistance to both. Combining two or more insecticides in a misguided attempt to avoid resistance can have all sorts of unintended consequences; don't do it.

Signal Words

By law, registered insecticides are organized into four toxicity classes, according to the hazard they pose to humans. The three most hazardous classes must be identified by a specific signal word, printed in capital letters on the product's label. Following the signal word is often a cautionary statement regarding actions you should take to avoid the hazard or to mitigate its effects. The signal words are as follows:

DANGER designates the highest toxicity class. These insecticides might burn the skin or cause eye irritation. They may be highly toxic to humans when inhaled or absorbed through the skin, or fatal when a small amount is swallowed. No insecticides from this group are described on these pages.

WARNING indicates that the insecticide is moderately toxic. It might be harmful if inhaled or absorbed through the skin and may be fatal to an adult who swallows up to 2 tablespoons (30 g).

CAUTION indicates an insecticide that is considered to be slightly toxic. It might be harmful or irritating if inhaled or absorbed through the skin and may be fatal to an adult who swallows more than 2 tablespoons (30 g).

No signal word is required for insecticides deemed to have low or no toxicity. While the legally required signal word offers some indication as to the hazard of using a particular insecticide, it doesn't necessarily reflect the accumulative effect of the product on the environment or on human and animal health, reproduction, or genetics.

Synthetic Insecticides

The use of insecticides in the United States is regulated by the Environmental Protection Agency, which has a mandate to ascertain that any licensed pesticide "will not pose unreasonable risks to human health or the environment." Additionally, each state has a separate agency that establishes pesticide laws and regulations, which differ from state to state.

Most licensed insecticides are not registered for use on or around poultry, because the various manufacturers have no economic incentive to conduct expensive tests to determine that their products work specifically against poultry pests and, if they do work, what the withdrawal times are for acceptable residues in chicken meat and eggs (see Withdrawal Time on page 180). Without providing the results of such tests, manufacturers cannot legally promote their products for poultry, leaving backyarders to decide whether to avoid them or use them "because everyone else does."

Compared to most natural insecticides, synthetic insecticides tend to be more persistent, which means they remain actively potent over a longer period of time. In some cases this persistence is cumulative; a product used frequently may become gradually more harmful to chickens, humans, or the environment than the same product used once or only occasionally.

SEVIN — Signal Word: WARNING

Carbaryl, sold under the brand name Sevin, is one of many forms of synthetic carbamate insecticides made from carbamic acid. Carbaryl is a wide-spectrum insecticide that is approved for use on a variety of crops, livestock, pets, and poultry. Formulations include dusts and granules, as well as powders and liquid concentrates designed to be sprayed.

Carbaryl works by disrupting the nervous system of insects. Technically it is a cholinesterase inhibitor, which is important to know to avoid using chemicals in the same class on resistant parasites. Cholinesterase is one of the enzymes needed for the proper functioning of the nervous systems of insects as well as those of vertebrates, including humans.

Carbaryl is relatively nontoxic to birds, moderately toxic to cats and dogs, and highly toxic to fish, as well as to honeybees and other beneficial insects. Although listed by the state of California as a potential carcinogen, carbaryl is considered to have low toxicity to humans when inhaled or absorbed through the skin. Humans, chickens, and most other animals rapidly excrete carbaryl in urine and feces.

As a treatment for individual chickens with lice or mites, 5 percent carbaryl powder is applied over the body every 2 weeks. As a spray for individual chickens, roosts, and coop cracks and crevices (but not nests), 4 ounces of 80 percent carbaryl is mixed in a 5-gallon bucket of water. Repeat in 4 weeks if necessary.

All pesticides, whether synthetic or natural, are toxic to some extent, or they wouldn't work. All, therefore, must be handled with care. Read labels and follow all the stated precautions. Keep children away while insecticides are being applied, and discourage them from handling chickens for several days afterward.

Before applying any insecticide, remove or cover feeders and drinkers, and gather eggs. Wear gloves and a face mask, and avoid inhaling sprays or dusts. If you get any on yourself, wash your skin and launder your clothing separately from other wash.

Keep insecticides in their original containers, both to avoid misidentification and to retain label instructions. Store them away from food, feed, children, pets, and livestock. Puncture empty containers so they can't be repurposed. Because of the increasing number of laws regarding disposal of toxic wastes, getting rid of empty containers can be problematic. Check with your local waste-disposal agency.

The withdrawal time for meat birds is 7 days. The label does not specify a withdrawal time for eggs.

MALATHION — Signal Word: CAUTION

Malathion is one of many organophosphates, a group of chemicals derived from phosphoric acid and originally developed as nerve gas for use in warfare. Malathion is the most common, and least toxic, organophosphate insecticide used in the United States. It is available in many forms that include concentrate, powder, and ready-mixed spray, used to control a range of insects, including mosquitoes, flies, chicken parasites, and human head lice.

Like carbamates, organophosphates are cholinesterase inhibitors that disrupt the nervous systems of insects as well as those of vertebrates, including humans. Malathion is stronger than carbaryl and is often used where pest populations have become resistant to carbaryl. Actually, the malathion itself is not nearly as toxic as malaoxon, a highly toxic chemical that develops when malathion is exposed to oxygen.

Malathion is considered moderately toxic to birds, highly toxic to some species of fish, and highly toxic to honeybees and other beneficial insects. How toxic it is to humans is the subject of heated debates. It is rapidly absorbed through the skin, as well as by way of the digestive and respiratory systems, but is also rapidly metabolized and excreted.

Although malathion is currently not approved for poultry, many Extension publications recommend it, listing 7 days as the withdrawal time for meat birds. No withdrawal time is specified for eggs.

Whether or not malathion should be applied directly to chickens is as controversial as the insecticide itself. As a coop spray to control lice, mites, ticks, and bedbugs, malathion is liberally applied to walls, ceilings, roosts, floors, nests, and litter. Housing is also sprayed on the outside, especially around doors and window openings.

PYRETHROIDS — Signal Word: CAUTION

Pyrethroids are synthetic versions of natural pyrethrins (described on page 153) that persist

APPLYING AN INSECTICIDAL POWDER

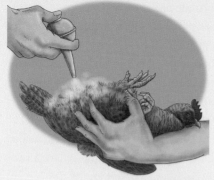

A baby nasal aspirator makes an inexpensive device for puffing insecticidal powder into vent fluff and other feathered areas.

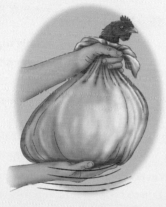

To completely coat a chicken with insecticidal powder, place the powder in a large plastic bag, enclose the chicken in the bag with only its head out, and bounce the bag to coat the chicken.

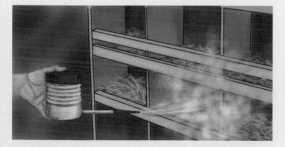

A lightweight garden duster comes in handy for getting insecticidal dust into a coop's nooks and crannies.

When applying a dust or powder directly to a chicken's body, avoid getting any on the chicken's face, especially in its eyes, and avoid breathing it yourself. One way to apply a powder into feathered areas is to put it into a shaker, a baby nasal aspirator, seedling sprayer, or squeeze bottle and puff it on.

Another option is to place a generous amount of powder in a large plastic bag, and insert the chicken into the bag with its head sticking out. Use one hand to hold the bag around the chicken's neck and with the other hand bounce the bag until the chicken is thoroughly coated with dust.

When applying an insecticidal powder inside the coop, a lightweight garden duster — such as Dustin-Mizer, Earthway Spritzer, or Pest Pistol — helps get the powder exactly where you want it. Shoo the chickens outside, wear a dust mask to avoid breathing in the powder, and wear goggles to keep the powder out of your eyes.

longer in the environment. Pyrethroids come in the form of a powder, spray, or dip and fall into two major groups: Type I, which works faster, and Type II, which kills better.

Both types work by paralyzing the insect's nervous system. Technically, pyrethroids are sodium channel blockers, the same mechanism that made DDT an effective insecticide. DDT is now banned in the United States because of its human health risks and adverse effects on the environment, while pyrethroids supposedly pose less of a risk to the environment and to the health of animals and humans.

Permethrin is a Type I pyrethroid approved for poultry that is typically more effective than either carbaryl or malathion. It has low toxicity for birds but is toxic to fish and honeybees and highly toxic to cats. It is an ingredient in shampoo used to treat head lice in humans.

For chickens permethrin is used against lice, mites, ticks, and bedbugs. It kills eggs and larvae as well as mature insects. As a spray, 3 ounces of 10 percent permethrin is mixed in a 5-gallon bucket of water and sprayed on chickens, roosts, walls, and nests. As a dust, 0.24 percent permethrin (trade name Prozap Poultry Dust) is dusted onto vents and under the wings of chickens. It is also added to bedding at the rate of 1 pound per 40 square feet, and applied to housing at the rate of 5 pounds per 1,000 square feet.

No withdrawal period is specified on the label. One study found that the maximum amount of permethrin in poultry meat peaks 1 day after treatment and in eggs 7 days after treatment, in both cases gradually diminishing. Traces of permethrin were still detected in egg yolks 21 days following treatment.

FIPRONIL — Signal Word: CAUTION

Fipronil (trade names Frontline, Pronyl) is a slow-acting wide-spectrum insecticide that is effective against bugs that have become resistant to both cholinesterase inhibitors (carbaryl and malathion) and sodium channel blockers (pyrethroids). It is sold for the control of fleas and ticks on dogs and cats and comes in the form of a spray or drops that are applied to the skin. Although fipronil is not approved for

WHEN CHICKENS GET POISONED

Chickens that overdose on an insecticide show signs within about 48 hours. They lose interest in normal avian activities, don't want to move much, and may have diarrhea. Chickens that have not been severely poisoned may recover on their own.

In the case of serious poisoning, chickens have trouble breathing and, if forced to move, appear to be stiff and uncoordinated. Some may become comatose. *Sometimes* you can revive a severely poisoned chicken by gently lofting it into the air, causing the bird to reflexively stretch out and flap its wings, which draws in oxygen and encourages the chicken's respiratory system to resume normal function.

Chickens not only may be poisoned directly by a pesticide but also by eating bugs that have been killed by an insecticide that is toxic to chickens. Don't take chances on insecticides that you don't know for certain are successfully used around chickens.

poultry or any other livestock, it is nevertheless widely used to rid backyard chickens of external parasites. Fipronil is also formulated as a bait for controlling filth flies.

Fipronil works by disrupting an insect's central nervous system. Technically it is a gamma-aminobutyric acid (GABA) inhibitor, meaning it blocks a key neurotransmitter in the central nervous system. It is more toxic to insects than to chickens or humans because it binds more readily to the nerve endings of insects. However, it is also highly toxic to honeybees and fish and generates a strong allergic reaction in some humans.

Fipronil is applied to the skin on the back of a chicken's neck, where the bird can't reach to preen. It is either spritzed from a sprayer or applied as three to four drops for large chickens, one to two drops for young (but fully feathered) birds and bantams. Some of the insecticide is rapidly excreted, while the remainder gravitates mostly to fatty tissue, from which it is slowly released to control parasites over an extended period.

Because fipronil is absorbed by fat tissue, it accumulates not only in body fat but also in egg yolks that are developing in a hen's ovary. No studies have been published that specify a suitable withdrawal time for table eggs or for meat. In countries where fipronil is approved for use on cattle, the withdrawal time for beef can be as long as 12 weeks.

Natural Pest Control

An increasing number of backyard chicken keepers, as well as those who seek organic certification, wish to avoid the use of synthetic insecticides. Integrated pest management (IPM) is an environmentally sensitive approach to insect control that involves, among other practices, limiting the use of pesticides to those that pose the least possible hazard to humans, other animals, and the environment. A growing body of information may be found online by doing a keyword search for "IPM poultry." The basic tenets of IPM parasite control are these:

- Correctly identify the parasite.

- Determine how serious the situation is.

- Take management measures to limit the parasite population.

- Use insecticides as a last resort, starting with the least toxic option that targets the specific parasite.

Chickens themselves are often an important component of IPM, since they actively eat insects in their environment. Many chicken keepers who practice IPM, especially those who are certified organic, use only naturally derived insecticides. "Natural" or "organic," however, does not necessarily mean "safe," so be cautious in your use of any insecticide.

PYRETHRINS — Signal Word: CAUTION

Pyrethrum is a natural insecticide produced by a white daisylike chrysanthemum (*Chrysanthemum cinerariaefolium*) grown commercially in East Africa and therefore sometimes called African chrysanthemum. The active components in pyrethrum are pyrethrin I and pyrethrin II, collectively known as pyrethrins. These pyrethrins are extracted and used to produce insecticidal powders, sprays, and shampoos that attack the nervous systems of insects in the same way that synthetic pyrethroids work.

PBO SYNERGY

Piperonyl butoxide (PBO) is a chemical that is synthesized from compounds related to natural safrole oil, derived from sassafras trees. Although PBO itself has mild insecticidal properties, as a synergist it is one of the most common ingredients added to both synthetic and natural insecticides to increase their potency. PBO is often added to natural pyrethrins (rendering them unacceptable for organic certification), as well as to synthetic carbamates and pyrethroids.

PBO works by inhibiting an insect's ability to use metabolic enzymes to detoxify an insecticide, increasing the insecticide's effectiveness and thus requiring less of it. Further, some insecticides, including pyrethrins, rapidly immobilize insects — an effect known as knock-down — but the effect may be only temporary. Insects that recover become resistant to the insecticide. The synergist ensures that insects die following knock-down.

PBO alone is toxic to fish and earthworms. It is categorized by the Environmental Protection Agency as a "possible human carcinogen" but otherwise is considered to have low toxicity for humans and other animals, including birds. However, most studies review the effects of PBO and active insecticidal ingredients separately. Few studies address their combined effect, which is greater than the sum of their separate effects.

Unlike synthetic pyrethroids, however, natural pyrethrins excite insects, causing them to move more rapidly and erratically. This intensified movement increases the insects' exposure to the insecticide, making it more rapidly effective. But pyrethrins rapidly degrade when exposed to sunlight and therefore do not provide the same lasting protection as pyrethroids.

Pyrethrins are highly toxic to fish, as well as to all insects, including honeybees and other beneficials. But they are much less toxic to humans and other mammals, and to birds, than most synthetic insecticides. They are usually allowed in organic production, unless they contain the synergist piperonyl butoxide (see PBO Synergy, above).

Pyrethrins do not kill larvae and eggs, only mature pests. The powder form is applied to a chicken's vent area to rid it of lice or mites. It is also dusted into nests, coop cracks and crevices, and bedding. As a spray it is spritzed onto a chicken's bottom or used to saturate the pests' hiding places in the coop. The concentrate comes in several different strengths, so read the label regarding dilution.

The amount of pyrethrins naturally released from flowers is minute compared to the concentration of commercially prepared insecticides, so homegrown blossoms have more of a repellent effect than insecticidal. To repel insects around your coop you might plant the flowers, called pyrethrum daisies in gardening circles. Unless the plants are outside the run, though, your chickens are as likely as not to eat them (without ill effect). Alternatively, you might grow the daisies in your garden, dry the flowers, and grind them into a repellent powder.

DIATOMACEOUS EARTH — Signal Word: CAUTION

Diatomite, diatomaceous earth, or DE, is a rock composed of the fossilized shells of diatoms, a type of algae. Diatom shells contain primarily the mineral silicon dioxide, or silica, most of which originates as volcanic ash. When a volcano erupts and its falling ash dissolves in a body of water, diatoms flourish. They use up the available ash until what remains can no longer support a large population of diatoms, and most of them die; their shells form a sediment deposit as diatomaceous earth. DE is found in large deposits in, among other places, the northwestern United States.

DE and related silica compounds make up 90 percent of the earth's crust. After oxygen, silicon is the second most prevalent element on earth (think sand). In fact, DE is composed of two oxygen atoms bound to one silicon atom. Depending on how the atoms are arranged, DE occurs naturally in two forms.

The atoms of amorphous silica are connected in a random network, giving the individual particles no clearly defined shape. Amorphous silica is powdery, mildly abrasive, and highly absorbent — properties that make it effective as an insecticide.

The atoms of crystalline silica are arranged in a regular pattern forming a three-dimensional lattice. The most common form of crystalline silica is quartz. Amorphous silica, processed with extreme heat, can be turned into crystalline silica. Called fused silica, calcined DE, or pool-grade DE, processed crystalline silica is used in swimming pool filters and similar applications.

Whether naturally derived or industrially processed, crystalline silica is nonabsorbent and therefore ineffective as an insecticide. Further, dust containing more than 1 percent crystalline silica poses a serious health hazard to livestock and humans breathing it over an extended period of time.

Naturally mined DE contains crystalline silica in varying minute amounts that are low enough not to pose a health hazard with ordinary use. Sold as fossil shell flour, food grade DE, or insecticidal DE, natural DE consists of approximately 85 percent amorphous silica, 5 percent sodium, and 2 percent iron, plus many other trace minerals, including boron, copper, manganese, titanium, and zirconium. It is relatively safe for animals and humans, and in fact is used as an abrasive in toothpaste and as an anticaking additive in a variety of foods. It is also used in gardens as a soil amendment and nontoxic insecticide.

Instead of poisoning insects, DE absorbs body fluids, killing insects through dehydration. But it works only as long as it remains dry. Once it gets wet, it softens and, of course, loses its ability to absorb additional moisture. However, when wet DE dries out, it can regain its insecticidal effectiveness.

As a means of controlling external parasites, DE is sprinkled into nests, bedding, and parasite hiding places around the coop. It is also dusted into the chickens' feathers.

DE marketed for insect control must be registered as an insecticide, and the label must include all the legally prescribed warnings. However, insecticidal DE is identical to food grade DE. The same product, when sold as a food, requires no safety warnings. It is used in the food industry to keep weevils and other insects out of stored grain, and does the same if you sprinkle a little into a bag or bucket of chicken scratch.

When purchasing DE to use on or around chickens, be sure the brand you buy doesn't include any other type of insecticide, such as pyrethrum or piperonyl butoxide. Since DE is not a toxin, no egg discard time or withdrawal time is required before eating eggs or chicken meat.

SULFUR — Signal Word: CAUTION

Pesticidal sulfur is labeled for treating fruit and vegetable plants and has been used for ages to control mites and lice on chickens. It is available as a liquid spray or as a powder.

When added to the chickens' dust bath, it is more effective than diatomaceous earth for two reasons. It has a residual effect, where DE does not. Also unlike DE, the effectiveness of sulfur rubs off onto chickens that don't themselves bathe in the sulfur-treated dust box.

Besides using it in a dust bath, sulfur may be added to bathing water (as described on page 162) or to chicken feed. Added to feed at the rate of 1½ to 2 ounces per 50 pounds (50 g per 20 kg), granular sulfur effectively controls mites without leaving any detectable residue in the chickens' meat or eggs. As a feed additive, sulfur also acidifies chicken poop, thus reducing ammonia fumes in the coop.

Sulfur may also be dusted directly on infested chickens. It is nontoxic to birds and mammals, including humans, but does irritate the skin and eyes.

Lime sulfur, made by boiling lime together with sulfur, is a horticultural spray and veterinary dip and is an old-time method of controlling chicken mites. However, it smells awful — like rotten eggs. It is also highly caustic and can burn the skin and eyes and if inhaled can irritate the lungs. Lime sulfur has been assigned the signal word WARNING, and the EPA recommends wearing goggles, gloves, and a respirator when using it.

CITRUS PEEL EXTRACTS — Signal Word: CAUTION

The peels of lemons, limes, oranges, and grapefruits contain the crude citrus oil d-limonene and the alcohol compound linalool, both of which are as potent as some synthetic pesticides. Citrus extract is a nerve toxin that causes overstimulation of an insect's nervous system, resulting in convulsions and paralysis. It is effective only on direct contact, and even then some insects recover. Commercial dips, sprays, and shampoos containing d-limonene or linalool therefore often include a chemical synergizer such as piperonyl butoxide.

Although citrus extract is a natural product — and at low concentrations is generally regarded as safe (a status granted by the United States Food and Drug Administration) — at high concentrations it can irritate the eyes, skin, and mucous membranes and may be toxic to birds and mammals, especially cats, although signs of toxicity are usually only temporary.

Little is known about the toxicity of unrefined citrus peel extract compared to commercially available dips, shampoos, and insecticidal soaps containing purified d-limonene or linalool. Using a homemade citrus peel extract directly on chickens is therefore not recommended. It may, however, be used inside the chicken coop to spray roosts and other areas.

To make 1 quart of citrus peel extract, grate the peel of four limes or two lemons, oranges, or grapefruits. Bring 1 quart of water to a boil, add the grated peels, and set it aside to steep for 24 hours. Use cheesecloth or a coffee filter to strain out the peel, and use the resulting liquid to spray inside the coop.

OIL TREATMENT

Linseed oil, neem oil, mineral oil, or any other natural nondrying oil can be applied with a paint brush to cleaned roosts, nests, and cracks in walls or floors. It is a messy but effective way to rid housing of parasites that spend part of their time off a bird's body.

Motor oil, especially recycled motor oil, was once commonly used for this purpose. However, motor oil contains potentially toxic additives. Used motor oil additionally contains heavy metals and is toxic to birds. Do not use motor oil in your chicken coop.

SPINOSAD — Signal Word: CAUTION

Spinosad (trade names Conserve and Entrust) is an insecticide derived from spinosyns, which are naturally occurring compounds with wide-range pesticidal properties produced by the fermentation activity of *Saccharopolyspora spinosa* bacteria. Spinosad is toxic to fish, as well as to honeybees and many other insects, but is relatively nontoxic to birds and mammals, including humans. It is, in fact, sold as a treatment for human head lice, although it can be irritating to the eyes.

Spinosad works by affecting an insect's nervous system, causing the insect to become overly active and resulting in paralysis and death, from sheer exhaustion, within a day or two. It has a residual effect of several weeks but degrades rapidly when exposed to sunlight.

The spinosad garden spray that's available in the United States is a 0.5 percent solution, and even at that low percentage a little goes a long way, since it is further diluted with water prior to use. However, it becomes unstable and begins losing effectiveness once mixed, so it should be mixed just prior to application, and any unused portion should be discarded.

Although spinosad is approved for the production of organic produce in the United States, it is not labeled for poultry. In some other countries it has been approved as a livestock dip against body parasites and as a spray to rid poultry housing of red mites, ticks, flies, and darkling beetles.

IVERMECTIN

Ivermectin is one of several drugs derived from avermectins, which are naturally occurring compounds with potent insecticidal and anthelmintic properties produced by the fermentation activity of *Streptomyces avermitilis* bacteria. Ivermectin is a liquid that may be formulated as a drench to be administered by mouth (trade name Ivomec) or as a pour-on applied to an animal's skin (Iver-On, Ivomec, Topline). An injectable form is also available that, for chickens, is used the same way as the oral form. Suitable dosages are the same as for deworming, as described on page 179.

Because ivermectin is a drug, not an insecticide, it has not been assigned a signal word. However, its overuse can result in resistant parasites, reducing its effectiveness for controlling internal as well as external parasites, and an excessive dose is toxic to chickens. Ivermectin is not recommended for chickens raised for meat or eggs, since no formulations are sold specifically for poultry and therefore no withdrawal period has been officially published; unofficially, the withdrawal time is 21 days.

DUST BATHING

One way to control external parasites is to ensure that a flock has access to dry dust or fine sand for bathing. Given the opportunity, chickens will instinctively hollow out bowls in loose dirt or dry litter, working it through their feathers by flapping their wings and kicking their legs. When they're done bathing, they stand up and shake themselves, and you can see the dust billowing out. Then the preening begins. Dust bathing helps chickens condition their feathers and rid themselves of external parasites, which they dislodge by pulling feathers through their beaks while preening.

Chickens with access to dry soil outdoors will create their own dust bowls. If their coop is bedded with deep litter, they will dust bathe indoors during hot or rainy weather. Otherwise they will appreciate a bin of fine soil, sand, or loose litter to bathe in, especially in a rainy climate. A bright light over the bin will encourage hens to use it for bathing instead of as a community nest for laying eggs.

Chicken keepers are fond of adding such things as wood ashes, diatomaceous earth, or sulfur garden powder to their chickens' dust hole or bin. Although adding such foreign materials can effectively control external parasites, it can also be harmful to the chickens' health.

Dust consists of particles of various sizes. The largest particles rapidly settle out. The remaining airborne particles may be categorized by particle size as either inhalable or respirable.

Inhalable dust particles are large enough to be trapped and filtered out by cilia in a chicken's windpipe, and therefore normally don't penetrate farther than the bronchi. Respirable dust is so small it can penetrate deep into the respiratory system, where it may be removed by scavenger cells. (See Respiratory Defenses, page 75.)

An excess of inhalable dust can overwhelm the cilia, rendering them ineffective. An excess of respirable dust can likewise overwhelm the lung's scavenger cells. Even when the scavenger cells can keep up with respirable dust removal, the particles are swept into the circulatory system. If the respirable dust contains toxins, the result can be decidedly detrimental to the chicken's health.

Some types of respirable dust physically stick to lung tissue and therefore cannot be removed by the scavenger cells. Respirable particles of crystalline silica in diatomaceous earth is an example of dust that sticks, causing scar tissue to form that impairs respiration. Although food grade diatomaceous earth contains less than 1 percent crystalline silica, and only a small percentage of that is respirable, it's still there.

Because the respiration rate of chickens is much faster than that of humans, and because the chicken's respiratory system includes delicate air sacs, chickens are more susceptible to respiratory problems than we humans. Regularly breathing in foreign materials with particle sizes and structures that different from ordinary dirt dust can make matters worse.

On the other hand, when chickens are seriously infested, the benefit of temporarily adding such materials may outweigh the potential danger. In such a case, if you expect your chickens to live long and prosper, make sure the dustbin is in a well-ventilated area — ideally, outdoors, where breezes can whisk away airborne dust. If the dustbin is inside the coop, ventilate the shelter well enough to prevent dust particles from hanging in the air.

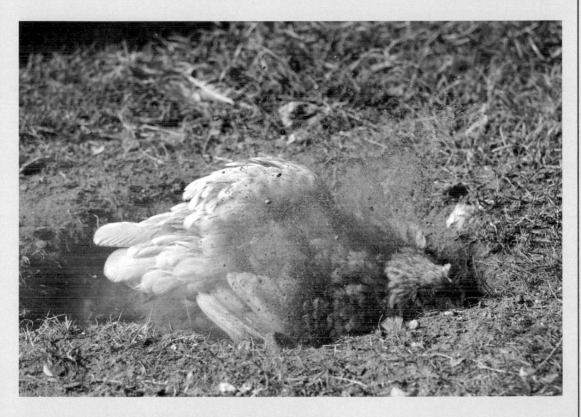

Chickens bathe by flapping their wings and kicking their legs to cover themselves with dust. The preening that follows helps control external parasites.

Zapping External Parasites

PRODUCT	BRAND(S)	RED MITES	FOWL MITES	LEG MITES	FEATHER MITES
Carbaryl synthetic	Sevin	X	X		X
Citrus peel extract		X			
Diatomaceous earth	(many)	X	X		X
Fipronil synthetic	Frontline, Pronyl				
Ivermectin	Iver-On, Ivomec, Topline	X	X	X	X
Linseed oil		X			
Malathion synthetic	(many)	X			
Petroleum jelly	Vaseline			X	
Pyrethrin	(many)	X	X		X
Pyrethroid synthetic	Permethrin	X	X		X
Spinosad	Conserve, Entrust	X			
Sulfur	(many)	X	X	X	X
VetRx	VetRx	X		X	

Usage varies with specific formulations; always consult the product's label.

LICE	STICKTIGHT FLEAS	TICKS	BEDBUGS	HOW TO USE*
X	X	X	X	Dust or spray chickens; dust bedding; spray housing
	X	X	X	Spray housing
X	X	X	X	Dust chickens, housing, bedding
	X	X		3–4 drops applied to skin at back of neck (or directly to face fleas)
X	X	X	X	Drops of pour-on applied to chicken's body; drops of oral given by mouth
				Coat roosts
X		X	X	Dust or spray housing and bedding
	X			Coat legs/face
X	X	X	X	Dust, dip, or spray chickens; dust bedding; dust or spray housing
X	X	X	X	Dust, dip, or spray chickens; dust bedding; dust or spray housing
	X	X		Spray housing
X	X	X		Dust chickens; add to dust bath or water bath; add to feed
				Coat legs and roosts

Shampoo Treatment

Shampooing individual chickens makes an excellent parasite-control option, especially if you bathe your chickens for exhibition anyway. Shampooing has the advantage of washing away parasite eggs and larvae, as well as mature pests.

You can use a commercial pet shampoo or flea dip, or any liquid dishwashing soap or detergent. Dishwashing liquid is safe and inexpensive and will control a wide range of parasites, provided the pests are thoroughly soaked. The main downside of using dishwashing liquid is that it lacks the residual effectiveness of a commercial pet shampoo. Also, if you have hard water, the minerals will neutralize the effectiveness of dishwashing soap but not detergent. On the other hand, a harsh detergent can make feathers brittle.

Use pet shampoo as directed on the label. When using dishwashing liquid, add 1 ounce, or about 2 tablespoons, to each gallon of warm water (8 mL/L). If your chickens are seriously infested, before adding the dishwashing liquid to the water, stir in 2 ounces (60 g) of sulfur powder per gallon, being careful not to inhale any.

Choose a warm, sunny day so your chickens will dry without getting a chill. Thoroughly soak each bird, and work a good lather among the feathers. Rinse the bird at least twice in fresh warm water. Pat the feathers dry with towels. Let the bird dry in a warm area, away from drafts, or hasten drying with a blow dryer.

Even when not bathing your chickens, you can make a reasonably effective insecticidal spray by adding 5 tablespoons of dishwashing liquid to a gallon of water (20 mL/L). Use it to spray or squirt onto the roosts and into the nooks and crannies of a thoroughly cleaned coop.

Shampooing a Chicken

I. In a tub large enough to hold 6 to 10 gallons of water and a chicken, slowly immerse the chicken to its neck, then thoroughly soak it by raising and lowering it and drawing it back and forth through the water. Rub in extra lather around the tail and vent. When the chicken is clean, lift it from the bath, and press out soapy water with your hands, working from head to tail.

2. Rinse the chicken in fresh warm water, letting it soak for a few minutes, until its feathers fan out or float, then move it back and forth in the water to work out remaining soap. Lift the chicken from the rinse, and press out excess water.

3. If any shampoo remains, the feathers will look dull and faded when they dry and the plumage won't fluff out properly, so rinse the bird once more in fresh warm water.

4. Squeeze out excess water from the feathers, and gently towel off the bird. Wrap the chicken in a fresh towel, and blot it to soak up remaining water.

5. Place the shampooed bird in a warm, draft-free area to dry.

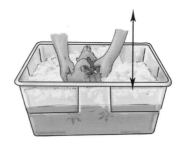

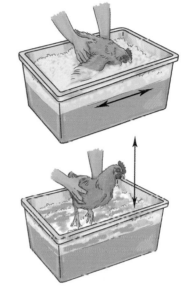

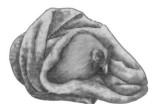

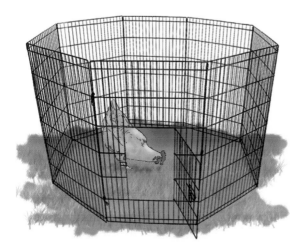

REPELLENT HERBS

Not a lot of scientific studies have been done to verify the use of herbs as insecticides or insect repellents. However, using herbs in the chicken coop by sprinkling them, fresh or dried, on bedding and into nests, and hanging small bunches from the roost, won't harm your chickens and just may discourage some of the external parasites that plague them. The following herbs have traditionally been used to repel insects of various kinds:

- Basil (*Ocimum basilicum*)
- Bay laurel (*Laurus nobilis*)
- California bay (*Umbellularia californica*)
- Catnip (*Nepeta cataria*)
- Citronella (lemongrass) (*Cymbopogon nardus*)
- Feverfew (*Tanacetum parthenium*)
- Garlic (*Allium sativum*) — see Garlic Juice Spray, page 388
- Lavender (*Lavandula angustifolia*)
- Lemon balm (*Melissa officinalis*)
- Marigold (*Tagetes* spp.)
- Mints of various kinds (Lamiaceae family spp.)
- Nasturtium (*Tropaeolum* spp.)
- Rosemary (*Rosmarinus officinalis*)
- Sage (*Salvia* spp.)
- Thyme (*Thymus vulgaris*)
- Wormwood (*Artemisia absinthium*)
- Yarrow (*Achillea millefolium*)

STEAM 'EM

For a completely nontoxic approach to ridding a chicken coop of hiding pests, a quality handheld steam cleaner comes in handy at coop clean-out time. First remove the bedding, scrape away poop and other debris, and vacuum up the resulting dust. Then thoroughly steam every crack, corner, nest, and roost. A good steaming, using only plain water, will kill parasite eggs as well as adult pests. It also loosens up dried poop that a scraper alone won't budge. When you're done, mop up excess moisture so the coop will dry out more quickly.

CHAPTER 6

When Chickens Get Wormy

WORMS DIFFER FROM other infectious pathogens in several ways. For one thing, most of them are easy to see without a microscope. They also do not multiply inside a chicken's body as do bacteria, fungi, protozoa, and viruses; instead their eggs or larvae are expelled in chicken poop, to be eaten by another chicken or other organism. How serious a chicken's worm load is, therefore, depends on how many infective eggs or larvae it eats.

Most chickens have worms somewhere in their bodies. Under good management the worms and chickens become balanced in peaceful coexistence, with the chickens showing few, if any, signs of having worms. A worm load becomes a problem, however, where chickens are kept in the same yard year after year.

Compared to other diseases, worm infections develop gradually and therefore tend to be chronic. A chicken infected with intestinal worms may gradually lose weight as the worms interfere with food absorption and other digestive processes. Worms that invade the respiratory system cause breathing difficulties and eventually block the airways. Less commonly, worms invade other parts of the body. In most cases, a serious infestation left untreated can result in a chicken's death.

Speaking of Parasitic Worms

ascariasis. Also called ascaridiasis: infested with roundworms

capillariasis. Infested with capillary worms

cestode. A tapeworm

cestodiasis. Infested by tapeworms

direct life cycle. A life cycle that does not involve an intermediate host

embryonate. To develop an embryo inside a parasitic worm egg

fecal-oral transmission. The spreading of an infection through ingesting contaminated poop; regarding parasitic worms, fecal-oral implies a direct life cycle

helminth. A parasitic worm

indirect life cycle. A life cycle that involves an intermediate host

intermediate host. Also called an alternate host; an animal in which a parasitic worm lives during an immature stage in its life cycle

natural host. Also called definitive host or primary host; an animal in which a parasitic worm matures and reproduces sexually

nematode. A roundworm

predator-prey transmission. The spreading of parasitic worms with an indirect life cycle

---

1. Roundworm eggs are passed in chicken's droppings

2. Worm eggs embryonate

3. Chicken eats infective worm eggs, becomes infected or reinfected

4. Roundworm-infested chicken

The Nature of Worms

Parasitic worms fall under the category of helminths, from the Greek word *helmins*, meaning "worm." Based on general body shapes, helminths are organized into two main groups, roundworms and flatworms. Similar to flatworms, but distantly related and relatively uncommon, is a third category, the thorny-headed worm. It is neither a nematode (roundworm) nor a cestode (flatworm), but an acanthocephalans. Although it does not fall into one of the two main categories, it does occasionally infect chickens.

Life Cycles

The life cycle of helminths occurs in three basic stages: adult, egg, and larva. The chicken is considered to be the definitive, natural, or primary host of worm species that mature and sexually reproduce inside a chicken's body. The mature worms expel eggs or larvae, which pass out of the chicken in its poop.

Direct Life Cycle of Roundworm

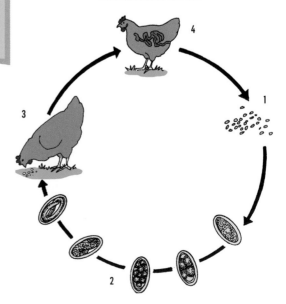

Depending on the species of worm involved, the larvae may infect new chickens in one of two ways: directly or indirectly. Eggs or larvae that are expelled by one chicken, then ingested by another (or the same) chicken have a direct life cycle. Because the eggs or larvae are expelled in feces, then eaten, the spreading of worms with a direct life cycle is also called fecal-oral transmission.

Some worm species require another step in their life cycles: The larva must be eaten by some other creature — such as a beetle or an earthworm — which in turn (worm larva and all) is eaten by a chicken. The intervening creature, in which the worm lives during an immature stage in its life cycle, is considered to be an intermediate or alternate host. A parasitic worm species requiring an intermediate host has an indirect life cycle. Because the chicken as predator eats the intermediate host, its prey, the spreading of worms with an indirect life cycle is also called predator-prey transmission.

More than half the roundworms and all the tapeworms that invade chickens require an intermediate host. Indirect-cycle parasites involving earthworms tend to be a greater problem in spring, when frequent rain brings earthworms to the soil's surface. Other indirect-cycle parasites may create greater problems in late summer, when beetles, grasshoppers, and similar intermediate hosts proliferate. Knowing which parasites have indirect life cycles, and which intermediate hosts they involve, is an important part of your parasite control program.

Roundworms

Roundworms are thin, threadlike worms also called nematodes, from the Greek words *nema*, meaning "thread," and *odes*, meaning "like." In the number of species involved and the damage they do to chickens, roundworms are the most significant parasitic worm. Different species invade different parts of a chicken's body, including the eye, windpipe, crop, stomach, gizzard, intestine, and ceca.

Indirect Life Cycle of Roundworm or Tapeworm

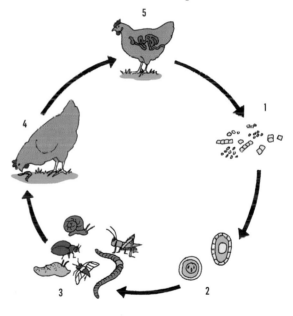

1. Roundworm eggs or tapeworm segments containing eggs are passed in chicken's droppings
2. Roundworm egg/tapeworm egg
3. Eggs eaten by intermediate host (beetle, fly, slug, earthworm, grasshopper, etc.)
4. Chicken acquires parasite by eating intermediate host
5. Roundworm- or tapeworm-infested chicken

Direct-cycle nematodes and those requiring an indoor-living intermediate host (such as cockroaches or beetles) are more of a problem in penned birds. Indirect-cycle nematodes requiring an outdoor-living intermediate host (such as grasshoppers and earthworms) are more of a problem in pastured flocks.

Roundworms may be identified in part by the organ they lodge in, and in part by their appearance. However, most nematode species have two sexes, and in some cases the male and female look so dissimilar that an untrained person might believe they are two different species.

For most worm species that affect backyard flocks, chickens are not the only natural hosts, which can be important to chicken keepers who raise multiple species of poultry. The table on pages 172 and 173 indicates which common barnyard birds besides chickens may be infected by each type of nematode.

Large Roundworm

The large roundworm (*Ascaridia galli*) is one of the most common poultry parasites. Roundworm or ascarid infection is called ascariasis or ascaridiasis. The large roundworm is approximately the same thickness as a pencil lead and grows as long as 4½ inches — big enough to be seen without a magnifying glass.

Adult large roundworms roam a chicken's small intestine. Occasionally one will migrate down the intestine to the cloaca, and from there up the oviduct, getting trapped inside a newly forming egg — a decidedly unappetizing occurrence. Such a worm easily may be detected by candling, which, if you sell eggs, is a good practice anyway.

Each female ascarid lives for several months, during which she lays up to 5,000 eggs. The eggs take 10 days or more to embryonate and can survive in the environment for a year or more. Ascarids are spread by direct cycle — embryonated eggs are picked up by a chicken from droppings, soil, feed, and water.

Birds that are older than 3 months are more resistant to ascaridiasis than younger birds. Heavier breeds such as Rhode Island Red and Plymouth Rock are more resistant than lighter breeds such as Leghorn and Minorca. The resistance of any breed may be increased by a diet that's high in calcium, vitamin A, and the B-complex vitamins.

Signs of ascaridiasis are pale head, droopiness, weight loss or slow growth, emaciation,

EMBRYONATION

Not all nematode eggs are infective when they are expelled from a chicken. Some must develop an embryo, or embryonate, to become infective. Some eggs embryonate in as little as 3 days; others require 30 days or more.

Some nematode eggs embryonate before leaving the chicken. Others must encounter just the right conditions of temperature and humidity in the environment. When conditions are less than favorable, embryonation may take longer or may not occur at all.

In general, nematode eggs embryonate more quickly under fairly warm, humid conditions. Minimizing moisture in the chickens' environment inhibits embryonation and slows the buildup of parasite loads in the flock.

and diarrhea with increased white urates. In a severe infection the intestines become plugged with worms, causing death. Even a somewhat mild infection may be devastating when combined with some other disease, such coccidiosis or infectious bronchitis.

The only drug approved for ascarids in poultry is piperazine, which has been used for so many years that ascarids are becoming resistant. Therefore more effective (but not approved) drugs are often used for backyard flocks, particularly exhibition birds and others not kept for meat or table eggs.

Capillary Worm

Six species of *Capillaria*, or capillarids, invade chickens, causing capillariasis. Capillarids are white, hairlike or threadlike worms; hence, they are commonly called hairworms or threadworms. Most capillary worms are too small to be seen with the naked eye but may be seen with the aid of a magnifying glass. Depending on the species, they burrow into tissue in a chicken's mouth, esophagus, crop, small intestines, or ceca.

Most capillary worms have an indirect cycle, with earthworms as the intermediate host. Some have a direct cycle. One species (*C. contorta*) can be either direct or indirect. Capillarid eggs are so small they are difficult to identify during fecal examination (see page 187), yet they survive well on pasture, especially where drainage is poor, and in housing litter, especially where ventilation is inadequate.

General signs of capillariasis are pale head, poor appetite, droopiness, weakness, emaciation, and sometimes diarrhea. Chickens may sit around with their heads drawn in. Postmortem examination (described in chapter 13) may reveal adult worms in thickened and inflamed mucous membranes of the capillarid species' preferred site of attachment.

Crop Worm

The crop worm (*Gongylonema ingluvicola*) is often confused with capillary crop worms. It is a threadlike worm that invades the crop, and sometimes the esophagus and proventriculus. Its indirect cycle involves beetles and cockroaches.

Unless they get out of hand, crop worms do little damage. Signs of a serious infection are droopiness, weakness, lack of activity, reduced appetite, and thickening of the crop wall. Crop worms may be contained by controlling beetles and cockroaches.

Cecal Worm

The cecal worm (*Heterakis gallinae*) is the most common parasitic worm in North American chickens. As its name implies, it invades a bird's ceca. Other than carrying blackhead, to which chickens are typically resistant, the cecal worm does not seriously affect a bird's health.

Cecal worms are slender, white, and about ½ inch long, making them easy to see. Their cycle is direct. Eggs survive for long periods under a wide range of environmental conditions.

Strongyloides avium is another parasite that invades the ceca. So far it has not appeared in chickens within the continental United States, but it is a problem in Puerto Rico. This worm is unusual for two reasons. First, rather than hatching in an animal host, *S. avium* eggs hatch in soil, where mature worms live and grow. Second, only the female worm parasitizes chickens. An infection can be deadly to young birds but may cause no signs in mature birds.

Stomach Worm

The stomach worm (*Tetrameres americana*) invades a chicken's proventriculus, causing anemia, emaciation, diarrhea, and, in a severe infection, death. This worm is such a bright red color that you can sometimes see it through the wall of an unopened stomach during postmortem examination. On close inspection you will find worms of two shapes: the long, thin ones are male; the round ones are female.

Roundworms

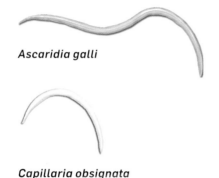

Ascaridia galli

Capillaria obsignata

Heterakis gallinarum

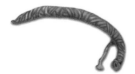

Syngamus trachea

A roundworm is long and thin, with an unsegmented tube-shape body and a digestive tract running the length of the body. The body cavity is filled with fluid that gives the worm its rigidity. Mature roundworms have two distinct sexes.

T. americana has an indirect cycle involving cockroaches and grasshoppers. Its near relative, *T. fissispina,* which is identical but considerably smaller and rarely affects chickens, is carried by the same intermediate hosts and also by earthworms and sand-hoppers. Controlling stomach worms involves controlling their intermediate hosts.

Eye Worm

Eye worm (*Oxyspirura mansoni*) occurs in the southeastern United States, southern Texas, Hawaii, and other tropical and subtropical areas where its intermediate host, the burrowing Surinam cockroach (*Pycnoscelus surinamensis*) is found. It is a small, slender white worm that's thinner at both ends than in the middle.

The worm lodges in the corner of a chicken's eye underneath the nictitating membrane. The membrane swells, causing the corners of the eye to slightly bulge beyond the eyelids, impairing the chicken's vision. Because of the discomfort, the nictitating membrane constantly blinks back and forth across the eye, and the chicken rubs or scratches its eye, trying to relieve the irritation. The eyelids may stick together, with white cheesy material accumulating underneath. The eye may turn cloudy, and eventually the chicken may go blind.

Worm eggs deposited in the eye pass into the tear duct, from which they are flushed into the chicken's mouth, swallowed, and expelled in droppings, which are then eaten by the burrowing cockroach. When a chicken eats an infective cockroach, worm larvae migrate from the crop up the esophagus to the mouth, through the nasal cavity, into the tear duct, and into the eye. This migration takes about 5 minutes. Wild birds are also infected by eye worm, and may help spread it to chicken flocks.

Eye worm is controlled by eradicating burrowing cockroaches around the henhouse. Treatment involves putting three drops of dewormer — ivermectin or levamisole — into the chicken's eyes every day for 3 days, or until the worms are gone. If the worms haven't been there long enough to do serious damage, the eyes should clear within 2 to 3 days. Frequent treatment may be needed where burrowing cockroaches cannot be controlled.

Gapeworm

The gapeworm (*Syngamus trachea*) buries its head in the lining of a bird's windpipe or other part of the respiratory system, causing an infected bird to continually yawn or gasp for air. Because of the constant opening of the mouth, or gaping, to gulp in air, the infection is called gapes, or the gapes, and the worm is commonly called the gapeworm. These worms, which are big enough to see without magnification, are also called red worms or forked worms — each blood-red female has a somewhat paler male permanently attached, forming the letter Y.

An infected chicken coughs up worm eggs, swallows them, and expels them in droppings. The cycle is direct but can also appear to be indirect, involving earthworms, flies, slugs, or snails. Although such intermediate hosts are not necessary for the completion of a gapeworm's life cycle, when eaten by one of these intermediate hosts an infective larvae can wrap itself in a cyst and hibernate for 4 years or more, until some unlucky chicken gobbles up the host. If the intermediate host is harboring numerous hibernating larvae, the chicken can appear to get the gapes virtually overnight.

Young chickens up to about 8 weeks of age are more susceptible than mature birds. Signs of gapes are yawning, grunting, gasping, sneezing, coughing (sometimes coughing up a detached worm), choking, loss of energy, loss of appetite, weakness, emaciation, closed eyes, head shaking, frequently stretching the head forward with mouth open to gasp for air, and convulsive shaking of the head (to dislodge worms from the windpipe). Gapeworms can rapidly clog the narrow windpipe of a chick or young growing bird, causing it to suffocate to death.

No drug is approved for poultry, although several nonapproved dewormers will work if started early. Gapeworms produce eggs within less than 3 weeks after infecting a chicken and, because their life cycle is direct, can quickly infect the entire flock. Once started, treatment must be repeated at least every 3 weeks to reduce worm loads in the flock and their environment. Fortunately, most people who think they have a chicken with the gapes are seeing a bird yawning for other reasons, perhaps as a nervous reaction to something unusual happening in its environment, because it has something caught in its throat, or as an early sign of respiratory disease.

Flatworms

Flatworms differ in appearance from roundworms in having bodies that are flattened and more ribbonlike than tubular. They come in two versions, ribbon-shape tapeworms (cestodes) and leaf-shape flukes (trematodes). Fortunately, flukes are not a problem for chickens in the United States and Canada, because fluke infection results from eating infected snails (or infected dragonflies), which are found primarily in moist environments — marshes, swamps, wetlands — not ideal places for keeping chickens.

Roundworms (Nematodes)

ORGAN AFFECTED	COMMON NAME/SCIENTIFIC NAME	APPEARANCE
Ceca, sometimes small intestine	Capillary worm; hairworm; threadworm *Capillaria anatis*	White, threadlike, 0.3–1" (8–28 mm) long
Ceca, sometimes small intestine	Common roundworm *Trichostrongylus tenuis*	White, thin; 0.2–0.4" (5.5–11 mm) long
Ceca, sometimes small intestine (Puerto Rico)	Cecal worm *Strongyloides avium*	White, tiny, 0.08" (2.2 mm) long
Ceca	Cecal worm**; pinworm *Heterakis gallinarum*	Yellowish-white, thin, 0.3–0.6" (7–15 mm) long
Ceca	Cecal worm *Subulura brumpti*	White, curved at one end, 0.3–0.6" (7–14 mm) long
Ceca	Cecal worm *Subulura strongylina*	White, 0.2–0.7" (4.5–18 mm) long

Reliable diagnosis involves positive identification of the nematode, usually requiring postmortem examination.

**The most common nematodes affecting chickens*

Tapeworms

Most backyard chickens are infected by tapeworms, a disease known as cestodiasis. Like roundworms, tapeworms come in many species. The eight species that invade chickens range in size from microscopic to 13½ inches (34 cm) long.

Most tapeworms are host specific: those infecting chickens invade only chickens and their close relatives. All tapeworms lodge in the intestinal tract, using four pairs of suckers to attach their heads to the intestine wall. Each species prefers a different portion of the intestine: duodenum, small intestine, or large intestine. General signs in young chickens include stunted growth. In mature chickens signs include weight loss and decreased laying. Rapid breathing and dry, ruffled feathers are additional signs.

A tapeworm's body is made up of individual segments, each of which has both male and female reproductive organs. As the segments farthest from the head mature, they become wider and fill with eggs until they break away and are expelled in chicken poop. In a severe infection you may see segments in droppings or clinging to the area around the vent, looking like bits (or sometimes strings) of flattened white rice. Each segment may contain hundreds of eggs — in its lifetime (which can be well over a year), each tapeworm releases millions of eggs, ensuring that some survive.

All tapeworms require an intermediate host — which may be an ant, a beetle, an earthworm, a fly, a slug, a snail, or a termite — that eats either individual worm eggs or a whole segment and in turn is eaten by a chicken. Caged chickens are most likely to be infected by worms with a cycle involving flies. Litter-raised flocks are likely to be infected by worms with a cycle involving beetles. Pastured chickens are likely to be infected by tapeworms with a cycle involving ants, earthworms, slugs, or snails.

INTERMEDIATE HOST	SIGNS*	SEVERITY	OTHER NATURAL HOSTS
Unknown	Weakness, emaciation, sometimes diarrhea, death	Moderate to severe	Duck, goose, pheasant, turkey
None	Paleness, weight loss, death (peaking in spring and fall)	Severe (rare in chickens)	Duck, goose, guinea, pigeon, turkey
Free living	None or thin and bloody cecal discharge, death	Mild in mature birds, severe in young	Goose, turkey
None	Weakness, weight loss (carries blackhead)	Mild	Duck, goose, guinea, pheasant, turkey
Beetle, cockroach, earwig, grasshopper	None	None	Dove, duck, guinea, pheasant, turkey
Beetle, cockroach, grasshopper	None	None	Guinea

NODULAR TAPEWORM DISEASE

The nodular tapeworm (*Raillietina echinobothrida*) invades the small intestine, where attachment sites develop into lumps that resemble tumors caused by tuberculosis, a condition known as nodular tapeworm disease. Although a heavy infestation can cause serious health problems, most infected chickens show few, if any, signs of illness other than possible slow weight gain in growing chickens and reduced laying in hens. Chickens with nodular tapeworm disease are rarely diagnosed unless a necropsy is performed, usually for other reasons.

Tapeworms

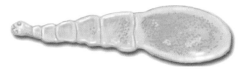

Davainea proglottina

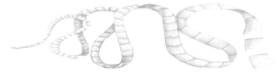

Raillietina echinobothrida

A tapeworm has a long, flat, ribbon-shape body made up of a head and neck followed by numerous independent segments, each of which contains both male and female organs. The worm has no interior digestive tract but absorbs nutrients through its porous skin.

During postmortem examination (described in chapter 13), most tapeworms may be seen easily without benefit of magnification. The exception is the microscopic tapeworm *Davainea proglottina*. Compared to the several dozen segments possessed by other species, *D. proglottina* has nine or fewer segments at a time; compared to other species that shed as many as a dozen segments each day, *D. proglottina* sheds only one. Ironically, this smallest species is also the most deadly, especially in young chickens. A microscopic tapeworm lives as long as 3 years, and as many as 3,000 have been found in a single chicken.

TAPEWORM CONTROL

The usual recommendation for controlling tapeworm is to control the intermediate host. Since signs are similar for most tapeworm species, you would have to know which species you're dealing with so you'll know which intermediate host(s) to look for. Furthermore, the idea of exterminating earthworms and beneficial beetles is troublesome. Your county Extension agent or state poultry specialist should have information on problem beetles and their control in your area.

Tapeworm infections are difficult to treat, and many common dewormers have no effect at

Tapeworms (Cestodes)

ORGAN AFFECTED	COMMON NAME/ SCIENTIFIC NAME	APPEARANCE*
Duodenum	Short tapeworm *Amoebotaenia cuneata*	Wedge-shaped, 25–30 segments, total length less than 0.16" (4 mm)
Duodenum	Microscopic tapeworm *Davainea proglottina*	Fewer than 9 segments, total length less than 0.16" (4 mm)
Duodenum	Threadlike tapeworm *Hymenolepis carioca*	Threadlike, up to 3" (80 mm)
Duodenum, jejunum	Large chicken tapeworm *Raillietina cesticillus*	Total length up to 6" (15 cm); sheds up to a dozen segments a day
Ileum	None *Raillietina tetragona*	Up to 0.12" (3 mm) wide, total length up to 10" (25 cm)
Small intestine	Branching tapeworm *Hymenolepis cantaniana*	Slender, total length up to 0.8" (20 mm); 100 or more per bird
Small intestine	Sawtooth tapeworm *Choanotaenia infundibulum*	About 30 segments, wider than long and widening toward rear, up to 0.12" (3 mm) wide, total length up to 9" (23 cm)
Small intestine	Nodular tapeworm *Raillietina echinobothrida*	Up to 0.16" (4 mm) wide, total length up to 13.5" (34 cm)

*In appearance, all tapeworms are white, flat, and segmented.

all. The benzimidazoles described on page 183 are commonly used to treat backyard chickens for tapeworm.

Thorny-Headed Worm

Wild birds are the natural hosts of the thorny-headed worm, which can also infect chickens but rarely does. Sometimes called spiny-headed worms or Acanthocephalans (their phylum), these parasites attach to a chicken's intestines, drawing nutrients and potentially causing anemia and weakness.

The thorny-headed worm is about ⅓ to ½ inch (9 to 15 mm) long and looks similar to a nematode in having a cylindrical body. However, in the way it functions it's more like a tapeworm, to which it is distantly related.

A characteristic feature of these worms is their retractable tubular sucking appendage, or proboscis, sporting curved spiny hooks, from which they derive their common names. The species most likely to infect chickens is *Prosthorhynchus formosus,* sometimes identified as *Plagiorhynchus formosus.*

INTERMEDIATE HOST	SIGNS	SEVERITY	OTHER NATURAL HOSTS
Earthworm	Possible weight loss, decreased laying	Mild	Turkey
Slug, snail	Lethargy, emaciation, dull feathers, labored breathing, bloody diarrhea, paralysis, death	Severe	None
Dung beetle, ground beetle, termite	Usually none	None to mild	Turkey
Beetle (several species)	Usually none, sometimes emaciation or slow growth, slimy diarrhea	Mild to moderate	Guinea, turkey
Ant	Emaciation, decreased laying	Mild to moderate	Guinea, peafowl, pigeon
Dung beetle	Usually none	None to mild	Peafowl, turkey
Beetle, housefly	Weight loss, decreased laying	Moderate	Turkey
Ant	Emaciation or slow growth, paleness, yellow slimy diarrhea, death	Moderate to severe	Turkey

The thorny-headed worm has an indirect life cycle that involves the pillbug (*Armadillidium vulgare*), also known as the woodlouse or roly-poly, which is identifiable by its penchant for rolling into a ball when disturbed. Pillbugs hide in moist environments during the day and are active at night, making them unlikely to be found by chickens under normal circumstances. An exception would be in a garden using natural pest control, where (for instance) boards are laid down for insects to hide under during the night, then turned over in the morning for chickens to have a feast.

Still, thorny-headed worms aren't a problem for mature chickens — but they can devastate chicks under 3 weeks of age. Prevention is simple enough: keep baby chicks away from areas where pillbugs congregate.

Controlling Worms

A chicken in a healthy environment becomes resistant to worms as it matures, unless some other condition triggers a parasite overload. Controlling parasitic worms in growing chickens therefore requires good management rather than constant medication. Not only can parasites become resistant to medication, but deworming becomes an expensive and never-ending cycle unless you take measures to eliminate, or at least minimize, sources of infection.

Reducing the need for deworming medications includes providing a proper diet: a diet that's high in vitamin A, the B-complex vitamins, and animal protein enhances immunity to roundworms. Good management also involves these sensible parasite control measures:

- Practice good housing sanitation, including proper bedding management.

- Clean feeders and drinkers often.

- Control intermediate hosts.

- Rotate the pasture of outdoor chickens, and mow or till the previous pasture.

- Avoid overcrowding, which can rapidly lead to a worm overload.

- Avoid mixing chickens of different ages from different sources.

- Raise turkeys separately from chickens.

Most worms spend part of their life cycles off the bird's body, offering a good handle on parasite prevention and control. To avoid direct-cycle parasites, design housing so chickens can't pick in droppings that accumulate under roosts, or regularly clean out the droppings. To avoid indirect-cycle parasites, keep intermediate hosts away from the coop. Take care when using insecticides, though, since chickens can be poisoned from eating poisoned insects. When possible, use an insecticide only in an unoccupied house, then thoroughly clean up before housing the flock.

Deworming

A healthy chicken can tolerate a certain amount of parasitic invasion. Avoid using a dewormer unless parasites cause your chickens to look scrawny and scruffy, lose weight, and lay fewer eggs. If worms get out of control and reach the point where they begin to affect the chicken's health, you may have no choice but to use a dewormer, more properly called an anthelmintic (from the Greek words *anti*, meaning "against," and *helmins*, meaning "worms") or a vermifuge (from the Latin words *vermis*, meaning "worm," and *fugare*, meaning "to drive away").

Earliest Age at Which a Chicken Is Infected by Mature Worms

WORM	CHICKEN AGE
Capillary worm	3 weeks
Cecal worm	8 weeks
Gapeworm	1 week
Roundworm	4 weeks
Tapeworm	5 weeks

After you've used one dewormer for a time, parasites will become resistant to it, which takes between eight and ten generations. To minimize the development of resistant strains, avoid always using the same anthelmintic. Don't switch too quickly, though, or the parasites may become resistant to *all* the dewormers you use. Since all the dewormers in the same chemical group work the same way, avoiding resistance involves rotating chemical groups, not just brand names.

In the old days anthelmintics worked against a narrow range of parasites. Today's more potent wormers work against a wider variety, and they work in two ways: by interfering with the parasite's feeding pattern (in other words, starving it) or by paralyzing the parasite so it is expelled live in the chicken's droppings. Different dewormers may be administered to chickens in the following ways:

- Orally, placed directly in the beak as a liquid or paste

- Applied as drops on the skin

- Injected under the skin

- Added to drinking water as a liquid or soluble powder

The first three methods require handling individual chickens, which is time consuming but more effective than treating the drinking water. The problem with adding a dewormer to the drinking water is that you have no way of knowing whether each bird gets an adequate dose. Some dewormers may be added to feed, either in powder form or as a liquid solution, which also results in some chickens getting more than an adequate dose and others getting less.

Withdrawal Time

All dewormers are transported throughout the chicken's body, metabolized, and eventually excreted. But different dewormers require different amounts of time before they disappear entirely from a bird's body. Any drug approved for use in poultry has an established withdrawal period — the amount of time it takes before the drug no longer shows up in the bird's meat or eggs.

The withdrawal period for the only dewormer approved for meat birds, piperazine, is 14 days. No dewormer is approved for table egg production, because the development of each egg, starting with maturing of the yolk

Parasitic worm eggs and larvae dry out fairly rapidly when exposed to air and sunlight. Rotating pasture and mowing the grass or tilling the soil of the previous pasture exposes worms, larvae, and eggs to sunlight, helping reduce the overall population. In a rainy climate, or where rainfall is higher than usual, worm eggs and larvae in the environment are protected from drying out by moisture and mud, allowing more to survive and increasing the potential for worm overloads in chickens.

in the ovary, occurs over such a long period of time that few studies have been done to establish exactly how many eggs must be laid before drugs no longer appear in the eggs.

Although the occasional inadvertent deworming probably wouldn't hurt most people, potentially serious problems can arise. Piperazine, for an example, is used to treat humans for roundworms and pinworms. Residual piperazine in meat or eggs could result in resistant roundworms and pinworms in humans who regularly eat such meat or eggs. (How the humans become infected with worms is another issue; they don't get the parasites from chickens.)

A second problem arises in someone who is allergic to the drug in question, or to a related medication. Again using piperazine as an example, anyone allergic to the solvent ethylenediamine may experience an allergic reaction to piperazine residue in meat or eggs.

A third issue is that a dewormer may interact with certain prescription medications. Such an interaction might increase the risk of side effects or cause some medical problems to become worse.

If you check online for information on a dewormer other than piperazine, you will likely find specific withdrawal times mentioned. Some of these withdrawal times are the result of guesswork or misinformation; others are established in countries where the drug in question is approved for use in poultry. Unfortunately, people who post this type of information don't always tell you what country they're in or where they obtained their information. The only way to determine a drug's withdrawal time is to check the label or visit the manufacturer's website.

Approved Dewormers

Among commercially available dewormers for backyard chickens, your options are limited. The only readily available FDA-approved drugs are piperazine and hygromycin-B.

Piperazine

Piperazine (trade name Wazine) is approved for large roundworms, the only helminth it affects. It is relatively nontoxic and therefore has a wide safety margin, although its continuing use over many years has led to widespread resistant strains of ascarids.

Piperazine is rapidly absorbed and rapidly excreted and requires a large dose to be effective. It acts as a narcotic, weakening and paralyzing mature worms and causing them to be expelled from the chicken, live, with a bird's digestive wastes. Chickens that are heavily infected may release an alarming number of worms, which die soon after being expelled. Since worms that are not completely paralyzed may not be released, some chicken keepers follow deworming with a flush (as described on page 392) to remove any worms that might have been left behind.

Piperazine works best as an oral dose of 50 mg per bird under 6 weeks of age; otherwise 100 mg per bird. The next most effective method, and one that's more practical for larger flocks, is to add piperazine water-wormer to the birds' sole source of drinking water at the rate of 1 ounce per gallon for 4 hours, by which time all the water should have been drunk and must be replaced with fresh water.

Piperazine affects only mature roundworms. When an embryonated egg hatches in a chicken's intestine, within 7 days the new young worm attaches itself to the bird's intestinal lining. Although this immature form does more damage than an adult roundworm, during the 10 days it remains embedded in the intestine, piperazine can't touch it. Whenever you deworm your flock, repeat the treatment in 7 to 10 days, giving young worms time to release their hold on the intestinal lining.

Piperazine comes in varying strengths, so always follow dosage recommendations on the label. The withdrawal period for meat birds is 14 days. Piperazine is not approved for hens laying eggs for human consumption.

Hygromycin-B

Hygromycin-B (trade names Hygromix 8, Rooster Booster Multi-Wormer) is sold as a multipurpose dewormer for controlling capillary worms, cecal worms, and large roundworms. It kills mature worms, reduces the ability of female worms to lay eggs, kills some larvae, and renders surviving larvae unable to reproduce when they mature. Controlling worms with hygromycin can therefore take several weeks.

As a feed additive, hygromycin is approved for all chickens, including laying hens. It has a low absorption rate and, according to the manufacturer, leaves "no significant residue" in eggs, therefore requires no egg discard period. The withdrawal time for meat birds is 3 days.

However, and this is a huge however for anyone concerned about the use of antibiotics in food production (see Antibiotic Caveats on page 244): hygromycin is an antibiotic. To repeat, so you can be certain this is not a misprint: hygromycin is an antibiotic.

Not only that, but Hygromix 8 contains a second antibiotic, tylosin phosphate, which is used in industrial chicken production as a feed additive to increase rate of weight gain, improve feed efficiency, and control chronic respiratory disease. Rooster Booster also contains a second antibiotic, bacitracin methylene disalicylate, a feed additive used to improve rate of weight gain, increase feed efficiency, and control different types of enteritis (intestinal diseases that generally result in diarrhea).

If you are concerned about the indiscriminate use of antibiotics in food production, you might want to think twice about deworming your chickens with hygromycin.

Off-Label Ivermectin and Levamisole

Many flock owners use drugs that are not approved. Such use is considered off-label or, when prescribed by a veterinarian, extra-label. Using any of them on chickens raised for the purpose of selling their eggs or meat is illegal.

Drug approval for chickens doesn't change often. Since industrially confined chickens aren't likely to be infected by parasites (they are not exposed to them), drug manufacturers do not recognize a lucrative market for new dewormers. However, with the increase in popularity of backyard chickens and the trend toward pasturing commercial flocks, that may change. Check with your state poultry specialist, veterinarian, or veterinary products supplier regarding the latest regulations. Carefully follow the label directions of any drug you use.

The following dewormers are those most commonly given to backyard flocks. Since their use on chickens is off-label, withdrawal periods either have not been established or have not been published for fear of appearing to imply approval.

Ivermectin (brand name Ivomec) is a systemic livestock and human dewormer that is effective against a wide variety of internal and external parasites, but it can be toxic to chickens in relatively small amounts. It works by paralyzing worms, which are then released in the chicken's poop. Most farm stores sell ivermectin as a cattle dewormer in one of three liquid forms: injectable, drench (administered by mouth), and pour-on. The injectable and drench forms may be either given to chickens individually by mouth at the rate of 0.25 cc per large breed or 6 to 7 eyedropper drops (0.1 cc) per bantam, or else added to drinking water at the rate of 4 cc (4 mL) per gallon for 2 days. The pour-on form has an oil base and is not suitable for internal use. Instead it is applied as drops to the skin at the back of the neck, and it gradually releases into the chicken's body: 1 eyedropper drop per tiny bantam, 3 drops per regular-size bantam, 4 per lightweight breed, 5 per heavy breed, and 6 for a mondo-size or especially fluffy chicken. Repeat in 2 weeks. Chicken keepers who regularly use ivermectin to control external parasites find that internal parasites eventually become resistant to it.

Levamisole, the active ingredient in tetramisole, is effective against a wide variety of roundworms. It acts on a worm's nervous system, paralyzing the worm and causing it to be expelled, live, with digestive wastes. Levamisole drench may be added to drinking water at the rate of 10 cc (10 mL) per gallon for 1 day only. Levamisole injectable is injected under the skin one time only at the rate of ¼ cc per 2 pounds of body weight (25 mg/kg). Levamisole should not be used on severely debilitated chickens, because it can decrease a bird's ability to fight infection. In humans it is used to treat colon cancer.

Off-Label Benzimidazoles

Benzimidazole is an aromatic compound used in creating a variety of organic medications with antimicrobial and anthelmintic properties, including several broad-spectrum dewormers with limited residual effect and a wide margin of safety. They kill worms by disrupting their energy metabolism and, unlike most other dewormers, are effective against tapeworms as well as roundworms. The following benzimidazoles are those most often used for poultry.

Albendazole (trade name Valbazen) is effective against all types of worms affecting chickens; it is also used on humans. Only a small amount is needed. To ensure the drug spreads adequately throughout the intestine, measure out the appropriate dosage (based on the bird's weight) in a 3 cc syringe, then draw in enough water to bring the total up to 1 cc. One dose should be enough to kill any type of worm, but to be certain, repeat treatment in 2 weeks.

Fenbendazole (brand names Panacur and Safe-Guard) is effective against most worm species that affect chickens. It comes as a powder, liquid, or a paste. The powder form is added to feed at the rate of 1 ounce per 15 to 20 pounds of feed (3 to 4 g/kg feed), dissolved in 1 cup (240 mL) water and mixed into the feed for 1 day. As a liquid it is added to drinking water at the rate of 3 cc (3 mL) per gallon of water. The paste is given individually to chickens, squeezed out in pea-size portions placed inside the beak; repeat in 10 days. Fenbendazole is approved for turkeys (but not for chickens), for which no withdrawal period is required.

Warning:

⚠ Excessive amounts of fenbendazole are toxic to birds. Since the drug metabolizes slowly, overuse can lead to toxicity. Deworming with fenbendazole during the molt can cause newly emerging feathers to be deformed. Deworming breeder cocks may reduce sperm quality.

EASY ORAL DEWORMING

For a small number of chickens, easier than catching each one to squirt dewormer in its beak is to cut a slice of bread into small pieces, soak the appropriate individual dose into each piece, and give one piece to each chicken; that is, assuming your chickens are civilized enough not to steal bread from their neighbor.

Chemical Dewormers

DEWORMER	BRAND NAME	Effective Against:				
		CAPILLARY WORM	CECAL WORM	GAPEWORM	ROUNDWORM	TAPEWORM
Albendazole	Valbazen	X	X	X	X	X
Fenbendazole (liquid)	Panacur, Safe-Guard	**	X	X	X	X
Fenbendazole (paste)	Panacur, Safe-Guard	**	X	X	X	X
Fenbendazole (powder)	Panacur, Safe-Guard	**	X	X	X	X
Ivermectic (drench or injectable)	Ivomec	X	X	X	X	—
Ivermectin (pour-on)	Ivomec	X	—	X	X	—
Levamisol (drench)	Prohibit	X	X	X	X	—
Levamisole (injectable)	Prohibit	X	X	X	X	—
Piperazine	Wazine	—	—	—	X	—
Piperazine	Wazine	—	—	—	X	—

Note: All dewormers except piperazine are off-label for chickens.

*Dosage may vary depending on the strength of the dewormer; always consult the product's label.

**Effective against some, but not all, capillary species

Natural Worm Control

Natural methods of worm control differ from chemical dewormers in not paralyzing or killing existing parasites but rather work by making the environment inside the chicken less attractive, or downright unpleasant, for parasites to take up residence. They are therefore more suited to preventing worms than to removing an existing worm load. In addition to a number of homeopathic and herbal preparations available on the market, following are some of the more popular methods of natural worm control.

BRASSICAS AND CUCURBITS

Some garden vegetables, fed raw, supposedly have vermifuge properties. Among them are brassicas, which include cabbage (as well as broccoli and cauliflower leaves), mustard, nasturtiums, horseradish, radishes, turnips. The sulfurous organic compound responsible for the pungent taste of vegetables in this group supposedly repels internal parasites.

Cucurbits options include cucumbers, pumpkins, and squash, especially the seeds. Raw seeds contain the amino acid cucurbitine, which is marginally effective against tapeworms

Orally, ¼ cc (mL)/bantam, ½ cc (mL)/large breed, repeat in 2 weeks
In water, 3 cc (mL)/gal for 3 days (for gapeworm repeat every 3 weeks)

Orally, pea-size dose/bird, repeat in 10 days (for gapeworm repeat every 3 weeks)

In feed, 1 oz dissolved in 1 cup (240 mL) water, mixed with 15–20 lb feed (3–4 g/kg feed) for 1 day

Orally, ¼ cc (mL)/large breed, 6–7 drops (0.1 cc)/bantam; in water, 4 cc (mL)/gal for 2 days

Drops to back of neck: 3/bantam, 4/lightweight breed, 5/heavy breed, 6/oversize chicken

Orally, ¼ cc (mL)/lb body weight; in water, 10 cc (mL)/gal for 1 day; repeat in 7 days and again in 7 days

Injected under skin, ¼ cc (mL)/2 lb body weight (25 mg/kg)

Orally, 50 mg/bird (<6 weeks of age) 100 mg/bird (≥6 weeks of age) or according to label; repeat in 7–10 days
In water, 3 cc (mL)/gallon, or according to label; repeat in 7 days

by causing degeneration of their reproductive organs. Most reports suggest grinding or chopping the seeds, which is unnecessary except maybe for really big pumpkin and squash seeds, which might be broken up by a quick whirl in a blender. Otherwise, just cut the fresh cucurbit in half and let the chickens work it over.

GARLIC

Garlic is another garden vegetable with potential vermifuge properties that supposedly prevent the eggs of some parasite species from developing into larvae. Garlic may be used in a number of different ways, the easiest of which is to sprinkle dried garlic powder on the chickens' feed.

Fresh garlic cloves may be crushed and fed free choice or added to the drinking water. One water method is to steep crushed garlic cloves in a jar of water for several hours, strain out the garlic, and include the steeped water when filling the drinker. Another water method is to place crushed cloves in a cheesecloth sack or nylon stocking and hang it in the drinker.

For more on garlic, see Garlic Guidelines, page 386.

How often your chickens need deworming, if they need it at all, depends in part on the way your flock is managed. Outdoor chickens may need deworming more often than chickens confined indoors. Caged chickens need deworming least often of all.

Chickens that are kept into old age in the same housing year after year are more likely to need deworming than a flock that is periodically replaced by younger birds following a complete coop cleanup. A flock in a warm, humid climate, where intermediate hosts are prevalent year-round, needs deworming more often than a flock in a cold climate, where intermediate hosts are dormant part of the year. The best way to determine if your chickens need deworming is with a fecal test, described starting on next page.

WORMWOOD

Many species of wormwood have vermifuge properties, which is where the plant gets its name. Some species, such as mugwort (*Artemisia vulgaris*), grow wild. Others, such as tarragon (*Artemisia dracunculus*), are garden herbs.

The active ingredient in wormwood is the oily organic compound thujone, which is a neurotoxin — a poison that affects the nervous system, causing muscle spasms. Used regularly, or in excessive amounts, it can cause convulsions and death, not just to the parasitic worms but also to the chicken.

Different species of wormwood vary in their amount of thujone, making the use of wormwood as a vermifuge potentially hazardous to the chickens' health in more than small amounts. A relatively safe way to use wormwood is to grow it at the edge of the chicken yard and let the birds regulate their own intake. Other herbs that contain thujone include sage, tansy, tarragon, and oregano, and the essential oils derived from these herbs.

DIATOMACEOUS EARTH

Diatomaceous earth (DE) is sometimes fed to chickens as a dewormer on the theory that it dehydrates internal parasites the same way it dehydrates garden insects and external poultry parasites (see Diatomaceous Earth — Signal Word: CAUTION, page 155). But think about it: after absorbing a chicken's saliva, DE becomes wet and no longer absorbent. Further, if it worked the same way on internal parasites as it does on garden insects, it would equally affect a chicken's innards.

Although no one has been able to explain how or why DE works as a vermifuge, many chicken keepers swear by it. *If* it works, one possible explanation might relate to its mineral content, especially calcium. DE contains about 19 percent calcium, and internal parasites are discouraged by a diet that's high in calcium. DE also contains a lot of trace minerals, so feeding it to chickens can be healthful, and the healthier a chicken is, the better able it is to fend off internal parasites.

If you choose to feed DE to your chickens, make sure it is not crystalline or calcined. Also, although DE used for insecticidal purposes is identical to food grade DE, when purchasing the former, make sure it contains no toxic additives.

The generally recognized acceptable rate for feeding diatomaceous earth to chickens is no more than 2 percent of the total feed. In practical terms, that amounts to about 2 cups per 50-pound bag of feed.

EFFECTIVENESS OF NATURAL OPTIONS

No definitive studies on the effectiveness of these natural methods of worm control have been forthcoming. However, many of these remedies provide nutrition in one form or another. So even if they don't — or only marginally — affect the internal parasite population, they still can be beneficial to a chicken's overall health.

At any rate, it's best not to rely entirely on natural methods unless you are certain your chickens are not suffering from an overload of worms, especially if you expect your birds to live into old age. The only way to determine their worm load is with regular fecal exams.

Giving a Fecal Exam

Some internal parasites may be identified by signs that appear in the infected bird's droppings. Examining droppings may therefore help you identify the parasite so you can determine appropriate management changes and/or treatment, and so you can avoid the unnecessary use of dewormers due to guesswork. You may discover that your chickens are not seriously infected with parasites, giving you reason to look for some other cause if your flock is experiencing health issues.

Checking droppings, or, more properly, conducting a fecal examination, can be done by any veterinarian, and even one who doesn't normally deal with chickens should be willing to run a fecal

test for you. You may, however, want to learn how to do your own testing. If you find something you aren't sure of, or that looks serious, you might then have your findings confirmed by a veterinarian before making drastic management changes or initiating potentially inappropriate treatment.

Handle with Care

⚠️ Chicken poop contains a variety of bacteria, as well as parasites, and should always be handled with care. To avoid the possibility of getting a bacterial infection, do not handle poop directly. Use an inverted plastic bag or a disposable wooden stick when collecting or transferring droppings. As an added precaution, wear disposable gloves. Afterward, wash your hands thoroughly. People who should never collect or examine chicken droppings (or any other kind of pet poop) include pregnant women, anyone who is immunosuppressed or fitted with a permanent catheter, and small children.

What You'll Learn

The most common type of fecal exam is a flotation test, which concentrates parasite eggs by mixing chicken poop with a liquid that has a specific gravity greater than the eggs but less than other fecal debris. The lighter eggs float to the top, while the heavier fecal debris sinks to the bottom. A flotation test will tell you if your chickens are infected by roundworms.

Another type of parasite egg that will be revealed by a flotation test is coccidial oocysts. A pictorial guide to help you identify coccidia may be found on page 202.

Most tapeworm eggs are not readily identifiable by flotation because they sink to the bottom with fecal debris. These eggs may be found using a different type of test that examines fecal sediment. On the other hand, since most tapeworms don't shed individual eggs but relatively large whole segments, the segments often may be seen in undiluted poop.

Thorny-headed worm eggs are also too heavy to be identified by flotation. These, too, require a sedimentation test, but are not likely to be found in a well-managed flock.

What You'll See

Conducting your own fecal examinations is not difficult. To get an idea of what's involved, take a fecal sample to your veterinarian and ask to have a look when the sample is placed under a microscope. The vet will help you identify anything that is found. Once you know what you're looking for, you will have an easier time identifying signs of parasites on your own.

The parasites in a bird's digestive tract release eggs, larvae, cysts, segments, and sometimes mature worms in the bird's droppings. Parasites in the respiratory system may be coughed up and swallowed, to appear in the bird's poop. Even external parasites, especially mites, are sometimes pecked by a bird and turn up in its droppings.

If you're checking the whole flock, collect about a dozen samples and mix them together, which may be done by sealing them in a plastic zipper bag and kneading the bag. You can collect droppings from the ground or floor, if you're certain they're fresh. The best samples are no older than about half an hour. Otherwise, storing the samples —well sealed, of course — in the refrigerator, but not the freezer, will help keep them fresh for a few hours. The sample need not be solid poop. Loose droppings and diarrhea may be floated just as readily as normal poop.

Examine the sample for clearly visible signs of dead worms or tapeworm segments. Whether or not you find anything, the next step is to examine the sample under a microscope. The most likely thing you'll see is parasite eggs. Some eggs are unique and easy to recognize. Others are quite similar within a group, making it difficult to tell one species from another. Either way, you'll need to consult a pictorial guide such as the one on pages 193 to 195.

Some things a bird eats that turn up in its poop may resemble parasites. Such pseudoparasites include air bubbles, hairs, mold spores, pollen grains, grain mites, and corn smut spores. The latter may easily be mistaken for tapeworm eggs.

What You'll Need

To conduct a fecal examination, besides a sample of fresh poop, you'll need the following items:

- **Flotation solution.** This solution allows the heavier fecal debris to settle to the bottom, while the lighter parasite eggs float to the top. Many different kinds of solutions are available, designed for detecting different kinds of parasites. A solution with a specific gravity of between 1.2 and 1.3 works best for most parasite eggs. Below 1.2 most eggs sink; above 1.3 fecal debris floats to the top right along with the parasite eggs.

  Most laboratories use a sodium nitrate solution (brand name Fecasol), which has an ideal specific gravity of 1.25. A readily available solution for home use is Sheather's Sugar Flotation Solution, which has a specific gravity of 1.27.

Taking a Single Fecal Sample

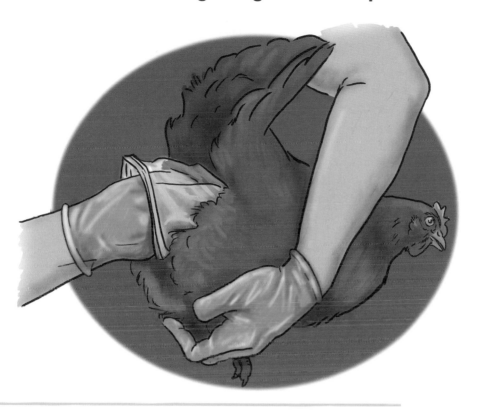

To obtain a sample from a single chicken (for example, a new one you plan to introduce into your flock), turn a plastic zipper bag inside out and place your hand inside it, gently press the abdomen to persuade the bird to do its duty into the bag, then roll up the bag around the sample and seal it.

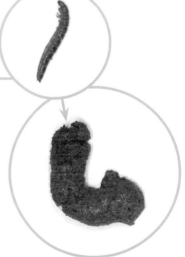

This nasty-looking critter found in a chicken's colon turns out to be a beetle larva eaten by the chicken and not well digested.

You can make your own flotation solution by dissolving magnesium sulfate (Epsom salt) in water at the rate of about 2 cups Epsom salt per quart of water (515 g/L). Half-fill a clean quart jar with warm water and stir in ¼ cup Epsom salt. Using a whisk helps the salt dissolve more rapidly. Continue adding salt and stirring until no more salt will dissolve, as indicated by some salt settling to the bottom of the jar. Sealed in the jar and left at room temperature, your solution will last for months. The specific gravity of this solution is 1.296.

- **A specimen cup and strainer.** The cup holds the poop and flotation solution, the strainer separates out the heavier particles while letting through the finer worm eggs. The most convenient type of cup and strainer is a fecal flotation device (brand name Fecalyzer), which is a combination specimen cup and a strainer. Fecalyzers are inexpensive and come in boxes of 50. If you don't need that many, you might get a few from a small-animal vet who uses them. Be sure to explain that you plan to do your own fecal exam so you don't get charged for an exam as well as the container. To dispose of the used Fecalyzer, snap on the lid and discard it.

- **Glass microscope slides and cover slips.** For viewing a fecal sample you'll need a glass slide and a cover slip. Blank microscope slides and cover slips are sold by the box, usually containing 50 or more. They are available at medical supply outlets, may be ordered by your local druggist, or may be purchased at greatscopes.com. The slides are 1 inch by 3 inches (25 by 76 mm). To fit a Fecalyzer you'll need 22 mm cover slips.

- **A microscope.** A good microscope is expensive but worth the price if you are serious about doing your own fecal exams. A microscope that magnifies 40X, 100X, and 400X is ideal, although a less expensive microscope that magnifies 40X, 100X, and 300X is sufficient. The platform on which the slide is placed is called the stage. A slide is easier to scan on a stage that can be moved back and forth mechanically, compared to a stationary stage that requires you to move the slide by hand. A good microscope is expensive but worth the price if you are serious about selecting a microscope is microscopes.org; a good place to get a decent one at a reasonable price is greatscopes.com.

- **An eyedropper.** Any kind of eyedropper is useful for adding flotation solution to the Fecalyzer.

- **Pincers or tweezers.** An ordinary pair of tweezers is handy for removing large pieces of fecal debris and for handling microscope cover slips. Some student microscopes come with a pair of tweezers.

- **A parasite egg identification guide.** Many parasitology books are available, although most of them include parasites that affect many different species, are rarely comprehensive for chickens only, and tend to be expensive. The parasite egg identification guide on pages 193 to 195 is offered to get you started. A similar guide for coccidial oocysts appears on page 202.

To speed up the separation of eggs from other fecal matter, veterinarians use a centrifuge, a machine that spins a container to separate particles of varying densities. At home, you'll just have to wait for the eggs to float to the top.

Flotation Method

The Fecalyzer consists of a white plastic cup with a lid, inside of which is a separate green plastic basketlike strainer. Small holes in the strainer allow parasite eggs and other fine material to float upward in the flotation solution while keeping larger pieces at the bottom of the container. At the bottom of the strainer is a poop-collection tube.

Pry the green strainer from the cup and use it to scoop up a blob of poop. Set the strainer into the cup without pressing down on it.

Pour in a little flotation solution (or squirt it in with your eyedropper) until the cup is about half full, as indicated by the arrow embossed on the side of the cup. Rotate the strainer back and forth a few times to thoroughly mix solution into the poop. Then turn the strainer until it hits a stop, and press down on it to lock it in place.

Place the Fecalyzer on a table or other solid surface, and use the eyedropper to add more solution until the cup is filled all the way to the top and then some. The solution should rise above the rim of the container but not overflow, creating a curved bulge of liquid called a meniscus. The eyedropper gives you good control to prevent overflow.

With a pair of tweezers, carefully set a cover slip on top of the meniscus, taking care not to leave an air bubble beneath the slip or jostle the Fecalyzer so it spills. To give parasite eggs (and oocysts) time to rise to the surface of the solution and stick to your cover slip, leave the cover slip in place for 15 to 20 minutes.

Using your tweezers, lift the cover slip straight upward off the solution. Gently place the slip, wet side down, in the center of a clean microscope slide. Any parasite eggs will be between the cover slip and the slide. Tap the cover slip gently with your fingernail or tweezers to remove air bubbles and excess solution, but avoid pressing or squeezing the cover onto the slide.

SIMPLE SEDIMENTATION TEST

A simple sedimentation test is used to find parasite eggs that are too heavy to float, which includes thorny-headed worm eggs, along with some tapeworm and some roundworm eggs. Use a tongue depressor or Popsicle stick to place a marble-size blob of poop into a paper cup. Add about ¼ cup (50 mL) of tap water, and stir thoroughly with the tongue depressor.

With a double layer of cheesecloth or a tea strainer that's used only for this purpose (it will no longer be usable for food purposes), strain the liquid into a second paper cup and discard the first cup, along with the strained-out solids. Set the second cup aside for about an hour, then use an eyedropper to carefully remove the liquid floating on the top.

Stir in about 1 teaspoon (5 mL) of tap water, and repeat the procedure. After siphoning off the floating liquid with an eyedropper, stir the remaining sediment, and place a few drops on a microscope slide. Place a cover slip over the sample, and systematically examine it at 100X total magnification.

Systematically examine the specimen, starting with your microscope set at 100X total magnification. Most parasite eggs are somewhat difficult to spot because they have little color. Reducing the brightness of your microscope's light helps increase contrast. Since not all parasite eggs are the same size, adjusting the focus as you scan is also helpful. If you spot something interesting, increase the microscope's light and increase the total magnification to 300X or 400X to get a closer look.

What You'll Find

Compare any eggs you find to the worm egg identification guide that starts on the next page. If you are looking for coccidiosis, consult the oocyst identification guide on page 202.

Finding a few parasite eggs is normal and not usually cause for alarm. An exception would be in a chicken that is already suffering from some other disease. Many otherwise healthy chickens carry a few parasites without being affected. Or a chicken might have a strong enough immune system to prevent the rapid replication of parasites (particularly coccidia), but not strong enough to eliminate them.

If, on the other hand, your chickens are showing signs of being infected by a parasite, but you find only a few eggs, or none, run another fecal exam 2 weeks to a month later. It's possible the chickens were so recently infected that the parasite hadn't yet started shedding eggs when the first test was done.

A count of more than 500 eggs per gram of feces (EPG) is considered a moderate infection, which translates into about a thousand eggs per sample. A count of more than a thousand EPG (or over 2,000 per sample) means prompt treatment is necessary. Of course, you would need a centrifuge to spin this many eggs from any sample, but you can see there's a vast difference between a few eggs on your slide and even a moderate infection.

If you find an alarming number of eggs, or you find signs of parasites that look like they fall into the severe category, take a fecal sample to a veterinarian or send a sample to a diagnostic laboratory for verification.

Worm Egg ID Guide

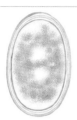

Ascaridia galli (large roundworm)

Length 70–80 μm

Width 45–50 μm

Slightly barrel-shaped with a thick, smooth, three-layer shell and unsegmented contents

Capillaria anatis (capillary worm)

Length 46–67 μm

Width 22–29 μm

Yellowish, rough, thick shell with a plug at each end

Capillaria annulata (capillary worm)

Length 60–65 μm

Width 25–28 μm

Colorless, thick, slightly ridged barrel-shaped shell with a plug at each end

Capillaria bursata (capillary worm)

Length 51–62 μm

Width 22–24 μm

Yellowish shell with fine longitudinal ridges and a plug at each end

Capillaria caudinflata (capillary worm)

Length 47–58 μm

Width 20–24 μm

Yellowish, finely sculptured, thick shell with a plug at each end

Capillaria contorta (capillary worm)

Length 55–66 μm

Width 26–28 μm

Yellowish shell with a plug at each end

Capillaria obsignata (capillary worm)

Length 44–46 µm

Width 22–29 µm

Brownish shell with a netlike pattern and a plug at each end

Cheilospirura hamulosa (gizzard worm)

Length 37–40 µm

Width 26–27 µm

Colorless, ellipsoidal, thick, smooth shell containing a developing larva

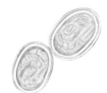

Dispharynx nasuta (spiral stomach worm)

Length 33–40 µm

Width 18–25 µm

Thick shell containing a developing larva

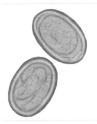

Gongylonema ingluvicola (crop worm)

Length 58 µm

Width 35 µm

Colorless, ellipsoidal, thick, smooth shell containing a developing larva

Heterakis gallinarum (cecal worm)

Length 59–75 µm

Width 31–48 µm

Thick, smooth shell with unsegmented contents; difficult to distinguish from *Ascaridia*

Oxyspirura mansoni (eye worm)

Length 50–65 µm

Width 45 µm

Egg contains a developing larva.

Worm Egg ID Guide

Strongyloides avium (cecal worm)

Length 47–65 μm

Width 25–26 μm

Colorless, thin, broadly elliptical shell containing a developing larva

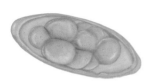

Syngamus trachea (gapeworm)

Length 78–100 μm

Width 43–60 μm

Smooth, slightly barrel-shaped shell, with rounded plugs at both ends, and containing several well-defined cells

Tetrameres americana (stomach worm)

Length 42–50 μm

Width 24 μm

Egg contains a developing larva.

Tetrameres fissispina (stomach worm)

Length 48–56 μm

Width 26–30 μm

Egg contains a developing larva.

Trichostrongylus tenuis (common roundworm)

Length 65–75 μm

Width 35–42 μm

Thin, smooth, oval shell with parallel sides and dissimilar ends

1 μm (micrometer or micron) = 1 millionth of a meter, or about 0.000039 inch

CHAPTER 7

Diseases Caused by Protozoa

Protozoa are single-cell animal-like creatures that live in damp habitats. They are considered to be like animals because they breathe, eat, and move around similarly to animals. They are the simplest members of the animal kingdom and also the smallest — too small to see without a microscope. Many protozoa are harmless, but others are parasites that cause serious illnesses. Luckily, the worst protozoan parasites are rare or not found in North America.

The most common protozoal diseases of chickens are caused by coccidia, which are microscopic. They have a life cycle involving both sexual and asexual reproduction and become infective as sporozoites, a stage that develops asexually outside the chicken. The coccidial disease coccidiosis is the most common of all chicken diseases. The less common coccidial diseases that affect chickens are cryptosporidiosis and toxoplasmosis. Two other less common protozoal diseases of chickens are blackhead and canker.

Coccidiosis

The most widely known protozoal disease of poultry, coccidiosis is caused by nine different species of protozoa known as coccidia in the genus *Eimeria*. Cocci is the most likely cause of death in growing birds, usually striking chicks 3 to 6 weeks of age. The worst cases typically occur at 4 to 5 weeks of age.

Coccidia are found wherever there are chickens. Even in the healthiest flock, coccidia are present in the intestines of most birds over 3 weeks old. Gradual exposure (or surviving an infection) confers immunity, and by maturity most chickens are immune to the coccidia in their immediate environment. An exception is chickens whose resistance has been reduced by some other disease. Marek's disease and infectious bursal disease are especially known to prevent chicks from developing the same immunities as healthy chicks normally do.

A flockwide infection with devastating consequences can occur when a large number of growing or mature birds are brought together from different sources, since they may not all have been exposed to the same species of coccidia and therefore may cross-infect each other. Infections also occur where sanitation is poor or birds are overly stressed because of crowding, a drastic change in rations, being moved, or some abrupt change in the weather.

Eimeria Life Cycle

Eimeria have short, direct life cycles. An infected chicken poops out egg cysts, or oocysts, each of which is basically a fertilized parasite egg encapsulated within a cyst. Fresh oocysts are initially noninfective, but given the right environment, they develop, or sporulate, and become infective.

Sporulation takes only a day or two and occurs in moist environments where the temperature ranges between 70°F and 90°F (21°C and 32°C). After sporulation each egg cyst contains four internal cysts, and each internal cyst encloses two infective sporozoites. Sporulated oocysts can remain in the environment for many months unless they are destroyed by freezing temperatures or hot (above 130°F/54°C), dry conditions.

Protozoal Diseases

DISEASE	GENERA	AFFECTS	PREVALENCE
Blackhead	*Histomonas*	Ceca and liver	Rare
Canker	*Trichomonas*	Mouth and throat	Uncommon
Coccidiosis	*Eimeria*	Intestine and/or ceca	Common
Cryptosporidiosis (intestinal)	*Cryptosporidium*	Digestive system, cloacal bursa, urinary tract	Common in confined chickens
Cryptosporidiosis (respiratory)	*Cryptosporidium*	Respiratory system	Uncommon
Toxoplasmosis	*Toxoplasma*	Central nervous system	Sporadic

When a chicken ingests a sporulated oocyst in feed or water or by pecking at the ground, the external cyst wall is crushed by the bird's gizzard, releasing the four internal cysts. When these cysts reach the chicken's duodenum, digestive enzymes break down the cyst walls to release the zoites, which then invade the intestinal lining. Different species of coccidia prefer different parts of the intestine.

Once they settle in, the zoites proliferate explosively by asexual reproduction through up to four generations (depending on their species) and eventually transform into sexually reproducing forms that produce hundreds of thousands of fertilized eggs, each of which is encased within a cyst. The oocysts break away from the intestinal wall and enter the environment in the chicken's poop, where they get spread around in the soil, bedding, feed, and water by the feet of birds, rodents, insects, and human caretakers. They also spread through the air in blown dust.

The entire cycle goes fast, taking a week or less from the time a sporulated oocyst enters a chicken's body until millions of fresh oocysts are generated and released. Infected and recovering birds thus shed countless oocysts that contaminate the flock's environment. As birds either die or recover and the infection plays out, the number of shed oocysts decreases but never dwindles to zero.

Since the life cycle quickly ends for the initially consumed oocysts, coccidiosis is a self-limiting disease with potentially inconsequential results. How seriously a bird is infected depends on the number of infective oocysts it ingests — in a highly contaminated environment, one chicken may consume as many as one million sporulated oocysts, causing extensive and perhaps irreparable damage to its intestinal wall. The survivor of a severe infection will recover in about 2 weeks but may never thrive.

By cycling through a chicken, coccidia cause intestinal damage that not only stimulates active immunity but also reduces the intestine's ability to absorb nutrients, affecting the growth rate of young birds and the laying ability of hens. Damaged intestines also increase the chicken's susceptibility to the fatal bacterial disease necrotic enteritis, as well as to other diseases involving the intestinal tract, including other species of coccidia than the one that produced the initial infection.

Eimeria Species

Eimeria protozoa come in many species that infect nearly every kind of livestock, but each is highly species specific, meaning the coccidia that invade chickens do not affect other species of livestock, and vice versa. Even different species of birds are infected by different species of coccidia.

Nine species of *Eimeria* protozoa invade chickens, but not all of them cause serious disease. The fact that a chicken may be infected with more than once species at a time increases the likelihood of a serious infection. Each species is identifiable by the following traits:

- The appearance of the oocysts — their size, shape, and color

- The minimum time required for sporulation under ideal conditions (12 to 30 hours)

- The amount of time that passes between ingestion of a sporulated oocyst and the appearance of sporozoites in the chicken's tissue (4 to 7 days)

- The preferred location in a chicken's intestinal tract

- The number of asexually reproduced generations within the chicken (2 to 4)

- Signs of infection (described in the table on page 200)

- Postmortem findings

- The protozoa's DNA sequence

The easiest traits for a backyard chicken keeper to identify are the signs exhibited by an infected chicken and the location of the infection within the intestinal tract of a dead chicken. The most likely cause of coccidiosis in North America is *Eimeria acervulina*. The species that produce the worst infections, which come on rapidly and can result in a high death rate, are *E. tenella* and *E. necatrix*. *E. tenella* generally infects chicks 3 to 6 weeks of age, while *E. necatrix* takes longer to develop and therefore is more likely to occur in chickens that are reaching maturity.

Signs of Cocci

Coccidia populations in a brooder take time to accumulate to dangerous levels, so chicks rarely become infected before they are 3 weeks old. As one of the first signs, chicks eat less at a time when you would expect growing chicks to gradually eat more. Other signs include slow growth, a change in the droppings (runny, off-color, sometimes tinged with blood), and dehydration due to diarrhea. The disease may come on slowly, or bloody diarrhea and death may come on fast, depending on the species of coccidia involved. (Don't confuse bloody droppings with normal sloughing of the intestinal lining, described as "pink tissue" on page 332.)

Speaking of Coccidiosis

acute. Having a severe and swift development

chronic. Describes a long-lasting disease that develops gradually and is difficult to treat

coccidia. Microscopic single-cell protozoa that have a life cycle involving both sexual and asexual reproduction, become infective in the asexually produced sporozoite stage, and multiply in the intestinal tract

nutraceutical. A food that provides health benefits, including the prevention and treatment of disease

oocyst. A tough membrane, or cyst, containing the fertile egg of a parasitic protozoa

protozoa. One-cell microscopic organisms with animal-like characteristics

self-limiting. Describes a disease that goes away without treatment

species specific. Associated with or affecting a single species

sporocyst. A tough membrane, or cyst, enclosing sporozoites within an oocyst

sporozoite. The infective stage of a parasitic protozoa

sporulate. The asexual development of sporozoites within an oocyst

unthrifty. Eating well while growing thin or laying poorly

virulence. The degree of infectiveness of a pathogen as indicated by the severity or harmfulness of the disease it produces

In hens reaching the age of lay, an early sign is slow or no egg production. Breeds with yellow shanks and skin may turn pale from the reduced ability of their intestines to absorb pigments from feeds. Maturing birds that are recovering and appear healthy become a source of infection for younger birds.

If you suspect coccidiosis, a fecal exam (described on page 187) will tell you whether

Identifying Coccidial Species by Signs*

SPECIES	PREVALANCE	SIGNS	DEATH RATE	USUAL AGE
E. acervulina	The most common	Long duration; slow growth; watery, whitish diarrhea	Usually low to none; varies with strain	2½–4 weeks
E. brunetti	Uncommon	Slow growth; bloody diarrhea	Moderate to high	Reaching maturity
E. hagani	Uncommon	Usually none; possible watery diarrhea	None	N/A
E. maxima	Common	Pale skin; bloody or off-color droppings	Low to moderate	3½–5 weeks
E. mitis	Common	Slow growth or weight loss	Usually none	Any age
E. mivati	Common	Slow growth	Low	3–5 weeks
E. necatrix	Common	Comes on fast; watery, bloody diarrhea; dehydration	Moderate to high	Reaching maturity
E. praecox	Uncommon	None or slow growth	Usually none	3–5 weeks
E. tenella	Common	Comes on fast; pale skin; bloody droppings	Moderate to the highest	4½–6 weeks

Different species of coccidia prefer different parts of a chicken's intestines. Cecal coccidiosis (E. tenella) causes acute infection, resulting in pale skin, bloody droppings, and often death. Intestinal coccidiosis (all other species) is more typically chronic and less likely to end in death. For postmortem identification of each species, see Identifying Coccidiosis by Intestinal Lesions on page 433.

LEVELS OF SEVERITY

Coccidiosis infection in chickens can result in one of three distinct levels of severity.

- **Acute coccidiosis** — The severest level causes bloody diarrhea and sometimes death. This level is most likely to occur in chicks brooded in an unsanitary environment or in chickens that are exposed to coccidia without having developed immunity.

- **Chronic coccidiosis** — A mild level that produces no readily identifiable signs other than affected chickens fail to thrive and lay well, a condition old-timers call unthrifty. This level is most likely to occur in chickens that forage in a large area or in rotated areas, where they avoid exposure to large numbers of oocysts.

- **Coccidiasis** — A condition that produces no detectable signs of infection. This level is most likely to occur in chickens that have developed immunity through gradual exposure. It may also result from exposure to species of coccidia that are associated with chickens but don't cause disease.

or not your birds are shedding oocysts and can help pinpoint the species. Several tests may be required to identify the species, since often more than one species is involved, and an infected chicken does not shed oocysts at a steady rate. If you conduct a postmortem examination (see chapter 13), do so immediately after death — within an hour tissue changes begin to occur that make diagnosis more difficult.

Damage to intestinal tissue typically occurs before the first signs become noticeable. Intestinal damage makes chicks more susceptible to a bacterial infection such as salmonellosis or necrotic enteritis. Conversely, coccidiosis is worse in a flock that's combating some other illness: for instance, coccidiosis often follows an outbreak of infectious bursal disease.

Chickens with damaged intestines may never become as productive as unaffected birds. A severe infection can destroy the intestinal lining, resulting in hemorrhaging and death. A wise move is to manage your chickens with cocci in mind, rather than waiting to treat the disease after it occurs.

Controlling Cocci

Coccidiosis cannot be eliminated from the environment of chickens. Therefore, controlling coccidia is the key to maintaining good health in your flock. Measures for controlling coccidiosis involve, in order of preference:

- Good management
- The use of drugs
- Vaccination

GOOD MANAGEMENT

The more chickens you have, the trickier coccidiosis can be to control. All chickens are exposed to infective oocysts throughout their lives. A well-managed flock develops resistance through gradual exposure, a concept known as trickle infection. The more naturally this immunity develops, the healthier your chickens will be (see The Dirt on Dirt, page 30).

Good management begins with adequate nutrition. Nutritional deficiencies of vitamins A, E, and K and in the mineral selenium can predispose chicks to coccidiosis. A good-quality chick starter should provide these nutrients. Other sources of vitamins A and K include dark leafy greens such as spinach, parsley, and Swiss chard. Additional sources of vitamin A are pumpkins and sweet potatoes. For vitamin E you couldn't find a better source than sunflower seeds. Providing a source of selenium can be problematic: Plants that grow in selenium-rich soils are high in selenium; plants that grow in selenium-deficient soils are low in selenium. And although selenium is a necessary micronutrient, too much can be toxic.

In addition to ensuring that your chickens get adequate nutrition, good management involves controlling coccidiosis by limiting the number of infective oocysts the chickens are exposed to while they develop immunity. The tricky part is getting the balance just right — chickens that are exposed to too many oocysts at once will get sick, while chickens that are insufficiently exposed to infective oocysts cannot develop immunity.

Control infective oocysts by keeping feed and drinking water free of droppings and making sure chicks never run out of feed, so they aren't tempted to peck in the bedding looking for something to eat. But even chicks brooded on wire, where their droppings fall through the floor, can succumb to coccidiosis if they ingest

Typical Signs in All Chickens

- Hunched up and inactive, with ruffled feathers

- Off-color or bloody droppings

- Eating less

- Drinking less

- Dehydration

Additional Signs in Growing Chickens

- Slow growth

- Severe diarrhea

- Numerous deaths

Additional Signs in Maturing Chickens

- Slow or no egg production

- Loss of pigment in skin and shanks

- Weight loss

Factors Influencing Susceptibility and Severity

- Chickens' age (rare in fully mature chickens)

- Status of acquired immunity

- Inherited resistance or susceptibility

- Nutritional balance of daily rations

- Other diseases occurring at the same time (reducing resistance)

- Number of infective oocysts consumed

- Virulence of the strain of coccidial species

NANOMETERS

10 20 30

E. acervulina

E. brunetti

E. hagani

E. maxima

E. mitis

E. mivati

E. necatrix

E. praecox

E. tenella

1 nanometer = 1 billionth of a meter

A fecal exam (as described on page 187) can help you determine if your chickens have coccidiosis and may reveal which species of coccidia is involved, based on the appearance of oocysts.

sufficient numbers of infective oocysts in contaminated feed or water.

Unless the brooder is overcrowded, though, chicks brooded on wire normally do not develop immunity through trickle infection. When they are later moved from the brooder, they lack immunity to ward off infection and can become seriously ill.

Control of infective oocysts in chicks brooded on bedding means providing adequate dry bedding. Even this seemingly simple concept can be tricky. Fresh litter can provide the perfect combination of temperature, moisture, and oxygen that allows fertilized oocysts to sporulate and become infective. On the other hand, aging litter accumulates a greater number of oocysts but also accumulates ammonia, bacteria, and molds that destroy oocysts. Some old-time farmers (as well as some modern-day chicken keepers) control coccidiosis by letting brooder house litter compost, then reusing it, combined with a little fresh bedding, from year to year to benefit from oocyst-eating microbes living in the compost.

Another tricky aspect of trickle infection is that it confers immunity only to the species of coccidia present in the chickens' environment. Chickens can still get coccidiosis if they are later exposed to other species to which they have not developed immunity.

Controlling coccidiosis is generally easier with free-range chickens and those raised on rotated pasture, compared to chickens that are confined to a limited area. Coccidiosis generally does not affect all chickens at precisely the same time but often starts with a few susceptible birds, which then infect the others. If you spot the early signs in a few chickens, and move the

entire flock to a new pasture or paddock, you can often prevent a serious infection.

Similarly, since oocysts take time to build up in brooder bedding, and they start to reach a peak level by about 3 weeks, simply moving chicks out of the brooder by the time they reach 3 weeks of age offers some measure of control. If moving your birds to fresh ground is not feasible, frequently cleaning and replacing litter will help prevent reinfection.

Preventing reinfection is important because coccidiosis is a self-limiting disease, meaning chickens will recover within a few weeks, with or without treatment. The primary purposes of medicating infected chickens are to minimize the number of coccidia they expel, thus reducing the chance of reinfection; to minimize the

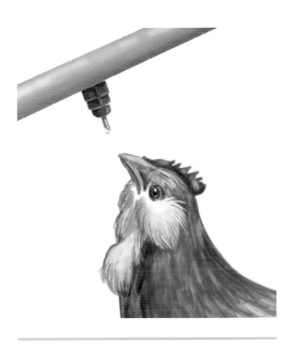

A nipple drinker, properly installed so it won't leak, eliminates the ingestion of oocysts from drinking water.

severity of damage to the intestine; to relieve diarrhea; and to prevent weakened birds from developing a potentially deadly bacterial infection.

NATURAL ANTICOCCIDIALS

A number of feed supplements have been identified as possibly helping chickens ward off a serious bout of coccidiosis. Such supplements include wheat bran, flaxseed oil, linseed oil, fish oil, the spice turmeric (*Curcuma longa*), the herb sweet wormwood (*Artemisia annua*), the herb oregano (*Origanum vulgare*), the herb echinacea (*Echinacea* spp.), neem (*Azadirachta indica*) fruit extract, green tea (*Camellia sinensis*) extract, citric extracts, prebiotics, and probiotics (for more information on prebiotics and probiotics, see page 378).

When using natural feed supplements to control coccidiosis, here are a few important things to keep in mind:

- Not all supplements are effective against all species of coccidia.

- A feed supplement can neither prevent chickens from becoming infected nor cure a serious infection, although supplements may help boost a chicken's immune system to reduce the possibility of a serious infection while the chicken is developing resistance.

GOOD HYGIENE IS GOOD PROTECTION

Here are some easy and commonsense ways to protect brooded chicks and young chickens from being infected with coccidiosis:

- Suspend or raise feeders and drinkers high enough to keep them from accumulating droppings and bedding.

- Clean feeders and drinkers as often as necessary to keep them free of bedding and droppings.

- Keep droppings from building up around feeders and drinkers by moving them often, as space allows.

- Take any measures necessary to prevent chicks from roosting on top of feeders and drinkers and getting their droppings in the feed and water.

- Keep bedding dry; place a wire platform under each drinker to keep drips out of bedding, or use nipple drinkers, properly installed so they don't leak.

- Keep bedding fresh; remove any packed or damp bedding and replace it with clean bedding.

- Make sure the brooder is ventilated well enough for moisture to evaporate rather than condense in the bedding — plastic tote brooders are especially notorious for accumulating excessive moisture.

- Feed supplements in their natural state are not standardized as to potency.

- Current knowledge does not include accurate information on effective amounts or doses of any of these feed supplements, therefore relying on such supplements as a sole means of controlling coccidiosis is not in the best interest of your chickens.

One natural antimicrobial that can be beneficial in preventing the spread of coccidiosis is vinegar, added to drinking water at the rate of 1 tablespoon per gallon (15 mL per 4 L); double the vinegar amount in alkaline water. By acidifying the drinking water, vinegar prevents any protozoa that land in the water from multiplying.

MILK FLUSH

Old-time poultry keepers used milk powder to control coccidiosis by treating infected chicks with a milk flush. Since chickens do not normally encounter lactose as part of their natural diet, when undigested lactose reaches the intestines, the chicken's body wants to flush it out. Accordingly, the intestines draw fluids from the bloodstream, and the influx of moisture results in diarrhea, which flushes out not only the lactose but also the coccidia.

The procedure is to add milk powder to the ration at the rate of 1 pound of milk powder per 3 pounds of ration for up to 7 days. Plenty of water must also be made available to prevent dehydration, since treated chickens drink three times more than usual.

Of course, the loose droppings make a huge mess of the litter, which must be cleaned out and replaced daily. Or if the birds are on pasture, they must be moved to new ground daily. Frequently removing the loose droppings, or moving the chicks away from the mess, keeps the birds from ingesting expelled coccidia, thus preventing reinfection until the disease runs its course.

Some modern chicken keepers believe that milk, offered occasionally or continuously, will prevent coccidiosis. Not so. Feeding an excessive amount of lactose to induce mild diarrhea is a method of *treating* an existing outbreak of coccidiosis.

But treating chickens with a milk flush is not without dangers. The bacterium *Escherichia coli*, which causes the group of infections collectively known as colibacillosis, considers lactose to be prime food. *E. coli* are normally present in small numbers in every chicken's gut, but during times of stress or illness the bacteria can proliferate out of control. Feeding milk to chickens at such times also feeds the *E. coli*, giving them extra nutrients in the form of lactose that allow them to multiply in even greater numbers.

ANTICOCCIDIAL DRUGS

The use of medication is not a substitute for good management. Nevertheless, several drugs are available to prevent or cure coccidiosis. Drugs used for prevention are called coccidiostats; those used for curing are coccidiocides.

Coccidiostats work by allowing a trickle infection to occur, giving chicks time to develop immunity as they grow. These drugs are most commonly used with chickens that are expected to mature into layers or breeders. Coccidiocides kill coccidia. They are most often used to treat an infection in progress but are also used for broilers that are barely old enough to develop immunity by the time they are big enough to be harvested.

Often the same drug may be used in a lower dose as a coccidiostat and in a higher dose or for a longer period as a coccidiocide. Two kinds of drugs are most often used for backyard poultry.

Amprolium is the drug most commonly used as a coccidiostat in medicated starter rations available at the local farm store. It may also be purchased as a liquid or soluble powder (trade names include Amprol and Corid) that is added to drinking water as either a coccidiostat or coccidiocide.

Amprolium is structurally similar to thiamin (vitamin B_1), which coccidia use a lot of to multiply within a chicken's body. By blocking thiamin uptake, amprolium reduces the ability of coccidia to multiply as rapidly as they would otherwise. Although amprolium is not as effective as some other drugs against all species of coccidia, it is relatively safe to use, has no withdrawal time, and is least likely to cause resistance.

In the same way amprolium keeps coccidia from absorbing as much thiamin as they need to replicate, it also limits the absorption of thiamin by the chickens, resulting in a deficiency. After a flock has been treated, offering a vitamin supplement designed for poultry is beneficial. Do not use a vitamin supplement while amprolium is in use, or it will counteract the benefit of the treatment.

Sulfa drugs (sulfonamides) are available in both powder and liquid form to be dissolved in drinking water to treat chickens showing signs of infection. Sulfas inhibit coccidia from replicating by preventing the absorption of folic acid (folate, or vitamin B_9), somewhat like amprolium blocks thiamin.

The safest sulfa for use with chickens is sulfadimethoxine (trade names Albon and Di-Methox). Two others commonly used for backyard flocks are sulfamethazine sodium (Sulmet) and a combination of three sulfonamides (PoultrySulfa); both treatments are effective primarily against *E. necatrix* and *E. tenella*. Since coccidiosis increases a chicken's susceptibility to bacterial infections, the advantage of using sulfas is their antibacterial properties, which help improve the rate of recovery.

However, sulfas can be toxic if used for too long or at too high a dose. The toxic level of sulfamethazine, for instance, is so close to the amount required for treatment that poisoning can occur at a normal dose if hot weather causes the chickens to drink more than usual. Signs of poisoning are depression, paleness, and slow growth. At temperatures above 80°F (27°C), poisoning may be avoided by using one-third the recommended dose.

Sulfa residues can appear in meat and eggs, and some people are allergic to sulfa drugs, so withdrawal times need to be considered (see the table on the next page). Sulfas are not approved for pullets more than 14 weeks old and should never be used for laying hens because the drugs can interfere with egg production. The

Coccidiosis Prevention and Treatment with Amprolium

PURPOSE	MEDICATION	FORM	DURATION	WITHDRAWAL
Prevention	Amprolium	Medicated starter ration	Continuous	None
Treatment	Amprolium	⅓ oz powder/gallon water	10–14 days	None

biggest problem with sulfas is the widespread development of resistance in various species of coccidia.

The use of drugs to prevent chickens from being infected with coccidiosis has these several drawbacks:

- Some drugs produce side effects or are toxic at high levels or after prolonged use.

- Some drugs arrest the development of immunity, paving the way for an infection when they are withdrawn.

- Chickens may not acquire adequate numbers of coccidia for natural immunity to develop.

- The continuous low dose of medication eventually leads to the development of drug-resistant strains of coccidia, requiring combining or rotating the drugs used.

- Broilers treated with an anticoccidial requiring withdrawal may become infected before the withdrawal time is up and the broilers may be safely harvested.

On the other hand, using drugs as a preventive measure has these advantages:

- Once a chicken is infected, its intestines may be severely damaged before signs of disease become noticeable.

- Once a full-blown infection occurs, no drug can stop it completely.

Never Mix, Never Worry

⚠ Anticoccidials work by killing some coccidia while letting others survive, as a way to limit intestinal damage while chickens develop immunity. Vaccines work by introducing a low dose of live coccidia early enough to stimulate an immune response before chicks become exposed to coccidia in sufficient numbers to cause infection. Medicating vaccinated chickens with an anticoccidial drug is counterproductive, because the drug would kill coccidia introduced by the vaccine, thus preventing the chickens from developing the natural immunity the vaccine is designed for. If your chicks have been vaccinated against coccidiosis, take great care not to feed them a medicated ration or medicate their water with any anticoccidial drug.

Anticoccidial Pharmaceuticals*

DRUG	COCCIDIOSTAT (PREVENTION)	COCCIDIOCIDE (TREATMENT)	WITHDRAWAL (DAYS)
Amprolium (Amprol/Corid)	X	X	0
Sulfas:			
Sulfadimethoxine (Albon/Di-Methox)		X	5
Sulfamethazine (Sulmet)		X	10
Triple sulfa combo (PoultrySulfa)		X	14

*Follow the manufacturer's label regarding dosage, length of treatment, and withdrawal time.

Adapted from The Merck Veterinary Manual

VACCINATION

Newly hatched chicks are not susceptible to coccidiosis for two reasons. One is that they are temporarily enjoying the benefit of maternal antibodies (as described in Passive Immunity, on page 28). The other reason is that their immature digestive systems have not yet developed conditions favorable for the replication of coccidia. Early exposure to coccidia therefore offers chicks a chance to develop an immune response.

Chicks that hatch under a hen are naturally exposed to coccidia in their environment right from the start. Chicks raised in a reused brooder may be similarly exposed. If the brooder is new or has been thoroughly sanitized, chicks may be exposed to coccidia by the introduction into the brooder of a little soil from the yard or bedding from a coop that houses a flock of healthy mature chickens. Chicks purchased from a hatchery may be exposed to coccidia by means of vaccine that is sprayed over the chicks and ingested by them during preening.

Vaccines contain a low dose of live, sporulated oocysts that produce a low level of infection. The original coccidia go through their normal life cycle, replicating and reinfecting the vaccinated chicks until the chicks develop immunity. The use of vaccines has these disadvantages:

- By introducing infection, vaccination causes temporary stress; chicks may become slightly droopy for a day or two within about a week of being vaccinated.

- A vaccine must include the species of coccidia to which your chickens are likely to be exposed. Most vaccines do not contain all possible species but do include the common ones. The vaccine Coccivac-B, for instance, contains four of the nine species, while Coccivac-D contains eight.

- Because vaccines rely on the natural cycling of coccidia, if conditions in the brooder are not conducive to the survival of infective oocysts, reinfection will not occur and the vaccine cannot do its job of encouraging an immune response. Appropriate conditions include a bedding moisture of 25 to 30 percent, as determined by squeezing a handful and then letting it go. If the bedding remains clumped together as it falls, moisture is too high (potentially resulting in an overload of infective oocysts); if the bedding releases dust, moisture is too low (resulting in the failure of oocysts to sporulate).

- Vaccinating a few chicks at home is not practical or economical, because the smallest available dose is enough to vaccinate 1,000 chicks, and once the vial is opened, the vaccine must be used right away.

On the other hand, the use of vaccines has these advantages:

- Vaccination is similar to natural exposure by means of a trickle infection.

- Since coccidiosis is self-limiting, the vaccine's low-level exposure prevents a massive buildup of oocysts that would cause a serious infection in growing chicks.

- Newly hatched chicks are relatively immune to a serious infection, so early vaccination gives them a head start in developing natural immunity.

- Vaccinated chicks develop protective immunity by the time they reach the age when nonvaccinated chicks are most likely to become infected.

Vaccine exposes chicks to a small amount of coccidia, causing stimulation of an immune response while also inducing coccidiosis, which is a self-limiting disease (that is, it runs a definite, limited course and then resolves on its own). Oocysts pass in the poop and are repeatedly ingested, increasing the chick's immune response and eventually resulting in naturally acquired immunity.

A chick that is not vaccinated may be exposed to a larger initial amount of coccidia. The same as with vaccination, oocysts induce disease and also pass in the poop to be repeatedly ingested, but in this case they started out so numerous they rapidly overwhelm the chick's immune response, causing the chick to become gravely ill or even die, before its system has time to develop immunity.

- Compared to the use of anticoccidial drugs, vaccination does not cause the development of drug-resistant strains of coccidia.

- A vaccine is not a drug; therefore, it may be used for organic or naturally raised chickens. However, if you are certified for raising organic poultry, confirm with your certifying agency before having chicks vaccinated.

Toxoplasmosis

Another coccidial protozoan, *Toxoplasma gondii,* can cause the disease toxoplasmosis, or toxo, in all warm-blooded animals, including chickens and humans. Toxo in humans is not well understood and in chickens is even less well understood, primarily because the disease rarely produces readily observable symptoms or signs.

Cats and their relatives are the only known animals in which these protozoal parasites sexually reproduce, making cats the primary source of infection. Despite the explosion of small flocks kept in the same yard as the family cat, no one can say just how common toxo might be in backyard chickens.

Toxo Life Cycle

T. gondii has a complex life cycle that allows chickens to become infected in a number of ways. The cycle starts when a cat, within about a month of being infected, poops out fertilized parasite egg cysts, or oocysts. An infected cat sheds egg cysts for only about 2 weeks but during that time can release millions of them. Once the infective stage passes, the cat usually stops shedding oocysts and becomes immune to future infections.

Meanwhile, the oocysts get spread around the environment on the feet of rodents, wild birds, flies, cockroaches, dung beetles, and similar vectors, and sometimes on the wind. In the environment the egg cysts begin subdividing by asexual reproduction and change into the infective sporozoite form. Within 1 to 4 days after leaving the cat, each oocyst contains eight zoites, which will infect any animal that inhales the oocysts in contaminated dust or ingests them from contaminated soil, plants, water, feed, or vectors.

Infective oocysts can survive for 18 months in water or warm, damp soil, but do not survive well in extremely cold climates or hot, dry climates. Toxo is more common in northeastern states than in western states, and more common yet in tropical climates. Contamination of soil by these microscopic parasites is difficult to determine by examining the soil, so ranging chickens on the soil in question and then testing the chickens for toxo antibodies is one way to determine if the soil is contaminated.

Other than cats, infected animals, including chickens, become intermediate hosts. Inside an intermediate host, each zoite rapidly multiplies via asexual reproduction and travels through lymph and blood to invade any part of the host's body. Within about 3 weeks reproduction slows, and the zoites become dormant inside tissue cysts. These cysts most often lodge in the chicken's muscle tissue, around the heart, and in the brain and eyes. Each tissue cyst contains as many as 2,000 zoites, which remain dormant for the life of the infected chicken, although

they will reactivate if ingested by an animal that hasn't previously been infected. In most cases the chicken shows no outward signs of having been infected.

The cycle begins again when a cat that isn't already immune becomes infected. A kitten may be born infected if its mother became infected while pregnant. A cat can become infected by eating an infective oocyst from the environment (such as while chewing on a blade of grass); eating an infected bird, rodent, or other intermediate host; or being fed raw or undercooked meat from an infected chicken. A chicken can become infected not only by ingesting oocysts from the environment, but by picking on the flesh of an infected chicken. Humans can be infected by eating undercooked meat from an infected chicken, as described on page 410.

Life Cycle of *Toxoplasma gondii*

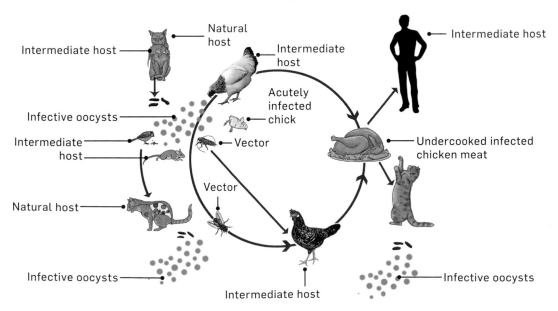

Toxo Signs and Control

While most chickens show no signs of having been infected with toxo, a chicken under the age of about 8 weeks, with its undeveloped immune system, or an older bird that's experiencing stress can develop an acute infection. Such an infection may affect the central nervous system, giving the appearance of Marek's disease or any similar disease that involves the nerves. Signs in acutely affected chickens include a drop in egg production and feed consumption, emaciation, white diarrhea, neck spasms, twisted neck, paralysis, blindness, and sudden death. No effective cure is known.

Control of toxoplasmosis in chickens includes keeping cats out of the chicken yard, not feeding raw or undercooked chicken meat to cats, and controlling filth flies, cockroaches, rodents, and wild birds. Since *T. gondii* thrives in moist environments, avoid puddles in the chicken yard and keep litter dry inside the coop.

Cryptosporidiosis

Cryptosporidiosis, or crypto, is caused by the coccidial protozoa *Cryptosporidium*. Of the many species that infect a variety of animals, including humans, the ones that affect chickens and other birds do not infect mammals or humans, although they may be spread from one flock of chickens to another on the feet of animals and humans.

Cryptosporidiosis is found largely in chickens raised in confinement, especially industrially raised broilers. How common it might be in chickens raised under other types of management has not been determined, as infection is usually mild — often producing no signs other than pale skin in yellow-skinned breeds — and therefore goes largely unnoticed. Because infection is usually not serious, and because infection results in immunity, crypto has not been studied as thoroughly as coccidiosis.

Crypto Species and Life Cycle

Three species of *Cryptosporidium* have been identified as affecting chickens. All three usually cause a mild and usually unnoticeable intestinal infection, although one species may invade the respiratory system and can be deadly.

C. baileyi infects either the respiratory tract or the cloaca and cloacal bursa of young chickens. A cloacal infection results in few visible signs, if any, but can cause atrophy of the cloacal bursa, resulting in immunosuppression and increased susceptibility to avian influenza. The protozoa may also migrate from the cloaca to infect the urinary tract.

A respiratory infection is less common but more severe than an intestinal infection and is likeliest to affect birds in the 4- to 17-week age group. Signs of respiratory infection, caused by inhaling *C. baileyi*, include sneezing, coughing, and other typical signs of a respiratory ailment that can last for up to 4 weeks. Signs of a serious infection include nasal discharge, swollen sinuses and eyelids, and stretching of the neck to facilitate breathing. A serious infection destroys the trachea's cilia, allowing mucus and dead cells to accumulate, resulting in airsacculitis and pneumonia. Survivors begin recovering in 2 to 3 weeks. *E. coli* often produces a secondary infection, and an existing infection with *E. coli* or infectious bronchitis virus makes respiratory cryptosporidiosis worse.

C. galli infects the proventriculus, or true stomach, of mature hens. Signs include ruffled feathers, tucking the head under a wing to sleep during the day, and general unthriftiness.

C. meleagridis infects the ileum of young birds, causing diarrhea and weight loss. This species primarily affects turkeys but sometimes also infects chickens.

Like other coccidial diseases, cryptosporidiosis is spread by oocysts, but each oocyst contains four (rather than eight) sporozoites that are not encapsulated within the oocyst. Crypto oocysts are therefore considerably smaller than those of other coccidia, and detecting them requires special laboratory techniques.

Another difference between crypto oocysts and other coccidial oocysts is that the former have sporulated, and therefore are already infective, when they leave the chicken's body. Some may not leave at all but remain and develop within the same host (called autoinfection). As few as 100 oocysts in one chicken can rapidly produce a serious infection. Like other coccidial oocysts, crypto oocysts can remain viable in the environment for many months and are resistant to most disinfectants but are sensitive to ammonia in litter.

Crypto Control

Cryptosporidiosis, like other coccidial infections, is a self-limiting disease that results in immunity. No means of prevention or treatment is known. Supportive therapy includes minimizing environmental stress and ensuring the chickens have plenty of clean, fresh drinking water. In the event of diarrhea, providing electrolytes (as described on page 385) is helpful.

No vaccine has been developed to prevent cryptosporidiosis. Natural immunity results from exposure to oocysts at low levels.

Blackhead (Histomoniasis)

The protozoan parasite *Histomonas meleagridis* causes a disease variously known as histomoniasis, infectious enterohepatitis, or blackhead. The term blackhead comes from the tendency of an infected bird's face to turn dark blue as a result of insufficient oxygen, although darkening of the head is neither a sure sign of the disease nor necessarily characteristic of it. The term enterohepatitis derives from a combination of the Greek words *enteron*, meaning "intestine," and *hepar*, meaning "liver." The microscopic histomonads first infect the ceca and may eventually migrate to the liver — especially in chickens already infected with *E. tenella* coccidiosis — causing acute disease in young chickens and chronic illness in older chickens.

Blackhead Transmission

H. meleagridis are found just about everywhere poultry are kept. An infected chicken sheds large numbers of histomonads in its droppings, causing the disease to spread rapidly. A chicken may become infected or reinfected in several different ways.

- **The chicken may eat a live histomonad.** The chicken might inadvertently eat a free-living histomonad while pecking in the soil or by eating a fly, beetle, sowbug, grasshopper, cricket, or other vector with a histomonad attached to its feet or other body part. This scenario is not highly likely, since a histomonad cannot survive long in the environment. Assuming it did survive long enough to be pecked up by a chicken, it normally could not survive the acid conditions within the chicken's digestive system. However, if the chicken has gone for several hours without eating — such as might occur first thing in the morning, or if the feeder goes empty — its digestive acids could be low enough to allow the histomonad to survive and reach the ceca.

- **The chicken may eat an infected cecal worm, larvae, or egg.** Parasitic cecal worms (*Heterakis gallinarum*) are common in chickens (see Cecal Worm, page 169). Although a histomonad shed in a chicken's droppings won't survive in the environment for long, one that enjoys the protection of the egg of a cecal worm can survive in the soil for as long as 3 years. Since cecal worms and histomonads both thrive in a chicken's ceca, histomonads have developed the survival strategy of invading cecal worms and their eggs, through which they find their way into another (or the same) chicken to continue replicating.

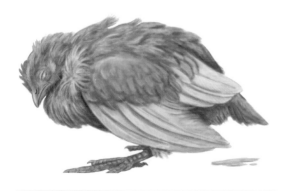

Among the typical signs of blackhead are droopy wings; dry, rumpled feathers; pale, shrunken comb and wattles; and sulfur-yellow cecal discharge.

- **The chicken may eat an infected earthworm.** An earthworm working its way through organic matter in the soil may eat an infected cecal worm egg. When a chicken chows down on the juicy tidbit, the earthworm becomes an intermediate host in spreading the disease.

Blackhead Signs and Control

Histomoniasis runs its course in about 4 weeks, usually without any sign of illness or long-term ill effect, although an infected chicken may shed large numbers of histomonads into the environment. In some cases the illness causes signs similar to those of coccidiosis. Typical signs of a serious infection include listlessness; droopy wings; dry, rumpled feathers; pale, shrunken comb and wattles; increased thirst; loss of appetite with accompanying weight loss or stunted growth; bloody droppings; sulfur-yellow cecal discharge. Watery or foamy sulfur-yellow droppings are a pretty clear indication of a blackhead infection.

Although all, or nearly all, the chickens in a flock may become infected, especially in birds just reaching maturity, most of them will recover. Chicks 4 to 6 weeks old are the most susceptible to histomonad infection. When deaths occur, they are most likely to happen between the ages of 6 and 16 weeks and will start within a few days of the first signs. Mature chickens may linger on, gradually becoming emaciated before dying. Recovered chickens continue shedding histomonads for another 6 weeks. Recovered hens may never lay as well as they once did.

In the past, blackhead was considered primarily a disease of turkeys, in which it is more commonly fatal than in chickens. Chickens are fairly resistant to the disease but are carriers that can readily infect turkeys. For this reason keeping turkeys with chickens or where chickens have been housed within the past 3 years is generally discouraged.

In recent years chickens seem to have become less resistant. Susceptibility usually results from depressed immunity from some other infection, particularly coccidiosis. Similarly, histomoniasis itself does not cause chickens to die. Rather, it opens the way for other pathogens, especially coccidial protozoa, *Escherichia coli,* and *Clostridium* bacteria. Histomonads, in fact, rely on bacteria to obtain the nutrients they need to thrive and become virulent.

No effective cure is available in the United States. Prevention includes good sanitation, especially avoiding damp bedding and muddy yards. Histomonads thrive in moist environments but are sensitive to heat, sunlight, dry air, and cold temperatures. Prevention also involves maintaining healthy chickens with robust immune systems, as well as controlling both coccidiosis and cecal worms.

Canker (Trichomoniasis)

The microscopic protozoan parasite *Trichomonas gallinae* occasionally infects chickens, causing sores in the mouth and throat. Known as canker, or sometimes roup, the disease primarily affects domestic pigeons and wild doves but may spread to chickens by way of drinking water contaminated with saliva from an infected bird's mouth or feed contaminated with infective saliva or droppings. The disease also potentially can spread to a chicken that pecks the infected flesh of another chicken, dead or alive.

T. gallinae lives in the upper digestive system of an estimated 80 percent or more of all pigeons, although not all infected pigeons show signs of illness. As chicken keeping has become popular in urban areas, where pigeons tend to congregate, canker has become more common in backyard poultry flocks. Trichomonads that invade a bird multiply rapidly but once shed into a dry environment cannot survive much more than a matter of minutes.

Signs of Canker

Canker first appears as small raised white or yellow buttonlike patches at the back of the mouth. The patches rapidly grow larger and more numerous, spreading down the throat and eventually reaching the proventriculus. The trichomonads feed on bacteria and dead cells and therefore thrive where a bacterial infection is already present. The more virulent strains release proteins and enzymes that eat through infected tissue. As masses of dead tissue accumulate, they block the upper digestive tract so the chicken can no longer swallow, and may also cause accumulated mucus to close off the windpipe so the chicken can't breathe.

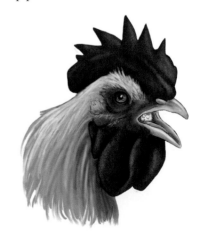

Canker first appears as small raised white or yellow buttonlike patches at the back of the mouth.

Canker Look-Alikes

CONDITIONS THAT CAN CAUSE
CANKER-LIKE MOUTH SORES

Capillary worms	Sour crop
Mycotoxicosis	Wet pox
Nutritional roup	

Signs of infection include breathing with the neck extended and mouth open; drooling and repeated swallowing; yellowish-white cheesy patches in the mouth and throat; asymmetrical appearance of the face, sometimes such that the two halves of the beak can't properly meet; difficulty eating, with accompanying weight loss or failure to gain; dehydration; pendulous crop; sometimes watery or sticky eyes; sometimes diarrhea; rarely wobbling and other nervous signs.

The disease can be mild or rapidly fatal, depending on the virulence of the protozoa. Death is often the result, not from the trichomonad infection, but from a secondary bacterial infection invading the damaged tissue and becoming septicemic. Recovered birds remain carriers but are immune to reinfection.

Identifying Trichomonads

Because canker can easily be mistaken for other diseases (see Canker Look-Alikes, above) the only way to definitively diagnose this disease is by examining a sample from the affected bird in a microscope using glass slides (described under What You'll Need on page 188). Take a fresh sample of poop, or a scraping from the edge of a mouth sore, and place it on a warm (not hot) slide. Work rapidly, because trichomonads don't live long once they leave the chicken.

Use an eyedropper to place a few drops of warm (not hot) saline solution on the sample (see Make a Saline Wound Wash on page 397). Having your slide and your saline solution at approximately the same temperature as your body will help keep the trichomonads alive long enough for you to get a look through your microscope. The saline solution and slide are the appropriate temperature if they feel neither warm nor cool when touched to the inside of your wrist.

Cover the slide with a cover slip, and examine the sample, using your microscope's most powerful setting, preferably 400X. If trichomonads are present, you will see colorless, nearly transparent creatures using their little tails to dart about erratically on the slide.

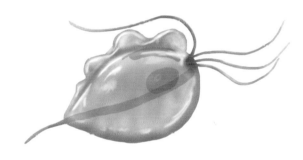

Trichomonas gallinae is a colorless, nearly transparent creature with four tiny tails that swims with decidedly jerky movements.

Treating Canker

Canker traditionally has been treated with a related group of antibiotic and antiprotozoal drugs that include metronidazole liquid or tablets (trade name Flagyl) and ronidazole powder (Ronivet). These drugs are effective and fairly safe, but because they are all chemically similar, many strains of trichomonads have become resistant to them. Further, these drugs are not legally approved for use with poultry and should never be used on chickens raised for meat.

Trichomonads prefer alkaline conditions with a pH of around 5 to 6 and do not survive well in an acidic environment. Because even a mildly acidic environment will kill them, adding vinegar to the drinking water or rinsing infected tissue with diluted vinegar will help keep the infection from spreading.

A Norwegian veterinarian has developed an effective alkaloid nutraceutical derived from the purified extracts of plants that include *Coptis japonica*, *Crocus sativus*, *Curcuma longa*, *Daucus carota*, *Hennae folium*, *Iridis rhizoma*, and *Vaccinium myrtillus*. This product, called Berimax, has a similar advantage to the traditional drugs in being effective not only against protozoa but also against *Clostridium* spp., *E. coli*, salmonella, and other bacteria.

Removing affected tissue from a chicken's mouth or throat is not a good idea, because it leaves a wound that can encourage a bacterial infection. However, if the bird can't breathe or swallow, it will likely die unless tissue masses are removed to clear the blockage. Use tweezers to pick them out without digging into the flesh. Although *T. gallinae* is not known to infect humans, wearing single-use disposable gloves when handling an infected chicken is a good idea. A chicken that has trouble eating will need supportive therapy to ensure that it gets sufficient nutrients.

Supportive therapy is any nonmedical treatment that helps an ailing chicken get better. In this case, it might mean stimulating the chicken's appetite with special treats, feeding moist or softened foods, or feeding the bird with an eyedropper or oral syringe.

Preventing Canker

Any chickens that have been in contact with an obviously infected chicken should be presumed to have been exposed to infection. Separate the exposed chickens from the infected chicken(s) to prevent further spread of the protozoa from the infected birds, and treat the exposed group with acidified copper sulfate (powdered bluestone). To make the acidified solution, combine ½ pound (225 g) copper sulfate with ½ cup (120 mL) vinegar and ½ gallon (2 L) water, and mix well. Add 1 tablespoon (½ ounce) of this solution per gallon of drinking water (15 mL per 4 L)for 4 to 7 days. Where chickens are frequently visited by pigeons or doves, this solution of acidified copper sulfate added to drinking water for 3 days once a month may help prevent infection.

To prevent the spread of canker, keep pigeons away from chickens. Locate chicken feeders and drinkers where wild birds can't gain ready access. Since canker spreads more readily in water than in feed, do not let chickens drink from a birdbath or from any source of stagnant water that may be visited by wild birds. Keep drinkers clean and sanitized, and acidify the drinking water with vinegar at the rate of 1 tablespoon per gallon (15 mL per 4 L); double the vinegar dose if the water is alkaline.

CHAPTER 8

Conditions Caused by Bacteria

BACTERIA ARE EVERYWHERE, including inside and on the human body. We humans carry around more bacteria than we have DNA cells. Most of these bacteria are either benign or beneficial. Chickens are no different in harboring multiple species of bacteria and other microbes in and on their bodies. Like the bacteria associated with humans, those associated with chickens can get out of control. By understanding how that happens, we can take measures to avoid bacterial diseases.

No one knows exactly how many species of bacteria exist, as new ones are constantly being discovered. Most species are harmless. Many are beneficial as part of the normal flora living on the skin or inside the body of a chicken (which is true of all animals, including humans). A few species of bacteria are either inherently pathogenic or are benign or beneficial bacteria that, given an opportunity, become pathogenic.

Speaking of Bacterial Diseases

acute. Having a severe and swift development

bacteria. One-cell microscopic organisms with plantlike characteristics

chronic. Description of a condition that develops gradually and lasts a long time

enteric disease. Any illness that causes inflammation of the intestines

pathogen. Any disease-causing organism

septicemia. A systemic infection that invades the body through the bloodstream; also called blood poisoning

systemic. Affecting the entire body

The Nature of Bacteria

Bacteria are single-cell microbes that are abundant in the soil, water, and air, as well as in the bodies of plants and animals, including chickens and humans. They are considered to be plantlike because of their basic structure and because they don't reproduce sexually, although like animals they are capable of independent movement. Most bacteria (such as salmonella) have tails that let them swim through liquids, although some bacteria (such as staphylococci) can move only on air or water currents.

Bacterial Growth Cycle

Most species of bacteria multiply by dividing themselves in half, a process called binary fission, from the Latin words *binarius*, meaning "two," and *fissio*, meaning "to split." Under ideal conditions bacteria multiply so rapidly that within a matter of hours one bacterium becomes millions. During this population explosion, a bacterial colony goes through four distinct metabolic phases.

1. **The lag phase** begins when bacteria encounter a suitable nutrient-rich environment and settle in to adapt to that environment. During this time they get busy synthesizing and storing the large amounts of protein they will need for a rapid growth in population. Depending on the species of bacteria and on the environment, the lag phase can last hours or days, during which the colony's population remains relatively stable.

2. **The log phase,** short for *logarithmic phase*, is a period of exponential growth. During this phase binary fission takes place and replication becomes ever more rapid — one bacterium becomes two, which become four, which become eight, and so forth — using available nutrients until one of the key nutrients is all used up. The amount of time required for the colony population to double, called the generation time, can range from about 20 minutes to 20 hours, depending on environmental conditions and the species. *E. coli,* for instance, can double in population every 20 minutes. Because a rapidly expanding colony is highly vulnerable during the log phase, many antibiotics are designed to inhibit replication.

3. **The stationary phase** is a transitional period during which the demands of an expanding colony exceed the available nutrients. As nutrients are depleted, the number of cells that die becomes equal to the number of new cells that develop. In addition to running out of nutrients, the colony begins swimming in its own dead cells and toxic wastes, and during this time other environmental conditions may become unfavorable.

4. **The decline phase** occurs when the number of cells that die exceeds the number of new ones that develop. Cells continue dying until either none are left or the few that remain can survive on whatever nutrients they can scavenge. If they can find enough nutrients, the cycle might start all over again. When an antibiotic has been used, and especially if it was discontinued too soon, the bacteria that survive are those that have the greatest resistance to the drug.

Bacteria and Disease

Pathogenic bacteria are those that are or become parasites, living on or in another organism, in this case a chicken, and surviving on nutrients obtained to the detriment of the host organism. Pathogenic bacteria cause infections, disease, and sometimes death. They enter the chicken's body through the digestive system, respiratory system, or cuts and wounds.

If they settle in an organ or tissue, the condition becomes long term, or chronic. If they travel throughout the body by means of the bloodstream — a disorder called septicemia or blood poisoning — the condition is short term, or acute, often ending in death.

Bacteria produce diseases in two ways: by causing mechanical damage to the body and by generating toxins that poison the body. Some bacterial diseases are caused by damage, some by poisoning, and some by both.

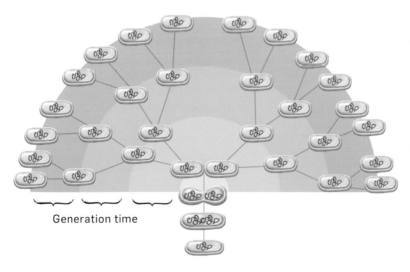

Generation time

Bacteria replicate by binary fission, or splitting in half. Depending on the species, how rapidly a colony's population doubles — the generation time — ranges from 20 minutes to 20 hours.

Infections Caused by Bacteria

CONDITION	CAUSE	AFFECTS	PREVALENCE
Air sac disease	*Mycoplasma gallisepticum, Escherichia coli*	Respiratory system	Common
Arizonosis	*Salmonella arizonae*	Intestines	Not common
Arthritis (staphylococcic)	*Staphylococcus aureus*	Joints or blood (septicemic)	Common
Avian tuberculosis	*Mycobacterium avium*	Respiratory system	Fairly common
Botulism	*Clostridium botulinum*	Nervous system	Sporadic
Breast blister	*Staphylococcus aureus, Mycoplasma synoviae, Pasteurella* spp.	Keel	Common
Bumblefoot	*Staphylococcus aureus*	Foot pad	Common
Campylobacteriosis	*Campylobacter jejuni*	Liver	Not common
Chlamydiosis	*Chlamydophila psittaci*	Respiratory system	Rare
Chronic respiratory disease	*Mycoplasma gallisepticum*	Respiratory system	Common
Egg peritonitis	*Escherichia coli*	Oviduct	Common
Erysipelas	*Erysipelothrix rhusiopathiae*	Blood (septicemic)	Rare
Fowl cholera, acute	*Pasteurella multocida*	Blood (septicemic)	Sporadic
Fowl cholera, chronic	*Pasteurella multocida*	Respiratory system	Common
Fowl typhoid	*Salmonella gallinarum*	Intestines or blood (septicemic)	Rare
Gangrenous cellulitis/dermatitis	*Clostridium septicum, C. perfringens, Staphylococcus aureus*	Skin	Sporadic
Infectious coryza	*Haemophilus paragallinarum*	Respiratory system	Common
Infectious synovitis	*Mycoplasma synoviae*	Joints, upper respiratory	Not common
Listeriosis	*Listeria monocytogenes*	Brain and heart or blood (septicemic)	Rare
Necrotic enteritis	*Clostridium perfringens*	Intestines	Rare
Omphalitis	*Escherichia coli, Staphylococcus aureus, Enterococcus faecalis*	Navel (chicks)	Common
Ornithobacteriosis	*Ornithobacterium rhinotracheale*	Respiratory, joints	Emerging
Paratyphoid	*Salmonella* spp.	Intestines or blood (septicemic)	Common
Pseudomonas	*Pseudomonas aeruginosa*	Blood (septicemic)	Rare
Pullorum	*Salmonella pullorum*	Intestines or blood (septicemic)	Rare
Spirochetosis	*Borrelia anserina*	Blood (septicemic)	Not common
Streptococcosis	*Streptococcus zooepidemicus*	Blood (septicemic)	Not common
Ulcerative enteritis	*Clostridium colinum*	Intestines	Not common

Many infections are caused by multiple species of bacteria, making them hard to diagnose and treat. Such infections may be identified as syndromes, meaning they consistently produce a set of signs that cannot be attributed to a single pathogen, or they might be identified by the location of inflammation. The terms "air sac syndrome" and "airsacculitis," for example, both refer to the same condition: infected air sacs, often caused by more than one type of bacteria.

Some backyard chicken keepers control bacteria by periodically replacing all their chickens and thoroughly cleaning and disinfecting the housing before bringing in new birds. Industrial poultry producers additionally use preventive antibiotics in rations, a practice that is unwise for reasons stated at the end of this chapter.

Staphylococcosis

Staphylococcus aureus bacteria commonly live on a chicken's skin or mucous membranes. Normally they increase the bird's resistance to other infections but will themselves cause infection if they get into the body through a break in the skin, such as might occur during a peck-order fight. Procedures such as dubbing and cropping (see page 300), spur trimming, and toe clipping also open the way to infection. Staph bacteria trapped in a wound thrive and multiply in the absence of oxygen.

If a chicken's immune system has been permanently damaged by a viral disease, such as infectious bursal disease or Marek's disease, staph may get into the bloodstream, causing sudden death. Crowded laying hens are particularly susceptible to acute death in hot weather. Ironically, mild stress increases a chicken's resistance to staph infections.

Bumblefoot

A common staph infection, especially among heavy breeds, is an abscess in the foot pad, resulting in lameness. This condition is known as bumblefoot, from the old British word "bumble," meaning "to walk unsteadily." Today the abscess core is sometimes referred to as a bumble.

An abscess may originate from such things as scratching in hard or rocky soil, jumping down from a too-high perch onto packed or splintery bedding, or spending too much time standing or walking on concrete or hardware cloth. As a result, the foot pad develops a bruise or cut through which staph bacteria enter.

The occasional bumblefoot may be the result of accident, much as a person might get a splinter. The frequent appearance of bumblefoot in a flock is a clear signal that management changes are needed.

Usually the first sign is that the chicken is reluctant to walk and limps when it does walk. The chicken's foot may look swollen and feel hot. At the bottom of the foot will be a callus-like lump, which may be either soft (if the infection is recent) or hard (if it's been going on for some time) and covered with a black scab.

If the infection has not progressed far, cleaning the foot, injecting the abscess with a suitable antibiotic, and moving the bird to a clean environment may be all that's needed. If the abscess has progressed to the hard, scabby stage, it won't go away unless you remove the core. You may get lucky and find a veterinarian willing to perform this surgery, but most likely you'll have to do it yourself.

Treating Bumblefoot

1. **Soften the abscess** by standing the chicken in warm water for about 10 minutes, gently massaging the foot to rinse off any clinging dirt. Epsom salt dissolved in the water will reduce inflammation and help soothe the foot. Don't let the chicken drink the water, as it will contain bacteria; also, if Epsom salts have been added, they are laxative.

2. **Press out the abscess core.** After a good soaking, the softened scab should pull off easily, along with some of the abscess's yellowish, cheesy, or waxy core. Once the scab has been removed, press the skin away from the sides of the abscess (don't squeeze) to encourage more of the core to come out. Use tweezers to pull out as much as you can. If the abscess is large and hard, use a sharp knife, such as a surgeon's scalpel or an X-Acto knife, to scrape or peel it out.

Repeat the soaking and core scraping as needed, working gently and taking your time until the abscess has been thoroughly cleaned.

3. **Rinse out the abscess with Betadine,** saline wound wash, or sodium hypochlorite (Dakin's Solution; see Wound Washes on page 396). After the abscess has been cleaned out, pack it with an antibacterial ointment, such as Neosporin.

4. **Cover the foot with a gauze pad,** secured with first-aid tape or thin strips of vet wrap, taking care not to make the wrap too tight.

Repeat this procedure every 2 or 3 days while the abscess heals. Meanwhile, house the chicken in a warm, safe, clean environment with plenty of water and adequate nutrition. Eliminating the possibility of roosting on a perch will prevent the chicken from jumping down and possibly reinjuring the foot.

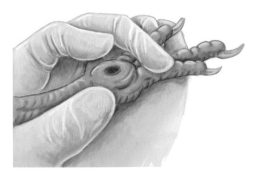

Press out the abscess core, and peel away the remaining edge.

Avoid Impetigo

⚠️ A human, especially a child or an elderly person, can potentially get a superficial skin infection (impetigo) while treating a chicken for bumblefoot or an infected breast blister. Although no case of a chicken infecting a person has ever been proven, wear disposable gloves during treatment. Take care in disposing of material removed from the abscess, as well as the dressings, as they are loaded with staphylococci. Disinfect all instruments after every use. And thoroughly wash your hands afterward.

Breast Blister

Breast blister is a swelling along a chicken's keel bone that is typically filled with a watery, clear or blood-tinged fluid. Blisters most commonly appear on cocks of the heavy breeds and are usually not discovered until affected birds are butchered for meat.

Cornish-cross broilers are particularly susceptible, because their sparse breast feathers provide little cushion. But blisters also occur on other heavy breeds and are associated with frequently resting on the keel, especially on a hard surface (such as dirt or packed bedding) or on hardware cloth (wire cage floor). Blisters are typically associated with leg weakness, which causes a bird to rest often, putting frequent pressure on its keel, and with injury, such as might occur when a heavy bird jumps down from a high perch and lands on its breastbone.

Breast blister is therefore primarily a management issue. The condition is not fatal and is usually not treated. Sometimes the blister pops on its own and heals over with scar tissue that can develop into a thick callus.

However, a breast blister can be infected, in which case it is filled with yellow creamy or cheeselike material instead of clear fluid. The most common cause of infection is *Staphylococcus aureus*, but a blister may also be infected by *Mycoplasma synoviae* or *Pasteurella* spp.

Such an infection is most likely to occur to a chicken suffering from a bacterial disease such as staphylococcic arthritis. Reluctant to move, the ailing chicken spends a lot of time resting with pressure against its breastbone, raising a blister that becomes infected with the same bacteria that made the bird ill in the first place. In this case, treatment is the same as for the underlying illness.

Staphylococcic Arthritis

Staphylococcosis can occur as an acute septicemic infection. Septicemia happens when the bacteria get into the bloodstream secondary to some other bacterial or viral infection, or as a result of decreased resistance due to a nutritional deficiency or drug toxicity. It may also occur in chickens that drink from a stagnant puddle teeming with staph bacteria that are ever present in the soil. Signs of an acute staph infection include listlessness, loss of appetite, reluctance to move, and foul-smelling, watery diarrhea.

Acute septicemia may settle into the joints, resulting in chronic arthritis. Signs include swollen joints that feel hot to the touch, limping, and weight loss. Because moving is painful, the arthritic chicken spends a lot of time resting on its hocks and breast and may develop a breast blister.

Staphylococci are resistant to many antibiotics. Successful treatment involves identifying the staph strain involved and determining a suitable antibiotic by means of laboratory sensitivity testing. Staph infection is an environmental issue that can be avoided through good management and proper nutrition, and by removing susceptible chickens from the breeder flock.

Infectious Coryza

One of the most common bacterial diseases of backyard chickens is infectious coryza, the chicken version of the common cold. This respiratory disease is caused by *Haemophilus paragallinarum* bacteria, which are particularly prevalent in the southeastern United States and in California.

Chickens are usually not susceptible to coryza until 3 to 4 months of age, and they become more susceptible as they get older. The disease can be difficult to recognize, because it resembles other respiratory diseases and often occurs in combination with them. The main signs are foul-smelling discharge from the nostrils; watery, sticky eyes; and swelling of the face. The characteristic putrid odor of the nasal discharge is a pretty good indication that the disease is indeed coryza.

Coryza is spread the same way as the common cold, in respiratory droplets coughed or sneezed by infected birds. Survivors of the disease remain carriers, as may other birds in the same flock, even if they never showed any signs. Coryza is therefore easily introduced into an established flock by unknowingly bringing in a carrier, and may be spread by such chickens entered into a poultry show or brought to a swap meet or live bird sale.

A vaccine is available, but it should be used only to prevent future outbreaks after coryza has been diagnosed. Once a flock has been vaccinated, the chickens must continue to be revaccinated twice a year.

Haemophilus paragallinarum bacteria do not survive long outside of chickens. The only way to rid the premises of infectious coryza once it has become established in a flock is to dispose of the chickens, disinfect the premises, and leave the housing vacant for at least 3 weeks before introducing new birds.

Infectious coryza is not transmitted through hatching eggs. It is therefore possible to preserve a flock's genetics by incubating eggs from infected breeders, provided you take great care to raise the chicks in an uncontaminated environment.

Mycoplasmosis

Mycoplasmosis is a complex of diseases caused by mycoplasma bacteria, the smallest living organisms capable of free existence. Although mycoplasmas are classified as bacteria, they are sometimes referred to as bacteria-like organisms.

They are about the same size as the largest viruses but (unlike a virus) can multiply outside a living cell, although they do not survive long away from a bird's body. Unlike most other kinds of bacteria, though, mycoplasmas lack a cell wall and therefore are not affected by antibiotics that work by inhibiting cell wall development (as described on page 239).

At one time, all chickens carried mycoplasma and became infectious in response to stress. Accordingly, mycoplasma infections were once known collectively as stress disease. Today mycoplasma-free chickens are available, although they can become infected if they are housed with infected chickens or with carriers. Some breeds and strains are more susceptible than others.

Diseases caused by mycoplasmas can be difficult to recognize without laboratory work, since they often occur in combination with other bacteria and with viruses. Survivors of infection become immune to future infection, but remain carriers that can spread the infection by direct contact or through hatching eggs. For this reason eliminating diseased chickens makes more sense than keeping them around to infect future generations. The National Poultry Improvement Plan (described on page 8) monitors for mycoplasmosis.

Chronic Respiratory Disease

Chronic respiratory disease (CRD), caused by *Mycoplasma gallisepticum,* is a contagious disease that usually comes on slowly and lasts a long time, sometimes appearing to recede, only to return. It primarily affects grown chickens, causing a 20 to 30 percent reduction in egg production, but rarely results in death. Chickens that recover generally are immune to further infection, but they continue to be carriers, spreading the disease to other chickens.

The first sign is weeping from one or both eyes, sometimes with minor swelling. This sign is not a definitive indication of CRD, as weepy eyes may also be caused by excessive dust, draftiness, or vitamin A deficiency. Treated with erythromycin eye ointment, the condition should clear up in a couple of days.

If the disease is left untreated, swelling increases around the eyes, they become foamy or sticky, and the chicken begins gasping for air. Other signs include nasal discharge with no odor, coughing, sneezing, and other respiratory sounds. A serious infection involves the air sacs (airsacculitis).

CRD often follows an acute respiratory virus, such as infectious bronchitis. It spreads by direct contact with infected birds or carriers and from hen to chicks via hatching eggs. Susceptibility increases in chickens that are subjected to cold temperatures or poor ventilation.

Infectious Synovitis

Less pathogenic than *Mycoplasma gallisepticum* is its relative, *M. synoviae,* which causes upper respiratory disease in growing and mature chickens. Affected birds may show no signs, or may have signs that are nearly identical to those of chronic respiratory disease and are more susceptible to viral infections.

In younger chickens, 4 to 12 weeks of age, *M. synoviae* may become systemic as infectious synovitis, the signs of which are lameness, swollen hocks, stilted gait, loss of weight, reluctance to move, and breast blisters. The appearance of greenish diarrhea is typical of chickens at death's door.

Salmonellosis

The salmonellae bacteria have been undergoing a major revision in classification. What formerly were considered thousands of different species have been reclassified into just three species, of which various bacteria within the species *Salmonella enterica* cause diseases in chickens. Evidence suggests that 75 percent of all chickens are infected with salmonellae at some time in their lives.

These bacteria create a serious problem for poultry keepers because chickens that appear perfectly healthy are often carriers. Signs may be triggered at any time by stress from crowding, molting, feed deprivation, drug treatment, or simply being moved from one place to another. Furthermore, some salmonellae affect humans as well as chickens.

How Salmonellae Spread

Hens transmit salmonellae bacteria to their off-spring through hatching eggs (a process called transovarian transmission) in one of two ways:

- The yolk may be infected as an egg is being formed in the body of an infected hen.

- The shell may be contaminated as the egg is laid or when it lands in a dirty nest; the bacteria then penetrate the shell (typically because the shell gets cracked or wet) and multiply within the egg.

During incubation, an infected embryo may die in the shell or may hatch into an infected chick. The disease spreads to healthy chicks or to chickens coming into contact with an infected bird or other infected animal (including a human). It spreads by means of contaminated droppings in litter, drinking water, and damp soil around drinkers. It is spread mechanically by flies, rodents, wild birds, used equipment, shoes, truck tires, and the like. Salmonellae may also be present in rations containing contaminated meat by-products.

Salmonellae generally enter a bird's body through its digestive system. Because the bacteria cause inflammation of the intestines, or enteritis, they are referred to as enteric bacteria. Acute enteritis is indicated by dripping diarrhea, sometimes smelly or containing blood. Signs of chronic enteritis are emaciation and persistent diarrhea, which may appear mucousy or bloody. If the disease becomes septicemic, the bird's head, comb, and wattles turn purplish. The four main diseases caused by salmonellae are so similar that laboratory identification is the only way to tell them apart with certainty.

Fowl Typhoid

Fowl typhoid is a contagious disease that is usually acute but may also be chronic. It is caused by *Salmonella* Gallinarum, which is not the same bacterium that causes typhoid in humans.

Unlike other salmonelloses, which are more likely to affect chicks, fowl typhoid is more likely to appear in mature chickens. Sometimes the first sign of fowl typhoid is sudden death. Other signs include loss of appetite, increased thirst, pale comb and wattles, and green or yellow diarrhea sticking to vent feathers.

Fowl typhoid is such a serious threat to the poultry industry that a huge effort was made to eradicate the disease in North America. Should it ever appear, most states require that it be reported to government authorities. (For information on reportable diseases, see page 418.)

Paratyphoid

In the United States and Canada, paratyphoid infection is the most common salmonellosis. Paratyphoid (from the Greek word *para*, meaning "near") is caused by numerous kinds of salmonellae that invade a large number of animal species, including birds, rodents, reptiles, and humans. Paratyphoid is the most important bacterial disease in the hatching industry, since it causes chicks to die and survivors to be stunted. This group of bacteria is also important in the meat and egg industry, since it is responsible for causing food poisoning in humans.

The most common paratyphoid bacteria to infect chickens is *Salmonella* Typhimurium; the most serious to humans is *Salmonella* Enteritidis. A sign in incubated eggs is numerous embryos dead in the shell, pipped or unpipped. Chicks 1 to 3 weeks old will be depressed, have decreased appetite and increased thirst, make chirping sounds of distress, huddle near heat, and have diarrhea with vent pasting. Mature chickens that are carriers exhibit no signs unless their immunity is suppressed.

Paratyphoid caused by *S.* Enteritidis is a human health risk. It is therefore reportable in most states.

Arizonosis

Like the paratyphoid group of salmonella bacteria, *S. enterica arizonae* bacteria infect a large number of animal species. These bacteria cause avian arizonosis, which occurs primarily in the western United States, as indicated by its name. It is more likely to appear in turkey poults than in chicks.

When chicks do come down with this disease, it is nearly identical to paratyphoid. One way to tell the difference is to have infected chickens tested for paratyphoid. A negative result is a pretty good indication of arizonosis. Since this disease can affect humans, it may be reportable in some states.

PULLORUM-TYPHOID TESTING

Many states require pullorum-typhoid-free certification for exhibition chickens entered into fairs or poultry shows, chickens sold at swap meets, or chickens transported from out of state. Annual testing is also required for National Poultry Improvement Plan (NPIP) membership. Pullorum-typhoid-free certification can generally be met in one of the following ways:

- The chickens came from an NPIP flock, either directly or through a hatchery or farm store, for which documentation is required.

- The chickens tested negative within 90 days of needing certification, are leg-banded for identification, and are accompanied by an official certificate.

The test involves drawing a bit of blood from under the chicken's wing and mixing it with an antigen containing a killed form of salmonella bacteria. Within minutes the blood will clump if the test is positive or fail to clump if the bird is pullorum-typhoid-free. Since *Salmonella* Pullorum and *Salmonella* Gallinarum react identically to the same antigen, a single test may be used to detect the presence of either bacteria. The results of the test are forwarded to a state lab. Each tested bird is assigned a numbered leg band and issued an official document that must be presented as proof of certification.

To cover the cost of expenses that include annually renewing the tester's license and purchasing antigen and leg bands, testers charge a fee that may be a small amount per bird for a few exhibition chickens or a per-hour charge for testing an entire flock to satisfy NPIP requirements. To find a tester, or to become one, contact your county Extension office.

Nearly every state is now classified as Pullorum-Typhoid Clean. You can find information on NPIP, including a directory of certified pullorum-free breeding flocks, by doing an online key word search for NPIP.

Pullorum

Salmonella Pullorum causes pullorum, a disease that affects only poultry, primarily chickens. Because it causes diarrhea topped with white caps, it was once called white diarrhea.

Pullorum is spread by infected breeders through hatching eggs, causing death to embryos in the shell or to chicks soon after they hatch. Survivors are stunted and remain carriers. Like fowl typhoid, pullorum is such a serious threat to the poultry industry that a major effort was made to eradicate it in North America, and should it ever appear, it is reportable in most states.

Controlling Salmonellae

Salmonellae readily survive and multiply in the environment, making their control difficult. They survive for years in infected droppings, feathers, dust, and hatchery fluff, and for almost a year in garden soil fertilized with infected droppings. The bacteria cannot survive long at 140°F (60°C), a temperature well below that of a heating compost pile. The bacteria thrive in fresh litter but cannot live long in built-up litter, because of the high pH of ammonia in old litter.

Antibiotics may be used to control salmonella, but disposing of infected chickens is preferable to treatment for at least the following three reasons:

- Antibiotics alter intestinal microflora, interfering with recovery.

- The use of antibiotics causes antibiotic-resistant strains of bacteria to develop.

- Survivors are carriers and continue to spread the disease in a never-ending cycle.

Clostridial Diseases

Clostridial diseases are caused by bacteria in the *Clostridium* group. They live naturally in soil and in the intestines of healthy animals — humans and chickens alike. They can make chickens sick in one of the following two ways:

- They invade a chicken's body tissues, replicating and producing tissue-destroying toxins. Gangrenous dermatitis and necrotic enteritis are two examples of this type of clostridial disease.

- They replicate in a rotting food item, producing toxins that poison any chicken that feeds on the contaminated matter. Botulism is an example of this type of clostridial disease.

Clostridium bacteria do not cause infection unless a chicken's immunity has been compromised for some other reason, such as internal parasites, coccidiosis or other illness, or nutritional issues. Although clostridial diseases can be deadly, they are unlikely to affect a properly managed flock.

Ulcerative Enteritis

Clostridium colinum causes ulcerative enteritis, an intestinal disease transmitted by infectious droppings in litter, feed, and water and spread by flies. The condition is commonly known as quail disease, because it was first identified in quail, the most susceptible of all avian species. Chickens are more resistant, unless their immunity has been reduced by stress — especially due to overcrowding — or some other disease such as coccidiosis or infectious bursal disease.

Ulcerative enteritis is most likely to affect layer pullets and can be either acute (causing sudden death) or chronic (resulting in gradual emaciation). Chickens acquire the bacteria by pecking in contaminated matter or drinking contaminated water. When the bacteria reach the intestines they settle in to cause inflammation and ulcers.

The usual first sign is loss of appetite, followed by diarrhea and other signs similar to those produced by coccidiosis (described on page 197), except that ulcerative enteritis does not cause bloody droppings. Although the disease is highly contagious, affected chickens usually recover within about 3 weeks, but remain carriers. This disease responds well to treatment with antibiotics, particularly bacitracin or streptomycin, although treated chickens may be susceptible to reinfection.

Once chickens become infected, the bacteria can survive in housing for years and are resistant to most disinfectants. Ulcerative enteritis may be avoided by raising chickens away from quail and other game birds, and by not introducing into your flock new chickens that may be carriers.

Necrotic Enteritis

Clostridium perfringens bacteria generate a potent toxin that causes necrotic enteritis in young, intensively raised chickens. The disease appears suddenly (often after a change in feed) and progresses rapidly, causing deaths within a few hours, sometimes without signs.

Necrotic enteritis is easy to treat with antibiotics and easy to avoid through good management, including maintaining proper sanitation, controlling coccidiosis and worms, and gradually making any changes in rations. The use of probiotics, as described on page 379, is also helpful.

Gangrenous Dermatitis

Gangrenous dermatitis is a skin infection that affects primarily young, intensively raised chickens. Gangrene refers to the death and decomposition of body tissue, in this case the chicken's skin. The word "gangrene" derives from the Greek *gangraina*, meaning "an eating sore," and dermatitis derives from the Greek word *derm*, meaning "skin," plus the suffix *itis*, referring to an inflammation.

SURVIVAL BY HIBERNATION

When clostridial bacteria encounter conditions that are unfavorable for survival — such as a shortage of suitable nutrients — they retreat into a dormant state by dehydrating and developing a tough triple-layer outer wall. A bacterium in this form is called an endospore, from the Greek words *endon*, meaning "internal," and *spora*, meaning "seed."

As an endospore a bacterium can hibernate for many years, even centuries, despite exposure to such environmental extremes as hot or cold temperatures, direct sunlight, dry conditions, and chemical disinfectants. When conditions again become favorable, the endospore rehydrates, absorbing moisture until its outer walls burst and release a potentially infectious bacterium back into the environment.

This infection comes on rapidly; often the first sign is sudden death. In less acute cases wattles may swell and become weepy, and dark patches of red, purple, or black skin appear on the wing tips, abdomen, breast, and thighs. Death follows within 24 hours.

Gangrenous dermatitis is typically caused by *Clostridium septicum, C. perfringens,* or *Staphylococcus aureus,* alone or in combination. It is most likely to occur in young chickens with reduced immunity caused by a serious bout of coccidiosis, a previous or current viral infection (especially infectious bursal disease), and/or a selenium–vitamin E deficiency. Bacteria enter the skin when a susceptible chicken rests on wet litter or has some injury, such as might occur from fighting or picking. This infection is easily avoided through good management, proper sanitation, and adequate nutrition.

Botulism

Clostridium botulinum, bacteria that commonly live in the intestines of chickens, are not themselves pathogenic. When they multiply in the carcasses of dead animals — environments that lack oxygen — they generate some of the world's most potent toxins. Botulism is therefore a poisoning rather than an infection.

Birds become poisoned after pecking at rotting organic matter or drinking contaminated water. The popular practice of hanging a rotting chunk of meat so maggots will fall into the chicken yard to provide the flock with a source of protein is an excellent way to poison the chickens. Feeding chickens a rotting head of unrefrigerated cabbage, or letting them scratch in compost, are other potential sources of *C. botulinum* poisoning.

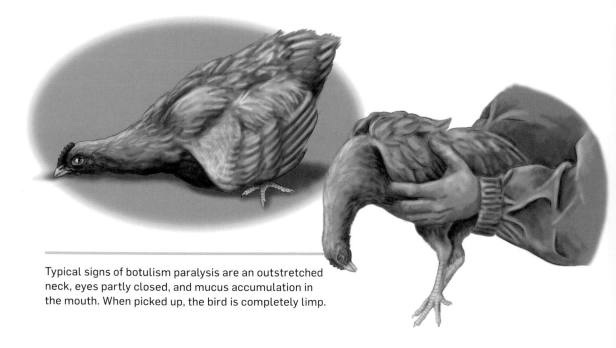

Typical signs of botulism paralysis are an outstretched neck, eyes partly closed, and mucus accumulation in the mouth. When picked up, the bird is completely limp.

A poisoned bird gradually becomes paralyzed from the feet up. Initially the bird sits around or limps if you make it move. As paralysis progresses through its body, its wings droop and its neck goes limp, giving the disease the common name limberneck. If you pick up an affected bird, it will hang loosely in your hands. By the time the eyelids are paralyzed, the bird looks dead, but it continues to live until either its heart or respiratory system become paralyzed.

A typical indication of botulism poisoning is finding healthy chickens, sick chickens, and dead chickens together in the same yard. A chicken that survives for 48 hours has not consumed a deadly dose and therefore is likely to recover. Of course, the first thing you should do is identify and remove the source of the toxin.

If a bird isn't too far gone, you might bring it around by squirting cool water and a molasses or Epsom salt solution into its crop (see Laxative Flushes, page 392). Treatment with an antibiotic such as bacitracin or chlortetracycline, along with a supplement of selenium and vitamins A, D, and E, may be helpful. Treatment with an antitoxin (available from a veterinarian) may be effective if administered in time; type C botulism is the toxin most commonly found in poultry. Botulism is easily avoided through good sanitation.

Colibacillosis

Colibacillosis is a collection of infectious conditions caused by one or more strains of *Escherichia coli,* which are among the so-called coliform bacteria (from the Latin word *coli,* meaning "of the colon"). Coliforms collectively consist of a large group of bacteria that inhabit the intestinal tracts of warm-blooded animals, including humans and chickens, and are commonly found in the environment worldwide. Many strains do not cause disease. Other strains are opportunistic, and still others are highly pathogenic.

E. coli can survive for long periods in dry litter and dust, and are spread through the droppings of infected rodents and infected chickens. A bird's susceptibility to *E. coli* invasion is increased by stress and by damage to its respiratory system from breathing ammonia fumes or dust. *E. coli* bacteria are of particular concern because they can affect humans as well as chickens, as described on page 416.

E. coli Infections

Illnesses caused by *E. coli* are varied and often complex. Susceptibility varies with a bird's strain and age; infection is more common in young birds than in older ones. The bacteria may be the sole infection or, more often, may combine with or follow other infections, especially chronic respiratory disease, infectious bronchitis, infectious synovitis, and Newcastle disease.

E. coli infections range from acute and severe to chronic and mild. The bacteria enter a chicken by way of either the digestive or the respiratory system, resulting in typical signs of any intestinal or respiratory disease. *E. coli* bacteria may eventually settle, and cause inflammation, in a bird's eye, heart, liver, navel, oviduct, leg joints, or wing joints. They may get into the bloodstream, causing acute septicemia and sudden deaths among apparently healthy chickens.

Respiratory colibacillosis may be prevented by minimizing stress, providing good ventilation, and keeping chickens free of mycoplasmal and viral infections. Intestinal colibacillosis is more difficult to avoid, but may be minimized by controlling rodents and keeping feed and drinking water free of droppings.

SALPINGITIS AND PERITONITIS

Salpingitis, or inflammation of the oviduct, derives its name from the Greek word *salpinx*, meaning "trumpet," in reference to the funnel shape of the opening to the oviduct. Salpingitis generally results from a bacterial infection, often due to one of the coliforms.

This infection typically affects high-producing hens, because the muscle separating their cloaca from the vagina tends to be more relaxed, allowing fecal bacteria to migrate up into the oviduct. The hen initially may show no sign of infection but eventually will lay fewer eggs or stop laying altogether.

Instead, the material that would normally develop into eggs accumulates and festers in the oviduct, which becomes filled with a mass that looks like cooked yolks, smells bad, and may include eggshells, membranes, or intact eggs.

Eventually the amassing material spills into the hen's body cavity. The hen's abdomen appears swollen, and the discomfort causes her to walk or stand with her rear end lowered. This development is called egg peritonitis, deriving from the Greek word *peritonaion*, meaning "abdominal membrane." The longer the infection goes on, the bigger the mass will be, until the hen eventually dies.

The signs of salpingitis are similar to those of egg binding, and in fact an early infection may cause egg binding. Because the oviduct stops functioning properly and the ovaries atrophy, a survivor will no longer lay. However, most affected hens die within 6 months of becoming infected.

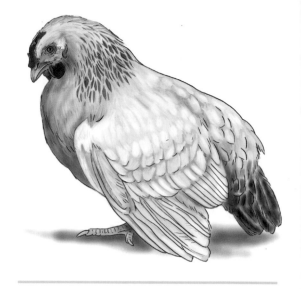

A hen suffering from egg peritonitis has a bulging abdomen and walks or stands with her rear end lowered.

Preventing salpingitis involves maintaining a healthful environment that includes good ventilation (to prevent weakening of a hen's immune system from respiratory illness) and good litter management (to minimize an accumulation of pathogenic bacteria in the coop). Using nipple drinkers, or changing the drinking water often, helps keep potentially infective droppings out of the water. Probiotics and prebiotics can help minimize pathogenic coliforms in the hens' digestive system, as explained under Competitive Exclusion on page 378.

Omphalitis

Omphalitis, from the Greek word *omphalos*, meaning "navel," plus the suffix *itis*, referring to an inflammation, is a condition in which an embryo's yolk sac isn't completely absorbed, so the navel can't heal properly. As a result bacteria invade through the navel, causing chicks to die at hatching time and for up to 2 weeks after-ward. Although *E. coli* is the usual cause of this infection, staphylococci or enterococci are often also involved.

This infection results from improper operation of an incubator, often combined with unsanitary practices. Causes include the following:

- Bacteria from an infected hen get into the egg before it is laid.

- Bacteria penetrate shells of soiled eggs before or during incubation.

- Incubator temperature is too low.

- Incubation or hatching humidity is too high.

- The incubator is inadequately ventilated.

- The incubator is contaminated by dirty eggs or by failure to clean and sanitize the unit between hatches.

- Newly hatched chicks are subjected to excessive chilling or heating.

Because chicks with omphalitis characteristically have large, moist, soft bodies, this condition is often called mushy chick disease. Other signs include a swollen, bluish-colored abdomen with an unhealed navel, and a bad odor. Affected chicks hang around the brooder heater, show little interest in eating or drinking, and may dribble diarrhea.

No effective treatment is known. When the infection is not septicemic, gently cleaning the navel with povidone iodine (brand name Betadine, among others) two or three times a day may help the chick survive.

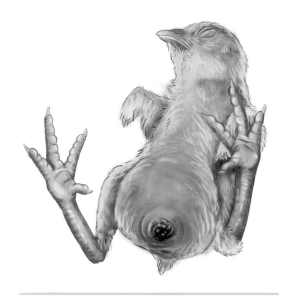

A chick with omphalitis has a large, moist, soft body with a swollen, bluish abdomen, an unhealed navel, and a bad odor.

Pasteurellosis

Pasteurellosis is a group of related illnesses caused by several species of pasteurella bacteria. In chickens various strains of *Pasteurella multocida* bacteria cause fowl cholera, one of the earliest studied diseases of poultry. Different strains, with varying degrees of virulence, result in two basic forms of cholera: acute and chronic. Although the two forms are quite distinct, signs may overlap, since survivors of the acute form often become chronic.

All domestic poultry and game birds, as well as wild birds, are susceptible to fowl cholera. Among domestic poultry, turkeys and waterfowl are more susceptible than chickens. Among chickens, mature birds are more susceptible than young ones, and any chicken that recovers remains a carrier.

Acute Cholera

Acute fowl cholera is among the most virulent and infectious diseases of poultry. It may appear in the most dramatic fashion — a hen enters a nest to lay an egg and drops dead. The cause is fast-acting blood poisoning by bacterial toxins. The result is a chicken that dies without showing any signs of illness.

In less dramatic acute cases, chickens appear lethargic with ruffled feathers, loss of appetite, diarrhea, rapid breathing, and mucus discharge from the mouth. Survivors may recover and either eventually die from emaciation and dehydration or develop chronic cholera.

Chronic Cholera

In contrast to the systemic and fast action of acute cholera, chronic cholera develops slowly and settles into specific body parts. Because infections remain localized, this condition is sometimes referred to as localized pasteurellosis. Because it's not nearly as dire as acute cholera, it's sometimes described as mild fowl cholera. It may develop in survivors of acute cholera, or may result from infection by a less virulent strain of pasteurella.

A typical sign of chronic cholera is abscessed wattles, swelling of the membranes around the eyes, and swelling of the face below the eyes (due to congested sinuses). Swelling may also occur in the joints and foot pads, causing lameness. If the infection settles in the head or ear, the chicken may have a twisted neck.

Preventing and Treating Cholera

P. multocida bacteria survive at least 1 month in droppings and up to 3 months in moist soil and in the bodies of decaying dead chickens. The bacteria are spread primarily through mucus discharged from the mouth, nose, and eyes of infected birds (including wild species). They may be either inhaled or ingested in contaminated feed or water and may be spread on contaminated equipment and shoes.

Antibiotic treatment may keep affected chickens from dying, but the disease usually returns when medication is discontinued. At one time cholera was extremely common. Today it is avoided through good management, which includes not bringing in older birds that might be carriers and not mixing birds of different ages from different sources.

FOWL CHOLERA BACTERINS

Bacterial vaccines, or bacterins, are available to prevent fowl cholera, but should be used *only* where fowl cholera poses a problem. The bacterins are of two types: inactivated and attenuated. The inactivated bacterin is effective against limited strains of fowl cholera. The attenuated vaccine is effective against more strains, but because it contains live bacteria that have been modified to make them less virulent, it carries the risk that the bacteria will revert to their original virulence. Vaccine types and methods of application are discussed in detail under Vaccination, starting on page 278.

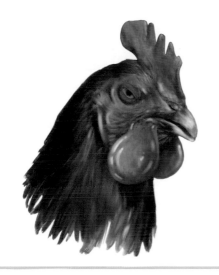

A classic sign of chronic fowl cholera is swollen wattles that abscess and burst, leaving scars.

Ornithobacteriosis

Identified in the mid-1990s, ornithobacteriosis is one of the most recently studied diseases of poultry. It is an emerging disease about which a lot of questions remain unanswered.

What is known is that it is caused by *Ornithobacterium rhinotracheale* bacteria, often abbreviated as ORT. It is similar to pasteurellosis in being either acute (resulting in sudden death) or chronic (causing either a respiratory or a joint infection). The severity of respiratory infection is influenced by environmental stressors, including overcrowding, poor sanitation, inadequate ventilation, and ammonia fumes.

Ornithobacteriosis affects many species of birds. Among domestic poultry it is a greater problem in turkeys than in chickens. Among chickens it affects mainly intensively raised and multiage flocks. The bacteria spread from bird to bird by being either inhaled or consumed in drinking water and are also transmitted through hatching eggs.

O. rhinotracheale infection is triggered by the presence of some other bacterial infection, notably colibacillosis or mycoplasmosis, or a viral disease, especially infectious bronchitis or Newcastle disease. Precisely because ORT bacteria take advantage of the presence of other pathogens, and because the other pathogens rapidly outnumber *O. rhinotracheale,* this disease is difficult to diagnose.

Making the identification of ORT even more difficult, it can take on one of several different forms. It is therefore sometimes referred to as *O. rhinotracheale* infections. Some of the known infections include these:

- Brain infection resulting in sudden death, primarily among young, intensively raised chickens

- A mild respiratory disease in young chickens or hens just starting to lay

- A severe respiratory disease in young chickens

- A joint infection in older chickens, often leading to lameness and paralysis

O. rhinotracheale has rapidly become resistant to most antibiotics, but remains sensitive to most disinfectants. A vaccine is available, used primarily for broiler breeders to pass immunity to intensively raised broiler chicks.

Avian Tuberculosis

One of the first poultry diseases to be investigated, avian tuberculosis is caused by *Mycobacterium avium,* bacteria that infect all species of birds, but more often chickens and captive exotic birds than other domestic poultry or wild species. The same bacteria also infect rabbits, pigs, and sheep, and to some extent people (although a different bacterium is usually responsible for human TB).

When hens are kept for eggs, and the flock is replaced annually to maximize egg production, avian tuberculosis is not an issue. But when chickens are kept as family pets, and are expected to have long lives, avian tuberculosis can be the sad outcome. It is a chronic disease that takes many months to develop and spreads slowly from one chicken to another. Although it can infect chickens of any age, TB takes such a long time to appear that it normally does not affect chickens less than 1 year old.

It spreads to birds that pick in soil, feed, or water contaminated by the droppings of infected chickens or other infected animals. It may also spread through cannibalism or by picking at the carcass of a dead chicken. It is especially prevalent in the midwestern states when chickens are allowed to free-range, are kept in multiage flocks, or are housed in contact with pigs.

Typical signs of TB are gradual weight loss while eating well — a condition known as going light — resulting in emaciation and eventually death. An infected bird may live for months or years, depending on how extensively the bacteria invade its body. No effective treatment is known.

Preventing TB entails not mixing chickens from different sources and of different ages, replacing each year's breeder or layer flock with young birds, keeping chickens away from housing or range that formerly held an infected flock, and housing chickens away from pigs and sheep. Since contaminated facilities are difficult to decontaminate, the safest approach in the face of a TB infection is to dispose of the flock and establish a new flock in a fresh environment.

Less Common Bacterial Infections

A number of bacterial diseases that may, but rarely do, infect chickens are notable because they can be shared with other animals, they can affect humans, or they are deadly and have no effective cure. In many cases the bacteria that cause these diseases are ever present, becoming pathogenic only in poorly managed flocks.

Campylobacteriosis

Campylobacter bacteria commonly dwell in the intestines of chickens, often without signs of disease, but are of concern because they can result in serious food poisoning in humans (see page 411). The species of greatest concern is *Campylobacter jejuni*, which is more likely to be a problem in intensively raised chickens than in backyard flocks.

These bacteria spread among chickens through infected droppings in feed and water. They are more prevalent in warm summer months, possibly spread by filth flies. Campylobacters are more likely to infect chickens that are stressed by some other condition, such as Marek's disease or internal parasites, or have experienced extreme environmental stress.

Because this infection affects the liver, campylobacteriosis is sometimes called liver disease or infectious hepatitis (from the Greek word *hepatos*, meaning "liver," plus the suffix *itis*, referring to an inflammation). The chief sign is a significant (up to 35 percent) drop in egg production. No effective treatment has been found.

Left untreated, chickens may naturally develop antibodies against campylobacter, causing the infection to resolve on its own. Campylobacters are also particularly sensitive to drying and may be effectively eliminated from housing with a thorough cleaning, followed by leaving the coop empty for at least a week.

Chlamydiosis

Chlamydophila psittaci is a bacterium that affects many species of birds. It is like a virus in that it multiplies only within the cell of another life form, but otherwise it behaves like a bacterium. It produces an infection commonly known as psittacosis or parrot fever, because it was first identified in psittacine birds (parrots). In poultry it is called chlamydiosis and is significant because it can infect humans and is potentially fatal (see Ornithosis, page 408).

This contagious disease is difficult to diagnose in chickens because it typically causes listlessness with no other signs of illness. Outbreaks are cyclical but rare in chickens, which are naturally resistant. Among poultry, chickens are less likely to fall victim to chlamydiosis than ducks, turkeys, or pigeons, and among all birds the disease is most likely to appear in parrots, parakeets, lovebirds, and other psittacines rather than in poultry. No treatment is effective, and survivors are likely to remain carriers.

Erysipelas

Erysipelas, caused by the *Erysipelothrix rhusiopathiae* bacterium, is significant as a disease chickens share with many birds and other vertebrates, notably turkeys, pigs, sheep, fish, and humans (see Erysipeloid, page 408). Chickens on pasture that previously held infected turkeys, sheep, or pigs may become infected through open wounds that result from fighting, cannibalism, or procedures such as dubbing or spur trimming.

This disease is difficult to diagnose. The most startling sign is the sudden death of apparently healthy chickens, while birds in nearby flocks (on uncontaminated soil) thrive. Some chickens may briefly become listless, lose interest in eating, develop diarrhea, have trouble walking, and either die or recover within about 24 hours. In rare instances chronic illness causes hemorrhaging under the skin, resulting in purplish-reddish blotchiness that gives this disease the occasionally used name of red skin.

Erysipelas may be treated with penicillin, but since survivors continue to shed *E. rhusiopathiae* bacteria, and since this disease poses a potentially serious health risk to humans, the only safe approach is to dispose of an infected flock and start a new flock on fresh ground. Erysipelas is not transmitted through hatching eggs, making it possible to start a new flock by hatching eggs from infected breeders, provided the new birds are raised away from contaminated soil.

Listeriosis

Listeria monocytogenes bacteria are common in the soil and intestines of birds and other animals living in temperate climates. They can cause listeriosis, a disease to which most chickens are resistant. It is mainly a disease of ruminants and can spread to or from chickens and cattle, goats, or sheep that share pasture. The chief importance of this disease is that it can infect humans that handle infected birds or eat their meat.

The bacteria may infect a young chicken's brain (encephalitic form), the main sign of which is arching of the head over the back. If the infection gets into the bloodstream (septicemic form), sudden death results. Chickens can, however, carry the bacteria without showing any signs.

L. monocytogenes may be treated with an appropriate vet-prescribed antibiotic. Where an infection occurs, the best course of action is to identify and eliminate the source. Aside from contaminated effluent from a neighboring food-producing animal operation, infection might result from feeding chickens contaminated foods such as deli meats, soft cheeses, or produce such as celery or commercially purchased sprouts (all of which would also sicken a human).

Pseudomonas

Pseudomonas aeruginosa bacteria live in soil, water, and other humid environments, waiting to infect young chickens, excessively stressed birds, and those with compromised immunity. Infection is extremely rare and typically occurs in combination with viruses or other bacteria, particularly mycoplasmas.

Pseudomonads are among the many bacteria that combine to produce omphalitis, which spreads from breeders to chicks through hatching eggs and causes deaths in embryos during late incubation or in chicks during early hatch. In growing chicks pseudomonads affect the respiratory system, resulting in incoordination, swelling, and rapid death. These infections may be prevented through good sanitation, avoiding excessive stress, and otherwise maintaining conditions designed to prevent any disease.

Spirochetosis

Spirochetosis is rare in North America, although the fowl tick that carries it is quite common in the Southwest. Signs include green diarrhea with large amounts of white urates, progressive limp paralysis, and a high rate of deaths. Survivors are immune. Control this disease by controlling fowl ticks and by keeping susceptible birds away from chickens that were recently exposed to fowl ticks.

Streptococcosis and Enterococcosis

Streptococcus and the closely related *Enterococcus* bacteria normally live within the intestines of chickens, infecting birds mainly if their resistance is low — usually because of an infection by some other pathogen. *S. zooepidemicus* can cause sudden death in mature chickens. *E. faecalis* is one of the causes of omphalitis, in which embryos die in the shell and chicks die soon after hatching. Avoid these infections by maintaining good sanitation and avoiding stressful conditions.

Antibacterial Agents

Some bacterial diseases may be effectively treated with antibacterial or antibiotic drugs. The distinction between antibacterials and antibiotics is murky; no two authorities seem to agree on a precise definition. Sometimes "antibiotic" is defined as a medicine and "antibacterial" as a disinfectant. In common usage antibacterials and antibiotics are the same thing — antimicrobial drugs that are not effective against viruses. Sometimes, however, an antibiotic is defined as any antimicrobial used to treat any infection. Elsewhere, antibiotics are defined as antibacterials derived solely from living organisms, which leaves out chemically synthesized drugs such as sulfonamides. What a confusing mess!

Since we're not cramming for a final exam here, let's avoid the quibbling and consider antibiotics to be basically the same as antibacterials. Let's define both as drugs that either kill or inhibit the growth of infectious bacteria while causing little or no harm to the infected host.

Action of Antibacterials at Normal Concentrations

BACTERICIDES	BACTERIOSTATS
Aminoglycosides	Erythromycin
Bacitricin	Spectinomycin
Penicillins	Sulfonamides
Sulfonamides	Tetracyclines

Antibiotics can be either bactericides or bacteriostats. A bactericide destroys bacteria, usually by disrupting cell wall synthesis. Bacitracin is an example of an antibiotic commonly used to treat chickens by inhibiting cell wall synthesis in certain types of bacteria.

A bacteriostat prevents bacteria from multiplying, usually by interfering with protein production or DNA replication. By retarding the growth of bacteria, a bacteriostat gives the chicken's immune system time to produce antibodies and otherwise rally its own defenses. Examples of bacteriostats used for treating chickens are tetracyclines, which interfere with protein synthesis, and sulfonamides, which disrupt bacterial metabolism. Many antibacterials are bactericidal in a high dose and bacteriostatic in a lower dose.

Spectrum Range

Some antibiotics are narrow spectrum, meaning they affect only one or a limited number of related bacterial species. Bacitracin is an example of a narrow-spectrum antibiotic, used to control strains of *Clostridium perfringens* bacteria that are susceptible to the drug. Other antibiotics are broad spectrum, meaning they affect several different species. Oxytetracycline is a

broad-spectrum antibiotic commonly used in chickens to control a variety of intestinal bacteria.

Whether an antibacterial is narrow spectrum or broad spectrum, its effectiveness will be reduced in a bird that has been infected for a long time or with its immunity weakened by poor sanitation, malnutrition, or the presence of a viral infection. Although antibacterials have no effect against viruses, they are often used in treating viral diseases to keep weakened birds from getting a secondary bacterial infection.

Antibiotics for Chickens

The word "antibiotic" comes from the Greek words *anti*, meaning "against," and *bios*, meaning "life." Some antibiotics are natural drugs

GRAM STAINING

Most species of bacteria are encased within a protective cell wall. Some have a thick wall consisting of many layers with no outer membrane; they are called gram positive. Others have a thin wall made up of fewer layers surrounded by an outer membrane; they are called gram negative. Gram refers to the process of Gram staining, named after Hans Christian Gram, the scientist who invented the technique of using dye to identify bacterial species.

When stained by this method, gram-positive bacteria turn blue or purple, while gram-negative bacteria turn pink or red. Some species of bacteria cannot be classified according to Gram staining; however, staining is the usual first step in categorizing pathogenic bacteria. The significance of Gram staining is that the two groups of bacteria react differently to different antibacterials — some drugs work only against gram-positive bacteria, while others are effective only against gram-negative bacteria.

Unless you are a microbiologist, you are unlikely to go around staining bacteria. A pathology report, however, may include the results of Gram staining as a preliminary step toward identifying the specific bacteria causing an infection, and this information will help your veterinarian determine what kind of drug to prescribe.

Gram-Stain Classification of Bacteria Affecting Chickens

GENUS	GRAM POSITIVE	GRAM NEGATIVE	NEITHER
Borrelia			X
Campylobacter		X	
Chlamydophila		X	
Clostridium	X		
Erysipelothrix	X		
Escherichia		X	
Haemophilus		X	
Listeria	X		
Mycobacterium			X
Mycoplasma			X
Ornithobacterium		X	
Pasteurella		X	
Pseudomonas		X	
Salmonella		X	
Staphylococcus	X		
Streptococcus	X		

derived from living microbes, including, ironically, bacteria themselves. Bacteria, along with fungi, naturally produce antibiotics as a defense against competing microbes. Tetracyclines, for instance, are produced by bacteria, and penicillin is produced by fungi.

Semisynthetic antibiotics are drugs produced by microbes, which are then modified to make them more effective (or to make them unique enough to be patented). Some antibiotics, including the sulfas, are entirely synthetic.

Of the many existing kinds of antibiotics, only a few are approved for use with poultry. The government agencies responsible for issuing their approval are interested solely in poultry raised for meat or eggs. Poultry products containing antibiotic residues can be hazardous to human health for a variety of reasons, including allergic reactions, possible toxic effects, and the development of bacterial resistance to antibiotics used to treat human infections.

The nonapproved use of any antibiotic is considered to be "off-label" or, when prescribed by a veterinarian, "extra-label." A veterinarian may prescribe an antibiotic that perhaps has not been tested for use with poultry, most likely because it offers no benefit to industrial poultry production or because it is too costly for industrial use. Nonapproved drugs might, for instance, be prescribed to treat chickens kept for show or as pets.

SULFA DRUGS

Sulfonamides, or sulfa drugs, are widely used because they are inexpensive and relatively broad spectrum. Since they were introduced in the 1930s, however, many bacteria have become resistant, particularly staphylococci, clostridia, and pseudomonas.

The sulfonamide group includes several related drugs, easily identified because their names almost always start with "sulf." They fall into these two categories:

- Rapidly absorbed and rapidly excreted, requiring treatment one to four times a day

- Rapidly absorbed and slowly excreted, allowing treatment only once every second or third day

Most sulfonamides are bacteriostatic, but some can be bactericidal, depending on the drug, the dose, and the bacteria involved. Sometimes three different sulfonamides are combined to create a more effective tablet or liquid triple sulfa medication.

Sulfas are typically used to treat bumblefoot, coryza, toxoplasmosis, a variety of respiratory infections, and systemic colibacillosis (often in combination with penicillin G). The sulfas work best when treatment starts in the early stages of infection. A chicken usually shows improvement within 3 days but should be treated for an additional 2 days after signs disappear.

In any case, sulfa treatment should not go on longer than 7 days or the result may be kidney damage (due to crystals forming in the kidneys) or vitamin K deficiency (interfering with blood clotting). Prolonged treatment is not only toxic but results in decreased laying. In addition, if a chicken does not drink enough water during treatment, its pH balance becomes too acidic. Should prolonged treatment be necessary, provide a vitamin K supplement, and add 1 tablespoon of sodium bicarbonate (baking soda) per gallon to the drinking water.

PENICILLINS

The penicillins are a large group of antibiotics derived from fungi and identified by names ending in "cillin." Penicillin was discovered in 1928 by bacteriologist Alexander Fleming, who wondered why bacteria fail to grow in the presence of mold. When penicillin was first used in 1941, it was considered a miracle drug and used so indiscriminately that many strains of bacteria are now resistant.

The penicillins may be bactericidal or bacteriostatic, depending on the sensitivity or resistance of the bacteria involved, and are used to treat a variety of acute infections. They fall into these two types:

- **Natural penicillin** (such as penicillin G) works against a narrow spectrum of bacteria, including some strains of staphylococci, streptococci, and *E. coli.* It is sensitive to light and heat, so it is usually mixed just before it is used. Natural penicillin is poorly absorbed by the intestine, so it must be administered by intramuscular injection.

- **Semisynthetic derivatives** (such as ampicillin and amoxicillin) absorb better than natural penicillins, so they may be given orally. They work against a broader spectrum of bacteria that have become resistant to natural penicillins, including most strains of *E. coli* and salmonella.

BACITRACIN

Bacitracin is similar in range to penicillin G, but does not absorb well in the intestine and is relatively toxic when given as an injection. It is sometimes added to drinking water to treat necrotic enteritis, but is more often used topically to treat superficial staphylococcal and streptococcal infections of the skin and mucous membranes. Common antibacterial ointments containing bacitracin are Polysporin and Neosporin; the difference between them is that the latter contains the additional antibiotic neomycin (described under Aminoglycosides on the next page).

TETRACYCLINES

The original tetracyclines were naturally derived from fungi, but newer versions are either modified or wholly synthetic. All tetracyclines are bacteriostatic, and all have names ending in "cycline."

All the tetracyclines target the same kinds of bacteria — some chlamydia, staphylococci, streptococci, mycoplasmas, spirochetes, and a few other groups (but not most strains of *E. coli*). They are most often used to treat chronic respiratory disease, infectious coryza, fowl cholera, and necrotic enteritis.

Despite their broad spectrum, tetracyclines work rather poorly, and as has occurred with other overused drugs, many strains of bacteria are now resistant. Chlortetracycline (trade name Aureomycin) was the first tetracycline to be identified (in 1945) and is now effective against only susceptible strains of bacteria as determined by a laboratory sensitivity test.

The tetracycline most often used for chickens is naturally derived oxytetracycline (trade names Agrimycin and Liquamycin), which comes either in injectable form or as a powder to be added to drinking water. Because the injectable form may cause muscle damage, the soluble form is more often used.

Since oxytetracycline works best in an acidic environment, its absorption rate may be improved by adding 1 cup of cranberry juice,

½ cup of vinegar, or 2 teaspoons of citric acid (from the canning department at a grocery store) to each gallon of drinking water. To further increase the drug's effectiveness, discontinue calcium supplements during treatment.

AMINOGLYCOSIDES

Aminoglycosides get their name from the fact that each contains at least one sugar (glycoside) attached to one or more amino groups. These drugs are not readily absorbed through the digestive system and therefore are most commonly used either topically or by injection. Aminoglycosides kill gram-negative bacteria that multiply rapidly — such as those causing enteric and septicemic diseases — after only brief contact, but when used internally these drugs must be treated with caution because they can be highly toxic. Aminoglycosides include the following drugs:

- Gentamicin is available as a spray or ointment to treat infected skin wounds, and is also available as an injectable to treat coryza and intestinal infections caused by salmonella and E. coli.

- Neomycin is used for staphylococcal skin infections, such as bumblefoot and infected breast blister. As a topical antibiotic, it comes in powder form (trade name Neo-Predef) or as an ointment (trade name Neosporin, among others). Neomycin sulfate soluble powder is also available to treat diarrhea caused by susceptible E. coli and salmonella.

- Streptomycin injectable works against a fairly narrow range of susceptible E. coli, Pasteurella, Pseudomonas, salmonella, and staphylococcal bacteria.

Aminoglycosides are often combined with penicillin or some other antibiotic to create synergism — a phenomenon whereby two drugs applied together have a greater total effect than the sum of their individual effects. Combining drugs without knowing which ones work synergistically can backfire, however, as some combinations cancel each other out or worse, with disastrous consequences for the chicken.

SPECTINOMYCIN

Spectinomycin (trade name Spectam) is a natural antibiotic in a group of drugs (aminocyclitols) that are structurally similar to the aminoglycosides, but much less toxic. As a soluble powder it is used to treat chronic respiratory disease and other conditions caused by mycoplasma bacteria. As an injectable it is used to control intestinal infections caused by E. coli and salmonella, but readily results in resistant strains.

Like its cousins the aminoglycosides, spectinomycin is poorly absorbed by the chicken's digestive system. When used in drinking water it is rapidly excreted in droppings. When used as an injectable it is rapidly excreted in urine.

ERYTHROMYCIN AND TYLOSIN

Erythromycin (trade name Gallimycin) and tylosin (Tylan) belong to a group of broad-spectrum drugs (macrolides) that are basically bacteriostatic but can be bacteriocidal at high doses or when used over a long period of time. These drugs are inactivated in an acidic environment, so do not add vinegar or other acidifiers to treated drinking water. Similarly, when taken orally these drugs absorb rather poorly because they are inactivated by digestive acids. Used in injectable form, they are absorbed rapidly but cause painful swelling.

Relative Effectiveness of Common Antibiotics Used for Chickens

ANTIBIOTIC	GRAM POSITIVE	GRAM NEGATIVE	MYCOPLASMAS
Bacitracin	Some	Few	None
Erythromycin	Many	Few	Some
Gentamicin	Some	Most	Many
Neomycin	Some	Most	Some
Penicillins, modified	Some	Some	None
Penicillins, natural	Some	Few	None
Spectinomycin	Few	Most	Many
Streptomycin	Few	Most	None
Sulfonamides	Some	Some	None
Tetracyclines	Many	Many	Many
Tylosin	Many	Some	Some

Erythromycin is so similar to penicillin that it is often considered an alternative against bacteria that are resist to penicillin, especially enterococci, staphylococci, and streptococci. It is most often used to treat coryza, chronic respiratory disease, and infectious synovitis.

Tylosin is similar to erythromycin and is used to treat the same conditions, but it is more effective against mycoplasmas. Compared to the relatively rapid resistance bacteria develop to erythromycin, resistance to tylosin develops much more slowly.

Antibiotic Caveats

Antibiotics can cause reactions that are as bad as, or worse than, the disease they are used to treat. Treating chickens with any antibiotic can prove problematic for the following reasons:

- If a disease is misidentified and the wrong antibiotic is used, the chicken's condition could become worse.

- An antibiotic can't tell the difference between beneficial and pathogenic bacteria. The indiscriminate use of an antibiotic, especially one that is broad in spectrum, damages the chicken's normal microflora, particularly in the digestive system, leaving the chicken more susceptible to diseases and parasites. A classic sign of microfloral disruption is diarrhea, which can be fatal if the drug is not immediately discontinued.

- The indiscriminate or incorrect use of an antibacterial can cause bacteria to become resistant to that particular drug or class of drugs. When diseased chickens are treated with a bactericide, strains that are sensitive to that drug are destroyed, while resistant strains survive — particularly if the drug is discontinued too soon. Exposure of the stronger bacteria to a drug causes them to raise defenses against that particular drug should it be encountered again in the future.

As a result, bacterial diseases, particularly fowl cholera, colibacillosis, pseudomonas, salmonellosis, and staphylococcosis, are becoming more difficult to treat. Successful treatment may require a sensitivity test to determine which drug will work against the strain causing the disease.

- Giving antibiotics routinely to chickens, particularly baby chicks, in a misguided effort to boost their immune systems often backfires because they interfere with the development of the birds' natural immunities.

- Some drugs are approved for use in meat birds. Although some of these drugs have no withdrawal period, many of them do have a specified withdrawal period, representing the amount of time that must pass after discontinuing treatment until drug residues in the meat reach an "acceptable" level. Eating chicken meat containing drug residues can affect your resistance to medical treatment with those or similar drugs.

- Antibiotic residues continue to be deposited in eggs for many weeks after a drug has been discontinued. For this reason few drugs are approved for treating laying hens.

- Antibiotics are excreted in droppings, some more rapidly than others. If you compost used bedding from your chicken coop, antibiotic residues will eventually get into your garden soil and from there into the body of anyone who eats vegetables from your garden.

- If you are allergic to a particular antibiotic or class of antibiotics, you can experience an allergic reaction just from handling the drug while treating your chickens.

Enough said?

Common Treatments for Bacterial Infections*

PATHOGEN	TREATMENT	DOSE	DURATION	WITHDRAWAL**
Bacterias	Chlortetracycline	1 gm/gallon water	2–8 weeks	5 days
	Oxytetracycline	1 gm/gallon water	2–8 weeks	5 days
	Sulfamethazine	2 tablespoons/gallon water	6 days	10 days
	Sulfaquinoxaline	2 tablespoons/gallon water	6 days	10 days
Mycoplasmas	Erythromycin	½ gm/gallon water	5 days	1 day
	Tylosin	2 gms/gallon water	2–3 days	1 day

*Not approved for hens kept for table eggs
**Withdrawal period for meat birds

CHAPTER 9

The Fungus Among Us

Fungi comprise a kingdom of organisms that include molds, mildews, yeasts, and mushrooms. These related organisms share the following characteristics:

- They have a nucleus, or core.

- They lack chlorophyll and thus are unable to produce their own food, but instead absorb nutrients from other organisms, living or dead.

- They are made up of either long branching filaments or, as in yeast, single cells.

- They have a cell wall made of chitin — the same substance that makes up an insect's shell.

- They all reproduce by means of spores.

The word "fungus" comes directly from the Latin word *fungus*, meaning "mushroom." The study of fungi is called mycology, from the Greek word *mykes*, meaning "mushroom."

Of the one-million-plus different species of fungi, most are either beneficial or harmless. Some, however, generate powerful poisons in the course of their normal metabolism, while others are parasites capable of invading a chicken's skin or internal organs.

Mycotoxicoses

Mycotoxicoses are caused by various kinds of mold that grow in grain and release toxins as part of their normal metabolic processes. These toxins can poison chickens in much the same way that pesticides do. Such illnesses nearly always result from eating moldy feed, although some toxins can poison chickens through skin contact or by being inhaled, but they do not spread directly from chicken to chicken.

The molds that produce mycotoxins grow naturally in grains, and some molds generate more than one kind of poison. But not all molds produce mycotoxins, and not all mycotoxins are poisonous to chickens. Penicillin, for instance, is a mycotoxin that poisons bacteria, so instead of calling it a toxin, we call it an antibiotic.

The severity of illness caused by mold toxins and the specific signs depend on the type of mold involved and how long the chickens are exposed to it. Their age and state of health also influence the degree of poisoning. Conversely, fungal poisoning can increase a chicken's susceptibility to other diseases.

Diagnosing Mold Poisoning

Molds are natural environmental contaminants that are commonly present in grains, but they cannot produce toxins unless conditions are favorable for their growth. Even then, mycotoxins are usually at such low levels that they remain undetected and rarely cause serious illness in chickens. Diagnosing an illness caused by a specific mycotoxin can prove difficult for these several reasons:

- Signs may not become readily apparent unless the chickens consume or inhale a toxin over a period of time.

- Not all mycotoxins produce readily identifiable signs of illness.

- Many mycotoxins produce signs that are similar to one another or to signs of other diseases.

- Mold is not always easy to detect in contaminated feed or litter, which may look and smell perfectly normal.

- Many mycotoxins remain stable during feed milling and storage, leaving active toxins after the molds that produced them have been destroyed.

- More than one toxin may be involved, resulting in a confusion of signs.

- Mycotoxicosis is not so common that it is the first thing anyone thinks of when chickens fall ill.

Speaking of Fungi

mycosis. Any infection caused by members of the fungus family

mycotoxicosis. Any illness caused by a mycotoxin

mycotoxin. Any poison generated by the mold members of the fungus family

opportunistic pathogen. An organism that normally doesn't cause disease except in a chicken with a weakened immune system

primary pathogen. An organism that can infect a chicken with a healthy immune system

superficial mycosis. A fungal infection of the skin or feather follicles

systemic mycosis. A fungal infection affecting the entire body

- Infectious diseases, internal parasites, and other stressors increase a chicken's susceptibility to fungal poisoning, which then may not be recognized or identified as contributing to the chicken's condition.

- Most mycotoxins increase a chicken's susceptibility to infectious diseases, which may be diagnosed without identifying mold poisoning as the underlying cause.

- Methods of analyzing feed or litter for mycotoxins are not always readily available to the backyard chicken keeper.

- By the time signs appear, the mold-contaminated feed or litter may have been used up or replaced, making a positive identification of a toxin impossible.

- Chickens that are not exposed to a lethal dose of toxin tend to recover on their own once the contaminated feed or litter is removed.

Suspect mycotoxicosis if chickens die with few, if any, signs of illness and you cannot determine the cause, especially if your chickens have been eating feed from other than the usual source. Of the many different mycotoxins, three groups are the most likely to affect backyard chickens: aflatoxins, fusariotoxins, and ochratoxins. A fourth mycotoxin, ergotism, can poison chickens foraging on cropland or wild grasses.

Aflatoxicosis

The most common mycotoxins affecting chickens and other poultry, aflatoxins were discovered in the 1960s, when thousands of turkeys died after eating contaminated peanut meal. Aflatoxins consist of four distinct poisonous compounds produced by *Aspergillus flavus* and other molds that readily contaminate feedstuffs grown in hot, dry weather; stored with

Mycotoxicoses (Fungal Poisoning)

ILLNESS	CAUSED BY	AFFECTS	GRAIN SOURCE	WEATHER CONDITIONS	STORAGE CONDITIONS
Aflatoxicosis	*Aspergillus flavus* and other molds	Liver, blood coagulation, immunity, fertility	All grains, seeds, and nuts	Hot and dry	Warm and humid
Ergotism	*Claviceps* spp.	Circulatory system, nervous system	Rye, wheat, and other cereal grains	Cool and damp	(Present at harvest; destroyed by heat)
Fusariotoxicosis	*Fusarium* spp. and other molds	Skin and mucous membranes, especially in mouth; immunity	Corn, barley, millet, oats, rye, sorghum, safflower seed, wheat	Cool and damp	Cold (present at harvest; destroyed by heat)
Ochratoxicosis	Several species of *Aspergillus* and *Penicillium*	Kidneys, immunity	Barley, corn, millet, sorghum, sunflower, wheat	Hot and dry	Warm and humid

a moisture content greater than 14 percent; or stored under humid conditions or for too long.

Aflatoxicosis is the resulting illness. How sick the chickens become depends on their age, how much contaminated feed they eat, and how long they eat it. Young chickens are more susceptible than older birds but are much less susceptible than ducklings or turkey poults.

SIGNS OF AFLATOXICOSIS

Aflatoxins are highly toxic, and acute aflatoxicosis is deadly. Signs of acute toxicity include loose droppings containing undigested seed or grain particles, pale comb and wattles, low egg production with reduced fertility and low hatchability, incoordination and paralysis, followed by a high death rate.

Chronic aflatoxicosis increases a bird's susceptibility to heat stress and infection, reduces egg production, and causes significant liver damage, which can lead to ascites (described on page 110). Although aflatoxins are known to cause cancer in humans, chickens have a shorter lifespan and rarely develop this type of tumor.

PREVENTING AFLATOXICOSIS

Aflatoxins are not stored in the chicken's body but are rapidly excreted in bile and urates. Replacing contaminated feed can therefore result in the rapid recovery of chickens that are not lethally poisoned.

These molds get into grain with the help of insects that attack growing or stored crops and break down the protective hull of individual kernels, opening the way to mold penetration. Grains that are deliberately cracked or crushed to make them easier for chickens to digest, when stored improperly or for too long, are also subject to mold contamination.

To avoid aflatoxicosis, do not feed your chickens grains or seeds that are visibly infested with insects or that show signs of insect damage — such as the presence of fine powder or kernels that are off-color, smaller than normal, or misshapen. Most commercially prepared pellets and crumbles contain mold inhibitors that prevent the development of aflatoxins. Sprinkling diatomaceous earth into fresh scratch grains helps inhibit insects.

Ergotism

A parasitic disease of cereal grains, ergot occurs when a fungus grows on a grain head in place of a grain kernel. It is so common that until the 1850s farmers thought ergot was a natural part of grain plants. It is caused by *Claviceps purpurea* and some 35 related mold species that grow naturally in rye, wheat, and other cereal grain crops and are harvested along with the grains.

Ergot contains several alkaloids that have been used to develop a number of prescription drugs, one of which is the infamous LSD. In its natural state ergot can be highly toxic, causing poisoning called ergotism — the oldest known

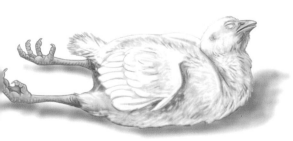

Chickens that die from acute aflatoxicosis are usually found lying prone with their feet stretched out behind them and head drawn back.

mycotoxicosis. Ergotism takes on one of two distinct forms.

- **The acute, or convulsive, form** affects a chicken's central nervous system, causing incoordination, trembling, neck twisting, convulsions, and death.

- **The chronic, or gangrenous, form** constricts the blood vessels that go to the chicken's extremities, causing a painful burning sensation and decomposition of the affected body tissue, usually the comb, wattles, beak, shanks, or toes.

Ergot favors wild grasses such as bluegrass, brome, and ryegrass, as well as cereal grains, including rye, barley, and wheat grown in cool climates, especially in wet weather. Ever since the cause of ergotism was discovered, however, cereal grains have been grown and harvested using methods designed to minimize the presence of ergot.

Ergotism in chickens and other farm animals today rarely comes from eating contaminated feed; it is more likely to result from foraging in fields containing ergot-infected grain crops or grassy weeds. However, given ergot's bitter taste, a chicken under normal circumstances would likely not eat enough to be seriously poisoned.

Fusariotoxicosis

Various species of *Fusarium*, along with several other molds, produce a number of mycotoxins that differ in the severity of their toxicity to chickens and in the types of resulting illnesses. A sizable group of these mycotoxins, the trichothecenes, occur worldwide in soil and in crops, especially in corn, oats, wheat, barley, rice, rye, sorghum, and safflower seed. Although not all trichothecenes are generated by *Fusarium* molds, the majority are, and the resulting illness is commonly called fusariotoxicosis.

Trichothecenes cause poisoning not only when eaten but also when inhaled or absorbed through the skin — features that make them of interest for biological warfare. Most of the mycotoxins in this group are highly caustic, causing a burning sensation on the skin; watery eyes and labored breathing when inhaled; and a burnlike irritation in the mouth and on the tongue when ingested. Chickens generally refuse to continue eating trichothecene-contaminated feed and therefore are likely to recover when provided with fresh, uncontaminated feed.

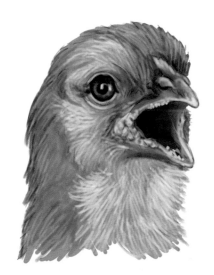

Trichothecenes cause a burnlike irritation to a chicken's mouth and tongue, along with a crusty accumulation along the edges of its beak.

Ochratoxicosis

Related poisons called ochratoxins are generated by several species of molds, including some of the same molds that produce aflatoxins. Ochratoxins and aflatoxins therefore may be present in the same grain. Fortunately, even though ochratoxins can be deadlier than aflatoxins, they are less common.

Ochratoxins are found in barley, oats, rye, wheat, and other grains. They mainly affect a chicken's kidneys, but they also increase susceptibility to infections and tumors. Moderate poisoning in growing birds reduces their growth rate and in layers affects egg production, fertility, and hatchability. Signs of severe poisoning are depression, huddling, reduced body temperature, diarrhea, rapid weight loss, and death from kidney failure.

Ochratoxins develop in stored feed and can be present at low levels without causing obvious signs of poisoning. Like aflatoxins, the molds that generate these toxins flourish at high temperatures, so in contrast to ergot and fusarium molds, they can occur in pelleted feed (which is produced under intense heat) unless the ration formula includes mold inhibitors. Since ochratoxins are rapidly excreted, chickens that are not lethally poisoned usually recover once the contaminated feed is replaced.

Treating Mold Poisoning

Once mold toxins contaminate grain or feed, nothing can remove them or neutralize their harmful effects in chickens that consume the feed. Most of the time, however, chickens will recover on their own, once the source of contamination has been removed.

All mycotoxins increase a chicken's need for vitamins, trace elements (especially selenium),
and protein. Supportive therapy during recovery therefore includes improving their ration's overall nutritional profile.

Aside from supportive therapy, no specific treatments have been found to hasten recovery. Minimizing stress during recovery is, of course, essential. The chickens may also need to be treated for any internal parasites or bacterial infection responsible for increasing their susceptibility to fungal poisoning (or that may have occurred from reduced immunity caused by fungal poisoning). If a bird is treated with an antibiotic that doesn't work as well as it should, so that more than the normal amount of antibiotic is needed, and the chicken takes longer to recover than would be considered normal, it's a clue that a mycotoxin may be involved in the chicken's bacterial illness.

Normal feathers   **Sign of toxicity**

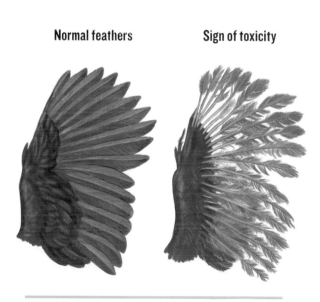

Ragged-looking feathers are among the signs of ochratoxicosis and other mycotoxicoses.

Technically speaking, mushroom poisoning is a type of mycotoxicosis. However, it is considered to be significantly different from other types of fungal poisoning because, unlike the microscopic fungi that cause mycotoxicoses, mushrooms are large and readily visible. (See Identifying an Amanita Mushroom on page 307.) A chicken therefore presumably chooses to peck at a mushroom, compared to inadvertently consuming microfungal toxins hidden in the ration.

At any rate, chickens are not likely to eat enough poisonous mushrooms to get sick, unless they are pretty hungry and have nothing else to eat. Even so, a mushroom of any kind would have a hard time growing in the average active chicken yard.

Preventing Mold Poisoning

Controlling mycotoxins mainly consists of prevention, which can be difficult, given that molds occur naturally in the environment. Ergot and fusaria, in particular, develop on growing crops and therefore may be present at harvest. Aflatoxins and ochratoxins, however, develop primarily after harvest, in grains that are stored under improper conditions.

Fungal poisoning largely can be avoided by using commercially prepared feeds containing mold inhibitors, although such additives may not affect toxins that are already present. Never give chickens feed that is insect ridden or has gone moldy. If you buy buggy or moldy feed, take it back and demand a refund.

Storing feed away from humid conditions is another helpful control measure, as is storing no more than about a 2-week supply at a time, so the feed doesn't sit around long enough to get moldy. Buying feed more often, rather than storing a lot at a time, has another advantage — should one batch contain mold toxins, your chickens are not likely to get sick enough to develop signs of toxicity by the time they are fed a fresh, mold-free batch.

Mycoses

In contrast to a mycotoxicosis, caused by poisons generated by a fungus, a mycosis is an infection occurring when a parasitic fungus invades a chicken's body tissue. Such an infection may result from an abnormal proliferation of fungi that commonly live on a chicken's skin or in its digestive tract, or it may be caused by a fungus that usually lives in the environment.

Fungi that normally coexist on or in a chicken's body can grow out of control and cause disease in a bird with any condition that suppresses its immune response, including stress, or that has been treated with an antibacterial drug. Fungal infections have gotten more common with the widespread and indiscriminate use of antibiotics, since these drugs destroy normal body flora, paving the way for pathogenic fungi to take over.

Disease-Causing Fungi

The fungi that cause disease are classified as being either opportunistic or primary. Opportunistic pathogenic fungi infect a chicken with an immune system that is in some way suppressed or impaired. Brooder pneumonia and sour crop are examples of diseases caused by opportunistic fungi. Primary pathogenic fungi can infect a healthy chicken with a normally functioning immune system. Ringworm is an example of a disease caused by a primary pathogen.

The diseases caused by fungi are classified as being either superficial or systemic. A superficial mycosis affects the skin or feather follicles and is caused by fungi that obtain nutrients from keratin, the protein that makes up feathers, claws, and the dead outer layer of skin. These fungi are known as dermatophytes, from the Greek words *derma*, meaning "skin," and *phyton*, meaning "growth." Ringworm, also known as dermatophytosis, is an example of a superficial mycosis that affects chickens.

A systemic mycosis infects internal organs, usually entering the chicken's body as inhaled spores and invading the lungs, but sometimes entering through an open wound. Such a fungus may travel through the chicken's body by means of the respiratory system or circulatory system to infect the nervous system or other internal organs. Brooder pneumonia and sour crop are examples of systemic mycoses.

Systemic fungal infections are usually caused by opportunistic fungi that typically grow in the soil and feed on decaying matter, but that take advantage of a chicken's low resistance due to stress or the presence of some other disease. Such an infection may be chronic but may also be fatal.

Treating a Fungal Infection

Although fungal diseases do not often infect chickens, they can be devastating to the chicken that does get infected. Yet because mycoses are less common in chickens than are bacterial and viral diseases, and because most mycoses are not contagious, methods for their control and treatment remain less advanced than those for diseases caused by bacteria and viruses.

Additionally, any fungal infection is difficult, if not impossible, to treat. For one thing, the cell structure of a fungus is more similar to that of a chicken, or a human, than to that of a bacterium. A drug that kills a fungus can therefore do harm to the patient.

Further, because opportunistic fungi target individuals with already weakened immune systems, the infected chicken has few reserves to help fend off the infection, even with the help of antifungal drugs. And even when such infections are successfully treated, the susceptible chicken may be readily reinfected in the future by fungi in the environment or by fungal colonies or spores remaining dormant in the chicken's body. For all these reasons, avoiding a fungal infection is far better than attempting to treat one.

Aspergillosis

Aspergillosis is a respiratory disease caused by the spores of several species of *Aspergillus* molds, the same fungi that cause aflatoxicosis. Evidence indicates that the toxins may contribute to a chicken's susceptibility to the infection.

These molds are readily found in the environment, especially in soil, grains, and decaying vegetation. They thrive at warm temperatures and therefore grow well in chicken coop litter and feed, as well as in brooders and incubators. Eggs with damaged shells may release mold spores during incubation that infect chicks as they hatch.

Inhaled spores cause acute pneumonia in chicks, commonly known as brooder

Mycoses (Fungal Diseases)

DISEASE	NATURE	CAUSE	AFFECTS	PREVALENCE
Aspergillosis (brooder pneumonia)	Opportunistic; not contagious	*Aspergillus* spp.	Respiratory system	Fairly common
Ringworm (favus)	Primary pathogen; contagious	*Microsporum gallinae*	Skin and feather follicles	Sporadic
Sour crop (thrush)	Opportunistic; not contagious	*Candida albicans*	Upper digestive tract	Common

pneumonia. Newly hatched chicks are especially susceptible to brooder pneumonia if they are subjected to cold stress, dusty conditions, or ammonia fumes from an accumulation of moist droppings in the brooder. A brooder made from a plastic storage tote can be particularly problematic because it readily accumulates moisture from chick respiration and spilled or splashed drinking water.

Older chickens are less seriously affected unless their immunity has been reduced by some other issue or they are heavily subjected to mold spores. A chicken that recovers from brooder pneumonia can develop chronic aspergillosis that gradually gets worse as the chicken matures and needs increasingly more oxygen as the infection increasingly weakens its respiratory system.

Diagnosing aspergillosis is difficult because it looks similar to any other respiratory disease. Suspect brooder pneumonia in chicks if they have a respiratory illness and are less than 2 weeks old. Suspect chronic aspergillosis

in an older chicken if it has trouble breathing but doesn't make the distress sounds typical of most other respiratory diseases.

A less common form of aspergillosis results in an eye infection in both chicks and mature chickens. Typically only one eye becomes swollen, with yellowish cheesy material accumulating underneath the nictitating membrane.

This infection is largely the result of mismanagement and may easily be prevented through good sanitation (especially in the incubator and brooder), providing good ventilation to minimize dust, managing litter to avoid ammonia fumes, and keeping overall stress to a minimum. Avoid moldy litter surrounding feeders and drinkers, and do not buy (or else discard) baled shavings that appear to have been wet — as indicated by a grayish or otherwise off color to the shavings, or visible condensation inside the bag.

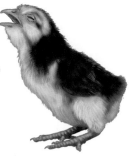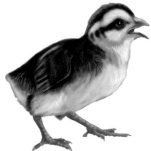

Gasping chicks under 2 weeks old may have brooder pneumonia; note the difference between gasping (left) and panting (right) caused by excessive brooder temperature.

Sour Crop

A yeast that normally lives in the digestive tract of chickens and other animals, including humans, *Candida albicans* can get out of control and infect a chicken's upper digestive tract. This disease — known variously as candidiasis, sour crop, or thrush — occurs either when a chicken's immune system has been weakened by some other condition, or the normal bacteria of the crop are somehow disrupted, such as through the use of a coccidiostat or antibiotic. As a result, candida proliferate and invade the mucous membranes of the upper digestive tract.

Sour crop primarily affects young chickens, and sometimes aging chickens, but may occur at any age. The most obvious signs are a sour or yeasty odor coming from the chicken's mouth (bad breath) and an enlarged crop that feels squishy and fluid-filled when you apply slight pressure. An affected chicken becomes generally lethargic, stops eating, and in an extreme case may die.

Treatment is not always successful, especially if the crop has been stretched beyond its normal elasticity. Further, unless you eliminate the underlying condition that allowed this infection to occur, the chicken will most likely have a relapse.

If an avian vet is available, having the crop surgically emptied and rinsed with an antiseptic solution is the safest option. A popular — but risky — method is to massage the crop to loosen its contents while briefly (no more than 20 seconds at a time) turning the chicken's head downward to try to drain out the contents, repeating the procedure once or twice until the crop is emptied. The chicken, however, runs the risk of inhaling regurgitated crop contents. For a more sensible treatment option, see Sour Crop Treatment, below.

SOUR CROP TREATMENT

Copper sulfate is commonly used to treat a chicken with sour crop, but an overdose is toxic. To avoid overdosing, first prepare a solution by mixing ½ pound copper sulfate plus ½ cup vinegar into ½ gallon of water. Clearly label this container as your stock solution. To each gallon of the chicken's drinking water, add 1 tablespoon of stock solution.

First flush the bird's digestive system with molasses or Epsom salts (see Laxative Flushes, page 392). Then feed as usual while using the stock solution to treat the chicken's drinking water until the infection is under control. During this time avoid using any antibiotics, which will make the condition worse.

As a follow-up treatment, nystatin oral antifungal may be helpful, as may also be using a probiotic to restore normal crop bacteria (see Probiotics, page 379). Adding vinegar to the drinking water at the rate of 1 tablespoon per gallon (15 mL per 4 L) — double the dose if the water is alkaline — can help prevent a recurrence of this infection in two ways: by discouraging the growth of candida in the drinking water, and by helping the chicken's crop maintain a pH that encourages beneficial bacteria to compete against candida and other potentially harmful microbes. Note that adding too little vinegar to the drinker can actively stimulate yeast growth.

To prevent sour crop, guard against coccidiosis and other diseases that reduce a chicken's overall immunity. Avoid prolonged or inappropriate use of coccidiostats, antibiotics, and other antimicrobials. Immediately treat any chicken with crop impaction, a condition that encourages the fermentation of feed lodged in the crop (see Pendulous Crop, page 79).

Ringworm

In chickens ringworm goes by many names, including dermatomycosis (from the Greek words *derma*, meaning "skin," and *mykes*, meaning "mushroom"), dermatophytosis (from the Greek words *derma*, meaning "skin," and *phyton*, meaning "growth"), favus (the Latin word *favus* means "honeycomb"), and white comb (plain English). The latter is the most descriptive term, as this skin disease initially looks like white flour clinging to the surface of the comb and wattles, and sometimes the face, eyelids, ear openings, and other parts of a chicken's head and neck. Left to spread, the infection will result in feather loss and a honeycomb appearance to the skin.

Ringworm is more likely to occur in chickens kept in a warm, humid, darkened environment than in chickens that spend a lot of time outdoors in the sunshine. Excessive bathing, or grooming of the comb and wattles, such as might be experienced by a frequently exhibited show bird, increases the possibility of infection by removing the skin's protective oils and proteins.

This infection is caused by the fungus *Microsporum gallinae*, which spreads slowly from chicken to chicken within a flock and can infect the chicken keeper as well. Some chickens recover on their own, but others continue to get worse as the fungus gradually spreads over the body, and the infected bird eventually loses interest in normal chicken activities. Shed scales contaminating the coop and run can infect any future chickens.

Treatment involves isolating the affected chicken and, wearing disposable gloves to avoid infecting yourself, applying an ointment containing the antifungal miconazole (brand name Monistat) every day until the infection is gone. An alternative treatment is to use garlic oil as an antifungal (see Garlic Oil, page 388).

Successful treatment takes time and patience, and there's always the possibility of reinfection. The best way to prevent this disease is to avoid introducing an infected chicken into your flock.

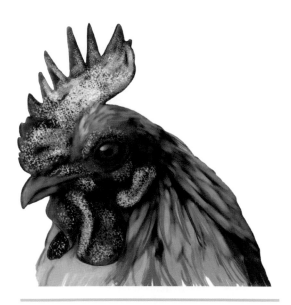

Ringworm (favus) looks like a white powder clinging to the surface of the comb, which, left untreated, crusts over, spreads to other parts of the face and body, and infects other chickens and possibly also the chicken keeper.

CHAPTER 10

Diseases Caused by Viruses

Viruses are the smallest known pathogens — so tiny they may be seen only through an electron microscope that magnifies them to 100,000 times. Not all viruses cause disease, and the diseases they do cause range widely, from mild to fatal.

Although viruses tend to be more host specific than bacteria, they are also more difficult to control for these reasons:

- Viruses remain viable in nature.

- They are easily transmitted from one location to another.

- They break down the defenses of a healthy bird (unlike bacteria, which tend to produce secondary infections).

- Once they invade a living cell, they reproduce rapidly.

- Some viruses constantly mutate.

- Viruses cannot be treated with antibiotics, but some may be prevented with vaccines.

Since they are so small, millions of viruses can travel on one speck of dust. Just think how many could be carried on the hair of a fly, a rat's foot, a feather, the sole of your shoe, or a used chicken carrier.

Virus Groups

Wherever life exists, viruses also exist. Outside the cell of another living organism, however, a virus has no life — it neither breathes nor eats. Its only known activity is to take over the cell of another life form for the purpose of making copies of itself.

A virus consists of a strand of hereditary information, or genome, which may be either DNA or RNA. One difference between them is that DNA viruses mutate less rapidly. Vaccines against DNA viruses are therefore effective for many years, while vaccines against RNA viruses must be constantly updated. Some tricky viruses contain DNA at one stage during their growth cycle and RNA at another stage.

For both types of virus the genome is enclosed in a protective protein coat, called a capsid. Some viruses have an outer layer, called an envelope, that protects the protein coat until the virus encounters a suitable living cell to invade. The envelope allows a virus to remain infective outside of a living cell so it can spread by horizontal transmission, as described in How Diseases Spread on page 4. The influenza virus, among others, uses this strategy.

DNA/RNA and Enveloped Viruses Affecting Chickens

VIRUS	CHICKEN DISEASE	DNA/RNA	ENVELOPED
Birnavirus	Infectious bursal disease	RNA	No
Coronavirus	Infectious bronchitis	RNA	Yes
Herpesvirus	Laryngotracheitis & Marek's disease	DNA	Yes
Orthomyxovirus	Avian influenza	RNA	Yes
Paramyxovirus	Newcastle disease	RNA	Yes
Picornavirus	Epidemic tremor	RNA	No
Poxvirus	Pox	DNA	Complex
Retrovirus	Lymphoid leukosis	RNA => DNA	Yes

Reportable Viral Diseases

⚠ Many viral diseases are so dire that when they occur they must be reported to your state veterinarian, as described on page 417. The following viral diseases are reportable:

- Avian influenza
- Epidemic tremor
- Fowl pox
- Infectious bronchitis
- Laryngotracheitis
- Marek's disease
- Newcastle disease
- Infectious bursal disease

Viral Growth Cycle

The specific details of the growth cycle vary among different viruses, but all viruses replicate following the same six basic phases. In simplified form, these phases are as follows:

1. **Attachment.** The virus binds to receptors on the surface of a suitable host cell. Specific viruses can bind only to specific receptors, as determined by the kind of cells in which the particular virus is able to replicate.

2. **Penetration**, also known as viral entry. Changes in the virus's outer surface, induced by attachment, allow the virus to invade the host cell.

3. **Uncoating.** Enzymes weaken the capsid, allowing the virus to release its genome into the host cell and thus take command of the cell's function.

4. **Replication.** The host cell continues to reproduce as usual, but instead of carrying on its normal function, it produces multiple copies of the virus's genome and protein.

5. **Self-assembly.** The viral proteins are modified into capsids, and each encloses a viral genome.

6. **Release.** Viruses leave the host cell. Enveloped viruses are released by budding, during which the envelope is derived from the host cell's membrane. Nonenveloped viruses rupture the host cell, thereby killing the cell.

Some sneaky viruses hide their genome by incorporating it into the host cell. Every time the cell undergoes division, a copy of the viral genome is included. When the virus is inspired to become active, it releases itself by rupturing the host cell.

Viral Growth Cycle

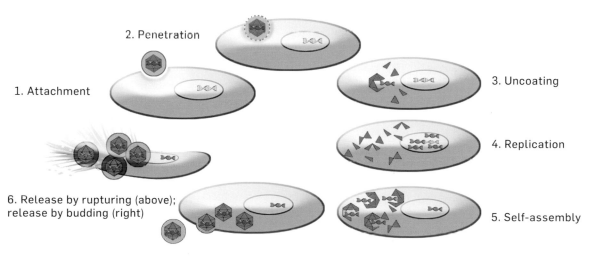

2. Penetration

1. Attachment

3. Uncoating

4. Replication

6. Release by rupturing (above); release by budding (right)

5. Self-assembly

Pathogenic Viruses

Virus is a Latin word meaning "poison." Pathogenic viruses usually get into a chicken's body by being inhaled or swallowed, but they may also enter through an eye or a wound (including an injection puncture). Sometimes viruses invade a cell and hide there for months or years before becoming active.

Viruses may take over cells near their point of entry, causing a skin disease such as pox. Or they may travel to another preferred site, most often the respiratory system, as in infectious bronchitis, or the nervous system, as occurs with Marek's disease. Sometimes they travel through the bird's body, producing a plaguelike infection, such as exotic Newcastle disease and lethal forms of avian influenza.

Usually when a bird is attacked by a virus, its immune system mobilizes to fight off the virus, which may take a few days to a few weeks. In the process the bird's body becomes sensitized to the virus, and it becomes immune to the disease caused by that virus. The bird may, however, continue shedding the virus, infecting other birds that haven't yet been exposed.

Some viruses, on the other hand, attack so fast the bird's body cannot respond before serious damage or death occurs. Other viruses weaken the immune system, leaving the bird open to attack by an opportunistic or secondary infection, usually bacterial, which may be the actual cause of a chicken's death. If a chicken has a viral infection when it is vaccinated against some other disease, the virus may interfere with the vaccine's ability to trigger immunity.

The 2,000-plus recognized virus species are taxonomically classified according to their size, their shape, and the type of disease they cause.

Prevalence of Viral Infections

CONDITION	VIRUS	SYSTEM AFFECTED	PREVALENCE
Avian influenza, high-path	Orthomyxovirus	Systemic	Very rare
Avian influenza, low-path	Orthomyxovirus	Respiratory system	Common
Epidemic tremor	Picornavirus	Nerves	Sporadic
Infectious bronchitis	Coronavirus	Respiratory system	Common
Infectious bursal disease	Birnavirus	Lymph tissue (cloacal bursa)	Common
Laryngotracheitis, acute	Herpesvirus	Upper respiratory tract	Not common
Laryngotracheitis, mild	Herpesvirus	Upper respiratory tract	Common
Lymphoid leukosis	Retrovirus	Liver and other organs	Common
Marek's disease	Herpesvirus	Nerves, organs, eyes, skin	Common
Newcastle disease, mild	Paramyxovirus	Respiratory system or intestines	Common
Newcastle disease, virulent	Paramyxovirus	Respiratory system, digestive tract, nerves, brain	Very rare
Pox, dry	Poxvirus	Skin	Common
Pox, wet	Poxvirus	Upper respiratory tract	Not common

Each group includes numerous members, and new viruses are constantly being discovered. Of the 395 established genera, only 7 are likely to affect backyard chickens.

Viral Tumors

Some viruses mimic the signals that tell a chicken's cell it's time to divide. Instead of dividing as normal, the cell multiplies out of control, causing a mass of cells that grow into a tumor.

Tumors can occur in any part of a chicken's body. They may be benign (developing and remaining in one place) or malignant (spreading to other parts of the body). External benign tumors may be removed surgically (assuming you are willing to undergo the expense); malignant tumors usually come back after surgery. Internal tumors, whether benign or malignant, are rarely discovered until after a bird dies.

In veterinary jargon a tumor is called a neoplasm, from the Greek words *neo*, meaning "new," and *plasma*, meaning "formation." Miscellaneous viruses can cause neoplasms in a hen's ovary or oviduct (most often in birds more than 1 year old) or along the back and thighs of a broiler (appearing as craterlike ulcers that may clump together).

By far the most important tumors in chickens are those in the avian leukosis complex. These interrelated viral diseases affect few other birds (or animals) besides chickens, and fall into two main categories.

- Marek's disease — named after veterinarian József Marek, who first described the disease — is caused by herpesviruses that primarily infect young and growing chickens but can also affect aging chickens.

- The leukosis/sarcoma group of viruses — leukosis is an excess of leukocytes, or white blood cells; sarcoma is a malignant tumor, its name derived from the Greek word *sarkoma*, meaning "fleshy substance" — are retroviruses that primarily affect chickens just reaching maturity.

Marek's Disease

Marek's disease is a complex condition that can take on many forms, from no apparent signs to temporary paralysis, to blindness in one eye or both, to sudden death. The virus switches off a chicken's tumor-blocking genes and also attacks the cells that produce antibodies, impairing the chicken's immune system and opening the door for other diseases. Marek's therefore often appears in combination with other diseases, particularly coccidiosis and *E. coli* respiratory infections.

THE MAREK'S VIRUS

Marek's is one of the most widely studied chicken diseases; entire books have been written about this one condition alone. It is so common that you can safely assume your chickens have the virus, even if they don't show any signs of infection. The virus can remain dormant in a chicken's body, becoming active as a result of stress caused by overcrowding, being moved, poor ventilation, an overload of worms, or even the natural process of maturing and beginning to lay. It can also cause slow-growing tumors that produce no other signs until they become so massive in an aging bird that the chicken cannot survive.

The virus is not transmitted by means of hatching eggs. In fact, a newly hatched chick is briefly protected if the mother hen transmits a high antibody level through her eggs. Chicks should be brooded away from mature birds,

Forms of Marek's Disease

EYE FORM (GRAY EYE)

- Rare
- Graying, shrunken iris
- Irregular-shape pupil
- Unequal-size pupils
- Blindness in one or both eyes
- Up to 25% mortality

NERVE FORM (NEURAL LEUKOSIS)

- Sporadic
- Lack of coordination or walking stilted
- Muscle spasms
- Progressive paralysis of neck, leg, or wing
- Weight loss
- Paleness
- Enlarged crop
- Gasping
- Up to 20% mortality

NERVE FORM, TRANSIENT (PSEUDOBOTULISM)

- Common
- Temporary limp paralysis of neck or legs
- 0% mortality

SKIN FORM

- Rare
- Enlarged feather follicles, especially on legs
- Reddened, bloody looking shanks
- 0% mortality

VISCERAL FORM (VISCERAL LEUKOSIS)

- Common
- Rapid loss of weight
- Sometimes greenish diarrhea
- Massive internal tumors
- 60–80% mortality

---

however, since the first few weeks of life are the most critical time for infection. Chicks that are isolated until the age of 5 months develop a natural immunity that helps them overcome the Marek's virus as adults.

Some chicken strains are genetically more resistant than others. Fayoumis, with their ultra-strong constitution, are resistant to Marek's and many other diseases. Sebrights and Silkies, on the other hand, tend to be particularly susceptible, as are some strains of Polish, among other exotic breeds.

MAREK'S VACCINE

Turkeys carry a related non-tumor-forming virus that prevents the Marek's virus from developing tumors, as described under Natural Vaccination on page 280. Marek's vaccine is derived from the turkey virus, usually combined with a weakened form of the Marek's virus. Although chickens may be vaccinated at any age, the vaccine won't be effective in a chicken already exposed to Marek's disease. Vaccination should therefore occur as soon after hatch as possible, and chicks should be isolated while their immunity develops.

Most hatcheries offer the option of having chicks vaccinated. If you hatch your own chicks, you can purchase vaccine and administer it on the day of hatch. Be aware that handling the vaccine may make your eyes itch for a couple of days.

Vaccination does not prevent the possibility that the chickens may become infected by and spread the Marek's virus, but it does prevent the virus from causing tumors and paralysis, and it reduces shedding of the virus by infected birds. However, shedding can increase at any time during the chickens' lives, if they are subjected to extreme stress.

Further, vaccination is not 100 percent foolproof — about 5 percent of vaccinated chickens succumb to Marek's disease anyway. Also, as the virus becomes progressively more virulent, the currently available vaccines become less effective.

Marek's disease in chickens has been used as a model for studying cancer in humans, and Marek's vaccine has become a model for developing a human cancer vaccine. However, no evidence has proven that the Marek's virus causes cancer, or any other disease, in humans.

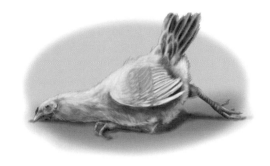

A typical sign of Marek's disease in young chickens is leg paralysis, resulting in one leg being stretched forward and the other back.

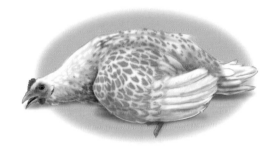

Highly virulent Marek's virus can cause temporary limp paralysis of the neck, resembling botulism.

Avian Leukosis Viruses

The leukosis/sarcoma group consists of several related retroviruses that mutate rapidly and affect primarily chickens, although they occasionally infect other poultry. They are referred to collectively as avian leukosis viruses or ALVs. Many strains have been identified, and periodically new ones appear. It's a pretty good bet your chickens are infected by one or more strains, even if they show no signs.

Lymphoid Leukosis vs. Marek's Disease

CHARACTERISTIC	LL	MD
Incubation period	14 weeks	2 weeks
Earliest age affected	14 weeks	4 weeks
Usual age affected	Over 6 months	Under 6 months
Peak ages affected	4–10 months	2–7 months
Peak ages for deaths	24–40 weeks	10–20 weeks
Paralysis	Possible	Common
Eye tumors	No	Possible
Skin tumors	Rare	Possible
Nerve tumors	No	Yes
Liver tumors	Yes	Yes
Heart tumors	Yes	Yes
Intestinal tumors	Yes	Yes
Lung tumors	Rare	Possible
Bursal tumors	Yes	No
Muscle tumors	Rare	Possible
Egg transmitted	Yes	No

In the environment, avian leukosis viruses don't survive long at normal temperatures and are easily killed by disinfectants. They can be transmitted to chicks through the egg, infecting the cloacal bursa during incubation. Not all the offspring of an infected hen will be infected, but the chicks that are infected will spread the disease in the brooder. Although an infected hen sheds the virus in her eggs, she may show no signs aside from laying fewer eggs of poorer quality.

Depending on the strain, these viruses can result in a number of tumor-causing diseases, which sometimes overlap. Some of the most typical ones are listed in the table Typical Diseases Caused by Avian Leukosis Viruses, on page 266.

By far the most common disease in this group is lymphoid leukosis, a close relative to Marek's disease. The two can be virtually indistinguishable from one another, especially when lymphoid leukosis results in paralysis in one or both legs, caused by kidney tumors pressing against a leg nerve.

HOW TO VACCINATE CHICKS AGAINST MAREK'S DISEASE

To vaccinate a newly hatched chick against Marek's disease, take a pinch of skin from the back of the chick's neck between your thumb and forefinger. Stick the needle into the skin and inject the vaccine, taking care not to poke the needle out the other side or stab your fingers.

Once mixed, Marek's vaccine has an extremely short life at normal room temperatures. Placing the vaccine in an ice bath will give you about an hour and a half to get all your chicks vaccinated.

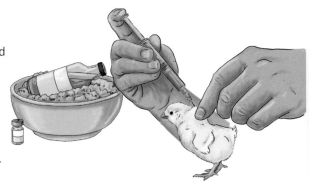

One distinguishing feature between the two diseases is that lymphoid leukosis has a longer incubation period and therefore typically strikes chickens just reaching maturity, while Marek's disease generally affects growing chickens. When it produces slow-growing tumors, Marek's can also affect aging birds.

Signs of lymphoid leukosis are not always obvious until a chicken is near death, at which time the bird becomes noticeably emaciated and depressed and may develop green diarrhea. Deaths rarely occur in chickens less than 14 weeks of age and tend to be more frequent around the time pullets start to lay.

Lymphoid leukosis is not as contagious as Marek's disease, and susceptibility decreases with age. In addition to being transmitted through the egg, it is spread via the droppings of infected birds and can be transmitted by blood-sucking insects. It starts as a tumor in the cloacal bursa and from there moves into other abdominal organs. Unlike Marek's disease, it cannot be prevented by vaccination. No treatment is known, and survivors may remain carriers.

Infectious Bronchitis

Infectious bronchitis, the most contagious disease of chickens, is a respiratory illness caused by a coronavirus that infects few other species besides chickens. It starts suddenly and spreads rapidly. It is characterized by coughing, sneezing, and rattling sounds in the throat that are more obvious in brooded chicks but may not be evident in older birds, except at night when they are on the roost. Deaths occur primarily in chicks.

Pullets that survive may have permanent ovary damage and may not lay well as mature hens. Infected hens lay fewer eggs; the shells tend to be rough, misshapen, and thin; and the albumen may be watery. Brown-egg layers may lay white-shell eggs, and the eggs of all infected hens hatch poorly. Recovered chickens continue to shed the virus for several days, then develop temporary immunity, only to become reinfected as their immunity declines or some other strain of the virus comes along.

A vaccine is available for use where bronchitis cannot be controlled any other way. Within about a week of vaccination, success is indicated by a mild reaction consisting of listlessness and coughing. Otherwise revaccination may be necessary. Even when the first round is successful, the vaccine is not foolproof, since it bestows immunity only against the strains contained in the vaccine, and new strains keep popping up. The only sure way to rid a flock of infectious bronchitis is to get rid of the infected chickens, clean up, disinfect, and start over.

Fowl Pox

Pox in chickens and other poultry — which is not the same disease as chicken pox in humans — appears in two forms: dry pox, affecting the skin (cutaneous form), and wet pox, affecting the mucous membranes of the upper respiratory tract (diphtheric form). Dry pox is usually temporary and resolves on its own. Wet pox is much more serious, sometimes ending in death. The two forms may follow one another, in either order, or may occur at the same time among different chickens in the same flock.

Dry pox is the more common form, typically occurring during warmer months when mosquitoes are busy. It is spread through wounds, such as from insect bites, fighting, dubbing, cannibalism, or injury from poorly designed facilities or equipment. It causes wart-like bumps on featherless skin, including the beak, comb, wattles, earlobes, and eyelids, and sometimes on the legs and feet and around the vent. The bumps eventually come together to form scabs that fall off, sometimes leaving scars.

Wet pox typically affects mature chickens, generally occurs during the cooler months, and is acquired by inhaling the virus from dust and dander. It causes yellowish curdlike bumps in the mouth and windpipe, which often accumulate until they affect the bird's ability to breathe and swallow, causing suffocation or starvation.

In either case, survivors recover in 4 to 5 weeks. In pox-prone areas this disease may be managed by controlling mites and mosquitoes and through annual vaccination. Vaccination is sometimes recommended for exhibition chickens, which requires vaccinating the entire flock, including any birds that are not shown.

Pox Vaccination

Injection with a live-virus vaccine gives chickens a mild case of pox, allowing them to develop immunity against reinfection. A vaccination kit consisting of fowl pox vaccine, diluent, and a two-prong wing-web stabber is available inexpensively from most poultry suppliers. The stabber is used to inject the mixed vaccine into the wing web of chickens at 12 and 16 weeks of age.

Typical Diseases Caused by Avian Leukosis Viruses

FORM	AFFECTS	INCUBATION PERIOD	PEAK AGE
Aleukemic myeloid leukosis	Skull, ribs, limb bones	3–11 weeks	Mature
Erythroid leukosis	Liver, spleen	3 weeks	3–6 months
Hemangioendothelioma	Blood vessels	1–4 months	6–9 months
Leukemic myeloid leukosis	Blood	10 days	Mature
Lymphoid leukosis	Liver and other organs	14 weeks	Early maturity
Ocular leukosis	Eyes	1–4 weeks	Early maturity
Osteopetrosis	Bones	4 weeks	8–12 weeks

*Signs for all ALVs are progressive weakness and emaciation, and diarrhea; death follows soon after signs become apparent, or may occur without any apparent signs.

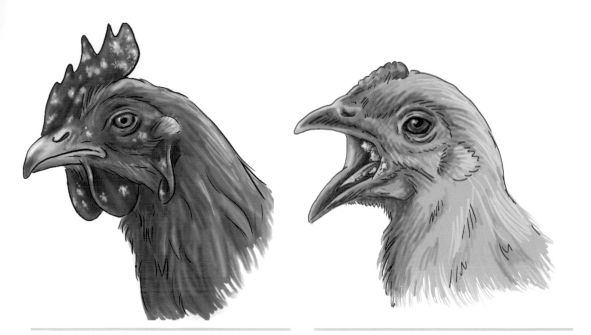

Dry pox appears as wartlike bumps on featherless skin that eventually form scabs.

Wet pox appears as yellowish curdlike bumps accumulating in the mouth and windpipe.

MORE SUSCEPTIBLE	SIGNS*	PREVALENCE
Female	Pale comb, tumors on head, breast, and shanks	Sporadic
Female	Bloody feather follicles	Uncommon
Female	Blood blisters on skin that may burst	Uncommon
Female	Pale comb, bloody feather follicles	Rare
Female	Pale and shriveled comb, enlarged abdomen, green diarrhea, death	Common
Female	Grayish pupil, blindness	Uncommon
Male	Stunted growth, thick leg bones, limping or stilted gait	Sporadic

The vaccine must be used right after it is mixed, and one vial is enough for up to a thousand chickens, so plan to do all your birds at the same time. Also round up a helper. While one person holds the chicken, the other stretches out a wing, locates the web underneath, and applies the injection by dipping the stabber into the vaccine, then firmly stabbing the wing web, forcing the tines of the stabber all the way through the web.

Take care to avoid getting vaccine on a chicken's head, particularly near its eyes and beak, which can cause sores serious enough to interfere with eating and drinking. For the same reason, vaccinate early in the day, when the chickens won't soon go to roost; a chicken that tucks its head under the vaccinated wing could get vaccine in its eyes. Sometimes a chicken will rest during the day with its head under a wing, so watch for pox sores, and be prepared to deal with them as described in Pox Treatment, below.

A week later examine the chickens for takes, or reactions indicating the vaccination was effective. A take consists of either a pimplelike swelling or a scab at the stab site. If a large percentage of chickens lack a take, revaccinate with a new batch of vaccine. Failure to take could mean one of the following:

- The vaccine was improperly applied (for instance, the web was not stabbed all the way through).

- The vaccine was improperly stored prior to use.

- The vaccine was past its expiration date.

- The chickens were already immune to fowl pox through previous vaccination or exposure to the virus. (If they don't "take" after a second round of vaccine, it's a pretty good indication that they are immune.)

A take that is larger than a pimple and is cheesy in the middle indicates contamination. Either the vaccine was contaminated during manufacture or the vaccination process was done in an unhygienic manner. Treat this as you would any other abscess or infected skin wound. See Treating Wounds on page 395.

Fowl pox vaccine can cause chickens to develop a fever within about 10 days after being vaccinated. They may be less active than usual, eat less, and have watery droppings for up to 3 weeks while their immunity kicks in.

Where pox is a problem and mosquitoes are prevalent all year, two rounds of vaccine may be needed. Chicks may be vaccinated as young as day-old for temporary immunity, then revaccinated as usual for permanent immunity. In such a case some chickens may still be protected from the first round and therefore may not take.

Pox Treatment

Since pox spreads slowly, you can further slow its spread by vaccinating as soon as you notice the disease is in progress. Hens that are vaccinated may stop laying during the fever stage. Otherwise, no treatment is effective against pox, other than keeping infected chickens as comfortable as possible while they recover.

Isolate, in uncrowded conditions, all birds that develop pox sores. The sores will usually heal on their own within about 4 weeks. To help dry them up and keep them from developing a bacterial infection, use a cotton swab to gently apply Betadine to each sore daily.

How to Vaccinate a Chicken against Pox

1. While a helper holds the chicken, stretch out a wing and locate the unfeathered skin of the wing web, or the chicken's "armpit."

2. Immerse the stabber in vaccine, and firmly stab through the featherless wing web (pulling a few feathers, if necessary, to avoid stabbing into feathers).

3. You can tell if the vaccination takes by watching for slight swelling and scabbing in about a week.

Supplies

- A pox vaccination kit, including the vaccine, diluent, and a two-prong wing-web stabber

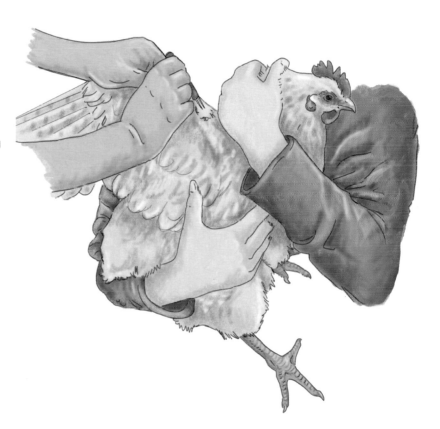

Sores around the mouth that inhibit eating may need to be softened with warm saline wound solution and, if necessary, removed with a cotton swab. Sores on the eyelids that prevent a chicken from seeing to eat may also need to be removed.

If thick discharge at the back of the mouth interferes with swallowing and breathing, try to clear the airway with cotton swab coated with Betadine, working gently to avoid excessive bleeding. A broad-spectrum antibiotic may be needed to prevent a bacterial infection.

While the disease is in progress, a sanitizer added to the drinking water will help keep the virus from spreading. Vinegar, added at the rate of 1 tablespoon per gallon of water (15 mL per 4 L), or double the amount of vinegar if the water is alkaline, is a good sanitizer, although it hastens rusting in a galvanized steel drinker. An alternative water sanitizer that does not react with metal is chlorine dioxide (brand name Oxine), which is not the same as chlorine bleach. Use chlorine dioxide at the rate of ¼ teaspoon per gallon of water (1 mL per 4 L), preparing a fresh batch daily.

During treatment the sores will first continue to grow, then gradually diminish until they fall off. Recovered birds become immune to pox, although some remain carriers and may become reinfected during molt or other times of stress.

After the flock has recovered, thoroughly clean housing to remove infective scabs, feathers, and dust, then disinfect with chlorine dioxide. Repeat the cleaning and disinfecting weekly for 4 weeks.

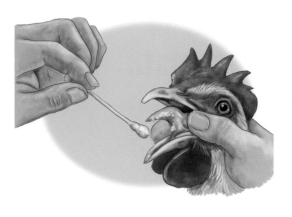

If wet pox interferes with eating and breathing, gently clear the accumulation with a cotton swab coated with Betadine.

Laryngotracheitis

Laryngotracheitis is a highly contagious disease of the larynx and trachea, hence the name (*laryngo* + *trache* + *itis*). Commonly called laryngo, it is caused by a virus in the herpes family.

This upper respiratory infection affects primarily chickens but can also infect pheasants. It affects chickens of all ages, although birds under 14 weeks of age are less susceptible than older birds, and illness tends to be more severe in mature birds.

Usually the first sign you'll notice is watery eyes, which may appear as tiny bubbles in the corner of the eye. Soon yellowish crusty material starts clinging to the area surrounding the eyes, and the infected bird has difficulty breathing.

Because laryngo interferes with breathing, infected chickens tend to be less active than usual. Instead of making normal chicken sounds, they cough and sneeze. They may shake their heads a lot and stretch out their necks while gulping for air.

Mild versus Acute Laryngo

Laryngotracheitis can be either mild or acute, depending on many factors, including the virulence of the virus. In the United States most cases are mild. Chickens may have swollen eyes and have difficulty breathing, as evidenced by moist respiratory sounds (gurgling, choking, rattling, whistling, or cawing). Hens may experience a slight decrease in laying. Few, if any, infected birds die.

By contrast, the acute form can be deadly, if the windpipe gets plugged so the bird can no longer breathe. A classic sign of acute laryngo is gasping for air with the neck stretched upward and beak open. Another typical sign is chickens that sneeze while shaking their heads, trying to dislodge a plug from the windpipe. As the windpipe suffers significant damage from this virus, the bird coughs up blood that may dry on its beak and feathers, as well as on feeders, drinkers, and the coop walls.

Acute laryngo can take up to 6 weeks to run its course, although survivors may continue to cough for another month or so. Survivors are carriers but do not spread the virus as readily as do acutely ill chickens.

No treatment has been found for laryngotracheitis, other than supportive therapy that includes removing windpipe plugs from gasping birds. On the other hand, because survivors may remain carriers that can infect other chickens or even become reinfected themselves, the recommended procedure is to dispose of infected chickens and start over. In fact, in some states doing so is mandatory (see Reportable Diseases, page 418).

Since this virus does not survive long off birds, thoroughly cleaning and disinfecting housing, and leaving it empty for 2 months, will rid the premises of future infection. Laryngo is not spread through hatching eggs, so you could maintain your original bloodlines by starting a new flock from infected breeders if you are careful about keeping them away from infectious housing until it is virus-free.

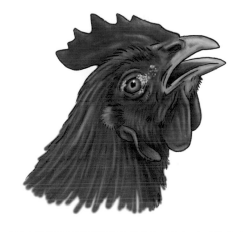

A typical first sign of laryngotracheitis is watery eyes surrounded by dried crusty material.

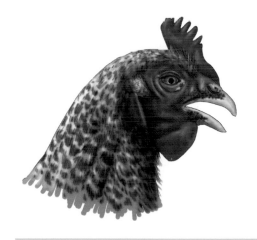

Typical signs of acute laryngo are open-mouth breathing and coughing up bloody mucus, which dries around the nostrils and lower beak.

Laryngo Vaccination

Vaccination against larygotracheitis is recommended where the disease is prevalent, where new chickens are regularly introduced to an existing flock, and for exhibition chickens. Additionally, vaccinating mature chickens at the beginning of an outbreak of laryngo can protect the chickens that haven't yet been infected. The following three types of vaccine are available:

Chicken embryo origin (CEO) vaccine. This vaccine is made by passing the virus through a series of developing chicken embryos, during which time the virus becomes increasingly less virulent. The resulting vaccine produces a higher level of infection than the other two types of vaccine, therefore it results in greater immunity. It can also cause severe signs of infection, and vaccinated chickens become carriers. Not only can these chickens infect unvaccinated chickens, but as the virus spreads, it eventually reverts back to its original virulence. This type of vaccine is used primarily to control outbreaks in industrial flocks and is unsuitable for use in backyard chickens. (CEO vaccine is sometimes referred to as vent-brush vaccine, because in the old days it was applied to the cloaca of individual chickens using a brush.)

Recombinant vaccine. This genetically engineered vaccine stimulates a chicken's immune system without producing disease. Vaccinated chickens may develop mild signs of laryngotracheitis, but they do not shed the virus. The vaccine is administered by subcutaneous injection and provides temporary immunity (up to 60 weeks). Its chief disadvantage is its high cost.

Tissue culture origin (TCO) vaccine. This vaccine is made from a virus that has been attenuated, or altered, to reduce its ability to cause disease. It is administered as an eyedrop. It produces a low-level infection and therefore low-level immunity. It has the advantage of not causing a severe reaction, although vaccinated chickens may shed the low-virulence virus for a short while.

Only tissue culture or recombinant vaccines are safe for use in backyard chickens. Tissue culture vaccine is most commonly used for exhibition chickens. To avoid spreading the virus to other chickens, birds should not be vaccinated within the 30 days preceding a show. The procedure for applying eyedrop vaccine is similar to Eye Treatment, illustrated on page 98.

Two Forms of Laryngotracheitis

VIRULENCE	USUAL AGE AFFECTED	SIGNS	PERCENT AFFECTED	DEATHS
Mild	Young	Mild respiratory distress, slight drop in laying	5%	Up to 2%
Acute	Mature	Severe respiratory distress, coughing blood, sharp drop in laying	90–100%	Up to 70%

Infectious Bursal Disease

A birnavirus causes infectious bursal disease by invading lymph tissue in young chickens and suppressing immunity by destroying immature lymphocytes in the thymus, the spleen, and especially the cloacal bursa. The disease is sometimes called Gumboro disease, because it was first identified in Gumboro, Delaware. The severity of illness varies with the affected chicken's age, level of maternal antibodies (which have a half-life of about 4 days), and the virulence of the particular birnavirus strain.

Chicks that are infected before 3 weeks of age, or are protected by maternal antibodies, or are infected with a low-virulence virus generally show no sign of disease, making it difficult to determine if the chicks have been infected. But the end result is atrophy of the cloacal bursa, giving such birds greater susceptibility to future infections, including from normally nonpathogenic microbes. Further, affected birds respond poorly to vaccines.

Chicks that are infected between 3 and 6 weeks of age become suddenly ill, with signs rapidly running through the flock. The first sign is watery or whitish diarrhea that clings to vent feathers, typically causing affected birds to pick their own vents. Other signs include lethargy, loss of appetite, huddling with ruffled feathers, slight trembling, reluctance to stand, and wobbly gait.

Depending on the virus's virulence, chicks may either recover or die. Usually the death rate is no greater than 20 percent, although a particularly virulent virus can cause a much higher rate of death. Generally deaths peak within about a week, and survivors recover rapidly thereafter.

Infectious bursal disease is highly contagious and difficult to get rid of in housing that once held an infected flock. But it is not egg transmitted, and survivors are not carriers. Chicks exposed to the virus before they are 2 weeks old develop natural immunity and, as mature breeders, pass antibodies to their offspring.

Vaccines are available, but their use is complicated because of the many differing types of vaccine, the wide range in virulence of different birnavirus strains, and the birds' level of maternal antibodies. Vaccination is recommended only where infectious bursal disease has become an issue and thus requires development of a customized vaccination plan.

Newcastle Disease

Named for the British town of Newcastle-upon-Tyne, one of the first places where it was studied, Newcastle disease is caused by several strains of paramyxovirus that infect many bird species. The different paramyxovirus strains are categorized as being highly virulent (velogenic), moderately virulent (mesogenic), or mildly virulent (lentogenic); most strains are either velogenic or lentogenic.

Velogenic strains are commonly grouped together as exotic Newcastle, a disease that appears suddenly, spreads rapidly — aided by infective droppings carried on the feet of mice and the shoes of humans — and causes numerous deaths. It is one of the top two most devastating diseases of poultry, second only to highly pathogenic avian influenza, with which it is easily confused.

Mesogenic strains are not as devastatingly deadly but are nonetheless virulent and quite serious, especially when they interfere with egg laying. They cause respiratory disease, and sometimes nervous conditions, that tend to be worse in young chickens than in older

Forms of Newcastle Disease (ND)
from Mildest to Most Lethal

FORM	TYPICAL AGE	AFFECTS	SIGNS	PERCENT AFFECTED	DEATHS
Asymptomatic enteric lentogenic ND	All ages	Intestines	Mild infection, no obvious signs	Up to 100%	None
Lentogenic ND	Young	Respiratory system	Mild respiratory distress	Up to 100%	Rare
Mesogenic ND	All ages	Respiratory system	Acute respiratory distress, drop in laying, possible partial paralysis	Up to 100%	Adults: rare Young: up to 10%
Neurotropic velogenic ND	All ages	Nerves & respiratory system	Appears suddenly; rapid drop in laying; gasping & coughing; partial paralysis	Up to 100%	Adults: up to 50% Young: up to 90%
Viscerotropic velogenic ND	All ages	Brain & digestive tract	Sudden death or rapid drop in laying, swollen head, greenish dark (bloody) diarrhea	Up to 100%	Nearly 100%

birds. Fortunately, both mesogenic and velogenic forms of Newcastle are rare in the United States and Canada, where authorities make a major effort to stamp them out whenever they do appear, typically introduced by illegally imported pet birds and fighting cocks that have not gone through official quarantine.

Lentogenic, or mild, forms of Newcastle, on the other hand, are quite common and not particularly serious, and chickens usually get better on their own with few, if any, deaths. Lentogenic Newcastle comes in two forms. One is a mild intestinal infection that rarely produces any apparent signs. The other is a respiratory infection that causes coughing, gasping, and rales and is often mistaken for any other disease of the respiratory system, except that Newcastle occasionally causes nerve disorders — such as paralysis of a leg or wing — in addition to respiratory signs.

Avian Influenza

Avian influenza, or bird flu, is caused by several different orthomyxoviruses, the same kind of virus that causes flu in humans, horses, pigs, and other animals. The type that causes avian influenza is known as type A. The natural hosts for type A influenza viruses are wild aquatic birds — seabirds (such as gulls and terns), shorebirds (such as plovers and sandpipers), and waterfowl (such as ducks and geese).

Although these birds do not typically show signs of disease, they can spread the virus among themselves and to other species, including humans (see Bird Flu, page 407). Chickens are not natural hosts for influenza viruses but have become susceptible, thanks to domesticated confinement.

Low-Path and High-Path Flu

Avian flu viruses have been around for many centuries, during which numerous strains have evolved among the various subtypes. All these viruses are grouped into two main categories according to whether they have low pathogenicity or high pathogenicity.

Most avian flu viruses are low-path. Low-path strains are common worldwide, including in the United States, and in most cases cause minor or no signs in chickens. But they have the potential to evolve into high-path viruses, which can occur when a low-path virus mutates as it spreads through a large number of chickens crowded in a confined area.

High-path avian influenza spreads more rapidly than low-path flu and produces illness that is much more serious, even fatal. In the United States, high-path strains have been periodically detected in intensively raised industrial flocks, which are then immediately quarantined and destroyed to prevent spread of the devastating disease.

The bird flu virus most commonly described in the news, H5N1, can have either low pathogenicity or high pathogenicity. The low-path virus is sometimes called North American H5N1. The high-path virus is sometimes called Asian H5N1. A virus is defined as high-path if it kills 6 out of 10 chicks inoculated in the laboratory. High-path H5N1 kills 10 out of 10 inoculated chicks.

How Flu Spreads

Avian flu comes in many forms, with signs that vary widely and may relate to respiration (coughing and sneezing), digestion (appetite loss and diarrhea), reproduction (drop in laying, reduced fertility, soft-shell eggs), or nerves (twisted neck, wing paralysis). When the virus is high-path, sometimes the first sign is numerous sudden deaths of apparently healthy birds.

The virus is shed and spread in secretions from the nostrils, mouth, and eyes and in the droppings of infected birds. It is transmitted

THE NUMBERS GAME

Type A influenza viruses that infect birds (as well as pigs, horses, and humans) are divided into subtypes according to combinations of their two main groups of surface proteins, the hemagglutinin, or H, proteins and the neuraminidase, or N, proteins. The 16 known H proteins are identified as H1 through H16, and the nine known N proteins are N1 through N9. These two groups combine to form 144 subtypes of the type A influenza virus.

Each subtype is identified by the two proteins it displays. The bird flu that swept through North America in 2015, for instance, is subtype H5N2, which has the fifth hemagglutinin and the second neuraminidase. All subtypes can infect birds.

Forms of Avian Influenza

VIRULENCE	SPREADS	AFFECTS	SIGNS	PERCENT AFFECTED	DEATHS
Low-path	Rapidly	Respiration, reproduction	No signs, or mild respiratory distress, drop in laying, sometimes diarrhea	Nearly 100%	Up to 5%
High-path	More rapidly	Nerves, cardiovascular, systemic	Sudden death, or reduced eating and drinking, rapid drop in laying, quivering or twisted neck, death within 48 hours	Nearly 100%	Nearly 100%

from bird to bird through direct contact, by sneezing and coughing, and through contact with infected droppings, which may be spread on contaminated equipment or the shoes of humans. Chickens that recover remain carriers.

Industrial poultry producers have long maintained that backyard free-range flocks are the chief concern with respect to controlling bird flu. The North American bird flu outbreak of 2015 provided a wake-up call that the real issue is lax biosecurity in the industry, along with the difficulties of rapidly disposing of millions of infected birds.

Epidemic Tremor

Avian encephalomyelitis is an infectious disease caused by a picornavirus that can infect pheasants, pigeons, quail, and turkeys, as well as chickens. Its chief signs are loss of coordination and rapid trembling of the head and neck, giving the disease its common name, epidemic tremor.

The disease may be brought into a flock through the introduction of an infected chicken showing no signs of disease. It is spread in droppings, replicates in the digestive tract, and travels through the bloodstream to the central nervous system. Infected birds shed, and

spread, the virus for about 2 weeks. Survivors become immune and are not carriers.

Infected chickens older than 3 weeks of age rarely show signs, other than that hens may experience a temporary slight drop in laying. Infection among mature chickens lasts less than a month. An infected hen sheds the virus in her eggs just before and during the period of reduced laying. If the eggs are incubated, about 25 percent more than usual of the embryos will die just before they would have hatched. Chicks that do hatch typically develop signs of infection between the ages of 1 and 3 weeks.

Usually the first noticeable sign is lack of interest in the usual chick activities, followed by loss of coordination, droopy wings, sitting on hocks, and falling over sideways. A characteristic sign is rapid trembling of the head and neck, and sometimes wings and legs — which may be easily observed by turning an infected chick onto its back and holding it in your cupped hands. Chicks may become paralyzed and die from inability to eat and drink.

Chicks that survive infection become immune to reinfection but may continue having coordination issues, and rarely grow to be good layers or breeders. Some recovered chicks may eventually develop cataracts, which appear as an opaque-looking, roundish pale blue or light gray spot in the eye, and may become blind.

This disease has no cure. A vaccine is available but must be used with caution, as described in Age at Vaccination on page 285.

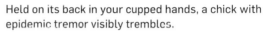

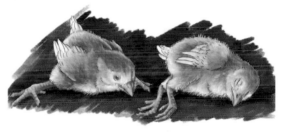

Held on its back in your cupped hands, a chick with epidemic tremor visibly trembles.

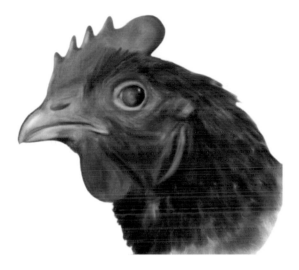

Chicks that survive epidemic tremor may eventually develop cataracts, appearing as a pale blue or grayish opaque area of the eye, and may become blind.

Chicks that are near death from epidemic tremor become prostrate (left) or fall over on their sides (right) and die from being trampled or from inability to eat and drink.

Antiviral Agents

Viruses are difficult to treat with drugs. To date no safe, broad-spectrum antiviral drug has been discovered. A virus in the environment neither eats nor breathes and is therefore unaffected by antivirals. Once a virus invades a cell in a chicken's body, any drug that harms the virus tends also to harm the infected cell.

Furthermore, the use of antivirals for poultry causes the development of resistant viral strains. In countries where antivirals have been given to poultry to prevent bird flu, strains of the H5N1 flu virus are now resistant to drugs typically prescribed to treat flu in humans.

Treatment of viral diseases therefore largely involves alleviating signs (in a respiratory infection, for example, using a product such as Vicks or VetRx to open up blocked airways) and keeping the bird warm, well fed, and as comfortable as possible while its immune system fights the virus.

Vaccination

The best way to prevent viral diseases is by maintaining good sanitation and observing proper biosecurity measures (as outlined in chapter 1). If your chickens are not at risk for exposure to viral diseases, vaccinating is unnecessary and may even be undesirable.

On the other hand, since most viral diseases have no treatment, vaccinating can help prevent or control viral diseases to which your chickens have been, or are likely to be, exposed. The most common viral disease in backyard flocks is Marek's. For chickens that are exhibited or swapped around, fowl pox and laryngotracheitis may also be of concern.

Be aware that in some states it is illegal to use certain live virus vaccines or to introduce viruses into the state by bringing in birds from another state that have been vaccinated with a live virus vaccine. Your veterinarian, Extension poultry specialist, or the avian pathologist at your state's diagnostic lab can help you work out a vaccination program based on your state's regulations, your method of flock management, and disease issues occurring in your area.

Establish a vaccination program only to solve specific problems: past problems your flock has experienced or the serious threat of a new problem. If you show your birds, if serious diseases have occurred on your place (in your own flock or in a previous owner's flock), or serious diseases infect nearby flocks (particularly if you live near a high concentration of commercial chickens), you may have good reason to vaccinate.

Do not vaccinate against diseases that do not endanger your flock. Doing so carries the risk of introducing diseases to which your chickens otherwise might not have been exposed.

The Nature of Vaccine

A vaccine is derived from live viruses and is used to trigger an immune response against the viruses from which it was derived. When a vaccine is administered, a chicken's body produces antibodies just as it would in a natural infection by the virus. If that virus should later infect the chicken, the antibodies thus produced will recognize the virus and be ready to mount a defense.

Most vaccines don't prevent disease but merely suppress signs or reduce the severity of illness. Vaccinated chickens, in most cases, still become infected and shed viruses, at least for a short while. In addition, not all vaccines are created equal. Some trigger a good immune response, others confer only a low level of immunity. Some produce a reaction that can be as serious as the disease itself.

To Vaccinate or Not to Vaccinate?

VACCINATING MAY BE UNNECESSARY IF:	CONSIDER VACCINATING IF:
You hatch your own replacement chickens or acquire new stock only as hatchlings from disease-free sources.	Your flock, or flocks in your area, have experienced diseases that may be prevented through vaccination.
You never introduce growing or mature chickens into your flock.	You periodically introduce growing or mature chickens into your flock.
Chickens that leave your property never return.	You exhibit your chickens at poultry shows or fairs.
Your long-term breeding program includes breeding for resistance.	Your chosen breed is especially susceptible to a disease that is preventable through vaccination.

The difference between an infection and a vaccination is that the viruses in a vaccine are selected for being particularly weak, have been modified to cause only a mild disease, or have been inactivated so they can't cause disease at all. A chicken's antibody-producing system can't tell the difference between the three basic vaccine forms: live, modified live, and inactivated.

LIVE VIRUS VACCINES

Live virus vaccines are the most effective in creating a strong immune response. Live virus vaccines are relatively inexpensive and easy to use, especially for mass application to large flocks. They cause immunity to develop through rapid replication, and they spread from successfully vaccinated birds to unsuccessfully vaccinated birds via the shedding of live viruses, offering those birds natural immunity.

A live vaccine has several disadvantages. It can easily be killed by heat and chemicals (such as alcohol used to sterilize a needle). It may be contaminated with other viruses during manufacture, spreading unintended diseases. Just as the virus can spread from successfully to unsuccessfully vaccinated birds, it can also spread to susceptible nearby unvaccinated flocks. The vaccine produces some of the symptoms of the disease

being vaccinated against, and if the chickens are stressed or infected with some other pathogen, vaccination can cause serious illness.

Because of these dangers, live vaccines are made from mild strains of virus or from less harmful viruses that are closely related to the pathogenic target virus. Therefore, revaccination is often required to induce an adequate immune response.

Live vaccines should be used only to prevent a serious disease already present that cannot be controlled any other way. Live virus vaccines are available against epidemic tremor, infectious bronchitis, infectious laryngotracheitis, Marek's disease, Newcastle, and pox.

MODIFIED LIVE VACCINES

Modified live vaccines contain viruses that have been altered, or attenuated, to make them less infectious. As a result, compared to live virus vaccines, they don't trigger quite as effective an immune response. Like live vaccines, however, modified vaccines do replicate, cause infection, and can result in shedding.

Also like a live vaccine, a modified live vaccine must be handled carefully to avoid killing the viruses, thus preventing them from triggering immunity. In addition, if the virus was incorrectly attenuated by the manufacturer, the vaccine may cause disease rather than immunity. Even if attenuation is correct, the vaccine may cause disease as a result of contamination by other pathogens or by interfering with the bird's immune response (making it susceptible to other diseases).

INACTIVATED VACCINES

Inactivated vaccines contain viruses that have been killed purposely by chemicals or heat. They therefore do not cause disease and do not result in shedding. The inducing of immunity relies on a larger number of virus particles to stimulate antibody production. These vaccines are the easiest to store and the safest to use.

On the other hand, they create a shorter-term and lower level of immunity than either live or modified live vaccines. To induce a higher, more uniform immune response, chickens are often primed with live vaccine first, to be followed by an inactivated booster.

Inactivated vaccines are both expensive and time consuming to administer, since they must be injected and require multiple doses. Although they produce few adverse reactions, the injection site may develop a lump caused by the fluid in which the killed viruses are suspended.

NATURAL VACCINATION

Before commercial vaccines became widely available, farmers practiced natural immunization by mixing young birds with older ones, thus exposing the young ones to any diseases the older ones may have been exposed to. Inducing disease by this method produces the same result as vaccination: causing the chickens to develop antibodies to fight future infection.

However, this method lacks the control offered by vaccination and can result in greater harm to the birds. Some may die, and among those that recover some may remain unthrifty and some may become carriers. On the other hand, you might eventually develop a genetically resistant flock by keeping the thus-immunized survivors as breeders and culling any birds that fail to fully recover, so they don't reproduce more weaklings.

Chicks may be naturally vaccinated for a variety of respiratory diseases, including chronic respiratory disease, infectious bronchitis, infectious coryza, and mild Newcastle. Signs that natural vaccination might be occurring include mild wheezing and watery eyes. In some cases you may not even realize your flock is being naturally immunized.

Natural vaccination can backfire, however, if chicks are exposed to massive amounts of pathogens before immunity is complete. At least one disease, Marek's, offers an alternative to gradual exposure to pathogens that cause disease in chickens. Turkeys carry a related, though harmless, virus that keeps the Marek's virus from causing tumors.

Chickens that are raised with turkeys develop some measure of immunity to Marek's (although keeping chickens and turkeys together creates other problems, such as the possibility of the turkeys getting blackhead from the chickens). To avoid keeping chickens and turkeys in the same yard, introduce the turkey virus by mixing a little soiled turkey bedding into the chicks' brooder bedding.

Vaccination Effectiveness

Whenever you use a vaccine, read and follow furnished instructions regarding storage and handling, method of application, dosage, recommended age of birds at the time of first vaccination, and the timing of any boosters. All these factors affect the degree, duration, and quality of the immunity conferred by the vaccine.

To ensure vaccination success, observe the following guidelines:

- Keep vaccines away from heat and sunlight. If you purchase vaccine in town, bring along a cooler to store it in until you get home. If you purchase vaccine by mail, use the shipper's tracking information to anticipate its arrival in your mailbox so you can retrieve it right away.

- Store vaccine in the refrigerator, freezer, or otherwise as directed, until you use it. Improperly stored vaccine deteriorates rapidly.

- Check the vaccine's expiration date. If it has long since passed, the vaccine may have deteriorated to the point of being no longer effective.

- Observe the recommended bird age for the type of vaccine being used.

- Make sure you use the right vaccine for your need. Not all vaccines protect against all strains of the same virus.

- Know the correct method for applying the vaccine. Each type of vaccine is designed to be administered in a specific way.

- Use the correct dosage. Underdosing is more common than overdosing.

- Handle vaccine in a hygienic manner.

- Vaccinate only healthy, parasite-free chickens. If your birds are wormy or otherwise in poor health, the results of vaccinating may be worse than not vaccinating at all. If you are vaccinating to control a persistent illness, do so only under the supervision of a veterinarian, who will positively identify the cause of the problem and recommend the appropriate vaccine.

- Try to schedule vaccinations for a time of year when weather conditions remain steady and the temperature is not much lower than 50°F or higher than 80°F (10–27°C). Chickens under stress from extreme heat or cold may not have an adequate immune response to the vaccine.

- Maintain good housing sanitation. Chickens that are using their immunity defenses to ward off opportunistic pathogens resulting from unsanitary conditions may have insufficient reserves to develop a good immune response to vaccine.

- Administer recommended boosters. Some antibodies, such as those induced by Newcastle-bronchitis vaccine, have a life expectancy of only a few months. Boosters increase antibody life expectancy, as well as increasing the total level of antibodies. Typically the first vaccination would be with a live virus, the booster with an inactivated vaccine.

- Dispose of used needles, empty vaccine vials, and unused vaccines responsibly, to avoid accidentally spreading live disease-causing viruses to unvaccinated poultry in the area.

Mishandled vaccines lose effectiveness, and the occasional bootleg vaccine has little or no effect to begin with. Purchase vaccines only from USDA-licensed manufacturers, as evidenced by an assigned code number stamped on the bottle. The best sources for licensed vaccines are well-known hatcheries and poultry suppliers and, of course, your veterinarian. In the event you should need to trace a source, record all vaccination dates, manufacturer's lot numbers, and any reactions your chickens experience.

No vaccine will protect your flock 100 percent; every vaccine has at least a 5 percent failure rate. In addition, disease can occur if you bring in new birds that are not on the same vaccination program as your old ones (a vaccine may cause your old birds or your new birds to shed pathogens). Then, too, you never know what disease may turn up next. Good management with an eye toward disease prevention remains your best defense.

Methods of Application

Vaccines are packaged for industrial use and therefore come in vials containing enough for 500 or 1,000 birds. Even if you can't use it all, the expense is usually still low in relation to the cost (and heartbreak) of losing birds to disease.

Vaccines may come as a ready-to-use liquid or as a powder or freeze-dried plug accompanied by a mixing solution, or diluent. Examples of the latter are Marek's and pox vaccines, which come in two vials, one containing the dry vaccine and the other a liquid diluent, usually saline. Once the two are mixed together, the vaccine is good for only a couple of hours, so you can't save it. Responsibly dispose of unused vaccine and empty vials.

Precise vaccination procedures vary with the type of vaccine used. Some methods of application involve handling each bird individually. Others are more suitable for vaccinating large flocks. Carefully read and follow the instructions that come with the vaccine.

INDIVIDUAL APPLICATION

Administering vaccine to chickens individually means you have to handle each bird. Depending on how many chickens you have to vaccinate, individual application can be time consuming, as well as stressful to both you and your chickens. Compared to whole-flock vaccination, the advantage is that you can be sure each bird gets an even dose. Vaccinating individual chickens may be done by several different methods.

Wing-web stab vaccination is used primarily for pox vaccine, as described on page 266. When using this method to vaccinate chickens of various ages, start with the oldest birds, then break one prong off the wing-web stabber to immunize chicks.

Intramuscularly injected vaccine is administered as a shot, usually into the breast muscle, taking care not to pass the needle through the muscle into the liver or other internal organ. Follow instructions carefully as to injection site and needle size. In most cases a ½-inch (12.5 mm) 19-gauge needle works best. Use each needle for no more than 200 birds — but take a

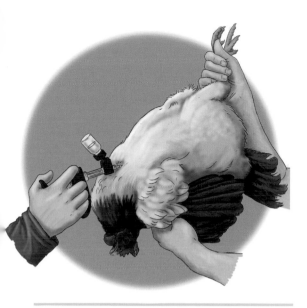

An automatic syringe is a time-saver for vaccinating a large number of chickens, and is especially helpful for vaccines with a short life.

fresh one if the needle doesn't stab well anymore. For vaccinating a large number of chickens, or using a mixed vaccine with a short life, an inexpensive automatic syringe will let you get the job done quicker. Just be sure the device is adjusted to deliver the appropriate dose.

Some vaccines must be applied intramuscularly; others must be applied subcutaneously. Still others may be administered by either method.

Subcutaneously injected vaccine is administered as a shot under loose skin over the breast or behind the neck, taking care not to release vaccine into feathers or fluff above the skin, or poke the needle through the skin and squirt vaccine into the air. To avoid a serious reaction, some vaccines must be administered only by subcutaneous injection. Newly hatched chicks are vaccinated against Marek's disease by subcutaneous injection, as described on page 264. As with

intramuscular application, using an automatic syringe will help you work faster.

Eyedrop or intraocular vaccine is administered into an eye, from which it passes into the Harderian gland behind the eye and from there into the respiratory tract. Eyedrop vaccine comes in a kit containing a vial of vaccine and a vial of dyed diluent with an eyedropper in the cap. After placing a drop in the eye and before letting the chicken go, wait until the bird blinks to make sure the vaccine stays in the eye rather than dripping out. The colored diluent is designed to verify proper vaccine placement — the dye stains the bird's tongue and nostrils when vaccination has been correctly done. The procedure for applying vaccine by eyedrop is similar to Eye Treatment, illustrated on page 98.

Nose drop or intranasal vaccinations are administered by placing a drop on a nostril and watching to make sure it is inhaled before releasing the chicken. This method is simpler than the eyedrop method, but less effective because the vaccine does not reach the Harderian gland behind the eye.

Vent-brush vaccination is applied to the mucous membrane of the cloaca, a method that is stressful for chickens and can easily lead to cross-contamination from one bird to another. Once a standard vaccination method, vent brushing is not as effective as other methods and is no longer recommended. Some old-timers, however, still prefer this outdated practice.

FLOCK APPLICATION

Flockwide vaccination is best suited to vaccinating a large number of birds at once. Compared to handling each chicken, this method is less time consuming and less stressful to both you and your birds, but has the disadvantage that you can't be sure each one gets an adequate dose. The vaccine may be delivered either in the drinking water or as an aerosol spray.

Drinking water vaccination is the most popular mass method. It may be used to target diseases involving not only the digestive system but also the respiratory system: the vaccine enters by way of the cleft in the roof of the chicken's mouth, which opens into the nasal cavity. It involves adding vaccine to the drinking water in a measured amount calculated to deliver an adequate dose, based on the amount of water the average bird is expected to drink within a 2-hour period, roughly the life span of live vaccine after it's been added to water. Since water consumption varies with age, feed, and weather, determine the exact amount of water your flock is likely to consume by measuring how much your birds drink the day before.

The vaccine may be rendered ineffective if the temperature is high or the water contains impurities, including sanitizers such as chlorine used to control bacteria or fungi. Do not use a water sanitizer within 48 hours of vaccinating. Clean waterers, and rinse them well, taking care to leave no disinfectant residue to inactivate the vaccine.

The vaccine may be somewhat stabilized by adding powdered milk to the water. Milk protein neutralizes chlorine and other sanitizers and prolongs the vaccine's life. About 20 minutes before adding the vaccine, stir in skim milk powder (nonfat dry milk) at the rate of 2 teaspoons per quart (2 g/L) of cool water.

Mix the vaccine with diluent, according to the manufacturer's directions. With clean hands submerge the opened vaccine vial in the measured water, and swish it around to make sure all the vaccine empties out. Then thoroughly stir the water to distribute the vaccine. If you have more than one drinker, mix the vaccine in a clean plastic bucket, then fill the drinkers from the bucket.

Remove drinking water at least 1 hour before vaccinating; in cold weather, when chickens drink less, withhold water for 2 hours. Provide vaccine-laden water immediately after mixing it. Since chickens drink the most at dawn and dusk, water vaccination is likely to be the most successful at one of those two times.

To ensure chickens drink the water, prohibit access to puddles or any other source of water. Feeding the chickens at the same time encourages them to drink the vaccine-laden water. For good immunization the chickens should drink all the vaccine solution within about 20 minutes.

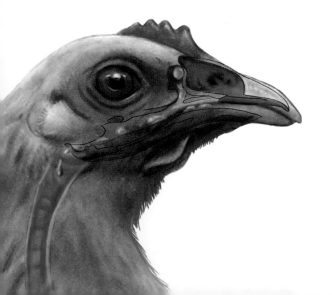

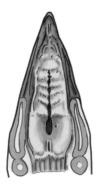

A vaccine added to drinking water targets diseases affecting not only the digestive system but also the respiratory system, which the vaccine enters through the nasal cavity by way of the cleft in the roof of the chicken's mouth.

Spray-on or aerosol vaccination offers an easy way to vaccinate large numbers of chickens in a short time, provided you have a spray device that produces liquid droplets just the right size for the type of vaccine being applied. Often a sprayer designed for horticulture may be used to spray vaccine either directly onto the chickens or into the air above them.

Day-old chicks are placed in a box or a small brooder and vaccinated with a coarse spray. The chicks are attracted to peck the shiny liquid droplets, thus swallowing the vaccine, although some vaccine enters through their eyes.

Older chickens are typically sprayed while confined inside their housing, with minimum lighting to reduce activity and ensure even distribution of the vaccine. The vaccine is sprayed in a fine mist, which the chickens inhale, although some vaccine may be swallowed or enter through their eyes.

Age at Vaccination

For their first 2 to 4 weeks of life, chicks benefit from parental immunity — antibodies passed by the hen, through the egg — against diseases to which the hen is immune. A vaccination administered while parental immunity is still at work partially neutralizes the vaccine's effect, and future boosters may be needed to maintain protective immunity.

As parental immunity wears off, chicks develop an increasing ability to produce their own antibodies. For consistent and long-lasting immunity, chicks should be vaccinated no younger than about 6 weeks of age. Vaccination against laryngotracheitis may be used earlier to control the spread of the virus in an already infected flock. Laryngo vaccine is one example of a vaccine that works best as a preventive after the age of 6 weeks, but may be used earlier as a method of control.

Marek's vaccine, on the other hand, *must be* administered before chicks are exposed to the Marek's virus, which can affect birds as young as 6 weeks old. So although chickens may be vaccinated against Marek's disease at any age, they are most commonly vaccinated on the day they hatch. A booster at 6 weeks of age helps increase resistance.

Vaccination against epidemic tremor is a bit trickier. Chicks may be vaccinated past the age of 8 weeks. Up to that time maternal antibodies may interfere with immune response, while vaccinated chicks lacking maternal antibodies may become ill. Pullets that are vaccinated

CHLORINATED TAP WATER

Chlorine is added to municipal water to kill microbes, so it stands to reason that chlorinated tap water is harmful to a vaccine. To get rid of the chlorine, you might leave the water in an open container for a few days to let the chlorine evaporate. Or you might boil the water, then cool it before adding the vaccine.

Neither of these options works if the source of chlorine in your local water supply is a derivative form called chloramine, which lacks free chlorine's distinctive odor and flavor. Chloramine can't be boiled, evaporated, or distilled out. The only ways to remove it are by using either a catalytic carbon filter or a reverse osmosis water filter system.

before they start laying will produce maternal antibodies that provide immunity to chicks hatched from their eggs. On the other hand, hens that are vaccinated after they start laying may transmit disease to their chicks. So epidemic tremor vaccine is best administered between the ages of 10 and 16 weeks.

Under normal circumstances mature chickens are rarely vaccinated or given boosters. A notable exception is Newcastle-bronchitis vaccine, which is typically administered to industrial breeder flocks to induce a high antibody level that transmits uniform parental immunity to the offspring. A backyard exception might occur if you introduce new chickens into your flock and either your flock or the new chickens have been vaccinated or exposed to a disease that results in viral shedding. In such a case, the unvaccinated or unexposed chickens may need to be protected by being vaccinated.

Vaccines at a Glance

RECOMMENDED AGE	VACCINE AGAINST	METHOD	COMMENT
At hatch	Marek's disease	Shot under skin at back of neck	Most hatcheries offer this vaccination as an option; a booster at 6 weeks increases resistance.
6 weeks	Laryngotracheitis (TCO vaccine)*†	Eyedrop, nose drop	State approval may be required. Annual boosters are recommended.
10–12 weeks (or at hatch with booster at 8 weeks)	Fowl pox*†	Wing web	Annual boosters are recommended.
10–16 weeks	Epidemic tremor	Drinking water	Vaccinate pullets at least 4 weeks before they start to lay.
12 weeks	Fowl cholera* (live attenuated)	Wing web	
	See Fowl Cholera Bacterins, page 234	Drinking water	
	Fowl cholera (inactivated)*†	Shot under skin	Limited immunity; requires 2 injections 4 weeks apart
SCENARIOS FOR VACCINATING AGAINST BRONCHITIS AND NEWCASTLE			
At hatch or at 10–35 days	Newcastle disease–infectious bronchitis	Drinking water, eyedrop, nose drop	Requires boosters every 3 months
14–18 weeks	Infectious bronchitis (inactivated)	Shot in muscle or under skin	Administer before start of lay
18–20 weeks	Newcastle disease* (inactivated)	Shot in muscle or under skin	Administer before start of lay. No booster required

*Vaccinate only where this disease is likely to occur.

†Vaccination can reduce the severity of an outbreak.

CHAPTER 11

Management
Issues

S OONER OR LATER every chicken keeper experiences
the same issues that have plagued humans since the first
fowl was domesticated. Although these problems usually can
be resolved with good management, they aren't necessarily an
indication of bad management. Bad stuff happens to the most
well-managed flocks; however, a lot of hazards can easily be
avoided if you are aware of the potential dangers and exercise
due diligence to avoid them. The intent of this chapter is to
help you deal with the following issues:

- Why chickens pick at each other and what you can do
  about it

- How to help your chickens avoid frostbitten combs
  and toes

- What causes scummy drinking water and how to
  prevent it

- Things to watch out for that might poison your
  chickens

- How to spot and eliminate hazards that endanger
  your birds

- Why hens stop laying and how to get them back in gear

Dealing with Rodents

Rodents are attracted to chicken houses by feed in troughs or spilled on the ground, ready availability of water, and protection from the elements. They can eat an amazing amount of feed, as well as spreading diseases on their feet and fur and through droppings left in feeders or storage bins. They can be especially numerous where the floor is raised above dirt, providing a darkened airspace underneath, or where wall cavities and trash piles provide attractive nesting sites. Rodents generally live outdoors during warm months, moving to indoor comfort during late fall or early winter as cold weather approaches.

Don't assume just because you rarely see rodents that you don't have them. Experts say that for every one you do see, many more are lurking nearby. Despite your best management efforts, always assume you have rodents. Make every effort to keep them away from your coop area, and step up your rodent control program if you spot any of these signs: holes through walls, tunnel openings (in soil, litter, or under floors), or droppings around stored feed.

Identifying Rodent Droppings

RODENT	DROPPINGS
House mouse (*Mus musculus*)	¼" long, ¹⁄₁₆" diameter, pointed ends, dark brown or black, found scattered and grouped in feeding areas
Norway rat (*Rattus norvegicus*)	¾" long, ¼" diameter, blunt ends, color varies, found in groupings
Roof rat (*Rattus rattus*)	½" long, ¼" diameter, curved with pointed ends, color varies (usually dark), found scattered

Since rodents are nocturnal, you are less likely to spot little furry creatures scurrying around than to see the droppings they leave behind. A rodent will drop about 50 pellets a day, which you will find around feed storage bins and trailing along the floor near a wall. The more droppings you see, the worse your infestation. Being able to identify rodents by the size and shape of their droppings will help you determine how to deal with the problem.

A Mouse in the (Chicken) House

A mouse is a small creature with large round ears and a nearly hairless tail that's as long as its body, which is generally 2½ to 4 inches (6 to 10 cm). The fur is light to dark grayish brown.

One mouse is adorable, but a pair of mice reproduces rapidly, having up to ten litters per year averaging six to eight young per litter. Each male may accompany several females, and in a protected environment they may live and reproduce for as long as 3 years. Since the offspring can reproduce at 2 months of age or less, you can see how fast mice might get out of control. Each mouse can gobble down a little over 2 pounds (1.0 kg) of chicken feed in a year.

Mice are most active at dusk and dawn, but they feed all day long and will travel an area up to 30 feet in diameter. They are nimble jumpers and climbers and can fit through openings as small as ¼ inch (6 mm). They are also good swimmers, but if one falls or jumps into a bucket of water from which it can't get out, it will drown from sheer exhaustion.

Chickens are the natural enemies of mice and will play keep-away with any mouse they can catch, although the agile little rodents are good at scurrying out of the way. Rats will also

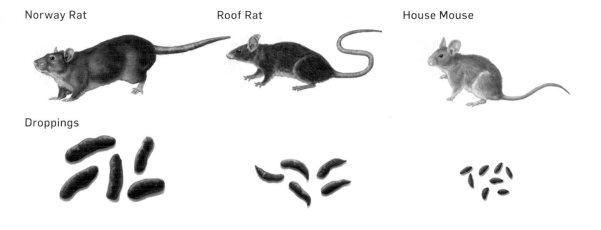

Norway Rat

Roof Rat

House Mouse

Droppings

A Norway rat has reddish-brown fur and a chunky body and ranges from 13 to 18 inches (33 to 45 cm) long, nose to tail. Its droppings are about ¾" (19 mm) long and capsule shaped.

A roof rat has dark fur and a slender body, ranges from about 13 to 18 inches (33 to 46 cm) long, and has a tail longer than the body. Its droppings are ½" (13 mm) long, pointy, and curved.

A mouse has grayish-brown fur and ranges from 5 to 8 inches (13 to 20 cm) long, nose to tail. Its tiny droppings are about ¼" (6 mm) long and concentrated in feeding areas.

kill and eat mice, so if you have rats you may not have mice. Instead, you have a bigger problem.

Rats

Rats eat eggs and sometimes attack chickens. If you find dead, chewed-up chicks in the morning, suspect rats.

These rodents are active at night, mostly shortly after sunset and shortly before sunrise, making them easy to spot with a flashlight. If you see a rat in the daytime, you have a *serious* rat problem — the rats have overpopulated, and the dominant ones are keeping the weaker ones away from feed, forcing them to eat during the day.

Feed loss is a serious consequence of a rat infestation. One rat will eat about 45 pounds (20 kg) of feed in a year. A pair of rats produces four to seven litters each year, mostly in spring and fall. Even though not all of the offspring reach breeding age, within a year one pair can easily become 1,500 rats.

According to the Centers for Disease Control and Prevention, rats in North America can transmit 10 diseases that infect humans, at least one of which — salmonellosis — infects chickens as well. Rats can also spread a variety of mites, lice, fleas, and ticks that affect chickens.

Two different rat species are commonly found in the United States and Canada. Norway rats (*Rattus norvegicus*) are widespread throughout the United States and subarctic Canada, with the exception of Alberta. Roof rats (*Rattus rattus*) prefer the warmer climates of the U.S. Southeast, the west coasts of the United States and Canada, and the Hawaiian Islands.

NORWAY RAT

The Norway rat goes by various names, including barn rat, basement rat, brown rat, common rat, gray rat, sewer rat, street rat, water rat, and wharf rat. It is most commonly called Norway rat because of the mistaken belief that it originated in Norway, which was disproved by the discovery that these rats existed in other countries before migrating to Norway.

A Norway rat may grow to a length of 18 inches (46 cm), can weigh up to 1 pound (0.5 kg), and may live as long as 3 years. Each female averages five litters a year, weaning some 20 offspring annually, and the young can begin reproducing at 5 weeks of age.

Norway rats are found nearly everywhere humans live. They are particularly numerous in cities, where they feast on garbage, although they also favor agricultural areas because of the ready availability of livestock feed and stored crops. They also thrive in sewers, along creeks, in thickets, and under woodpiles.

They are excellent swimmers but poor climbers. They live in social groups that excavate multilevel underground burrows, often starting a new burrow next to a wall or foundation, where the entrance will be protected. Each burrow has one or more escape exits.

ROOF RAT

The roof rat is known variously as the black rat, fruit rat, house rat, ship rat, or tree rat. Unlike the Norway rat, it is an agile climber and often travels along pipes, utility lines, or fence tops. This species prefers to live in trees or in a building's upper level, resulting in its most common name. Roof rats are known to start fires by gnawing the tough insulation off electrical wiring in an attempt to keep their teeth filed down.

A female roof rat makes a spherical nest of shredded paper, cloth, leaves, and sticks. She'll have three or four litters a year, with five to eight young per litter. The offspring begin reproducing as young as 2 months of age.

Roof rats have a much less extensive geographic range than Norway rats, and they occupy a different ecological niche. However, the two species may coexist in the same area — the Norway rat living underground and the roof rat living higher up in an attic, garage, woodpile, vine-covered fence, barn loft, tree, or cliff.

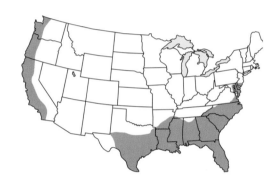

Roof rat range

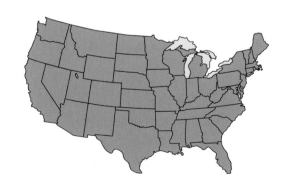

Norway rat range

Unlike Norway rats, roof rats do not live in social groups, and the two species do not interbreed. In fact, they don't even get along. In a fight the Norway rat will kill the roof rat.

Besides preferring different habitats, the two species may be distinguished from one another by size and shape. A roof rat is slenderer than a Norway rat, reaching a maximum weight of about ¾ pound (340 g). Although its total length is similar to that of a Norway rat, the roof rat has a longer tail in relation to the length of its body, as well as bigger eyes and ears.

Rodent Control

Despite all our modern technology, we still haven't found a truly better mousetrap. By far the best way to discourage rodents is to make the chicken area unattractive to them. Since rats and mice shun open spaces, keep the land around your coop clear of weeds, loose lumber, and debris.

If the coop floor is raised, make sure it's at least 1 foot (30 cm) above ground so rodents won't feel protected underneath. If you use a droppings pit, clean it out regularly, as an undisturbed pit provides an ideal place where rodents are protected from the chickens and have ready access to feed and water while the chickens are roosting at night.

Norway Rat versus Roof Rat

TRAIT	NORWAY RAT (*RATTUS NORVEGICUS*)	ROOF RAT (*RATTUS RATTUS*)
Body length	7–10" (18–25 cm)	6–8" (15–20 cm)
Hind foot	1.7" (43 mm)	1.3" (33 mm)
Tail length	6–8" (15–20 cm); shorter than head and body	7–10" (18–25 cm); longer than head and body
Weight	10–18 oz (283–510 g)	6–12 oz (170–340 g)
Appearance	Thick, stocky	Slender, graceful
Belly color	White with gray underfur	All white, all buff, or all gray
Ears	Short, close to head	Large, creased, upright
Eyes	Small	Large
Fur	Coarse	Smooth
Fur color	Reddish brown to gray to black	Black to brownish gray
Muzzle	Broad, blunt	Narrow, pointed
Tail	Thick, naked, scaly, pink or tan	Thin with fine scales; dark gray; prehensile
Climber	Clumsy	Agile
Swimmer	Powerful	Poor
Travels	Deliberately	Rapidly
Geographic range	All states, most of Canada	Warm coastal areas
Habitat	Underground	Aboveground

Use hanging feeders. Compared to trough feeders, hanging feeders are more difficult for rodents to reach. Store feed in containers with tight-fitting lids. Some chicken keepers have had rats chew through plastic containers, in which case galvanized cans will solve the problem. When filling storage containers, immediately sweep up any spills.

Eliminating sources of drinking water may encourage rats to move elsewhere. An adult rat needs about 3 tablespoons of water each day, which it may get from your chicken's waterer. If you remove or empty drinkers overnight, and no other water source is handily available, rats will soon go looking for a more favorable location where they can find water to drink. Making the chickens' drinkers unavailable to rats also helps prevent the spread of disease from rats to chickens.

Keep a dog. A terrier is a small dog with lots of energy that enjoys digging up rodent tunnels to retrieve the occupants. A rat terrier is, of course, the quintessential ratter, and so is the Russell terrier. Actually, just about any member of the terrier family enjoys going after rodents, as do also the dachshund and the German pinscher, provided the dog is discipline-trained to leave your chickens alone.

Keep a cat. But don't overfeed your cat or it will lose interest in rodent patrol. A young female cat may catch a fair amount of mice, and maybe young rats as well, but most cats are not much interested in tangling with a mature rat. On the other hand, cats may hunt baby chicks, and dogs may kill grown chickens. So if pets have access to the area where the chickens live, they may not be the best solution. Also, eating a mouse or rat can have undesirable consequences for a cat or dog, including contracting intestinal worms or the disease toxoplasmosis, and secondary rat bait poisoning.

Flooding the burrows of Norway rats and tunneling mice with a garden hose can be effective. Since rat tunnels are multilevel, flooding could take a fair amount of water. Afterward, fill in the entrances with dirt and cover them with something heavy, like a flat rock or a concrete block. Watch for the tunnel to be reopened, and reflood it as needed.

A number of devices are available on the market for dealing with rodents. Some work better than others. Don't waste money on glue boards, odor repellents, and electronic, magnetic, ultrasound, or vibration devices. The tried and true methods for dealing with rodents are trapping and, when all else fails, poisoning.

TRAPPING RODENTS

If you have a rodent problem, set traps. Trapping has these several advantages over poison:

- It's cheaper, because traps can be reused, while bait must be replaced frequently.

- It's nontoxic and therefore won't inadvertently poison your chickens or other animals or children (but keep your children and animals away from them anyway).

- A trap that kills immediately is more humane than slow poisoning.

- You can readily find and dispose of the bodies before they stink up the place.

- You can easily gauge how well your rodent control program is going, because you have clear evidence.

How to Place Snap Traps for Greatest Success

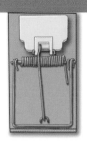 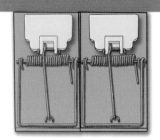 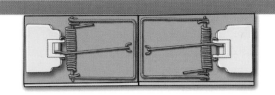

Single trap perpendicular to wall, trigger next to wall

Double traps, side by side, set as for single traps

Double traps set end to end, triggers on the outsides

Despite all the modern gadgets hawked as rodent traps, wooden snap traps remain the most effective type. They are also the most humane, because they nearly always kill the rodent immediately. Snap traps come in small sizes for mice and larger sizes for rats.

Set traps along well-used runways. Rodents feel protected running alongside walls, which is where you'll find most of their travel routes. These runways usually can be identified by stains and droppings, but if you have trouble finding them, a light dusting with flour will help you spot tracks.

Once you identify a runway, place a single trap at right angles to the wall, with the trigger and bait close to the wall and the trap touching the wall. To increase your success, place two traps together, either side by side at right angles to the wall or end to end and parallel to the wall, with the triggers to the outside.

For mice set traps every 10 feet (3 m); for rats set them no farther apart than 50 feet (15 m). Using more traps than you feel is necessary will increase your success rate.

Since mice and roof rats also run along sills, rafters, and other high places, set traps high as well as on the ground. Rats are suspicious of anything new and may avoid the traps for several days. Once you find a successful location, keep resetting the trap in the same spot.

Traps that are properly placed along runways usually work fine without bait, but trap-shy rodents can be attracted with a tasty bait. The best bait to use is something that will stick to the bait tray without rolling off, such as peanut butter. Sometimes a wily rodent will manage to eat the bait without tripping the trigger. Rebait, and try again.

In the event a rodent is caught but not killed — for instance, the trap snags a leg or tail — anchor traps down so they won't disappear into a tunnel, never to be seen again. One method is to drill a hole in a corner of the trap, where it won't interfere with the trigger, thread a wire through the hole (or staple the wire to the trap), and fasten the wire to the wall or floor.

Be careful when setting rat traps, as they can be strong enough to break a finger.

(Firmly warn curious children to stay away.) Since rodents are not bothered by the scent of humans, you needn't scrub traps between uses. But for your own protection, wear disposable gloves when handling used traps or dead rodents and deeply bury or, where legal, incinerate the bodies.

PROBLEMS WITH POISON

Poisoning rodents can be dangerous to any chickens, pets, wildlife, and children having access to the poison bait. With some poisons, secondary poisoning is a risk for any chicken or any other nontarget animal that might eat a poisoned rodent.

Further, rodents are smart and wary and therefore can be hard to kill with poison. Rats, especially, are suspicious of anything new and may not take bait for several days or weeks. Even then, they may taste only a little at a time. The bait therefore has to be highly lethal in small amounts but slow acting so rodents don't learn to associate the bait with illness or death.

Another big problem with poisoning rodents is that they tend to hide to die, and the resulting odor is anything but pleasant. And the smell is worse in warm weather. For this reason, if you feel you must use poison, wait until cooler weather. By the time spring rolls around, the rodent carcasses will have dried out enough not to smell.

Although poison can effectively reduce a large population of rats, any rats that remain will rapidly rebuild the population. Further, rats may be attracted to repopulate empty burrows by the presence of residual pheromones, which can linger for years.

Cannibalism

Cannibalism is the nasty habit chickens have of pecking at one another. It often starts with one bird that draws blood, attracting others to join in. The initial trigger may be a bleeding injury or missing feathers that attract flesh picking. Sometimes a whole flock gangs up on one unfortunate individual and pecks it to death. Identifying and removing the original offenders may stop the problem before it gets too far along, but preventing it in the first place is far easier than trying to stop it once it gets rolling.

No one is sure exactly what causes cannibalism. Since eating is one of the chicken's main activities, and a chicken's mode of eating is to peck and swallow, cannibalism quite likely stems from a chicken's inherent need to peck. A bird that is not kept busy pecking to satisfy hunger will keep itself busy pecking to make mischief. Frustration and stress increase the problem. Any of the following conditions, alone or in combination, can trigger cannibalism:

- Chicks reared in a brooder rather than under a mother hen

- Chicks raised in a brooder with a hardware cloth floor

- Crowding, especially with fast-growing chicks that overfill available space

- Excessive heat without adequate ventilation

- Bright lights on 24/7

- Insufficient roosting space

- Lack of exercise opportunities

- Frequent disruptions to the pecking order

- Feeders and drinkers too few or too close together

- Abrupt changes in ration palatability

- Ration too low in salt or protein

- Ration high in calories and low in fiber

- Ration in the form of pellets

- External parasites

- Bleeding injuries

- Too few or improperly designed nests

Forms of Cannibalism

FORM	LIKELY GROUP
Toe picking	Chicks
Feather picking	Growing birds
Tail pulling	Growing birds
Head picking	Cocks; any birds in adjoining cages
Vent picking	Pullets
Egg eating	Hens

Toe Picking

Cannibalism often starts with toe picking, a common problem among chicks, especially those reared on paper to prevent litter eating. Chicks looking for something on the floor to peck may peck their own toes. Manure balls clinging to toes can also attract picking.

Toe picking can be a problem among chicks brooded on hardware cloth — sharp wire edges cut their toes, and the bleeding attracts toe pickers. Toe picking may start when chicks can't find anything else to eat because the feeder is poorly designed, too high, too far from the heat source, or too small for the number of chicks involved.

To get chicks picking at feed instead of feet, sprinkle a little starter ration on paper, or place shallow containers of starter close to (but not under) the heat source where the chicks can easily find it. If toes are injured from picking, light the brooder with a red light so chicks can't easily detect blood while the toes heal.

Feather Picking

Feather picking occurs most often among growing birds that are just developing their full plumage coat. It is common in young birds that are crowded and frustrated, or that are brooded on hardware cloth, which offers no opportunity for normal scratch-and-peck behavior.

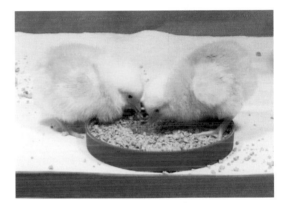

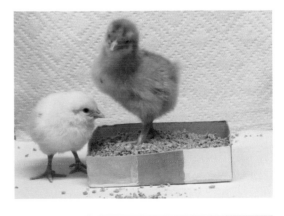

Starter ration placed in a shallow container such as a large jar lid (top) or a cut-off tissue box (bottom) helps baby chicks learn to peck feed instead of feet.

Not all feather loss is a sign of feather picking. Layers often have broken or missing feathers, especially on their necks and tails, that were rubbed off on feeders and nests. Mating cocks wear the feathers off a hen's back by treading. A broody hen will remove feathers from her breast to line her nest. A predator attack can result in missing feathers, often from the back or tail.

The annual molt causes regularly scheduled feather loss, which sometimes can be extreme (see Protective Feathers on page 62). During the molt, or any time a bird experiences extreme feather loss, encourage feather regrowth and discourage feather picking by increasing dietary protein (see Upping Protein on page 48).

Evidence of feather picking is bare patches on a bird's neck, breast, back, or below the vent. In growing birds, feathers are most likely to be picked from the back at the base of the tail, where newly emerging blood-filled feathers are especially tantalizing. Feather picking can quickly escalate to flesh pecking, opening bleeding wounds at the tail base.

In older birds an infestation of external parasites can cause a pecking frenzy. Lice and mites irritate the skin and feathers, causing chickens to peck at themselves in trying to relieve the itch, and the resulting injured skin invites pecking by other chickens. Likewise, hens that are missing feathers because of treading may have a hard time growing new feathers if their flock mates keep pulling out feathers that are regrowing.

Tail Pulling

Tail-feather pulling is a type of feather picking that is especially common in growing birds, particularly when they are too crowded, too hot, frustrated, or bored. This type of cannibalism is easy to spot, since the picked-on chickens lack tail feathers and the long feathers litter the coop floor. Picked birds must continually grow new tail feathers, causing the same stress reactions as are associated with molting.

If you keep different poultry species together, tail pulling may not necessarily be initiated by the chickens. Guinea fowl, for instance, are more active and somewhat more aggressive than most chicken breeds and may pull out the chickens' tail feathers — whether for fiber, protein, or pure sport.

Head Picking

Sometimes one chicken appears to be grooming another by gently pecking the tips of the second bird's head and neck feathers, while the second bird relaxes, often with closed eyes. This behavior is normal and is not a problem unless the groomer becomes obsessive about pecking the same feathers for hours on end.

Cannibalistic head picking more often occurs when one bird is going through a hard molt, leaving the head and neck skin bare. Another pecking trigger is a bloody comb or bloody wattles resulting from a fight or frostbite.

Two cocks or two hens housed in adjoining cages may pick each other's heads, as might be seen in show birds being coop trained for exhibition. When possible, space cages far enough apart to prevent picking. Cardboard or a feed sack wedged between cages is not always the best answer, since a solid barrier reduces air circulation, which can cause the caged birds to suffer in warm weather.

Vent Picking

Vent picking is the worst form of cannibalism. It can start if nests get too much light, so that a laying hen's everted vent attracts the attention of flock mates and gets picked. Locating nests in a darkened area of the coop should prevent this type of picking.

Vent picking more commonly occurs among pullets just coming into lay, usually after one tears tissue or prolapses while passing an egg that's larger than her maturing equipment is ready to handle. Other chickens, attracted to the protruding tissue, pick until they pull out the hapless hen's intestines. For more information, see Prolapse page 93. Using controlled lighting to push pullets to early maturity encourages this type of vent picking.

Vent picking can also get started when one chicken wanders beneath a roost where another chicken is resting, looks up, and takes one peck and then another. To avoid this attraction, place the lowest perch at least 18 inches (45 cm) above the floor.

Egg Eating

Egg eating occurs when not enough nests are provided, nests are too brightly lit, housing is too light in general, or hens are crowded and bored. Egg eating is also encouraged by anything that causes egg breakage: eggs aren't collected often, have soft or thin shells, or become cracked because of inadequate nesting material. Once chickens find out how good eggs taste, they will purposely break them to eat them.

The way to stop egg eating and keep it from spreading is to remove the culprit early. Identify instigators by checking for egg yolk smeared on beaks or by catching the eaters in the act. To discourage activities in the nests other than laying, darken nests by tacking or stapling curtains in front, pinning up one edge for a few days until the hens learn to go behind the curtains.

A nutritional deficiency, especially vitamin D or calcium, can cause soft shells that lead to egg eating. A laying hen's calcium needs are increased by warm weather and by age. Appropriate nutritional supplements include free-choice feeding of limestone or ground oyster shell, or adding vitamin AD&E powder to drinking water three times a week.

Preventing Cannibalism

Since cannibalism often begins in the brooder, head it off before it starts by keeping the brooder from becoming overheated or crowded. Use an infrared heater panel instead of lights for warmth, so after the first week you can turn off lights at night. Use a brooder with a solid floor. Increase living space and ventilation as the birds grow and become more active, and when the weather turns warm.

Furnishing adequate perch space helps prevent pecking by giving chickens more places to get away from one another. Pecking from below can be discouraged by making sure the bottom perch is no closer to the floor than about 18 inches (45 cm).

Providing suitable areas for dust bathing both helps minimize external parasites and gives chickens something to do besides peck each other. In general, establishing a rich environment that encourages normal exploring, nesting, grooming, and foraging behavior discourages cannibalistic pecking.

Patrol your chicken house and yard regularly, and repair broken wire or protruding nails that could cause bleeding wounds. Isolate and treat any chicken that's been injured or has reddened skin irritated by parasites. Similarly, remove any chicken from the flock that is lame, ill, or not growing well, as chickens tend to peck at weaker birds.

While chicks are growing, do not combine vastly different age groups, as the stronger, older birds will peck the weaker, younger ones. Avoid continually introducing new birds to your flock. Constantly disrupting the pecking order leads to frequent fighting, which can escalate into cannibalism.

Chickens are less likely to become cannibalistic when their diet is high in sources of insoluble fiber, such as grains, bran, seeds, and dark leafy greens. Feeding crumbles rather than pellets helps deter cannibalism, because crumbles take longer to eat. Feeding mash is even better, because chickens spend time searching through the ground-up particles for their favorite tidbits, thus taking longer to eat and having less time to peck each other. Protein deficiency can lead to cannibalism, and protein requirements change with age and season, so take care to adjust rations as needed to ensure your chickens are getting sufficient protein.

Provide a large enough feeder to ensure each chicken has a chance to eat its fill (see Feeder Space on page 59). If your flock size requires two or more feeders, space them far enough apart to avoid crowding and jostling. The same goes for drinkers.

Controlling Cannibalism

At the first sign of picking, remove the injured bird(s). Then try to identify and remove the instigator(s). If you can't catch them in the act, look for birds with blood or egg yolk on their beaks and face feathers.

Switch to red lightbulbs in the brooder or coop. If the problem is caused by bright sunlight coming through a window, cover the pane with clear red plastic (imitation stained glass). Red lighting gives everything a rosy hue, making bloody sores more difficult for birds to identify.

Change bright lightbulbs to dimmer lights. A good guideline for dimming the lights is to provide just enough light so you can barely read a newspaper. If the temperature inside the housing is hot, open windows or turn on a fan to stir the air and reduce the temperature. Like people, chickens get irritable when they're too hot.

Alleviate boredom by feeding less at a time and feeding more often, or by letting chickens spend time outdoors, where they will keep busy exploring and finding things to peck besides each other. At times when they must be confined indoors, provide toys such as shiny aluminum pie tins attached to the wall at head height for them to peck at or swinging perches for them to play on. Straw bales give chickens something interesting to explore and also attract insects for them to peck at. Feeding a portion of the ration as grains, table scraps, or garden greens scattered over the litter or across the yard gives them something to hunt for and peck.

Feather-pulling chickens that subsequently eat the feathers quite likely are seeking needed fiber. Providing pasture forage is an easy way to solve that problem. Oats are another good source of fiber.

Some breeds, and strains within a breed, tend more toward cannibalism than others. Breeds with the strongest foraging instincts have the strongest tendency toward cannibalism if they have inadequate opportunities to satisfy their need to forage, both as an activity for its own sake (something to do) and as source of dietary fiber. Light, high-strung breeds that frighten easily, especially Leghorns and other Mediterraneans, are also likely to develop cannibalistic behavior — attempting to relieve stress by pecking each other. Highly territorial aggressive birds that constantly engage in peck-order fighting also tend toward cannibalism.

Chickens of the same strain may be cannibalistic when raised in one place but not cannibalistic when raised in a different place, indicating that the problem can be controlled through good management. Still, if you experience cannibalism with a certain breed or strain, avoid perpetuating the problem by not hatching chicks from birds that behave aggressively, pull out each other's feathers, or otherwise engage in undesirable behavior. Choosing your breeding stock from among the better-natured individuals can resolve the issue in just a generation or two.

Since most of a chicken's body sodium is in its blood, salt deficiency can cause chickens to crave blood. This issue can be easily resolved by adding 1 tablespoon of salt per gallon (18 g/4L) of water in the drinker for one morning, then repeating the salt treatment 3 days later. At all other times provide plenty of fresh, unsalted water.

Pine tar and various other preparations — such as Blu-Kote, Hot Pick, or Pick-No-More — have been devised or recommended for smearing on wounds to make them unpalatable. Some of these products work for a short time, especially when picking first starts, but they must be reapplied frequently. None of them works really well after picking has become serious.

Blinders, specs, or so-called peepers are designed to prevent or control cannibalism by keeping chickens from seeing directly ahead to aim a peck. The chief disadvantage to using specs, aside from their looking ridiculous, is that they can lead to eye disorders.

Bottom line: no method of attempting to stop cannibalism once it starts is as effective as managing your flock to prevent it in the first place.

Frostbite

Frostbitten combs can be a problem for chickens that hang out in damp, drafty conditions during freezing weather. Large single combs, especially on cocks, are more likely to be frostbitten than small combs or combs that lie close to the head.

Toes can also be frostbitten, but not as commonly as combs and wattles, especially when chickens have a place to rest where their feet are not in direct contact with a frozen surface. Chickens on a properly constructed roost, for instance, can keep their feet warm by covering their feet with their bodies. (See Preventing Frostbite, page 302.)

Treating Frostbite

If you discover the condition while the part is still frozen, slowly warm the frozen area. Do not use a heat lamp, heating pad, or other form of direct heat that warms rapidly, which would increase the pain. And do not rub the affected area, which would increase the damage.

To thaw a frozen foot, place the foot in warm water (100°F/38°C) for 20 minutes. To thaw a frozen comb or wattle, carefully apply a damp, warm cloth to the frozen part for 15 minutes, rewarming the cloth as needed.

After the part has thawed, gently apply a hydrogel (water-based) wound treatment. A spray (such as Vetericyn) is easy to apply without putting pressure on the affected part. Isolate the bird in a clean, warm facility, and keep an eye on it to see that the wound heals properly. Use feeders and drinkers of a style that won't rub against the affected part. If the feet are involved, use soft bedding, and if necessary, protect the toes with vet wrap or a protective shoe (such as Birdy Bootie).

Frostbite is more likely to be discovered after the part has thawed and become swollen and painful. The bird appears listless and loses appetite. Since the part has already thawed, warming it is no longer necessary. Coat the part with a hydrogel spray, and isolate the bird so the damaged area has a chance to heal without getting pecked by flock mates. If the chicken won't eat or otherwise appears listless, it is likely in pain. See Aspirin for Pain on page 395.

After the swelling goes down, the skin may peel, the part may itch, and it may be sensitive to cold for a while. It may turn scabby, develop blisters, turn black as the tissue dies (dry gangrene), and eventually slough off — resulting in permanent disfigurement. Don't be tempted to pop blisters or remove blackened tissue, both of which aid healing.

Infection (wet gangrene) can be a serious and even life-threatening complication of frostbite. A sign of infection is bad-smelling fluid leaking from a wound that isn't healing. To prevent the spread of infection, the affected part may have to be surgically removed.

Dubbing and Cropping

The amputation of a comb (a procedure called dubbing) or wattles (cropping) is stressful and painful and should be done under the supervision of a veterinarian, who will use an anesthetic and prescribe a suitable antibiotic. Some chicken keepers dub and crop to prevent frostbite; others do it to hasten healing after a chicken has been frostbitten, and still others undertake the procedure only if the frostbitten comb or wattles become infected.

You will need a pair of sharp scissors, such as those designed for dubbing and cropping and available from many poultry suppliers. Alternatives include 6-inch curved surgical scissors, small tin snips, or leathercraft scissors.

Have a helper hold the chicken, or wrap it in a towel to control struggling. Disinfect both the scissors and the comb or wattles with rubbing alcohol, and snip off the affected parts with decisive cuts, leaving about ½ inch of the comb above the head. When amputating a wattle, avoid pulling on it, which can result in cutting off more than you intend.

If bleeding occurs, apply a wound powder such as McKillip's, or sprinkle on a little flour to stop the bleeding. If blood has dripped down into the bird's nostrils, use a cotton swab to clear it away. Treat the amputation as you would treat any wound, as described under Wound Care on page 399.

PROGRESSIVE SIGNS OF FROSTBITE

Frostbite occurs when fluid freezes in the cells of the comb, wattles, or toes, depriving the cells of oxygen. After a short period of freezing, the affected part may recover. If the part doesn't thaw in a timely manner, the cells die and may become infected.

Signs of frostbite include the following:

- Pale, gray, or white tips of comb or edges of wattles

- Reddening of the feet or toes

- Subsequent swelling of comb, wattles, or toes

- Blistering within a day or so

- Blackening of comb tips, edges of wattles, patches on feet

- Loss of interest in eating and other normal activities

Signs of Frostbite

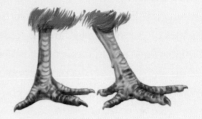

Toes redden.

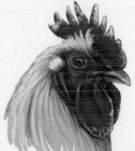

Pale edges appear around comb and wattles.

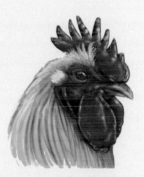

Comb and wattles become swollen.

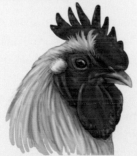

Comb tips and wattle edges blacken.

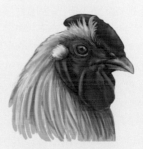

Dead tissue eventually sloughs off.

To prevent infection, either inject ½ cc penicillin into the bird's breast muscle daily for 10 days or add 1 teaspoon (5 mL) Tetracycline or Bacitracin per gallon (4 L) to the drinking water for 10 days. The comb and wattles should heal within about a month.

Toes rarely need to be amputated. Usually the dead tissue eventually sloughs off on its own, leaving the chicken with permanently missing toes or perhaps an entire foot. Chickens are adaptable and can get around well despite the missing limb, although a cock may not be able to mate effectively without all his toes. And of course, a chicken with missing parts is not suitable for exhibition.

Preventing Frostbite

The easiest way to prevent frostbitten combs and wattles is to opt for a breed with tight-fitting headgear, such as cushion, rose, or walnut combs. To prevent frostbitten feet, use wide roosts constructed from 2×4 lumber with the wide surface facing upward, so your chickens can sleep with their feet entirely covered by their bodies.

Placing roosts close to the coop's ceiling, or designing the coop with a low ceiling, is also beneficial, as the ceiling traps warmth from the chicken's bodies. Where roosts are more than 2 feet from the ceiling, a flat-panel radiant heater attached to the ceiling might be used to provide gentle heat. (Check the heater's specs for how far away the roosts should be placed.) Don't be tempted to heat the entire coop, however, which can be detrimental to flock health. And be sure to place the heater in such a way that chickens don't have to roost under it if they prefer not to.

A small, uninsulated coop doesn't hold heat well, especially one made of plastic, and the few chickens such coops are designed to house may not generate enough heat to keep each other warm. If your chickens live in portable prefab housing, consider protecting them from severe weather by moving the whole shebang inside a garage or other outbuilding for the duration.

Controlling humidity within the coop is an important frostbite prevention measure. During cold weather ambient humidity is usually low. Inside a coop, however, humidity can be high

THE VASELINE CONTROVERSY

Coating combs and wattles with petroleum jelly (Vaseline) to prevent frostbite is a matter of some controversy. Whether or not it works depends on just how low the temperature drops and for how long.

The coating works in three ways: First, it helps conserve heat that might otherwise dissipate from the comb and wattles. Second, since moisture is what causes frostbite, the coating insulates the comb from moisture and thus

from freezing. Third, petroleum jelly freezes at a slightly lower temperature than the cell fluid in a comb or wattles and therefore protects these parts from freezing at temperatures hovering around the freezing point. Note, however, that if the temperature dips much below the freezing point (32°F/0°C), especially for a prolonged period, petroleum jelly *will* freeze and therefore become useless at preventing frostbite.

thanks to damp litter, fresh droppings, and respiration — especially when chickens spend more time inside than out.

Keeping litter dry involves fixing or replacing leaky drinkers, protecting doorways from falling rain and snow, and keeping the outside of doorways cleared of snow so it won't get tracked inside. Deep litter that's stirred or topped off frequently absorbs moisture from fresh droppings. Deep sand, instead of litter, not only makes fresh droppings easy to rake off daily but also retains daytime heat to keep the coop somewhat warmer at night. Another option is to use a droppings board and frequently scrape off accumulated droppings.

Humidity released by respiration can be controlled only through good ventilation. If the insides of your coop windows drip moisture, ventilation needs to be improved.

A coop will remain drier if the chickens spend their daytime hours outdoors. Encourage wintertime outdoor activities by providing a windbreak where your chickens can get out of icy winds and blowing snow. Establishing a covered outdoor area bedded with straw or shavings will give the chickens a place to loll without resting on snow or ice. But let the chickens decide for themselves if they'd rather be outdoors or in.

Controlling Biofilm

That yucky thin layer of smelly slime sticking to the insides of drinkers and water lines during warm summer months is biofilm. The two most common kinds of biofilm in poultry drinkers are caused by algae and iron. If the slime is green, it's algae biofilm. If it's rust colored, it's iron biofilm. Neither one is good.

Algae Biofilm

Green algae biofilm itself isn't harmful, and some people maintain it's actually beneficial because it filters water by removing organic waste matter. But the presence of algae indicates that the water is polluted with the type of nutrients algae thrive on. And if the biofilm is left long enough for the algae to start dying, they'll release pollutants back into the water. Living or dead, algae can impart an odor and flavor to the water that your birds may not like, and anything that discourages drinking is unhealthful to the flock.

Green algae need four things to grow: water, nutrients (fertilizer), light (for photosynthesis), and heat. Because algae like heat, their growth in drinkers is a greater problem in summer than in the cooler winter months.

Algae biofilm is common in plastic drinkers because the plastic lets in light; galvanized drinkers, on the other hand, block light, and algae can't grow in the dark. Minimizing the amount of light that falls on plastic drinkers helps control algae. Outdoor drinkers should be kept in the shade. Even indoor drinkers will develop algae if the lights are on more than 8 hours a day. Wrapping a drinker is cumbersome and temporary (since the chickens most likely will eventually peck it to pieces), but doing so to block light helps discourage algal growth. Using galvanized drinkers resolves the light issue.

Nutrients may be furnished by your birds — in the form of poop or feed residue — or may already be in your water supply. If you're battling algae in your drinkers, the first thing to do is examine your water source. Although the chlorine in municipal tap water should discourage algae, you can find out what else is in your water by obtaining a water quality report from the office of your local water district. If your water comes from a well, have the water tested, particularly for phosphorus and nitrogen — the two nutrients algae like best.

Chickens may furnish nutrients by way of scratching litter into the drinker, pooping in the water, or dropping feed from their beaks into the water. Using nipple waterers prevents these issues. Hanging bell waterers or placing them on platforms with the trough part about the height of the chickens' backs reduces the chances of nutrients getting into the water from scratching or pooping. Putting some distance between feeders and drinkers reduces the amount of feed that gets into the water.

Copper is toxic to algae, so putting a piece of scrap copper plumbing or a few copper-plated zinc pennies into the drinker is another way to discourage algae. Since they prefer a low-oxygen environment, the ideal way to control algae is to avoid letting the water get stagnant by frequently emptying and scrubbing drinkers and refilling them with fresh water.

Of the many species of algae, some are indifferent to the water's pH, some prefer a low pH (acidic water), and some prefer a high pH (alkaline water). Most species, however, don't do well in acidified water with a pH less than 5.5. Adding 1 tablespoon of vinegar to each gallon of drinking water (double the vinegar dose if you have hard water) helps control algae.

Iron Biofilm

Iron biofilm needs three things to grow: a low-flow water supply, a rough surface, and dissolved iron. This biofilm grows best at a temperature range between 43°F and 77°F (6°C and 25°C) but can tolerate temperatures as low as freezing and as high as 104°F (0°C to 40°C).

Unaffected by light one way or the other, it can grow in complete darkness. In the poultry yard it is most likely to be found in dark places where drinking water is relatively undisturbed: coating the insides of reduced-pressure water pipes leading to automatic drinkers and the inside surfaces of galvanized metal bell drinkers.

Since the chlorine in tap water helps control it to some extent, iron biofilm is associated with well water that has a high mineral content. It starts as a flaky deposit called scale, caused by the minerals in hard water. Hard scale is crusty and results from iron and manganese. Soft scale is light and spongy, therefore easier to remove, and is caused by calcium and magnesium. You can tell your water is high in mineral content if it leaves yellow or rust-colored stains around drains or discolors laundered white clothing. Such water also has an unpleasant metallic taste.

Scale accumulates more rapidly on the rough surfaces of copper plumbing and galvanized drinkers than on the smooth surfaces of PVC plumbing and plastic drinkers. Its presence in turn increases the roughness of the surface, creating pits that give silt and other fine particles in the water a place to stick and that give microbes from the water a place to hide.

Among the first microbes to take advantage of this environment are iron bacteria, which grow into an active colony through cell division and by recruiting more iron bacteria. The bacteria produce a gelatinous slime that both protects the growing colony and traps more silt and other sediment to protect the colony.

Iron bacteria themselves don't cause disease. Their chief claim to fame is their ability to absorb and accumulate dissolved iron, and sometimes manganese, from water. They live and reproduce by deriving energy from iron and manganese, and they deposit iron and manganese salts around their cells. The resulting rust-red slime has an unpleasant swampy-rot odor and gives the water a bad taste. Chickens don't like bad-tasting water, and hens that don't get enough to drink don't lay well. Chunks of biofilm that break away inside a water pipe can clog automatic drinkers, causing them to fail or leak.

A greater problem can occur if the iron bacteria colony attracts other microbes that otherwise wouldn't stick to plumbing and drinker walls but that take advantage of the protective environment created by the iron bacteria. These moochers may include such pathogenic bacteria as campylobacter, clostridia, *E. coli,* listeria, salmonella, and staphylococci that can spread disease through your flock. Outbreaks of botulism in broiler flocks have been associated with iron-rich drinking water.

Organic matter — especially sugar, vitamins, and some medications that are added to drinking water — clings to the slime and provides its inhabitants with nutrients. Left undisturbed, a colony can grow fairly rapidly. In a matter of weeks, one can reduce the inside diameter of a 6-inch water pipe down to 2 inches. Even inside a frequently refilled bell drinker, a colony can develop quickly if the inside of the drinker is not regularly scrubbed.

Chlorine and other disinfectants have no effect on bacteria embedded in biofilm. The slime must be removed before a disinfectant has any effect. Flushing water pipes with pressure, where feasible, and scrubbing the inside walls of drinkers at least once a week will control iron biofilm. In warmer weather, which encourages a rapid increase of pathogenic microbes, daily scrubbing may be needed.

Aside from treating your well, which is best left to a professional, you can reduce the development of iron biofilm by installing a water filter. Most common household water filters will remove dirt and sediment, including iron, but not bacteria or other microorganisms that might be in the water.

Water filters are rated in microns, a metric measurement equivalent to one-millionth of a meter. The micron rating indicates the ability of the filter to remove contaminants by the size of its particles. Most water filters are in the 5 to 25 micron range. The lower the micron rating, the finer the filtration. The finer the filtration, the better the filter works but the more rapidly it will clog and need to be replaced.

Scale forms faster in water with a pH higher than 7. Below 7, minerals tend to settle out as sludge. Iron bacteria prefer a pH range of around 6.5, but can get along in the 5.5 to 8.2 range. An acidifier that reduces the water's pH below 5.5 can therefore help discourage the development of scale and iron biofilm. Vinegar makes a good acidifier, added at the rate of 1 tablespoon per gallon of drinking water (double the vinegar dose if you have hard water). Note, however, that an acidifier cannot penetrate and remove an existing iron biofilm.

Prevent Poisoning

Poisoning is relatively unusual in backyard poultry, especially if you use common sense in keeping your flock away from such toxins as pesticides, herbicides, rodenticides, disinfectants, fertilizers, fungicide-treated seeds (intended for planting), wood preservatives, rock salt, oil, and antifreeze. Poisoning may be the result of misguided management.

Common sense tells you not to put mothballs in your hens' nests in an effort to repel lice and mites, since naphthalene is toxic. And not to spray for cockroaches or other pests where your chickens might eat the poisoned insects. And not to put out bait to kill garden pests such as slugs, snails, or earwigs where your birds might find it. But even without our help, the environment contains plenty of potential poisons.

Natural Toxins

Some weeds found in pasture can be toxic but should not be a problem if your flock has plenty to eat. Most toxic plants don't taste good and therefore are not tempting to eat, except to a starving bird. Since birds nibble here and there to get a variety in their diet, if they do get a bite or two of a toxic leaf or seed, it's unlikely to create a problem. Then, too, whether or not a specific plant is toxic can vary with its stage of maturity, growing conditions (including drought), and other environmental factors.

Even if a bird does get a potentially toxic dose, the effect depends on its age and state of health. The table on page 308 lists common plants that potentially pose a danger.

Some mushrooms are toxic as well, but mushrooms would have a hard time getting a foothold where chickens are active. Still, since amanita mushrooms are deadly, it's important to be able to recognize them and make sure they don't grow where your chickens can take a taste.

Toxins in Grains

Toxic seeds are sometimes accidentally harvested along with feed grains. Such seeds include the following:

- **Corn cockle** (*Argrostemma githago*). Causes diarrhea, weakness, reduced breathing and heart rate

- **Crotalaria,** also known as showy crotalaria or rattlebox (*Crotalaria spectabilis*). Causes a rapid drop in egg production, emaciation, and death in laying hens and droopiness, huddling, and death in growing birds; postmortem signs include swollen liver, internal bleeding, and ascites.

- **Coffee weed,** also known as coffeepod or sicklepod (*Senna obtusifolia*). Causes a drop in egg production in laying hens and reduced weight gain in growing birds; no postmortem signs

- **Coffee senna** (*Senna occidentalis*). Causes weight loss, diarrhea, muscle degeneration, paralysis, and death

TOXINS IN EGGS

Toxins, as well as some drugs, tend to accumulate in body fat. Egg yolks are drawn from body fat. Therefore eggs can continue to be toxic long after a toxin has passed through the hen's digestive system. No definitive studies have been published on how long any given toxin continues to be deposited in eggs until it is entirely cleared from the hen's body, which is why few medications and chemical products are approved for use with laying hens.

- **Jimsom weed** (*Datura stramonium*). Causes excitability, loss of appetite, convulsions, coma, or sudden death

- **Sorghum,** also known as milo (*Sorghum bicolor*). High-tannin strains depress appetite, resulting in a reduced growth rate in young birds and reduced egg production in layers.

- **Fungal poisoning** can result from by-products generated in moldy feed. A number of poisons, or mycotoxins, are produced by molds that grow naturally in grains. For details see Mycotoxicoses on page 247.

Go Easy on Kitchen Scraps

Most kitchen scraps are good for chickens and add variety to their diet when fed in moderation. With the exception of rotting produce and meat, even potentially problematic items — such as avocados, onions, and potatoes — are nonissues when offered as occasional treats.

Avocado peels and pits, as well as leaves from the trees, contain the natural fungicide persin, which is highly toxic to birds. The flesh is fine, if you care to share your guacamole with your chickens, but leave out the pits and peels. Signs of toxicity include labored breathing, increased heart rate, listlessness, or sudden death. That said, a chicken would have to eat a great many peels or pits to experience a problem.

Identifying an Amanita Mushroom

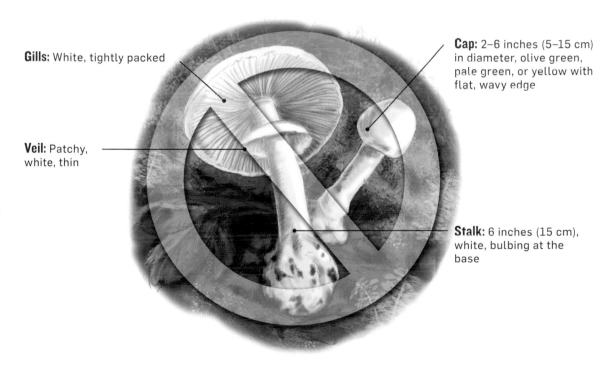

Gills: White, tightly packed

Cap: 2–6 inches (5–15 cm) in diameter, olive green, pale green, or yellow with flat, wavy edge

Veil: Patchy, white, thin

Stalk: 6 inches (15 cm), white, bulbing at the base

Plants Potentially Toxic to Chickens*

COMMON NAME	BOTANICAL NAME	TOXIC PARTS
Black locust	*Robinia pseudoacacia*	Sprouts, leaves, pods, seeds
Black nightshade	*Solanum nigrum*	Immature berries
Bladderpod, bagpod	*Sesbania vesicaria*	Seeds
Camas, death camas, black snakeroot	*Zygadenus* spp.	Leaves, flower, stem, bulb
Castor bean	*Ricinus communis*	All parts, but especially seeds
Coffee senna	*Senna occidentalis*	Seeds
Coffee weed, coffeepod, or sicklepod	*Senna obtusifolia*	Seeds
Corn cockle	*Agrostemma githago*	Seeds
Cottonseed	*Gossypium* spp.	Seeds
Crotalaria, showy rattlebox	*Crotalaria spectabilis*	Seeds, leaves, stems
Death cap, destroying angel	*Amanita* spp.	Mushroom
Horsenettle	*Solanum carolinense*	Berries, leaves
Jimson weed, thornapple	*Datura stramonium*	All parts
Milkweed	*Asclepias* spp.	Leaves
Monkshood, Indian hemp, dogbane	*Aconitum napellus*	All parts
Oak	*Quercus* spp.	Leaves, acorns
Oleander	*Nerium oleander*	All parts
Onion, green	*Allium ascalonicum*	All parts
Parsley	*Petroselinum crispum*	Leaves
Poison hemlock	*Conium maculatum*	All parts
Pokeberry	*Phytolacca americana*	Berries
Potato	*Solanum tuberosum*	Green tubers, peels, sprouts
Rapeseed	*Brassica napus*	Seeds
Rattlebox, Spanish gold	*Sesbania punicea*	Seeds
Rosary pea	*Abrus precatorius*	Seeds
Tobacco	*Nicotiana* spp.	Leaves, stems
Vetch	*Vicia* spp.	Seeds
Water hemlock, cowbane	*Cicuta* spp.	All parts
Yew	*Taxus* spp.	All parts

*This table is far from comprehensive; do not assume a plant is not toxic to chickens just because it is not listed here.

SIGNS

Weakness, depression, bloody diarrhea, paralysis, death

Dilated pupils, diarrhea, incoordination, paralysis

Bluish comb and wattles, bloody diarrhea, shock, death

Diarrhea, salivation, muscle weakness, coma, death

Gradual paralysis, slow heart rate, diarrhea, emaciation, convulsions, death

Weight loss, diarrhea, paralysis, death

Weight loss, reduced laying

Rough feathers, diarrhea, slow growth, slow respiration and heart rate

Bluish comb and wattles, emaciation, liver failure, heart failure

Depression, rapid heart rate, emaciation, bright yellow-green urates, death

Coma, death

Slobbering, diarrhea, weakness, slow breathing, death

Excitability, loss of appetite, convulsions, coma, death

Rapid heart rate, labored breathing, incoordination, convulsions, death or recovery

Diarrhea, labored breathing, convulsions, paralysis, death

Diarrhea, decreased appetite, increased thirst, dark diarrhea, death

Weakness, bloody diarrhea, heart muscle degeneration, sudden death

Sudden death

Sunburn in unfeathered areas

Diarrhea, incoordination, slow breathing and heart rate, paralysis, death

Slobbering, bloody diarrhea, incoordination, convulsions, death

Incoordination, coma

Fishy odor and flavor in brown-shell eggs, anemia, sudden death

Diarrhea, depression, respiratory failure

Convulsions, death

Stunted chicks, reduced egg production in hens

Excitability, labored breathing, convulsions, sudden death

Incoordination, paralysis, death

Bluish combs and wattles, labored breathing, incoordination, coma, sudden death

Onions, like garlic, contain sulfur compounds that break down into thiosulfinates, which in turn decompose into a number of disulfides — oxidizing agents that can cause red blood cells to rupture, resulting in hemolytic anemia. Compared to garlic, which contains only trace amounts of thiosulfinates, onions contain a much higher concentration.

Signs of thiosulfinate toxicity include diarrhea, loss of appetite, listlessness, paleness, difficulty breathing, and red-tinged urates. Whether the onions are raw or cooked makes no difference, and poisoning can occur whether a chicken eats a lot of onions at once or lesser amounts over a long period of time. However, because red blood cells are continually being replaced anyway, kitchen scraps containing the occasional bit of onion may be fed with no problem.

Potatoes are extremely nutritious, and any way you might cook them to serve at your table is safe to feed to chickens. Raw potatoes, however, contains starches that don't digest well. They also contain antinutrients — concentrated in the skin — that inhibit the activity of certain enzymes needed to break down proteins for digestion. A few scraps of raw potato or raw skins won't harm your chickens, but too much at once can cause digestive discomfort. Better to cook them first.

The parts of the potato plant that grow aboveground contain toxic alkaloids that protect the growing plant from insects and fungi. Normally these colorless alkaloids appear in insignificant amounts in the potato tuber, unless it has been bruised or otherwise damaged, exposed to light long enough to develop green patches of chlorophyll, or stored for so long it begins to sprout. Bruising, as well as the presence of sprouts and chlorophyll, are indications that the tuber is accumulating protective alkaloids, the most problematic of which is the nerve toxin solanine.

Solanine is concentrated in and directly under the skin, tastes bitter, and is not deactivated by cooking. Digested in small amounts, it is poorly absorbed and rapidly excreted. Excessive amounts can cause diarrhea, paralysis, and death. Toxicity is easily avoided by peeling away green parts of the skin and flesh, and removing any sprouting eyes, before cooking potatoes to feed to your chickens (or to yourself).

Botulism, one of the world's most potent toxins, can poison chickens that are fed rotting organic matter or fly larvae from contaminated meat. It can also occur when chickens drink water that has been contaminated by rotting organic matter. For details see Botulism on page 230.

Preventing poisoning caused by feeding chickens inappropriate kitchen scraps is largely a matter of common sense. Don't feed your chickens anything you wouldn't eat yourself, and don't feed them a whole lot of any one thing.

FLUSH OUT TOXINS

When a chicken suffers from food poisoning, you can hasten its recovery by flushing its system with a laxative that absorbs the toxins and removes them from the body. For details see Laxative Flushes on page 392.

Things Toxic to Chicks

Chicks are especially susceptible to certain toxins. The most common include the following:

- **Carbon monoxide** from a poorly maintained gas heater in the brooder, or from being transported in a poorly ventilated vehicle (chicks die)

- **Disinfectant** overuse, especially in a poorly ventilated brooder (chicks huddle with ruffled feathers)

- **Fungicides** on coated seeds intended for planting (chicks rest on hocks or walk stiff-legged)

- **Pesticides** used to rid housing of insects (chicks die)

- **Rose chafers** (*Macrodactylus subspinosus*), a beetle found in late spring and early summer in eastern and central North America (chicks appear drowsy, go into convulsions, and die or recover within 24 hours)

- **Nitrofurazone,** an antibiotic used to treat some bacterial diseases (chicks squawk loudly, move rapidly, fall forward)

- **Coccidiostats** (nicarbazin, monensin, sulfaquinoxaline) added to water in warm weather, when chicks drink more and may obtain a fatal dose

Although chicks, being smaller, are much more susceptible to toxins than mature birds, brooding them in a properly managed environment will protect them from being poisoned.

Coop and Run Hazards

Maintaining a safe environment for your chickens would seem to be a no-brainer; however, things are not always simple. Common hazards inside the coop include ammonia fumes, vinyl floor, Styrofoam insulation, and gas-emitting lightbulbs. Out in the run chickens might eat sharp metal objects or contaminated soil.

Ammonia Fumes

Chickens, with their highly efficient respiratory systems, are especially sensitive to inhaled toxins, including ammonia. Bacteria that thrive in damp litter release ammonia gas in the process of decomposing droppings. Damp litter is especially common during the heat of summer, when chickens drink more than usual and their droppings are looser than usual, and in the cold of winter, when chickens spend more time indoors and ventilation is reduced to keep the flock from becoming chilled.

Chickens start to suffer when ammonia levels in the air reach 25 parts per million. Luckily, your nose can detect the pungent gas at less than 10 ppm, giving you plenty of notice that corrective measures are needed. For details see Ammonia Check on page 15.

Piling and Suffocation

Chickens that are cold or frightened tend to crowd into a corner and pile on top of each other, suffocating the ones unfortunate enough to be at the bottom of the heap. Piling commonly occurs when chickens are moved to a new coop, especially if other chickens are already in residence and don't take kindly to the newcomers. Other causes of piling include a prowling predator or a nighttime power failure in a coop or brooder where the lights are on 24/7.

Finding one or more flattened, dead chickens in a corner of the coop or brooder is a reliable indicator that piling occurred sometime during the night. To eliminate possible causes of the piling, before moving birds to new quarters, check the new facility to make sure predators can't get in during the night. After transferring the chickens or after introducing new chickens into an existing flock, check before going to bed to make sure all the birds are tucked in safe and sound. If piling is in progress, stir up the birds to get them spread apart.

Piling is most likely to occur in the evening, as the chickens bed down and while they still have light. After dark they are less likely to move around, therefore less likely to pile. They may still pile, but spreading them apart after dark (or, if the facility is lighted overnight, after they settle down for the night) reduces the chance.

Hatchlings in a drafty or chilly brooder may pile together in an effort to get warm. In a brooder that is too hot, chicks may pile into a corner away from the heat source. Along with carefully monitoring the brooder temperature, fitting the brooder with a circular cardboard corral for the first week or so will cut drafts, as well as eliminating corners to prevent piling and suffocation.

Vinyl Flooring

Today's chicken keepers are fond of covering coop floors with linoleum and often find that their chickens enjoy pecking holes in the flooring. Although real linoleum is relatively nontoxic, vinyl (PVC) is often passed off as linoleum. Vinyl flooring may contain lead and other heavy metals, which are highly toxic. If vinyl is eaten the eventual result is gastrointestinal and neurological problems in the chickens and in any person who regularly eats their eggs. To make matters worse, vinyl gets its flexibility and durability from plasticizers called phthalates, which are also toxic.

Even with safe linoleum, if you glue it down, the adhesive could be problematic. The most likely sign of adhesive toxicity is digestive upset, indicated by diarrhea. Before gluing linoleum to your coop floor, do an online search for the Material Safety Data Sheet for the type of adhesive you intend to use to determine what's in it and whether or not it's toxic.

Foam Board Insulation

Chickens are notorious for chowing down on foam board insulation, which consists of a little plastic — polystyrene, polyurethane,

HARDWARE DISEASE

Small objects carelessly tossed into a poultry yard can cause injury or death. Cigarette filters, for instance, can cause impaction. Birds are attracted to small shiny objects like nails, pop-tops, and bits of glass or wire. Eating such a sharp object may simply irritate the bird and cause depression, or it may result in a blockage that interferes with digestion, or it can cause an internal tear that becomes infected, leading to the bird's death. Prevent such possibilities by meticulously picking up objects scattered in your poultry yard, and ask visitors not to toss discards on the ground.

or polyisocyanurate — and a lot of air. These types of plastic do not readily biodegrade and therefore are likely to pass through the chicken without causing any harm.

A problem could occur, however, if the chicken were hungry enough to pack its crop full of plastic bits, preventing anything nutritious from getting through. In such a case, the chicken would need to be treated for crop impaction, as described under Crop Binding on page 79.

Although a little foam board won't cause the chicken any harm, a few chickens can quickly destroy the foam board's insulation value. If you insulate your coop walls or ceiling with foam board, don't leave it exposed for long before you cover it with plywood or other siding.

Teflon Lightbulbs

You might think shatter-resistant lightbulbs would be a safe bet in the chicken coop, but exactly the opposite is true. Such bulbs are coated with polytetrafluoroethylene (PTFE) — commonly known by one of several brand names, Teflon — which encloses the glass in the event the bulb breaks. When in use, the bulb heats up and the PTFE emits a gas that is lethally toxic to birds.

Inhaling the fumes damages a chicken's respiratory system, causing body fluids to leak into the lungs and essentially drown the bird. An older chicken, depending on how far it is from the source, may die suddenly or may gasp for air before dying. Chicks in a brooder heated with a shatterproof lamp will die quickly.

These bulbs — sold in a variety of forms, including heat lamps, floodlights, and rough-service work lights — absolutely have no place in a coop or brooder. Neither should they be used anywhere chickens might be kept, including inside your house or garage.

Lead Contamination

With backyard flocks moving into urban areas, lead poisoning from contaminated soil has become a concern. Lead is naturally present in all soil but occurs in higher than normal concentrations in certain areas. Unfortunately, lead doesn't move through the soil and eventually filter out but instead persists in contaminated soil for hundreds of years.

The usual source of urban contamination is paint chips or dust from lead-based paints, which have been banned from residential use since 1978 but still may be flaking off older buildings or may have contaminated surrounding soil during removal by sanding or sandblasting. Former industrial sites may be contaminated with heavy metals, including lead.

But lead poisoning isn't just an urban issue. In rural areas the fungicide lead arsenate was used as an orchard spray until it was banned in 1988. Auto emissions of tetraethyl lead, added to gasoline as an antiknock ingredient prior to being banned for automotive use in 1995, contaminate soils along highly traveled roads. Chickens also may be poisoned by eating lead shotgun pellets, which lodge in their gizzards and release lead over a long period of time. And chickens can also be poisoned by inhaling lead dust while dust bathing.

If you have reason to believe your chickens are exposed to lead contamination, have your soil tested. Look online or in your local phone book for a soil testing laboratory, or contact your county Extension office for information. Although home test kits are available for detecting soil contamination, they are not reliable enough for this purpose.

The Extension office can also help you find a toxicology lab that will test eggs for lead.

Because lead remains concentrated near the soil's surface, you may be told to cover contaminated soil with sand, gravel, mulch, or low-lead soil. However, unless the cover layer is extremely deep, chickens are likely to uncover the contaminated soil while digging their sometimes sizable hollows for dust bathing. The better option is to have the surface soil entirely removed and, if necessary, replaced with low-lead soil. Aside from this drastic, and expensive, measure, other ways to protect your flock include housing them away from areas that are likely to be highly contaminated — such as old buildings, an old orchard, or alongside a highway — and don't let them forage there.

Above all, don't panic. If you feel you have reason to be concerned, have your soil tested. You will then have the information you need either to stop worrying or to develop a suitable remediation plan. Should the latter prove necessary, the National Lead Information Center (www2.epa.gov/lead or 1-800-424-5323) can help you locate a certified contractor and possibly also financial assistance.

Salt Poisoning

Chickens have a relatively low requirement for salt, and an excessive dose can be toxic. They can be poisoned after pecking rock salt used to deice a sidewalk or driveway or after eating a salt supplement intended for other livestock.

Chickens that do not have access to water at all times may be poisoned by even a normal amount of salt in the ration. In warm weather, when chickens need more water than usual, make sure they never run out; in winter take care to furnish unfrozen drinking water.

Poisoning can occur when a flock has no source of drinking water other than highly saline water. Some protein supplements — including fish meal, sunflower meal, and whey — may contain excessive amounts of salt, resulting in toxicity when combined with a normal salt-fortified ration.

Chicks are more susceptible to salt poisoning than are mature chickens. Signs include increased thirst, increased urine output (resulting in loose droppings and soggy litter), weak muscles, convulsions, and death. A lethal dose of salt is 0.06 ounce per pound (4.0 g/kg) of body weight, which for a 5-pound chicken amounts to about 1/3 ounce, or 1 1/2 teaspoons.

SIGNS OF LEAD POISONING

Signs of lead poisoning may not be apparent, or may include listlessness, increased thirst, decreased appetite, emaciation, and green-tinged droppings. As the affected chicken grows weaker, its wings may droop down. Young birds die more quickly than older chickens.

Even when chickens show no signs of lead poisoning, hens may pass lead into their eggs. The more lead the hens are exposed to, the more they deposit in their eggs, endangering humans — especially children and pregnant women — who regularly eat the contaminated eggs.

When Hens Stop Laying

Often the first sign of disease is a slowdown in laying, but low egg production is not necessarily a sign of disease. A hen doesn't have to lay eggs to remain healthy. From the hen's point of view, egg laying is strictly for procreation. For that purpose the hen needs to lay only as many eggs as she can cover with her body and hatch. That today's hens lay many more eggs than are needed for reproduction is entirely for the culinary satisfaction of the chicken keeper.

The number of eggs a hen does lay and their size, shape, and internal quality — as well as shell color, texture, and strength — is influenced by a variety of factors. Being able to determine the reason for slow, or no, egg production helps you decide whether some management issue needs to be addressed or you are receiving an early warning of impending disease.

Nonlayers

Like some people, some hens are simply lazy. A slacker reduces overall egg numbers, leaving the impression the entire flock isn't laying well.

Before looking for other problems, determine that all your hens are doing their fair share of the work. The best way to determine if a hen is laying is to examine her vent and pubic bones.

Vent. The vent of a good layer is large, moist, and oval. A nonlayer's is tight, dry, and puckered.

Pubic bones. The pair of pointy bones located between the keel and the vent should have enough room between them for you to place three or more fingers for most breeds, at least two fingers for small breeds. The space between the pubic bones and keel should accommodate at least four fingers. A hen that's tight and nonflexible in these areas is not laying.

A hen that is a nonlayer might actually be laying, but instead of the yolk traveling down the oviduct and coming out wrapped in a shell, it gets dropped into the body cavity. The occasional internally laid egg is fairly common, and such a yolk is resorbed by the hen's body without problems, but a persistent internal layer is an unhealthy hen. For details see Internal Layer on page 94.

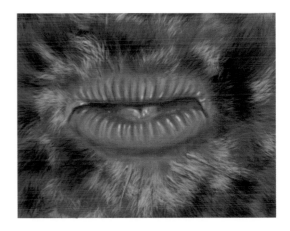

A nonlayer has a tight, dry, round vent.

A good layer has a large, moist, oval vent.

Breed

Some breeds lay better than others. The better layers are, quite naturally, more persistent layers. All hens lay a certain number of eggs, collectively known as a clutch, and then take a break for a day or two. The better layers produce larger clutches and therefore take fewer breaks.

White Leghorns and other production hens are selectively bred to lay as many eggs as possible per clutch. A top producer can lay an egg a day for the better part of a year before taking a break. Most breeds don't lay nearly that well.

If your hens are laying like gangbusters, then one day you don't get as many eggs as you think you should, several hens may be taking their break at the same time — especially if they are all the same age. If production doesn't pick up within a couple of days, look for other reasons.

Day Length

In autumn, when the number of daylight hours falls below 12, most hens take a break until spring brings longer days and a more favorable season for raising chicks. On the two equinoxes — about March 20 and September 22 — day length everywhere in the world is exactly 12 hours. Starting on June 22, the summer solstice, day length gradually decreases, and on December 22, the winter solstice, day length begins to increase gradually.

To get eggs from hens that don't normally lay during short winter days, you have to trick them into thinking the season remains right for reproduction year-round, which you can do by using lights to compensate for decreasing amounts of natural daylight. To ensure that light hours never fall below 12, a typical plan is to provide a constant 14 to 16 hours of combined natural and artificial light. Although 14

hours is adequate, when the weather is bitter cold, 16 hours lets hens get more nutritional energy by giving them more time to eat.

The farther you live from the equator, where day length is constant, the bigger your seasonal swing will be from longest to shortest days and back again. Courtesy of the United States Naval Observatory, you can find a month-by-month table of daylight hours for any location in the world at this website: aa.usno.navy.mil/data/docs/Dur_OneYear.php.

Start augmenting natural light when decreasing day length approaches 14 hours. Continue the lighting program throughout the winter and into spring, until natural daylight is back up to 14 hours a day. By setting a timer to go on for a few hours at the same time every morning, and again for a few hours in the evening, you can bracket the changing daylight hours to create a constant 14-hour day.

Don't be tempted to leave the coop lights on all the time. Besides being wasteful, 24/7 lighting encourages hens to spend more time inside during the day instead of being out in the fresh air. It also doesn't give them the 6 to 8 hours of rest per 24 they need to maintain a healthy immune system.

Molting

Short day lengths signal chickens that it's time to renew plumage, or molt, in preparation for cold weather. Molting occurs over a period of weeks, so most chickens never look completely naked — although one occasionally comes close. Under natural circumstances a chicken molts during late summer and early fall.

The best layers molt late and fast. They lay for a year or more before molting and take only 2 to 3 months to finish the molt. The poorest layers start early and molt slowly. They may lay for only a few months before going into a molt, and the molt may take as long as 6 months. These hens are easy to identify because they start molting before September and drop their wings' primary flight feathers one at a time.

During a molt, nutrients needed to produce eggs are channeled into producing feathers. As a result, most hens slow down, or stop laying altogether, until the molt is complete.

An out-of-season molt may result from disease or stress, such as chilling or going without water or feed. A stress-induced molt is usually rapid and partial and does not always cause a drop in laying.

Equinox and Solstice

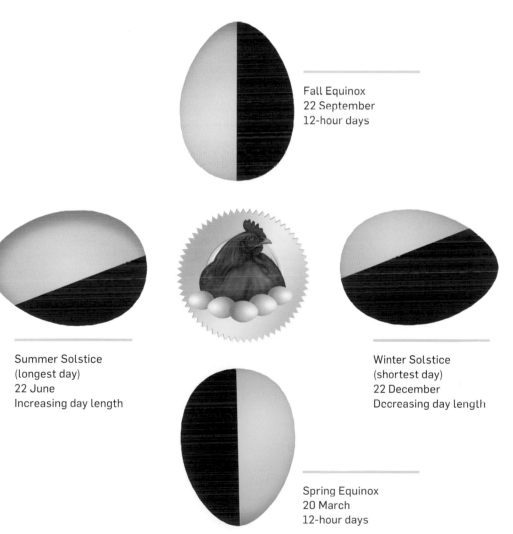

Fall Equinox
22 September
12-hour days

Summer Solstice
(longest day)
22 June
Increasing day length

Winter Solstice
(shortest day)
22 December
Decreasing day length

Spring Equinox
20 March
12-hour days

Broodiness

A hen that doesn't want to leave the nest, and pecks or growls at you when you try to move her or take her eggs, isn't sick. She's broody, which means she wants to hatch out some chicks to mother. The instinct to hatch eggs is triggered by increasing day length. When a hen gets broody, her pituitary gland releases the hormone prolactin, which tells her to stop laying.

Hens of some breeds, such as production Leghorns, rarely brood, while hens of other breeds, notably Cochins and Silkies, seem to think of nothing else. Most breeds lie somewhere in between, with some individuals tending toward broodiness and others having no interest at all in motherhood. As a general rule, the more eggs you can expect from your chosen breed, the less likely the hens are to brood; conversely, the fewer eggs you can expect from your hens, the more likely they are to brood.

Persistent broodiness poses a health risk. A setting hen eats about one-fifth of the amount she normally eats, and some days she won't eat at all. As a result, she can lose as much as 20 percent of her normal weight. A persistent broody with a nest full of infertile eggs that never hatch, or one that hatches clutch after clutch without a break, could eventually starve to death. For this reason chicken keepers who value their broody hens discourage them from brooding more than once a year.

Age

A healthy hen should lay for some 10 to 12 years, but at that age won't lay as well as she did as a young hen. Indeed, occasionally you hear about a hen that's still laying at the ripe old age of 20 — doing well to pump out one egg a week.

Depending on the breed, pullets start laying at 4 to 5 months of age and reach peak production at 7 or 8 months of age. From there, laying gradually declines until the hens molt, at the age of about 18 months. After the molt they resume laying.

As hens age, the pattern continues. Following the annual molt, production is greater than it was at the end of the previous year but not as good as it was at the beginning of the previous year. A hen that doesn't follow this pattern has something else going on. She may have become an internal layer, as described on page 94, or she may be obese.

Obesity

Some hens gradually accumulate fat as they age — especially when fed too much grain and other treats by a well-meaning keeper — which significantly impairs their ability to lay. Breeds that are known to be cold hardy are especially disposed to obesity because their natural tendency is to put on extra fat for the winter. For signs to help you determine if your hens are too fat, see Avoid Obesity on page 43.

One of the health hazards of obesity is prolapse, which can cause permanent damage or even death. For more on this subject, see Prolapse on page 93.

Stress

Excessive stress affects not only egg production but also a hen's overall health. A chicken's life is inherently stressful, so anything you do to keep your hens as calm and content as possible keeps the eggs coming by enhancing the birds' quality of life. For details on minimizing your flock's general stress level, see Stress Management on page 23. For details on reducing stress caused by high temperatures, see Heat Stress on page 103.

Effect of a Hen's Age on Laying

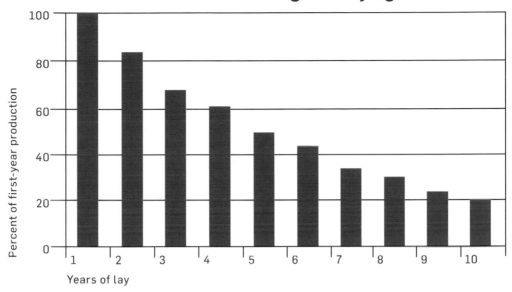

From: "Factors Affecting Egg Production in Backyard Chicken Flocks,"
University of Florida Institute of Food and Agricultural Sciences, 2013 (Publication PS-35)

Temperature

Hens lay best when the temperature is between 45°F and 80°F (7°C and 27°C). Any colder or warmer than that, production slows down.

In winter, when hens need extra energy to stay warm, they may not get enough to eat to both maintain body heat and continue laying well. One solution is to supplement the layer ration with a little scratch grain — no more than the hens can polish off within 15 to 20 minutes. Another solution is to give them more time to eat by lighting the coop to provide a combined total of natural and artificial light of no more than 16 hours, which still leaves the hens 8 hours for uninterrupted sleep.

Since chickens eat to meet their energy needs, layers naturally eat less in summer than in winter. If their summer ration contains the same amount of protein as their winter ration, they'll get less total protein and therefore won't lay as well. When temperatures rise, using a layer ration with 18 percent or more protein will give a boost to heat-stressed hens that eat too little.

Nutrition

Improper nutrition can cause a drop in laying. Hens may get too little feed or may be fed rations containing too little carbohydrate, protein, or calcium. Imbalanced rations often result from feeding hens too many table scraps or too much scratch, or from failure to offer a free-choice calcium supplement. Inadequate nutrition can also result from feeding old, stale rations.

Low temperatures increase a chicken's requirement for carbohydrates, and unless rations are adjusted accordingly, low production may result. Anything that causes hens to eat less than they should — such as high summer temperatures or inadequate feeder space — also causes them to lay less than usual.

ODD EGGS

Eggs with unusual shells can be a sign of disease but may also be perfectly normal. When oddball eggs appear, consider all the possible reasons before jumping to conclusions about the health of your hens.

Bloody shells can be a sign of coccidiosis, which causes intestinal bleeding. This disease does not often infect mature hens, but if it does you'll likely see bloody droppings as well as bloody shells. Other reasons for bloody shells include excess protein in the lay ration and pullets beginning to lay before their bodies are ready, causing tissue to tear.

Thin shells can be a sign of some disease, notably infectious bronchitis. A more common cause is warm weather — panting leads to a reduction in calcium mobilization, resulting in eggs with thin shells. Other possibilities include aging (older hens lay larger eggs with thinner shells), imbalanced ration (too little calcium or too much phosphorus), or a hereditary defect.

Soft shells can be a sign of a serious viral disease, especially when accompanied by a drop in production. More commonly, the occasional soft or missing shell occurs when a hen reaches peak production and her egg-making apparatus can't keep up. Other causes include stress (induced by fright or excitement), a nutritional deficiency (especially of vitamin D or calcium), warm weather (when a hen eats less and therefore gets less calcium from her ration), and age.

Pale shells can result from a respiratory disease — such as chronic respiratory disease, infectious bronchitis, or Newcastle — which can damage the shell gland. Excessive stress can cause brown-shell layers to produce eggs that are a lighter color than usual. Perfectly healthy aging brown-shell layers typically produce eggs with paler shells than those they laid when younger.

Miniature yolkless eggs, usually round, typically occur as a pullet's first effort, produced before her reproductive system is fully geared up. Sometimes a mature hen lays a tiny yolkless egg at the beginning or end of her laying cycle. Such an egg likely results when a bit of reproductive tissue breaks away, stimulating the egg-producing glands to treat it like a yolk and wrap it in albumen, membranes, and a shell as if it were a normal egg. In place of a yolk, this egg contains a small particle of grayish tissue.

The occasional appearance of such an egg is perfectly normal.

Weirdly shaped eggs may result from a viral disease. They may also occur after old hens or maturing pullets have been vaccinated for a respiratory disease. Occasional variations in shape, especially seasonal, are normal. Flat-sided or wrinkled eggs may be laid by a hen that has been handled roughly or, for instance, that recently flew down from a high place, landing hard and damaging a developing egg.

Runny egg white can be the result of a disease, notably infectious bronchitis, or a fungal toxin in moldy feed. More commonly it results from storing eggs for too long, especially at high temperatures. Aging hens may also lay eggs with thinner than normal albumen.

Tiny yolkless eggs can appear at the beginning or end of a hen's laying cycle.

Dehydration

Worse than letting the feeder go empty is letting the drinker go dry. A hen drinks a little at a time but drinks often. A hen therefore needs access to fresh drinking water at all times for her egg-laying apparatus to function properly.

Birds may suffer water deprivation if the water quality is poor or they just don't like the taste. In summer, water deprivation occurs when a hen's need for water increases but the water supply doesn't. In winter, drinkers may freeze. Drinkers that aren't cleaned regularly may develop bad-tasting biofilm that discourages drinking. Going without adequate water for even a short period affects a hen's overall health, as well as her ability to lay.

Disappearing Eggs

You may get too few eggs if your hens hide their eggs where you can't find them or if a hen lays her eggs, then turns around and eats them. Egg eating is a form of cannibalism, as discussed on page 297.

An egg eater may not necessarily come from within your flock. It may be a wily predator that has breached your security system.

Toxins

Aflatoxin and other mycotoxins in moldy feed can reduce egg production by interfering with the absorption or metabolism of nutrients or by disrupting a hen's hormones. Botulism poisoning (from pecking at decaying organic matter), salt poisoning, or any of the other toxins described on pages 305 to 311 can detrimentally affect egg production.

Parasites

Parasites, both external and internal, can depress laying. As bloodsuckers, northern fowl mites can cause a reduction in laying, as well as a reduction in overall immunity to disease. Lice and sticktight fleas cause irritability, often resulting in a drop in egg production.

Roundworms and tapeworms interfere with nutrient absorption, reducing egg production as well as immunity to disease. Coccidiosis doesn't normally affect mature hens, but when it does it can depress egg production, as can some of the anticoccidials — which shouldn't be given to layers anyway.

Disease

If you can find no other cause for a slump in laying, consider the possibility your hens are coming down with a disease, especially if several hens are involved. A reduction in laying is often the first general sign of disease, soon accompanied by lethargy, loss of appetite, and weight loss. Other signs that a disease may be involved include the sudden appearance of egg oddities, especially eggs with thinner, paler shells; irregular shapes; and watery whites.

CHAPTER 12

Diagnostic Guides

B EING ABLE TO recognize early signs of illness is an important first step toward treating any illness. No one who keeps chickens likes to lose a bird. Even more, no one wants one sick chicken to spread disease to the rest of the flock. The ability to make at least a tentative diagnosis allows you to be ready to take fast action.

Even if you have access to a veterinarian who will accept a chicken as a patient, it's good to be a knowledgeable first responder. You may find you can handle the situation yourself without the need to involve a veterinarian. On the other hand, should you need to consult a vet, any information you gather in advance will bring your vet that much closer to helping you solve the problem in a timely fashion.

Trying to figure out what is ailing your chickens involves these four basic steps:

1. Examine your flock's history.

2. Consider all the signs.

3. Conduct a postmortem examination.

4. Perform laboratory procedures.

Speaking of Diagnostics

brachial. The main vein of the wing

cull. To permanently remove an undesirable chicken from its flock

cyanosis. A bluish discoloration of the skin resulting from low blood oxygen

depopulate. To dispose of an entire flock

diarrhea. Droppings with the fecal portion too loose to retain its shape

feces. The solid brownish or grayish portion of a poop consisting of digestive waste

gaping. Opening the mouth wide while stretching the neck to get a good gulp of air; the chicken version of a yawn

gasping. Short, rapid inhaling due to the inability to take a deep breath

gurgling. An intermittent, low-pitched bubbling sound at the beginning of inspiration and sometimes during expiration

local infection. An infection confined to a limited area of the body

rales. A brief, intermittent rattling sound caused when air is forced through respiratory passages narrowed by fluid or mucus

septicemia. A systemic infection that invades the body through the bloodstream

sign. A readily observable indication of illness

systemic. Affecting the entire body

torticollis. Twisting of the neck

urates. Off-white, cream-colored, or yellowish cap on poop; the chicken version of urine

Home Diagnostics

If your chickens have a fairly common ailment, you may arrive at a diagnosis without the need for a postmortem or lab procedures. In this chapter you'll find details on maintaining a flock history, along with diagnostic guides to help you make sense of the signs you observe in your flock.

Should a postmortem become necessary, you will find an overview in chapter 13. Home laboratory procedures are pretty much limited to investigating internal parasites, as described under Giving a Fecal Exam on page 187.

Consider enlisting the help of a veterinarian if, after going through these steps, you're still not sure what ailment you're dealing with. If you do not have access to an avian vet, contact your state pathology laboratory. To find your state lab, and understand its procedure, see page 352.

Key to Age Designations
(Chapters 12 & 13)

DESIGNATION	APPROXIMATE AGE RANGE
Hatchling	Emerging from the egg or freshly emerged
Chick	Still downy, up to about 2 weeks
Young	Feathering out, up to about 8 weeks
Growing	Filling out, up to about 20 weeks
Maturing	20 to 25 weeks; pullets start laying
Mature	25 weeks or older
Aging	More than 2 years old

Taking Blood Samples

Your veterinarian or pathologist may ask you to furnish blood samples from ailing birds. Blood samples are usually taken from a main wing vein, or brachial.

Note: If the lab needs a whole blood sample (rather than one in which waterlike serum separates from the blood), your veterinarian or pathologist will give you an anticoagulant to keep the blood from separating.

1. Pull a few feathers from the depression in the upper part of the underside of the wing to expose the main vein.

2. Disinfect the skin with alcohol.

3. In one hand hold both wings over the chicken's back so it can't flap. Insert the needle into the vein with the needle pointing away from the chicken's body and toward the wing tip.

4. Starting with the plunger pulled back slightly to allow an initial air space in the syringe, slowly but steadily pull back on the plunger until the syringe contains at least 2 mL of blood.

5. Withdraw the needle from the wing and replace the protective cap.

6. Without rotating or jostling the syringe, place it in the clean container where it will remain horizontal.

7. Do not refrigerate or freeze it, but take the sample to the lab for analysis the same day it was drawn.

Supplies

- 70 percent alcohol (common rubbing alcohol)

- Sharp 20-gauge needle (¾ inch for chicks, 2 inch for mature birds)

- Clean container that fits the needle and syringe horizontally

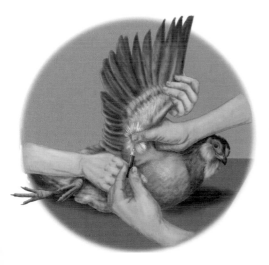

Insert the needle into the main wing vein (brachial), and slowly withdraw a blood sample of at least 2 mL.

Flock History

When you experience a problem, suddenly all those little details you thought you'd never forget, but now can't quite remember, become immensely important. You'll be happy now if you took a few moments to write down events as they occurred. If you neglected to keep accurate records as you went along, try to reconstruct your flock's history based on the accompanying table.

The Sick Bird Look

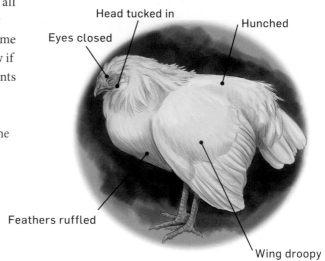

Head tucked in

Eyes closed

Hunched

Feathers ruffled

Wing droopy

Flock History

RECORDING THIS	CAN HELP YOU DETERMINE THIS
Ailing flocks nearby	Diseases in your area that could spread to your flock
Previous illness in your flock	Diseases already present on your property
Contacts	Diseases possibly brought in by new chickens, visitors, borrowed or purchased used equipment, etc.
Flock age	Diagnosis based on age group involved (approximation only)
Time of year	Relationship to weather or to mosquitoes and other carriers
Feed changes	Illness due to improper nutrition or toxins in feed
Duration of illness	Diagnosis based on how long signs last
Rate of spread	Diagnosis based on how rapidly chickens are falling ill
Past vaccinations	Diseases not likely to be involved because of vaccination, or occurring as a result of vaccination
Medications used in the past	Identification of possibly resistant pathogens
Medications used recently	Diagnosis based on flock response to meds
Percentage involved	Diagnosis based on percentage of sick birds
Mortality rate	Diagnosis based on percentage of dead birds
Appearance at death	Diagnosis based on carcass position and location

Signs of Illness

Signs are clearly visible indications of illness. To readily recognize signs, you need to be thoroughly familiar with how a healthy flock looks, acts, and smells.

Be observant when you tend your flock. Each time you enter your coop, stand quietly for a moment, watch, and listen. *Any* change you detect, including a change in the personality of individual birds and their desire (or ability) to actively remain with the rest of the flock, the amount of feed they eat, the amount of water they drink, or how energetic they are (or aren't), may be the first sign of disease.

Signs of Health and Illness

OBSERVE	HEALTHY	EARLY WARNING	SERIOUS
Posture	Erect, head and tail held high	Squatting, head tucked in, tail droopy	Hunched, head and tail hanging down
Movement	Consistent	Limping, lame	Reluctant to move, paralyzed
Activity	Active, alert, busy	Uninterested	Inactive, seeking solitude
Comb & wattles	Bright red, full, waxy	Pale	Dark, swollen, or shriveled
Face	Filled out	Shrunken	Sunken in or swollen
Eyes	Bright, shiny, alert	Dull, watery, partly closed	Swollen, crusty, closed
Nostrils	Clean	Dirty	Caked, crusty
Breathing	Quiet	Labored	Noisy, gasping
Beak	Clean, usually closed	Open	Wide open, with or without discharge
Breast	Plump	Thin	Shrunken
Abdomen	Firm but not hard	Swollen	Bulging, hard
Feathers	Smooth, clean	Dull or off-color; stained around nose, eyes, vent	Rough, ruffled, broken
Vent	Clean, slightly moist	Stained	Dry, shriveled
Shanks	Clean, smooth, waxy	Enlarged, crusty scales	Enlarged, warm joints
Appetite	Consistent	Increased or decreased	Loss of appetite
Thirst	Consistent	Increased or decreased	Excessive drinking
Weight	Consistent	Weight loss	Emaciation
Egg laying	Consistent	Decreased	Drastically decreased or stopped
Droppings	Firm, gray-brown with white caps; occasional sticky cecal dropping	Soft or loose	Runny, smelly, or off-color

Identifying Signs

If you notice anything unusual in your flock, follow these steps in identifying signs of disease:

1. Watch from a distance to see what each bird is doing, how it moves, and how it stands when still. Check droppings on the ground. Note unusual smells. Listen for unusual sounds: if you whistle, the birds will stop their activities to listen, and you can more easily hear respiratory sounds.

2. Count the number of affected birds. Come back a few hours later, and count again. How fast the illness sweeps or creeps through a flock can provide an important clue as to what the disease might be. Since different diseases progress at different rates, if more than one disease is involved, how fast individual signs move through a flock can be especially important.

3. Keep track of the number of birds that die. Note how and where they die, and how soon they die after showing first signs.

4. For a closer look, catch chickens with a minimum of fuss; signs can change when you pick up a bird, especially if the bird has to be chased to be caught. Check body openings for unusual excretions: discharge from the mouth, clogged nostrils, sticky eyes, diarrhea. Note any unusual smell coming from these discharges.

5. Check for wounds, swellings, external parasites. See chapter 5 for instructions on checking for parasites. Check for blindness. See How to Tell If a Chicken Is Blind on page 97.

6. Use the diagnostic charts in this chapter to help you identify the disease. Look up each possibility in the alphabetic list in Quick Guide to Diseases and Disorders starting on page 417 (or, in the case of possible parasites, chapters 5, 6, and 7), and find the condition with a combination of signs that most closely match those of your flock.

SYNDROMES

A syndrome consists of a group of signs that typically occur together and appear as a specific disease. The word derives from the Greek word *syndromos*, meaning "a place where several roads meet."

In most cases an illness described as a syndrome is poorly defined — its signs are not always precisely the same, its cause has yet to be identified, or it may have several different and generally unrelated causes. The following syndromes are described in the Quick Guide to Diseases and Disorders starting on page 417:

Air sac disease (also known as air sac syndrome)

Ascites (a.k.a. pulmonary hypertension syndrome)

Epididymal lithiasis (a.k.a. premature low fertility syndrome)

Fatty liver syndrome

Sudden death syndrome

Matching Signs to Disease

General signs appear in nearly any illness, whether it results from an infection, a parasitic invasion, nutritional deficiency, or poisoning. General signs include droopiness, ruffled feathers, weight loss, and reduced egg production.

Each disease group has its own set of general signs as well. Coughing, sneezing, and labored breathing are general signs of respiratory diseases (otherwise known as pulmonary disorders). Diarrhea, increased thirst, and dehydration are general signs of intestinal diseases (enteric disorders). Twitching, trembling, convulsions, and incoordination are general signs of illnesses that attack the nervous system (neurologic disorders).

Specific signs are produced by specific diseases and are considered diagnostic, meaning when you see such signs you can be pretty sure which disease is involved. Facial swelling with reddish, bad-smelling nasal discharge is specific to infectious coryza. An inflamed foot with a hard, swollen abscess at the bottom is specific to bumblefoot. Distended abdomen and an unhealed or mushy navel in newly hatched chicks are specific to omphalitis.

Your chickens may not have all the signs listed under the disease you suspect, or your flock may have signs in addition to those listed. Some diseases are caused by different strains of the same pathogen, affecting different birds in different ways. Some pathogens affect different birds in different parts of their bodies. Diseases may occur in combinations of two or more, causing a confusing array of signs.

Even veterinarians and pathologists go through the following three steps to arrive at a diagnosis:

1. **Differential diagnosis.** List all possible illnesses that fit the accumulation of signs.

2. **Tentative diagnosis.** Eliminate any illnesses that don't match all the signs. By deciding what the problem is not, you may be able to determine what it most likely is.

3. **Final (or positive) diagnosis.** Laboratory tests, requiring blood or tissue samples, may be needed before a final diagnosis can be reached.

Always start with the obvious. Consider management errors causing your birds to run out of feed or water, get too hot or too cold, become injured, or be attacked by a predator. If your chickens seem a little droopy or they aren't growing well, they may have worms, external parasites, or coccidiosis. Before considering rare diseases, eliminate the most common illnesses as the probable cause.

Respiratory Disorders

A chicken normally breathes with its beak closed. A chicken breathing with an open beak is either ill or under stress — perhaps from excessive heat or anxiety. A respiratory illness usually includes additional signs, such as sneezing, coughing, a runny nose, or sticky eyes. If the illness is severe, the chicken may gasp for air and cough up mucus. Sometimes a respiratory disease comes on so fast the chicken dies before you have time to notice any signs at all.

Mucus in the windpipe is a sign of respiratory inflammation but is not necessarily a sign of infection. It may also be caused by a chemical irritant, such as the overuse of disinfectants, or ammonia fumes caused by poor litter maintenance. Or it may be a reaction to dust, most likely due to inadequate ventilation. Look for additional signs to ascertain whether or not an infection is involved.

A general discussion of respiratory diseases and their signs appears on page 78. Although all respiratory diseases look pretty much alike, each has a distinctive combination of signs, as indicated in the table below. Sorting them out can become problematic when a chicken is suffering from more than one respiratory ailment at the same time.

Most respiratory infections are highly contagious. If you choose not to cull (individual birds) or depopulate (your entire flock), you take on the responsibility to not spread the illness to other people's chickens. Your surviving chickens will likely need continuing medical treatment, supportive therapy, and possibly vaccination.

Look-Alike Diseases Affecting Respiration

SIGN	MORE COMMON						LESS COMMON					
	CRD	FP	IB	IC	LT	MD	AC	AI	FC	IS	ND	ORT
Bluish-purple face/wattles	O	O	O	O	O	O	O	X	*	O	X	O
Conjunctivitis	X	O	O	X	X	O	X	X	X	O	X	O
Coughing	X	X	O	O	X	O	X	X	O	O	X	X
Diarrhea, general	X	O	O	X	X	X	X	X	X	O	X	X
Diarrhea, greenish	O	O	O	O	O	X	X	O	X	X	X	O
Eye discharge	X	X	X	X	X	O	O	X	X	X	X	O
Gaping	X	O	X	O	X	O	O	O	O	O	O	O
Gasping	X	X	X	O	X	X	X	O	X	O	X	X
Gurgling	X	O	X	X	X	O	O	O	O	O	O	O
Head shaking	X	O	O	X	X	X	X	O	O	X	X	O
Lameness	O	O	O	O	O	X	O	O	X	X	X	X
Mouth discharge	O	O	O	O	X	O	O	O	X	O	O	X
Mouth discharge, bloody	O	O	O	O	X	O	O	O	O	O	O	O
Nasal discharge	X	O	X	X	X	O	X	O	X	X	X	X
Nasal discharge, smelly	O	O	O	X	O	O	O	O	O	O	O	O
Paralysis	O	O	O	O	O	X	O	O	O	O	O	X
Prostration	X	O	O	O	X	X	O	O	O	O	X	X

Look-Alike Diseases Affecting Respiration

SIGN	MORE COMMON						LESS COMMON					
	CRD	FP	IB	IC	LT	MD	AC	AI	FC	IS	ND	ORT
Rales	X	X	X	X	X	O	X	X	X	X	X	X
Retarded growth	X	X	O	X	X	X	X	O	X	X	X	X
Sneezing	X	X	X	X	X	O	X	X	O	X	X	X
Spotted legs & comb	O	O	O	O	O	O	O	X	O	O	O	X
Sudden death	O	O	O	O	X	O	O	O	X	O	O	X
Swollen face	X	O	O	X	X	X	X	X	X	X	X	X
Swollen footpads	O	O	O	O	O	O	O	O	X	O	O	O
Swollen joints	O	O	O	O	O	O	O	O	X	X	O	X
Swollen wattles	O	O	O	X	O	X	O	X	X	O	O	O
Twisted head/neck	O	O	O	O	O	X	O	O	X	O	X	O
Warts/scabs	O	X	O	O	O	O	O	O	O	O	X	X

*At death

AC = Avian chlamydiosis (bacteria)
AI = Avian influenza (virus)
CRD = Chronic respiratory disease (bacteria)
FC = Fowl cholera (bacteria)

FP = Fowl pox (virus)
IB = Infectious bronchitis (virus)
IC = Infectious coryza (bacteria)
IS = Infectious synovitis (bacteria)

LT = Laryngotracheitis (virus)
MD = Marek's disease (virus)
ND = Newcastle disease (virus)
ORT = Ornithobacterosis (bacteria)

Intestinal Disorders

One of the first signs of an intestinal disease is any unusual appearance or odor in a chicken's droppings. Based on the disease involved, the poop may be watery, foamy, bloody, sticky, pasty, off-colored, smelly, or any combination thereof. Suspect a disease if more than one chicken is affected.

So many different conditions can influence a chicken's digestion that it is often impossible to identify a specific cause without laboratory tests or necropsy. But the occasional appearance of an odd poop is not necessarily a sign of disease, especially where only one chicken is involved.

Normal Poops

To be able to identify what is unusual, you first need to be familiar with what is usual. These five basic kinds of poop are perfectly normal:

Regular droppings. A normal intestinal dropping consists of feces and urates. Digestive waste, or feces, is the solid brownish or grayish portion of chicken poop that is usually firm enough to hold its shape. The feces are capped with white urine salts, or urates. A healthy chicken passes this normal poop 12 or more times a day, including during the night.

Cecal droppings. Pasty cecal droppings are usually light or dark brown (but may be greenish), often lack the whitish caps of regular droppings, and are usually smelly. They result from cellulose fermentation in the ceca, which empty their contents two or three times a day. The frequency of cecal droppings, and their appearance among regular droppings, tells you the chicken's digestive system is functioning normally. A chicken that passes only sticky droppings has a problem, most likely a dietary issue, such as eating hard-to-digest feeds.

Broody poop. This one looks just like regular poop only three or four times bigger. A broody hen holds in her poop so she won't foul her nest, then releases it all at once when she makes a brief excursion away from the nest. Larger than normal droppings released by a nonbrooding chicken may be caused by a diet that is unusually high in roughage.

Watery droppings. A chicken that drinks a lot, for instance during hot weather, or enjoys moist treats such as watermelon or tomatoes, may pass looser than normal poop. Unless the cause is readily apparent, consider excessive dietary protein, salt poisoning, kidney damage, or disease.

Pink tissue in droppings. Small pieces of pink tissue may occasionally appear in droppings. This scary-looking poop is normal and shouldn't be confused with bloody droppings that are an indication of coccidiosis or some other intestinal disease. A chicken's intestinal lining is constantly regenerating, causing bits of tissue to slough into the poop. Larger chunks of tissue, however, can be an early warning sign.

Regularly checking out your chickens' droppings is a good way to remain alert to a problem in the making. Some chicken keepers, especially those keeping only a few birds, install a droppings board beneath the roost, which they clean every morning so they can examine the overnight deposits.

THE EFFECT OF DIET

The exact color of the feces can vary with the chicken's diet. Greenish droppings may result from low feed intake (insufficient to dilute bile) or from eating a lot of green vegetables, including succulent spring forage; dark, nearly black droppings may come from eating a lot of blueberries or blackberries; reddish droppings may be the result of eating certain fruits, such as strawberries; orange-tinged mucous droppings can result from yellow corn.

Normal Droppings

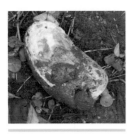

Regular

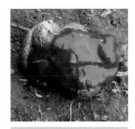

Cecal

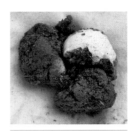

Broody

Is It Diarrhea?

Any departure in the firmness of a chicken's regular poop, causing it to lose shape after being deposited, is usually considered diarrhea. However, not all soft poop is diarrhea. Cecal droppings, for instance, are not diarrhea. Some medications can loosen the consistency of a chicken's poop.

Sometimes a chicken produces more liquid urine than usual. This urine may dilute solid feces in the chicken's cloaca, looking like diarrhea when it comes out. Chickens under stress often produce more liquid urine than usual, because stress increases blood pressure. That's why a chicken that's being chased, or grabbed without warning, typically releases a runny poop. Chickens that drink a lot of water during hot weather also produce more liquid urine than usual, as do chickens that eat a lot of juicy fruits or vegetables. These droppings often appear as a pool of liquid surrounding solid matter that's slightly greenish in color.

Occasionally a chicken will pass clear liquid urine, or semisolid whitish urates, without the usual accompanying feces. A chicken that regularly passes only urates or liquid urine may be suffering from chronic stress, a metabolic disorder, or an infection. An excessive amount of white urates is a typical sign that the kidneys are not functioning properly, perhaps because the chicken has a kidney disease or simply isn't getting enough to drink.

If you suspect one of your chickens is passing irregular poops, but you aren't sure which bird it might be, you can find out by placing each chicken in an elevated cage away from other chickens for up to 24 hours. During this time furnish the bird its normal feed and water. Place a split-open feed sack, with the plain inside facing upward, or a piece of brown paper beneath the cage, where the chicken's poop will accumulate for your inspection.

Diseases Causing Sores in Mouth and Throat

SIGN	CONDITION
Burnlike blisters	Fusariotoxicosis
	Sour crop
Red spots in roof of mouth	Red mites
Yellowish white patches	Canker
	Pox (wet)
	Roup (nutritional)

Conditions Affecting Appearance of Poop

APPEARANCE	AGE	CONDITION	PREVALENCE
Pasting	Chick	Stress	Common
	Chick	Paratyphoid	Common
	Chick	Arizonosis	Rare
Droppings, white, hard	Mature	Sour crop	Common
Droppings, green	All	Lead poisoning	Uncommon
Diarrhea	All	Avian influenza (low path)	Common
	Aging	Avian tuberculosis	Common
	Growing	Colibacillosis	Common
	Growing	Cryptosporidiosis (intestinal)	Common
	All	Infectious coryza	Common
	Mature	Lymphoid leukosis	Common
	All	Newcastle (lentogenic)	Common
	Chick	Omphalitis	Common
	Mature	Paratyphoid	Common
	Growing	Roundworms	Common
	Growing	Canker	Uncommon
	Growing	Ulcerative enteritis	Uncommon
	Growing	Ochratoxicosis	Uncommon
	Growing	Ornithobacteriosis	Emerging
	All	Ergotism	Rare
	Growing	Listeriosis	Rare
	Growing	Pseudomonas	Rare
Diarrhea, bloody	Growing	Coccidiosis	Common
	Growing	Infectious bursal disease	Common
	Growing	Fusariotoxicosis	Uncommon
	All	Chlamydiosis	Rare
	Growing	Blackhead	Rare
Diarrhea, smelly, dark (bloody)	Growing	Necrotic enteritis	Rare
Diarrhea, smelly	All	Cloacitis	Common
	All	Staphylococcosis	Common
Diarrhea, foamy	Mature	Colibacillosis	Common
Diarrhea, watery	Growing	Coccidiosis	Common
	Mature	Colibacillosis	Common
	Growing	Infectious bursal disease	Common

Conditions Affecting Appearance of Poop

APPEARANCE	AGE	CONDITION	PREVALENCE
Diarrhea, watery	Chick	Paratyphoid	Common
	All	Salt poisoning	Uncommon
Diarrhea, watery, dark	All	Newcastle (velogenic)	Rare
Diarrhea, watery, white	Growing	Fowl cholera	Uncommon
	All	Newcastle (velogenic)	Rare
Diarrhea, white, pasty	Growing; mature	Infectious bronchitis	Common
	Growing	Infectious bursal disease	Common
	Growing; mature	Gout (visceral)	Common
	Chick	Stress (chilling)	Common
	Chick	Pullorum	Rare
	Growing	Toxoplasmosis	Rare
Diarrhea, tan, pasty	Growing	Coccidiosis	Common
Diarrhea, yellow	Mature	Colibacillosis	Common
	Mature	Ochratoxicosis	Uncommon
	Mature	Streptococcosis	Uncommon
Diarrhea, yellow, slimy	All	Nodular tapeworm	Unknown
Diarrhea, greenish-yellow	Growing	Sour crop	Common
	Growing	Fowl cholera	Uncommon
	All	Erysipelas	Rare
	Growing	Fowl typhoid	Rare
Diarrhea, greenish	Maturing	Lymphoid leukosis	Common
	Growing	Marek's disease	Common
	All	Avian influenza (high path)	Rare
	All	Newcastle (velogenic)	Rare
	Mature	Pullorum	Rare
Diarrhea, greenish, excess urates	Growing	Infectious synovitis	Uncommon
	All	Spirochetosis	Rare
Cecal dropping, sulfur yellow	Growing	Blackhead	Rare
Urates, dry	All	Dehydration	Uncommon
Urates, watery	Growing	Infectious bursal disease	Common
Urates, excessive	Growing	Ochratoxicosis	Uncommon
Urates, yellow or lime green	All	Chlamydiosis	Rare
	All	Any liver disease	Varies
Urates, red	All	Lead poisoning	Uncommon

What's That Funny Smell?

Every coop has a characteristic odor resulting from a combination of the number of chickens housed and their age(s), the ration they are fed, the type and amount of bedding used, the degree of ventilation, and any herbs or products used to ward off insects. A departure from your flock's familiar odor could be an important early warning sign.

Normal fresh chicken poop doesn't have much of an odor. The smell associated with normal chicken droppings develops when the droppings are allowed to accumulate in a moist or humid environment, which means either the litter is damp or too many birds are housed in a too-small coop. Bad-smelling fresh droppings are commonly associated with diarrhea and may be a sign of an intestinal infection or septicemia (blood poisoning).

Chickens don't normally have bad breath. When they do, it may be a sign of an upper digestive disorder. A bad odor coming from the nose indicates a respiratory infection. A bad smell coming from the skin may result from a fungal infection (ringworm), an abscess or tumor, or an infected wound. The nature of the odor usually offers a good clue as to where to look for other signs that will help you reach a diagnosis.

Causes of Off Odors

SOURCE	CAUSE	AGE	PREVALENCE
Cecal discharge, yellow and smelly	Blackhead	Young	Sporadic
Coop, pungent ammonia	Management issue	All	Common
Diarrhea, dark and smelly	Necrotic enteritis	Growing	Rare
Diarrhea, smelly	Cloacitis	All	Common
	Coccidiosis	All	Common
	Staphylococcosis	All	Common
Mouth odor, sour	Sour crop	Growing; mature	Common
	Canker	Young; growing	Uncommon
Mouth odor, sweet	Pseudomonas	Chick; young; growing	Rare
Mushy chick, smelly	Omphalitis	Newly hatched chick	Common
Nasal discharge, sweet	Mycoplasmosis	All	Common
Nasal discharge, fetid	Infectious coryza	Growing; mature	Common
Skin scabs, moldy smelling	Ringworm	Growing; mature	Sporadic

Neurologic Disorders

A condition that affects a chicken's nerves, brain, or spinal cord triggers certain recognizable signs, including incoordination, neck twisting, and partial or complete paralysis. For a general discussion of the nervous system and signs of illness, see Nervous System on page 95.

Not all conditions that affect the nervous system are diseases. Inadequate nutrition can cause nervous disorders, as can toxic plants and other poisons, including many pesticides. In an aging hen, egg peritonitis or abdominal tumors pressing on a nerve can cause paralysis, usually involving one leg.

If you suspect a poison may be involved, after removing the potential source you might try treating affected chickens with charcoal or one of the laxative flushes described on page 392. A nutritional disorder may be reversed by correcting the birds' diet.

Bacterial, protozoal, and viral conditions defy treatment, with or without the help of a veterinarian. Luckily, all such conditions are relatively uncommon, and the one common disorder — Marek's disease — may be prevented through vaccination, as described on page 263. Vaccines are also available against epidemic tremor and Newcastle disease, but should be used only under veterinary supervision.

Neurologic Conditions

TYPICAL SIGN	AGE	CONDITION	CAUSE	PREVALENCE
One leg forward, one back	All	Marek's disease	Virus	Common
Toes curled under foot	Chick	Curled toe paralysis	Nutritional	Uncommon
Progressive limp paralysis	All	Botulism	Toxin	Sporadic
Trembling of head and neck	Chick	Epidemic tremor	Virus	Sporadic
Head over back, beak upward	Chick	Stargazing	Unknown	Sporadic
Jerking of head and neck	All	Toxoplasmosis	Protozoa	Sporadic
Partial paralysis	Chick	Encephalomalacia	Nutritional	Rare
Convulsions, inability to stand	All	Ergotism (convulsive)	Toxin	Rare
Head arching over back	All	Listeriosis	Bacteria	Rare
Paralysis with respiratory signs	All	Newcastle disease (mesogenic, velogenic)	Virus	Rare

NECK TWISTING

Twisting of the neck is a clear neurological sign. Sometimes called crookneck or wry neck, its technical term is torticollis, from the Latin words *torquere*, meaning "to twist," and *collum*, meaning "neck." Below are some common configurations resulting from torticollis.

Torticollis is often associated with painful muscle spasms commonly called stargazing, but technically known as opisthotonos, a Greek word meaning "drawn backward." It looks similar to the form of torticollis in which the head and neck pull backward over the bird's back — also called stargazing — except opisthotonos is not a steady pull but occurs in spasms.

Not always caused by disease, torticollis may result from a blow to the head or neck. Head injuries are fairly common in crested breeds, which tend to have less-bony skulls than noncrested breeds. If the crested skull bone doesn't entirely enclose the brain — due either to genetics or to injury — a blow can cause the brain to swell and press through the skull's gap.

A chicken with a head injury may tuck its head down between its legs and perhaps move backward until the bird backs into an obstacle, such as the coop or brooder wall. Depending on the extent of the injury, the condition may be temporary or permanent. In the case of a head injury, an anti-inflammatory may be helpful; see Aspirin for Pain on page 395. A veterinarian may prescribe something more specifically targeted to this type of inflammation, such as prednisone.

In chicks torticollis can be caused, though rarely is, by a deficiency of vitamin E or vitamin B_1 (thiamin). The starter ration may be old and stale or improperly formulated, or may contain vitamin-destroying mycotoxins. Excessive use of the coccidiostat amprolium can have the same effect. Changing to fresh, quality feed and providing a vitamin supplement usually solves this problem.

Congenital loco is a little-understood condition causing opisthotonos in newly hatched chicks. It is sometimes called stargazing, although a similar but apparently unrelated condition appearing in chicks at several days of age is also called stargazing. For more on these conditions, see Stargazing on page 97.

 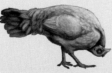 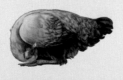 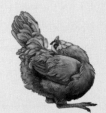

| Tucking the head between the legs | Neck twisted all the way around, head upside down | Sideways crooking of the neck and head | Sideways tilting of the neck and head | Stretching of the neck and head over the back |

Conditions Causing Torticollis

CONDITION	CAUSE	AGE	PREVALENCE
Fowl cholera (chronic)	Bacteria	Mature	Common
Marek's disease	Virus	All	Common
Marek's disease vaccine	Wrong procedure	Chick	Management issue
Aspergillosis (chronic)	Fungus	Mature	Uncommon
Blow to head or neck	Injury	All	Sporadic
Botulism	Bacteria	All	Sporadic
Toxoplasmosis	Protozoa	All	Sporadic
Avian influenza (high path)	Virus	All	Rare
Arizonosis	Bacteria	Chick	Rare
Encephalomalacia	Nutritional	Chick	Rare
Ergotism	Fungus	All	Rare
Listeriosis (encephalitic)	Bacteria	Growing	Rare
Newcastle (mesogenic & velogenic)	Virus	All	Rare
Vitamin B$_1$ (thiamin) deficiency	Nutritional	Chick	Rare
Congenital loco	Unknown	Hatchling	Unknown
Stargazing	Unknown	Chick	Unknown

Hock Resting

A chicken may rest on its hocks for any number of reasons. It could have an infection, a muscle disorder, a damaged ligament or nerve, or a bone fracture.

Cornish-cross broilers typically rest on their hocks, simply because the growth of their heavy muscles outpaces their skeletal growth. Birds that have to push and shove to get feed or water — because too few feeders or drinkers are provided for the flock size —can develop hock disorders because of the constant stress on their legs.

A chicken experiencing foot pain, such as might result from curled-toe paralysis or bumblefoot, may rest on its hocks to relieve the pain. In the rare case in which a slipped tendon affects both legs, the chicken will rest on its hocks.

Chickens that sit or rest on their hocks usually are reluctant to move or may refuse to move altogether. Sometimes when an affected chicken is inspired to move, it will use its wings for balance, like a pair of crutches, to help it scoot along.

Conditions Causing Hock Resting			
DISEASE	AGE	CAUSE	PREVALENCE
Arthritis (staphylococcic)	All	Bacteria	Common
Bumblefoot	Maturing; mature	Bacteria	Common
Curled-toe paralysis	Chick	Nutritional	Uncommon
Infectious synovitis	Growing	Bacteria	Uncommon
Slipped tendon	Growing	Nutritional	Uncommon
Epidemic tremor	Chick	Virus	Sporadic
Spirochetosis	All	Bacteria	Rare

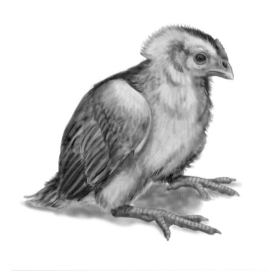

Hock resting, also known as dog sitting, can be a sign of infection, a muscle disorder, ligament or nerve damage, or a bone fracture.

Disorders Affecting Eyes

A number of different conditions can affect a chicken's eyes, not all of which are signs of infection. An eye may be injured. A bird can get dust or bits of feather fluff in its eye. Ammonia and other strong chemical fumes can cause inflammation.

One of the first signs of an eye disorder is avoiding light. The chicken wants to sit in a dark corner with its eyes closed and doesn't want to be out in the sunshine. Bumping into things and missing the target when pecking are clear signs that a chicken has a vision problem. Other signs include excessive blinking, swelling, redness, and any type of discharge from the eye. Inflammation of the eye's internal structure, left untreated, can develop into cataracts and eventual blindness.

Because a chicken that can't see well has a decided disadvantage, any eye disorder should be considered serious until proven otherwise. Some conditions are curable, others are permanent, and still others indicate a more serious underlying affliction. For a discussion on eye anatomy, treating eye disorders, and diagnosing blindness, see Eyes on page 96.

Conditions Affecting Eyes

APPEARANCE	AGE	CONDITION	PREVALENCE
Black eye	Mature	Newcastle (velogenic)	Rare
Blind	Chick	Paratyphoid	Common
	Growing	Marek's disease	Common
	Maturing	Lymphoid leukosis	Common
	Mature	Colibacillosis	Common
	All	Conjunctivitis (ammonia)	Common
	Chick	Epidemic tremor	Sporadic
	Young	Toxoplasmosis	Sporadic
Bloodshot	Maturing	Lymphoid leukosis	Common
Cheesy	Chick	Roup (nutritional)	Uncommon
	All	Aspergillosis	Uncommon
	All	Pox (wet)	Uncommon
Cloudy	Growing	Marek's disease	Common
	All	Conjunctivitis (ammonia)	Common
	Mature	Epidemic tremor	Sporadic
	All	Genetic	Rare
	All	Newcastle (mesogenic)	Rare
	Aging	Old age	Common
Distorted	Growing	Marek's disease	Common
Dull	Chick	Epidemic tremor	Sporadic
Foamy	Growing; mature	Chronic respiratory disease	Common
Gray	Growing	Marek's disease	Common
Irregular shape	Growing	Marek's disease	Common
Mucus discharge	Young; growing	Cryptosporidiosis (respiratory)	Uncommon
	Growing; mature	Infectious synovitis	Uncommon
	Mature	Roup (nutritional)	Uncommon
	All	Pox (wet)	Uncommon
Scabby	All	Pox (dry)	Common
Sticky	All	Infectious coryza	Common
	Young; growing	Canker	Uncommon
	All	Roup (nutritional)	Uncommon

Conditions Affecting Eyes *Continued*

APPEARANCE	AGE	CONDITION	PREVALENCE
	Mature	Laryngotracheitis	Sporadic
	Mature	Newcastle (velogenic)	Rare
Sunken*	All	Dehydration	Uncommon
Swollen	Chick	Paratyphoid	Common
	Growing; mature	Chronic respiratory disease	Common
	Mature	Fowl cholera (chronic)	Common
	All	Infectious coryza	Common
	All	Avian influenza (low path)	Common
	Chick	Roup (nutritional)	Uncommon
	Growing; mature	Eyeworm	Uncommon
	Young; growing	Cryptosporidiosis (respiratory)	Uncommon
	All	Aspergillosis	Uncommon
	Mature	Laryngotracheitis	Sporadic
	Mature	Newcastle (velogenic)	Rare
	All	Chlamydiosis	Rare
Watery	Chick	Infectious bronchitis	Common
	Young	Air sac disease	Common
	Growing; mature	Chronic respiratory disease	Common
	Mature	Fowl cholera (chronic)	Common
	All	Avian influenza (low path)	Common
	All	Infectious coryza	Common
	Growing; mature	Eyeworm	Uncommon
	Chick	Roup (nutritional)	Uncommon
	Young; growing	Canker	Uncommon
	Mature	Laryngotracheitis	Sporadic

Eyes may appear sunken because of facial swelling, a common sign for most respiratory diseases.

Conditions Affecting Egg Production

A hen stops laying for a variety of reasons not necessarily related to disease. However, the average hen isn't able to generate enough energy to both lay eggs and fend off disease, so one of the first signs of illness is a reduction in laying. Similarly, a number of conditions, many of which are disease related, can affect an egg's shell and internal qualities.

Since the membrane lining a hen's shell gland is similar to the membrane lining the windpipe, pathogens that attack the respiratory system can also affect the shell gland, where an egg acquires the hard outer shell and its color. Accordingly, respiratory diseases often cause a hen that normally lays brown-shell eggs to lay pale or even white-shell eggs, and the shell may be abnormally thin or missing altogether, resulting in a laid egg being covered only by rubbery membranes.

The following table lists egg problems and their most likely disease and nondisease causes. For more information on reproductive issues see Reproductive Disorders of the Hen on page 91 and When Hens Stop Laying on page 315.

Conditions Affecting Egg Production

PROBLEM	POSSIBLE CAUSE	PREVALENCE
Notable drop in laying	Broody	Normal
	Molting	Normal
	Reduced day length (winter)	Normal
	Obesity	Management issue
	Parasites, internal or external	Management issue
	Water deprivation	Management issue
	Nutritional (esp. calcium) deficiency	Management issue
	Chronic respiratory disease	Common
	Egg peritonitis	Common
	Gout (visceral)	Common
	Infectious bronchitis	Common
	Infectious coryza	Common
	Lymphoid leukosis	Common
	Coccidiosis	Common in pullets
	Fatty liver syndrome	Common in obese hens
	Avian tuberculosis	Common in aging hens

PROBLEM	POSSIBLE CAUSE	PREVALENCE
Notable drop in laying	Osteoporosis	Common in aging hens
	Campylobacteriosis	Uncommon
	Streptococcosis	Uncommon
	Mycotoxicosis	Sporadic
	Laryngotracheitis	Sporadic
	Avian influenza (high path)	Rare
	Chlamydiosis	Rare
	Erysipelas	Rare
	Newcastle (velogenic)	Rare
	Ornithobacteriosis	Rare
	Spirochetosis	Rare
Small egg	Beginning/end of laying cycle	Normal
	Fowl cholera (chronic)	Common
	Infectious bronchitis	Common
	Aflatoxicosis	Rare
	Ornithobacteriosis	Rare
	Spirochetosis	Rare
Thin shell	Heat stress	Common
	Infectious bronchitis	Common
	Osteoporosis	Common in aging hens
	Laryngotracheitis	Sporadic
	Mycotoxicosis	Sporadic
Soft shell	Stress	Management issue
	Infectious bronchitis	Common
	Avian influenza (high path)	Rare
	Newcastle (mesogenic, velogenic)	Rare
	Ornithobacteriosis	Rare
No shell	Stress	Management issue
	Avian influenza (high path)	Rare
Bloody shell	Vent picking	Management issue
	Immature pullet	Uncommon

Conditions Affecting Egg Production

PROBLEM	POSSIBLE CAUSE	PREVALENCE
Poop-stained shell	Spirochetosis	Rare
Rough shell	Infectious bronchitis	Common
	Newcastle (mesogenic)	Rare
Ridged/wrinkled shell	Stress or injury	Management issue
	Infectious bronchitis	Common
Misshapen shell	Occasional glitch in the system	Normal
	Infectious bronchitis	Common
	Newcastle (mesogenic, velogenic)	Rare
	Ornithobacteriosis	Rare
Pale shell	Aging hen (lays larger egg)	Normal
	Infectious bronchitis	Common
Watery whites	Aging hen	Normal
	Eggs stored too long or too warm	Management issue
	Poor ventilation (ammonia fumes)	Management issue
	Sulfa drugs	Management issue
	Heat stress	Common
	Infectious bronchitis	Common
	Laryngotracheitis	Sporadic
	Newcastle (velogenic)	Rare
Blood spot	Occasional glitch in the system	Common
	Genetics	Common
	Fowl cholera (chronic)	Common
	Roup (nutritional)	Uncommon
	Ochratoxicosis	Sporadic
Bloody yolk	Newcastle (velogenic)	Rare
Discolored yolk	Eating pigmented weeds or seeds	Management issue
	Excessive use of piperazine dewormer	Management issue
Pale yolk	Lack of green forage or yellow corn	Management issue
	Coccidiosis	Rare
Worm in egg	Roundworm overload	Management issue

Conditions Causing Discolored Skin

Some breeds naturally have pale or white skin. Paleness in other breeds may be a sign of either a reduction in red blood cells (see Anemia on page 100) or insufficient blood flow.

Restricted blood flow can result from cold exposure and frostbite or from shock, which is a reaction to dangerously low blood pressure. Shock occurs when the blood pressure gets too low to deliver sufficient blood to the chicken's body tissues, which therefore receive insufficient oxygen — a life-threatening situation. Causes of shock include a weak heart (see Heart Failure on page 109), low blood volume, and dilated blood vessels.

Shocking Conditions

Low blood volume means the chicken's heart gets too little blood to circulate throughout its body. It may be caused by excessive external or internal bleeding, an overload of bloodsucking parasites, loss of body fluids (from diarrhea, for example), or insufficient water consumption (dehydration).

Dilated blood vessels have a greater than normal capacity, allowing blood to flow faster than usual, thereby decreasing the amount of oxygen the blood distributes throughout the body. Causes of dilated blood vessels include severe bacterial infection and long-term use of antibiotics.

Signs of Shock

⚠ Signs of shock due to heart failure or low blood volume include lethargy, rapid breathing, and bluish, pale skin; sometimes a bluish network of blood vessels is visible through the skin. A sign of shock caused by dilated blood vessels is reddening of the skin, which may feel warmer than usual. Left untreated, shock is usually fatal (see Treating Shock on page 400).

Feeling Bluish

In a healthy chicken most of the red blood cells carry oxygen most of the time. Blood cells carrying a full supply of oxygen are bright red, giving the chicken's skin its hardy glow. Red cells that carry insufficient oxygen turn a dark bluish red, causing the chicken's skin and mucous membranes to take on a bluish hue. This condition is known as cyanosis, from the Greek word *kyanos*, meaning "dark blue."

Cyanosis can come on suddenly, such as might occur from rapid external or internal bleeding. Or it may develop over a long period of time; for instance, in the case of a chronic heart, lung, or kidney condition.

Not all conditions causing a chicken's skin to appear bluish are caused by cyanosis. A young chicken that hasn't yet developed much body fat may have bluish-looking skin, as will any chicken that lacks a subcutaneous layer of fat.

Some breeds naturally have dark or black skin. Among breeds that have black skin, Silkies are the most commonly found in North America.

Conditions Causing External Discoloring

BODY PART	COLOR	CONDITION	AGE	PREVALENCE
Head	Dark	Chronic respiratory disease	Growing; mature	Common
		Gout (visceral)	Growing; mature	Common
		Blackhead	Young	Rare
Head, comb, wattles	Dark	Avian influenza (high path)	All	Rare
	Pale	Parasites (internal & external)	All	Common
	Purplish	Paratyphoid	Mature	Common
Comb, wattles	Black	Frostbite (late sign)	Mature	Common
	Bluish	Fowl cholera (acute)	Growing (at death)	Sporadic
		Fusariotoxicosis	Hen	Sporadic
	Dark	Ergotism	All	Rare
	Pale	Molting	Hen	Normal
		Avian tuberculosis	Aging	Common
		Fatty liver syndrome	Hen (obese)	Common
		Streptococcosis	Mature	Uncommon
		Blackhead	Young	Sporadic
		Fowl typhoid	Growing	Rare
	Purplish	Spirochetosis	All	Rare
	White	Frostbite (early sign)	Mature	Common
	White, powdery	Ringworm	All	Sporadic
	White or yellow bumps	Pox (dry)	All	Common
Comb	Bluish	Ascites	Broiler	Common
		Lymphoid leukosis	Maturing	Common
		Aspergillosis (chronic)	Mature	Uncommon
	Pale	Coccidiosis (intestinal)	All	Common
		Kidney stone	Pullet; hen	Common
		Lymphoid leukosis	Maturing	Common
		Roup (nutritional)	Young	Uncommon
		Infectious synovitis	Young	Uncommon
		Toxoplasmosis	Young	Rare
		Pullorum	Mature	Rare

BODY PART	COLOR	CONDITION	AGE	PREVALENCE
Beak	Dark	Ergotism	All	Rare
Skin	Bluish	Omphalitis	Chick	Common
		Ascites	Broiler	Common
		Exudative diathesis	Chick	Rare
	Blood-blistered	Lymphoid leukosis	Maturing	Common
	Blotchy	Erysipelas	All	Rare
		Gangrenous dermatitis	Growing	Sporadic
	Dark	Aspergillosis (chronic)	Mature	Uncommon
	Pale	Coccidiosis (intestinal)	All	Common
		Coccidiosis (cecal)	Chick	Common
		Marek's disease	Maturing	Common
		Cryptosporidiosis (intestinal)	Young	Uncommon
	Scabby	Marek's disease	Maturing	Common
		Pox (dry)	All	Common
	Scaly	Ringworm	All	Sporadic
	White bumps	Marek's disease	Maturing	Common
Shanks	Blistered	Ergotism	All	Rare
	Bloody red	Marek's disease	Maturing	Common
	Dark	Gout (visceral)	Growing; mature	Common
	Pale	Coccidiosis (intestinal)	All	Common
		Aflatoxicosis	Hen	Sporadic
	Reddened	Avian influence (high path)	All	Rare
	White, powdery	Ringworm	All	Sporadic
Feet	Bluish	Ascites	Broiler	Common

Conditions Characterized by Untimely Death

As distressing as the death of a precious chicken may be, an infrequent loss does not necessarily mean some terrible disease is sweeping through your flock. It's not uncommon for the occasional chicken of any age to die for no immediately obvious reason. If, however, you find several chickens dead or dying within a short time, you have good reason for concern.

Death can occur as a result of organ failure due to a local infection (an infection affecting one area of the body) or due to a systemic infection (one that invades the entire body). Examples of local diseases that can result in death include enteric diseases that cause degeneration of the intestines, respiratory diseases that cause death by blocking off the airways, and neurological diseases that cause paralysis and death from an inability to eat or breathe. An example of a systemic disease that can result in death is avian influenza, which can spread throughout a chicken's body by invading lymph tissue.

Not all diseases that become systemic start out that way. A local infection can become systemic by entering the bloodstream for distribution throughout the body. This type of systemic infection is called septicemia, from the Greek words *septikos*, meaning "putrefaction," and *haima*, meaning "blood." Septicemia is also known as blood poisoning. All septicemias are systemic, but not all systemic diseases are septic.

An infection that becomes septic can begin anywhere in or on the chicken's body.

Bumblefoot, for example, may start out as an infected callus on the bottom of a chicken's foot that, left untreated, becomes septic. Breast blister may start out as an uninfected swelling on a chicken's keel that develops into an infection and eventually becomes septic. Even a seemingly simple skin wound that becomes infected can result in septicemia.

All bacteria and their toxins have the ability to become septic, developing into a potentially life-threatening condition. Fungi and, to a much lesser extent, viruses may also become septic.

Because septicemia may originate in any part of a chicken's body, the signs are not always the same. General signs of septicemia include weakness, listlessness, lack of appetite, and a dark or purplish head. Other signs include rapid breathing, diarrhea, prostration, and death. Most septicemic diseases result in reduced appetite and loss of weight before death. The cause of death often is the failure of one or more organs, a result of blood clotting caused by septicemia. Clotting leads to organ failure by reducing blood flow, thereby depriving various body tissues of nutrients and oxygen.

Acute septicemia occurs when reduced blood flow leads to dangerously low blood pressure, causing the rapid failure of multiple organs. Also called septic shock, acute septicemia hits a bird so fast it literally drops in its tracks. The classic indication of acute septicemia is the sudden death of an apparently healthy chicken in good flesh and with a full crop, indicating it had a normal appetite right up to the time of death.

Conditions Causing Multiple Deaths

AGE	CONDITION	CAUSE	PREVALENCE
Chick	Infectious bronchitis	Virus	Common
	Epidemic tremor	Virus	Uncommon
	Arizonosis	Bacteria	Rare
	Encephalomalacia	Nutritional	Rare
	Exudative diathesis	Nutritional	Rare
	Pullorum	Bacteria	Rare
Young	Air sac disease	Bacteria	Common
	Coccidiosis (cecal)	Protozoa	Common
	Infectious bursal disease	Virus	Common
	Toxoplasmosis (acute)	Protozoa	Uncommon
	Fowl typhoid	Bacteria	Rare
	Necrotic enteritis	Bacteria	Rare
	Roup (nutritional)	Nutritional	Rare
Growing	Cryptosporidiosis (respiratory)	Protozoa	Uncommon
	Aflatoxicosis (acute)	Fungus	Sporadic
	Fowl cholera (acute)	Bacteria	Sporadic
	Pseudomonas	Bacteria	Rare
Maturing	Marek's disease (acute)	Virus	Common
Mature	Laryngotracheitis (acute)	Virus	Uncommon
	Streptococcosis	Bacteria	Uncommon
All	Colibacillosis (acute)	Bacteria	Common
	Gout (visceral)	Kidney failure	Common
	PTFE-coated lightbulb	Poison	Management issue
	Campylobacteriosis (acute)	Bacteria	Uncommon
	Pox (wet)	Virus	Uncommon
	Botulism	Bacterial toxin	Sporadic
	Avian influenza (high path)	Virus	Rare
	Erysipelas	Bacteria	Rare
	Newcastle disease (velogenic)	Virus	Rare
	Spirochetosis	Bacteria	Rare

Conditions Causing Sudden Death

AGE	CONDITION	CAUSE	PREVALENCE
Chick	PTFE-coated brooding bulb	Poison	Management issue
	Arizonosis	Bacteria	Rare
Young	Ornithobacillosis (acute)	Bacteria	Emerging
	Necrotic enteritis	Bacteria	Rare
Broiler	Ascites	Heart failure	Common
	Sudden death syndrome	Heart attack	Common
Growing	Gangrenous dermatitis	Bacteria	Uncommon
	Aflatoxicosis (acute)	Fungus	Sporadic
Maturing	Lymphoid leukosis	Virus	Common
	Ulcerative enteritis (acute)	Bacteria	Uncommon
Mature	Gout (visceral)	Kidney failure	Common
	Fowl cholera (acute)	Bacteria	Uncommon
	Streptococcosis (acute)	Bacteria	Uncommon
Hen	Sudden death syndrome	Heart attack	Common
Hen, aging	Ascites	Heart failure	Common
Hen, obese	Fatty liver syndrome	Liver failure	Common
All	Colibacillosis (acute)	Bacteria	Common
	Marek's disease	Virus	Common
	Staphylococcosis (acute)	Bacteria	Common
	Poisoning, pesticide (see page 153)	Poison	Management issue
	Poisoning, plant (see page 308)	Poison	Management issue
	Botulism	Bacterial toxin	Sporadic
	Toxoplasmosis	Protozoa	Sporadic
	Avian influenza (high path)	Virus	Rare
	Erysipelas	Bacteria	Rare
	Listeriosis (acute)	Bacteria	Rare
	Newcastle disease (velogenic)	Virus	Rare

CHAPTER 13

What's Going on Inside

Ｆ YOU FIND several diseased or dead birds within a short time, to get a rapid diagnosis take some birds to your state poultry pathology laboratory. To locate your nearest lab call your county Extension office, do an Internet key word search for "Your-State-Name poultry pathology laboratory," or visit this website: metzerfarms.com/PoultryLabs.cfm.

The website also offers tips for shipping or transporting specimens to a lab. Requirements vary, so always call ahead to determine the requirements of the lab you will use. Some labs accept live birds; others do not. When you call the lab, you might want to ask about their fees as well.

The pathologist will be interested in the disease's progression. The best way to provide that information is to submit three birds in various stages of illness. For example, you might submit one bird that recently died, one that is seriously ill, and one just beginning to show signs of illness.

The pathologist will identify the illness so you can treat your remaining birds. Even when a lab takes in live birds, none will leave the lab. Not only must a bird be dead before its innards can be examined, but you wouldn't want the bird back after it has been exposed to all the pathogens floating around the average pathology lab, some of which may be worse than what your chickens already have.

Submitting Specimens

When submitting a freshly dead bird for examination, wet the feathers with cold water and a little detergent, taking care not to get any into the bird's mouth or nose. Bag the chicken in plastic, and refrigerate it until you're ready to leave for the lab. Whether you're submitting dead or live birds, identify each with a numbered leg band or wrap a piece of tape several times around its leg and write a number on it with an indelible marker.

Write a detailed history of the disease, how it affected each bird you are submitting, and anything else about your chickens you think might be important. The lab will provide a form for you to fill out. Attach your history to the form. If at all possible, the person who takes the birds to the lab should be familiar with the chickens and their history, in case the pathologist has additional questions.

If the lab is far from your home, you may wish to ship your birds. Call first for shipping instructions. You may be asked to consult your veterinarian and get a referral to the lab. If no veterinarians are nearby, or your vet is not willing to examine chickens, say so when you call the lab.

Many veterinarians know little about chickens. Even if you're lucky enough to find one with poultry experience, the fee may be more than the cost of starting over with new, healthy chickens. State poultry pathology laboratories, on the other hand, usually charge little or nothing for an initial examination.

Speaking of Posting

diagnosis. The identification of the nature and cause of a disease by examining external and internal signs

differential diagnosis. A preliminary list of possible causes of a disease

necropsy. A postmortem examination (equivalent to a human autopsy)

pathologist. A veterinarian who specializes in diagnosing diseases, primarily as a consultant

pathology. The science of studying the nature of diseases and their causes and consequences

WHY POST?

Many diseases, in addition to causing observable signs, result in less obvious changes inside the body. Scrutinizing the insides of a bird for signs of disease is called a postmortem examination (from the Latin words *post*, meaning "after," and *mortem*, meaning "death"). Scientifically, a postmortem is called a necropsy (from the Greek words *nekros*, meaning "corpse," and *opsis*, meaning "appearance") — the animal equivalent of an autopsy. But conducting a postmortem is more handily known as posting.

The bird in question may have recently died or, when several chickens are sick, one may be deliberately killed so you can look for clues to determine the cause. Posting will reveal such things as the progression of an infectious disease, tumors, abscesses, toxic reactions, foreign materials, nutritional deficiencies, and parasite overloads. It is less apt to reveal management issues such as overcrowding, poor ventilation, unsanitary conditions, or an environment that's too hot or too cold.

A pathologist can often make a differential diagnosis — or a preliminary list of possible causes — by studying a carefully prepared complete history of your chickens. When you submit a sample to a diagnostic laboratory, provide the following minimum information:

☐ Your name, address, and phone number

☐ Information on how your chickens are housed (such as cage, coop, pasture)

☐ The sources and types of feed you use

☐ Any recent changes in feeding behavior or feed consumption

☐ How much your chickens normally weigh and any changes in body weight

☐ Any recent changes in egg production

☐ Your chicken's breed(s)

☐ How many chickens are in your flock

☐ How old your chickens are

☐ Where you obtained your chickens

☐ Signs of disease you have observed

☐ The date when you first noticed these signs

☐ Approximately how many chickens are sick

☐ How many chickens have died

☐ When, where, and how they died

☐ Approximate number of days from the first signs to the first death

☐ Any vaccinations or medications you have used

☐ Recent management changes (such as new rations, new chickens brought in, potentially toxic spraying in your area)

☐ Any previous disease problems in your flock or on your property

☐ Locations of any nearby poultry flocks

☐ If chicks are involved, include your procedures for hatching and brooding

What to Expect

Within a few days the pathologist will call you with a preliminary report, then follow up with a written report. Don't be bashful about asking questions if you don't understand something; pathologists tend to use words only a veterinarian or other trained person can understand. If you submit your birds under a veterinarian's referral, your vet can explain the report to you.

Not all path labs are equipped to diagnose all poultry diseases. If the initial report is inconclusive, the pathologist may make an educated guess and ask if you want the diagnosis confirmed by further laboratory tests such as tissue examination, bacterial cultures, virus isolation, or sensitivity tests (to determine which drug, if any, will kill the particular pathogen in question). These tests can be expensive and time consuming, some taking as long as 6 weeks.

The function of a pathologist is to diagnose diseases, not recommend treatments. You should, however, be given enough information to obtain details on treatment options from your veterinarian, your state poultry Extension veterinarian, or your state Extension poultry specialist.

Armed with this information, you can decide whether to treat the remainder of your chickens or dispose of them, clean up their housing, and start over. On the other hand, if your chickens are beloved family pets, you may wish to spare no expense to identify and treat whatever ails them.

Do-It-Yourself Posting

Running to the path lab with every dead bird you find is neither feasible nor even necessary. An occasional death, sad as it might be, is normal. Still, it's a good idea to examine dead birds and record the results in your flock history. You may see an emerging pattern that can help you discover and treat a disease in its early stages of development.

Every flock includes weak birds that have lower resistance than others to disease as a result of stress, genetic factors, or insufficient nourishment because they are far down in the peck order. These weaker birds become indicators of approaching problems. If you do find signs of a disease in progress, you can take future samples to a qualified pathologist for a confirmed diagnosis.

Even when you prefer to go directly to the path lab, if the lab is particularly busy, the pathologist may not get back to you for several days or even weeks. Meanwhile, if your chickens

are getting sicker or are dying fast, by posting one or more chickens yourself, you might tentatively identify the problem and take appropriate timely action. The lab report, when it comes, will then serve as a confirming diagnosis.

Posting a chicken makes sense only if you know what the insides of a healthy bird look like — something you can easily learn if you regularly butcher chickens for eating. When you post a sick bird, your goal is to find abnormalities such as abscesses, tumors, swelling, fluid accumulation, foreign materials, changes in muscle or bone color or texture, and irregularities in the size, shape, or color of internal organs that offer clues as to what's going on. The more often you examine the innards of chickens, the quicker you will become at noticing anything unusual.

Use Caution

⚠️ If you suspect a chicken has chlamydiosis, erysipelas, or any other disease that is contagious to humans (see Zoonoses on page 407), *do not post it yourself*. Take it to the state pathology laboratory, where personnel are trained to deal with hazardous diseases.

What You'll Need

Equipment for performing a basic necropsy is quite simple and readily available. The first requirement is a suitable place to work in, and a flat surface on which to work. Conduct your postmortem outdoors or in a garage or carport, using a table or the tailgate of a pickup truck as your work surface. Never post a diseased bird in a kitchen where food is prepared.

SUPPLIES AND SETUP

- A flat work surface covered with clean paper

- Disposable plastic gloves, apron, and face mask (optional)

- Basin or bucket of wash water and clean towels

- Sharp knife, such as a surgeon's scalpel or an X-Acto knife, and a pair of surgical scissors, kitchen shears, tin snips, or other heavy-duty shears

- Disinfectant or clean water mixed with a little detergent to dampen the bird's feathers so they won't blow around. Dip the freshly euthanized bird into a bucket (easiest) or apply the wetting agent with a spray bottle or a cloth or towel

- Pencil and paper (or voice recorder or digital camera) to record your findings as you go along

If you're not sure of the proper terminology, just write down what you see. If you know something doesn't look right, but you don't know what it is, note the location and describe it as abnormal. If you don't know whether you've found a tumor or an abscess, call it a lump. Trying to use specific words when you're not sure can cause confusion if you later submit your notes to a veterinarian or pathologist. A digital camera makes a good recording tool, especially if you don't know how to describe your findings.

Preparing the Bird

When dealing with a flockwide disease, examine not just chickens you find dead, but at least one that recently began showing signs and one in which the disease is quite far along. Examining birds in various stages of illness shows how this particular disease progresses, which may help you determine what the disease might be. Checking more than one bird also helps you identify which signs are specific to individuals (thus possibly insignificant) and which are flockwide (thus likely signs of the disease in progress).

Do not post a bird that has been lying around dead for more than a few hours, since natural decomposition can change body tissues and muddle your findings. If a bird dies and you can't post it immediately, seal it in a plastic bag and store it in the refrigerator until you can get to it.

EUTHANIZING

When you want to post a chicken that is not dead, you will have to euthanize it. If that sounds like a drastic measure, remember you're doing it out of concern for the rest of your chickens. If a serious illness is gripping your flock, this and other birds may die anyway. Your goal is to determine the cause so you can prevent additional deaths.

Before euthanizing a sick chicken, check its general appearance for abnormalities such as deviations from normal weight; an unnatural posture or gait; changes in the color of the skin, comb, or shanks; changes in the color, texture, or odor of droppings; ruffled feathers; presence of external parasites; any injuries or deformities; respiration rate and any unusual sounds made during breathing; inflammation (indicated by reddening and swelling), mucus, or discoloration of the eyes; odor or discharge from the nose. Record any irregularities you notice.

To humanely euthanize a chicken for posting, stretch its neck, which painlessly breaks the neck and spinal cord, causing immediate death. Hold the bird's feet with one hand. Grasp the bird's head with the other hand, your thumb behind its comb and your fingers beneath its beak. Tilt the head back while pulling steadily until the head separates from the neck. You can feel when it slips, and as a reflexive reaction the bird will momentarily flap its wings.

Euthanizing a young bird takes little strength. The head separates from the neck rather quickly, and the skin is quite delicate, so you have to be careful not to pull the head off.

If the chicken is a mature rooster or older hen — especially of a larger breed — euthanizing by hand may take more strength than you can muster. In that case, using an emasculatome will give you a mechanical advantage. This device is designed for emasculating (castrating) young goats, sheep, or cattle and is available from a farm store or livestock supplier. Since you probably wouldn't need to use it often, instead of buying one you might find a livestock-raising neighbor who will let you borrow one. Have a helper hold the chicken while you clamp the device's jaws around the chicken's neck and squeeze them together as hard as you can.

If the bird is euthanized by hand, keep its head oriented upward until it stops flapping. If an emasculatome is used, keep the jaws clamped shut until the flapping stops. You don't want crop contents spilling into the mouth and down the windpipe, which can mimic a disease that causes foreign matter to accumulate in the respiratory system.

Wait a few minutes while blood collects and clots beneath the neck skin, and the body tissues firm up. Meantime, once again examine external openings (eyes, nose, mouth, ears, and vent) for unusual secretions, and run your

hands over feathered areas to find lumps, deformities, or other irregularities.

Necropsy Procedure

Begin by wetting the feathers so they won't blow around; spray the feathers or dip the whole bird (except for beak and nostrils) in a bucketful of clean water with a squirt of detergent. Lay the bird on its back with its feet toward you. Then begin your examination as following.

MUSCLES

Take a pinch of skin over the abdomen and pull it up, making a small tent just below the keel. Use the X-Acto knife to slit through the skin, taking care not to cut into the body cavity, then carefully cut away all the skin between the neck and cloaca, as well as the skin covering the legs.

To stabilize the body on the table, grasp both legs and press downward and outward

Internal Organs of a Chicken

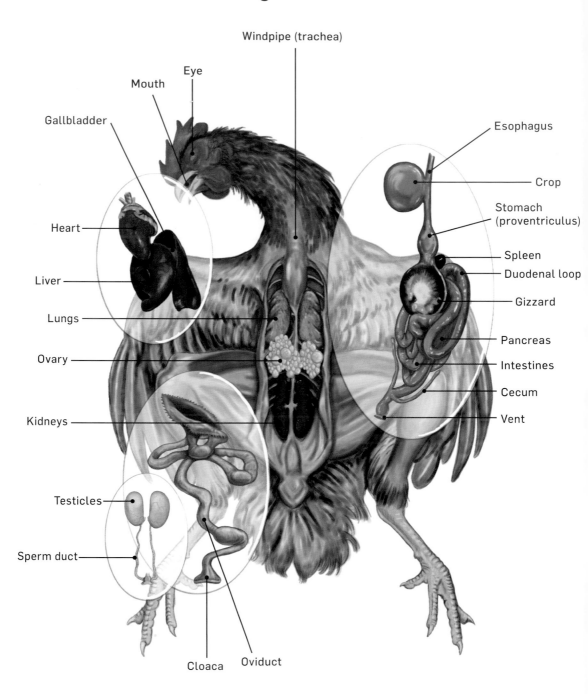

Windpipe (trachea)

Eye

Mouth

Gallbladder

Esophagus

Crop

Stomach
(proventriculus)

Heart

Spleen

Duodenal loop

Liver

Gizzard

Lungs

Pancreas

Ovary

Intestines

Cecum

Kidneys

Vent

Testicles

Sperm duct

Cloaca   Oviduct

to loosen the hip joints. When you hear them snap, the legs will lie flat against the table and keep the body from rolling side to side.

Examine the breast muscle to determine if it is unusually pale (indicating anemia), bruised, or spotted with pinpoint hemorrhages (indicating capillary fragility, such as might be caused by mycotoxins). The breast muscle should be not so round that it obscures the keel (indicating obesity), flat, or concave (indicating atrophy or emaciation). Examine the leg muscles for atrophy and pinpoint hemorrhages.

MOUTH AND WINDPIPE

Cut into one corner of the mouth and extend the cut down the length of the windpipe (trachea). This white or pale tan stiff tube consists of a series of regular rings of cartilage that keep the windpipe rigid and prevent it from collapsing when the chicken breathes. Irregularity in the rings, lumps, and discoloration are signs of respiratory disease. Bloody mucus inside the trachea may be a sign of laryngotracheitis; cheesy material may be a sign of any number of respiratory conditions, including aspergillosis, laryngotracheitis, or wet pox.

ESOPHAGUS

The esophagus is a thin, flexible tube running down the left side of the neck from the mouth to the crop and from the crop to the stomach. It should be smooth and pink. Cut down the length of the esophagus and spread it open. Look for small bumps or signs of injury (such as from any small, sharp material the chicken might have eaten).

CROP

At the lower end of the esophagus is the crop. Cut it open, and note if it contains abnormal feed material or smells sour. Rinse away the contents so you can see if the crop lining has any patchy, thickened areas (necrotic ulcers) or a Turkish-towel appearance (a possible sign of crop mycosis). Make a small cut into the crop lining, slowly peel it away, and examine the base of the tear for capillary worms, which will look like tiny, hairlike fibers.

AIR SACS

Normal air sacs appear to be covered with tiny bubbles or plastic wrap, although they turn somewhat cloudy soon after a bird dies. Diseased air sacs may be opaque, thicker than normal, or covered with mucus. Typically the air sacs will be torn when the breastplate is removed to examine the body cavity, but if you have excellent light you might get a peek at them by carefully lifting the keel and peeking underneath during the next step.

BODY CAVITY

Before cutting into the body cavity, note the abdomen's contour. It should be flat or concave. A bulging abdomen may indicate the presence of excessive body fat (the body wall appears soft and yellow) or fluid filling the body cavity (ascites, appearing firm and bluish). It may also result from an accumulation of putrefying yolks due to internal laying.

About halfway between the keel and the pubic bones, make a crosswise cut through the body wall from one leg joint to the other. Take care not to cut into or otherwise disturb the internal organs.

Using heavy shears, cut upward along one side, through the rib cage and other bones. Then angle the shears toward the joint where the wing attaches to the body. Do the same on the other side, noting how easy or difficult the bones are to cut — an indication of their condition; healthy bones snap when broken.

If you have trouble finding the ribs and wing joints, cut away the breast muscle to get a better view. Slice through the wing joints and carefully lift off the breastplate, revealing the internal organs in their natural positions. If the organs are covered by a layer of fat, carefully trim it away to get a better view.

HEART

The heart lies in the upper part of the body cavity. Note any irregularities, such as a cloudy thickening of the surface membrane; any excessive fluid between the outer membrane and the heart; any irregularity in the heart's size or shape. Remove the heart.

SYRINX

Beneath where the heart was, follow the windpipe to the point where it narrows and branches into an upside-down Y. That is the syrinx — the chicken's voice box. It should be clean and free of secretions, moldiness, and worms.

LIVER

The liver is a dark reddish-brown, two-lobed organ lying in the middle of the body cavity. Examine it for abnormal consistency (it shouldn't be mushy), size (it should not extend below the keel), and color (an extremely yellow liver is an indication of fatty liver disease); white, yellow, or red spots; abscesses; or tumors. Cut into the liver, and look for scar tissue and grayish (dead) tissue.

Between the two lobes is a dark green sac filled with bile — the gallbladder. Try not to break it open, which would contaminate nearby organs before you have a chance to inspect them. An enlarged gallbladder could be a sign of aflatoxicosis. A slight green discoloration of the liver or other organs adjacent to the gallbladder is normal.

BODY FAT

A healthy, well-fed chicken has some fat throughout its tissues, as well as a fatty deposit, or fat pad, lining its abdomen. Chickens evolved with the ability to develop a fat pad for use as reserve energy during times when forage is scarce. Most young chickens, especially active pastured birds, have a relatively thin fat pad. An exception is commercial-strain broilers fed for rapid growth; any excess feed they don't convert into muscle (meat) metabolizes into fat.

An older chicken generally has a thicker fat pad than a younger chicken, and a hen has a thicker fat pad than a cock of the same age. Old hens, especially inactive hens fed too much corn or other grain, can accumulate enormous quantities of fat, to the point that the abdominal cavity is nearly solid fat.

Most chickens have yellow fat, although it may also be white, pinkish, or grayish. The precise color of the fat is influenced by the chicken's breed, age, diet, and state of health.

SPLEEN

The spleen is a smooth, roundish, dark-red organ next to the liver. Check the spleen for swelling, hemorrhages, and anything else unusual. Remove the liver and spleen.

DIGESTIVE SYSTEM

Now you have a good view of the digestive organs. Note any abnormal lumps or hemorrhages. Work your way under the stomach, gizzard, and intestines to loosen them as one bundle. The pancreas will come along with this bundle; it is the pale pinkish organ cradled within the duodenal loop of the small intestine. Cut around the cloaca and cloacal bursa to remove the digestive bundle.

To examine the interior of the digestive system, use your shears to cut down the length of the stomach, gizzard, small intestine, large intestine, and ceca. Note any parasites present. Digestive glands, appearing as a series of bumps, run along the inside wall (mucosa) of the digestive system. The mucosa should not be thickened, discolored, bloody, or wormy. For details on typical changes in digestive contents as they pass through the system, see page 82.

STOMACH

The stomach, or proventriculus, is the enlarged area between the esophagus and the gizzard. It should be somewhat bulging, shiny, and tan. The interior digestive glands give the exterior something of a honeycomb appearance. Note any hemorrhages or a white coating on the lining (possibly indicating canker).

GIZZARD

The gizzard, or ventriculus, is a thick, firm organ shaped something like a clamshell. Open it, and examine the contents for anything unusual. Rinse it out, and examine the inner lining for unusual roughness or lesions. The tough yellow lining should be easy to peel away from the underlying muscles.

INTESTINES

The intestine should be pinkish, smooth, and shiny on the outside, with no clearly defined bulges, and soft and velvety on the inside. Look for the presence of worms, blood, and excess mucus. Check the lining for inflammation, ulcers, or hemorrhages. Also note any unusual odor. If you find anything amiss, make a note of which part of the intestine you found it in (duodenum, jejunum, ileum, or colon).

CECA

The ceca are two blind-end tubes occurring at the juncture of the small and large intestine. In a mature chicken they are about 5 inches long and filled with pasty material that may be dark brown, mustard yellow, or greenish, but should not contain cheesy cores, worms, or blood. If you see blood, rinse and examine the lining for scarring and cecal worms.

Where each cecum branches off from the intestine is a small but clearly visible lump of tissue known as a cecal tonsil. The pair of cecal tonsils consists of lymphoid tissue and has a similar role to the cloacal bursa as part of the chicken's immune system. They should be the same color as surrounding tissue, not bluish or bloody looking, and not swollen.

IDENTIFYING TAPEWORMS

To identify the point of attachment of a tapeworm, use scissors to carefully cut open the intestine down its length. Spread the cut-open intestine in water, and the loose end of the tapeworm will float away from intestinal tissue, showing you where the head is attached. This technique is especially helpful for spotting the microscopic *Davainea proglottina* in the duodenum. The Tapeworms (Cestodes) table on page 176 indicates what each species looks like and what part of a chicken's intestine each prefers.

If you find large tapeworms in the lower portion of the small intestine, and a swelling or lump at the site of each head attachment, you have found the nodular tapeworm, *Raillietina echinobothrida.* This parasite causes nodular tapeworm disease, resulting in tumorlike swellings that can be as large in diameter as ¼ inch (6 mm). If you find lumps, but no tapeworms, you could be looking at tuberculosis.

CLOACAL BURSA

On the top side of the cloaca is a round, grape-shaped organ — the cloacal bursa. The older the chicken, the smaller this bursa will be. Cut the bursa in half. It should be a cream color and have parallel folds on its inner surface that, when the bursa is opened out, have the appearance of a rosebud. Swelling, atrophy, or off-color are signs of disease.

REPRODUCTIVE ORGANS

Lying close to the backbone are the chicken's reproductive organs — a hen's single ovary and oviduct or a cock's paired testicles and sperm ducts. Only the hen's left ovary should be developed. The vestigial right ovary is commonly cystic — appearing as a fluid-filled balloon that may be tiny or grow to a diameter of 5 inches in diameter. A cystic right ovary is rarely significant to the hen's health or ability to lay eggs, but may indicate that the hen once had infectious bronchitis.

The functioning oviduct runs from the left ovary over the left side of the kidney to the cloaca. Occasionally an oviduct will be filled with masses of yolk, sometimes mixed with albumen, shell membrane, and (rarely) whole eggs. Tumors, perhaps caused by Marek's disease or lymphoid leukosis, are a fairly common cause of death in older hens.

The testicles lie above and at the top end of the liver. They should be off-white and bean shaped, and will be larger in cocks than in cockerels and larger during breeding season than in the off-season. Testicular tumors are fairly common, usually appearing as round white or yellow firm masses of tissue, sometimes containing fluid. Misshapen, bloody-looking testicles may be an indication of bacterial infection.

KIDNEYS AND URETERS

The kidneys are a pair of elongated, three-lobed dark-brown organs embedded in the pelvic bones of the lower back. The ureters are ducts through which urine passes from the kidneys to the cloaca. Look for swelling or whitish salt deposits — indications of kidney disease or dehydration.

LUNGS AND BRONCHIAL TUBES

The lungs are two organs lying one on each side of the backbone between the ribs. They are normally bright pink, but turn dark red in a bird that has inhaled blood (after being euthanized with a knife or ax) or in a chicken that has been dead for long. The lungs may be gently worked out of the rib cage for a close examination. Note any off colors, tumors, or excessive amounts of mucus.

NERVES

The sciatic (hip) nerve is a thin fiber extending from the spinal cord under the middle lobe of the kidney and along the thighbone into the lower leg, one on each side. These nerves should be smooth, creamy white, the same size on both sides, and free of swelling. Enlargement of the sciatic nerve may be a sign of Marek's disease.

LEG BONES

If the bird was lame or paralyzed, cut through the ligaments of one hock joint and twist the leg until the joint pops open. Break the leg bone, to examine the marrow cavity for any anomalies — such as tumors (possibly indicating lymphoid leukosis), pale marrow (fusariotoxicosis), or sparse medullary bone (osteoporosis) — and to test the bone's strength. A healthy bone makes a snapping sound when broken.

KNEE AND HOCK JOINTS

Cut through the joints at the knee and hock. They should be shiny and white, with a little clear, sticky fluid inside. Signs of disease are excess fluid, yellow or white thick fluid, or blood.

ONLINE VISUAL AIDS

A comprehensive video on how to perform a thorough necropsy may be purchased or viewed online at partnersah.vet.cornell.edu/veterinarians/avian-necropsy-examination. In Cornell's *Atlas of Avian Diseases*, online at partnersah.vet.cornell.edu/avian-atlas/, you can search photo archives based on your exam findings, lesion location, or the name of a disease you suspect. You can also find examples of what normal organs should look like.

Potential Diagnoses Based on Postmortem Findings

BODY PART	FINDING	AGE/SEX	POTENTIAL CAUSE
Bone	Fragile, thin, or soft	Hen	Osteoporosis
	Thickened	All	Osteopetrosis
	Sparse medullary	Hen	Hypocalcemia, osteoporosis
Bone marrow	Tumorous marrow	2 years and up	Tuberculosis
		All	Lymphoid leukosis
	Pale	Young	Infectious bursal disease
		All	Fusariotoxicosis
Body cavity	Broken yolk	Pullet, hen	Bronchitis, colibacillosis, cholera, egg peritonitis, influenza, Newcastle (velogenic), yolk peritonitis
	Unabsorbed yolk	Chick	Omphalitis
	Fluid filled	Broiler, aging hen	Ascites, aspergillosis, cholera
	Blood clots	Hen	Fatty liver, sudden death
Breast	Pale muscles	Young	Coccidiosis (cecal)
	Gray or tan muscles	Young, growing	Gangrenous dermatitis
	Off-color tenders	Broiler	Green muscle disease
	Thin	Young to maturing	Coccidiosis (intestinal)
	Shriveled	Young	Infectious bursal disease, ulcerative enteritis
		Pullet, hen	Kidney stones
		Growing or mature	Gout (visceral)
		Aging	Tuberculosis
	Blood spotted	Young	Infectious bursal disease
		Mature	Erysipelas
	Fluid under skin	Chick	Exudative diathesis
	Blistered keel	All	Breast blister, arthritis (staphylococcic), infectious synovitis
Ceca	Cheesy core	Chick	Pullorum
		Young	Blackhead, coccidiosis (cecal)
		All	Arizonosis, paratyphoid
	Bloody core	Chick	Coccidiosis (cecal)
	Yellow nodules	Young, growing	Ulcerative enteritis

Potential Diagnoses Based on Postmortem Findings

BODY PART	FINDING	AGE/SEX	POTENTIAL CAUSE
Cloacal bursa	Swollen, yellow	Young	Infectious bursal disease
	Shriveled	Young, growing	Gangrenous dermatitis
	Shriveled, gray	Young	Infectious bursal disease
	Tumorous	Maturing	Lymphoid leukosis
Crop	Empty of feed, thick lining	Young, growing	Canker
	Thick Turkish-towel lining	All	Sour crop
	Full at death	Growing, mature	Colibacillosis, sudden death syndrome
	Packed with feed	Mature	Crop binding
	Filled with feed and water	Mature	Pendulous crop
	Sores in lining	Young, growing	Canker, fusariotoxicosis
	Contains maggots	All	Botulism
Heart	Pale	All	Marek's disease
	Swollen	All	Chlamydiosis, ergotism, pullorum
	Swollen, pale	All	Listeriosis
	Swollen, bloody	Broiler, hen	Sudden death syndrome
	Swollen right side	Broiler, aging hen	Ascites
	Blood flecked	Growing	Cholera
	Chalky coating	All	Gout (vesicular)
	Tumorous	Maturing	Lymphoid leukosis
Intestines	Bloody	Growing	Coccidiosis
		Mature	Newcastle (velogenic)
	Mucus filled	Young	Infectious bursal disease
		All	Ochratoxicosis
	Mucus, bloody	Growing	Cholera
		All	Colibacillosis
	Mucus, greenish	All	Spirochetosis
	Mucus, sticky	Growing	Coccidiosis
		Mature	Erysipelas
	Watery contents	Chick	Omphalitis
	Cauliflower lining	Young	Necrotic enteritis

BODY PART	FINDING	AGE/SEX	POTENTIAL CAUSE
	Yellowish buttons	Young, growing	Ulcerative enteritis
	Swollen	Mature	Paratyphoid
	Swollen, slimy (duodenum)	Growing	Typhoid
	Feed filled	Broiler, hen	Sudden death syndrome
	Tumorous	Growing, mature	Nodular tapeworm
		Aging	Tuberculosis
Kidneys	Swollen	Chick	Salmonellosis
		Young, growing	Gangrenous dermatitis
		Mature	Streptococcosis
	Swollen, pale	Young	Infectious bursal disease
		Growing, mature	Infectious bronchitis
		All	Spirochetosis
	Swollen, pale, hard	Growing, mature	Ochratoxicosis
	Swollen, pale, mottled	All	Infectious synovitis
	Pale	Broiler, hen	Sudden death syndrome
	Partially shriveled, partially swollen and pale	Pullet, hen	Gout (visceral), kidney stones
	Swollen, blood spots	Growing	Pseudomonas
	Swollen, gray spots	All	Colibacillosis
	Swollen, tumorous	Maturing	Lymphoid leukosis
		All	Marek's disease
	Chalky coating	All	Gout (visceral)
Liver	Film covered	All	Campylobacteriosis, colibacillosis
	Mottled	All	Fusariotoxicosis
	Swollen	Young, growing	Gangrenous dermatitis
		Maturing	Lymphoid leukosis
		Mature	Erysipelas
	Swollen, dark	Chick	Omphalitis
	Swollen, yellow, mottled	Chick	Arizonosis, paratyphoid
	Swollen, yellow, spotted	All	Ochratoxicosis
	Swollen, yellow, soft	All	Aflatoxicosis

Potential Diagnoses Based on Postmortem Findings

BODY PART	FINDING	AGE/SEX	POTENTIAL CAUSE
		Mature	Fatty liver syndrome
	Swollen, bloody, mottled	Broiler, hen	Ascites, fatty liver syndrome
	Swollen, blood spotted	All	Spirochetosis
	Swollen, cooked looking	Growing	Cholera
	Swollen, gray, crumbly	Maturing	Lymphoid leukosis
	Swollen, gray spotted	All	Marek's, pullorum, spirochetosis
	Swollen, metallic	Growing	Typhoid
	Swollen, greenish	All	Colibacillosis, infectious synovitis, listeriosis
	Swollen, spotted	Growing	Pseudomonas
		All	Chlamydiosis
	Swollen, patchy	Young, growing	Ulcerative enteritis
		Mature	Streptococcosis
	Swollen, dished spots	Young	Blackhead
	Swollen, star spots	All	Campylobacteriosis
	Shriveled, pale	Broiler, hen	Ascites
	Shriveled, firm	All	Aflatoxicosis
	Blistered	Broiler, hen	Ascites
	Patchy gray spots	All	Listeriosis
	Mushy, yellow	Hen	Aflatoxicosis, fatty liver syndrome
	Chalky coating	All	Gout (visceral)
	Tumorous	Maturing	Lymphoid leukosis
		All	Marek's disease
		Aging	Tuberculosis
Lungs	Film covered	All	Colibacillosis
	Pale, gray	Broiler, hen	Ascites
	Grayish yellow	Chick	Brooder pneumonia
	Bloody	Young, growing	Gangrenous dermatitis
		Broiler, hen	Ascites, sudden death syndrome
	Cheesy contents	Chick	Brooder pneumonia, infectious bronchitis
		Growing, mature	Chronic respiratory disease

BODY PART	FINDING	AGE/SEX	POTENTIAL CAUSE
		Mature	Aspergillosis
		All	Influenza
	Tumorous	Maturing	Lymphoid leukosis
	Solidified	All	Marek's disease
Muscles	Dark red	Broiler, hen	Ascites
	Pale	Chick	Coccidiosis
	Spotted	Young	Infectious bursal disease
		Growing	Typhoid
		Mature	Erysipelas
	Shriveled	Chick	Exudative diathesis
		Young, growing	Ulcerative enteritis
		Mature	Kidney stones
		Aging	Tuberculosis
		All	Gout (visceral), water deprivation
	Shriveled, dark	Young	Infectious bursal disease
	Cooked looking	Young, growing	Gangrenous dermatitis
	Cystic	All	Toxoplasmosis
Skin	Pale	Chick	Coccidiosis
		Growing	Cryptosporidiosis, Marek's disease
	Bluish	Chick	Omphalitis
		Broiler, hen	Ascites
	Dark	Mature	Aspergillosis
	Blotchy	Young, growing	Gangrenous dermatitis
		Mature	Erysipelas
	Burnlike sores	Growing, mature	Fusariotoxicosis
	Scabby	All	Pox (dry)
	Scaly	All	Ringworm
	Air/gas underneath	Young, growing	Gangrenous dermatitis
		All	Ruptured air sac
	Fluid underneath	Chick	Omphalitis, exudative diathesis
		Young, growing	Gangrenous dermatitis, pseudomonas

Potential Diagnoses Based on Postmortem Findings

BODY PART	FINDING	AGE/SEX	POTENTIAL CAUSE
		All	Influenza
	Off odor	Young, growing	Gangrenous dermatitis, pseudomonas
	Tumorous	Growing	Marek's disease
Spleen	Swollen	Young, growing	Gangrenous dermatitis
		Growing	Cholera
		Mature	Erysipelas
		Growing, mature	Listeriosis
		Mature	Streptococcosis
	Swollen, spotted	Young	Infectious bursal disease
		Growing	Pseudomonas
		All	Colibacillosis, Marek's disease, pullorum
	Swollen, mottled	Young, growing	Typhoid, ulcerative enteritis
		All	Spirochetosis
	Swollen, dark, soft	All	Chlamydiosis
	Shriveled	Growing, mature	Fusariotoxicosis
	Tumorous	Maturing	Lymphoid leukosis
		Aging	Tuberculosis
Ureters	Blocked with crystals	All	Gout (visceral), spirochetosis, water deprivation
		Young	Infectious bursal disease
		Growing, mature	Infectious bronchitis, ochratoxicosis
		Mature	Kidney stones
Windpipe	Swollen, red	Growing, mature	Chronic respiratory disease
	Mucus filled	All	Newcastle (mesogenic)
	Cheesy contents	Chick	Bronchitis
		Young	Cryptosporidiosis
		Growing, mature	Chronic respiratory disease
		Mature	Laryngotracheitis
		All	Pox (wet)
	White semifluid contents	Cock	Gout (articular)
	Blood spots	Mature	Laryngotracheitis
	Moldy	Mature	Aspergillosis

Disposing of Dead Birds

Legal methods for disposing of animal bodies vary from place to place. For public health reasons, unceremoniously depositing them in a Dumpster or local landfill is illegal nearly everywhere. Some landfill operators, though, may give you permission to deposit a dead bird, which they will immediately cover with sanitary fill.

In some areas the sanitation department will pick up a carcass curbside, usually with certain stipulations — such as how the carcass is to be wrapped and identified as being a dead animal. If your next curbside pickup is more than 24 hours away, place the well-wrapped dead bird in the freezer for the duration.

Do not bury a diseased chicken in your backyard compost pile. The warm, moist environment may provide perfect conditions for pathogens to multiply, flies and rodents may spread the disease, and stray dogs or marauding wildlife may dig up and make off with the diseased carcass.

To dispose of the body of a diseased bird, you must use a method that prevents the spread of infection or toxins. The two best disposal methods are deep burial and burning.

Deep Burial

Bury a body deeply enough that it can't be dug up by dogs or wild animals. Find a spot far from a well, stream, or other water source. Some state statutes mandate these guidelines:

- Bury the body within 24 hours of death.

- Dig the burial pit deep enough to cover with at least 3 feet of soil.

- The burial site must be no closer than 100 feet from the nearest well and 300 feet from the nearest stream or other body of water.

- Make sure the bottom of the pit is at least 5 feet above the water table or bedrock.

Besides burying the diseased bird, bury all contaminated litter, feed, and droppings associated with it. Before backfilling the pit, cover everything with calcium hydroxide, sold at farm stores and builder supply outlets as hydrated lime, builder's lime, mason's lime, or slaked lime. Hydrated lime is an organic alkaline compound with low solubility in water. It effectively sterilizes the buried matter by increasing the pH level to the point of destroying pathogens and preventing their regrowth.

Note that hydrated lime (calcium hydroxide) is *not* the same as quicklime (calcium oxide) or agricultural lime (calcium carbonate). Unlike ag lime, which is pale gray, hydrated lime is pure white. Also unlike ag lime, hydrated lime is extremely caustic. Wear gloves when handling it, and take care not to breathe in the dust.

Cremation

Cremation may be necessary where the water table is high, the soil is rocky or frozen, or burying is prohibited by law but burning is not. Burning is relatively easy and extremely sanitary, and the ashes do not attract insects and rodents.

Cremation requires accumulating a heap of combustible materials such as scrap wood or tree prunings, along with dry straw or hay to get a hot blaze going. Choose a site well away from any combustibles, or use a backyard incinerator if you have one. After the carcass has fully burned and cooled, bury the ashes, scatter them, or add them to your compost pile.

Some areas have pet cremation services, and some veterinarians offer cremation services. Most of the time you can, if you so choose, obtain the ashes afterward.

CHAPTER 14

Treatments and Therapies

GOING BY THE philosophy of "whatever works," our family uses both conventional and traditional, or so-called alternative, remedies on our human selves. Sometimes the alternative methods are more effective and have fewer side effects than prescription drugs. So we are open to using alternatives on our livestock as well.

When dealing with a sick chicken, however, we tend to be more cautious about trying alternatives that may or may not work. One reason is that chickens hide their pain as long as they can. By the time a chicken exhibits signs of not being well, it needs help fast. Since a chicken can't tell us if it's feeling better, unless a treatment works fast, we can't tell if it's working at all.

We therefore limit alternative livestock therapies to their use as immunity enhancers. Happily, this plan has resulted in healthier chickens that haven't required any other type of veterinary treatment.

Treating a Sick Bird

Any time you treat a diseased bird, isolate it away from the rest of the flock. Once it has been moved, avoid moving it again to minimize stress. When you tend your flock, take care of healthy birds first, so you won't spread disease from the sick ones to the healthy ones.

Be sure recovering birds get plenty of clean water and fresh feed. Since many diseases cause a chicken to eat less, feeding often will help to stimulate appetites. Encourage drinking by providing cool water in summer and warm water in winter.

In cool weather supply additional heat, especially if the birds are young. Pay special attention to sanitation so the population of pathogens doesn't build up and reduce the birds' resistance even further — keep droppings out of feed and water, and make sure litter is deep and clean.

Some chicken diseases can be cured if treatment starts early. Others are irreversible or fatal. Chickens, being prey animals, instinctively avoid showing signs of weakness. So by the time you notice obvious signs of illness, the disease is usually pretty far along. Recognizing a disease as soon as it starts is the first step toward curing the ones that are curable and dealing effectively with those that are permanent or irreversible. The longer you wait before you take action, the more difficult treatment or control becomes and the more likely you are to lose the ailing bird or have the disease spread to others.

Attempting to treat a flock without knowing exactly what's wrong can be costly, may result in continuing losses, and could make the disease worse. Illnesses that have similar signs may require entirely different treatments.

Once you know what the problem is, you have to make the hard choice between culling the affected birds or embarking on a suitable course of therapy and hoping for the best. In this context, cull means kill. When a condition is serious, sometimes the only humane approach is to not prolong the suffering and put the bird out of its misery.

Some serious diseases should not be cured because recovered birds will be carriers, continuing to spread the disease intermittently or continuously for the rest of their lives. Other diseases are so contagious that the only way to keep them from spreading is to destroy the entire flock — depopulate, in veterinary parlance.

If you are raising chickens to get healthful meat, you may prefer to cull diseased birds and start over, rather than run the risk of eating meat containing drug residue or disease-causing microbes, some of which are harmful to humans.

If your chickens have become beloved pets, you may wish to do everything possible to try to save them. Decide in advance how much you're willing to spend. You could spend hundreds of dollars on veterinary care on a single chicken, only to lose the bird in the end.

If you're raising an endangered or exhibition breed, you'll likely wish to preserve the gene pool by keeping breeders going until you can hatch enough eggs to perpetuate the flock, an approach that works only if the disease does not spread through hatched eggs. You must, of course, raise the new chicks away from diseased adults, cull the diseased breeders as soon as possible, and meticulously clean up their housing with an appropriate disinfectant.

Waiting until the problem goes away works only if the disease is self-limiting, meaning it naturally runs its course in a short time and birds recover on their own. Few diseases fall into this category. A good number of diseases lie somewhere between serious and self-limiting and can be effectively treated.

Drug Use

Many nonprescription drugs are available from farm and feed stores and through mail-order catalogs. Such over-the-counter drugs are considered safe when they are used according to directions on the label. Whether you obtain a drug over the counter or by a veterinarian's prescription, it will be effective only if you have selected the right drug for the disease and know when to use it, how to use it, how often to use it, and how much to use. Additional sound drug-use practices include the following:

- Avoid out-of-date drugs.

- Store drugs at 35°F to 55°F (1.7°C to 12.8°C), away from sunlight.

- Administer a drug only as directed. If it's supposed to be given by mouth, for example, it may be toxic as an injection.

- Observe the safe dosage level. The drug won't be effective in an amount less than the label specifies, and may be toxic in greater amounts.

- Observe the withdrawal time when treating meat birds; if the drug is approved for laying hens, observe the egg discard period (see Avoiding Drug Residues on page 377).

- Do not combine drugs or use more than one at a time, unless such a combination is approved by a veterinarian.

Administering Drugs

For a drug to be effective, it must reach the infectious microbes in sufficient quantity and remain in contact long enough to do the job. Most drugs should be administered for at least 3 days, or for 2 days after the signs disappear,

Antimicrobials

An antimicrobial is any agent that either kills microorganisms or inhibits their growth. Another word for antimicrobial is antibiotic, although the word "antibiotic" is often used to mean the same as antibacterial — the largest group of antimicrobials. The five basic categories of antimicrobials are as follows:

Anthelmintic: against worms (see chapter 6)

Antibacterial: against bacteria (see chapter 8)

Antifungal: against mold and fungi (see chapter 9)

Antiprotozoal: against protozoa (see chapter 7)

Antiviral: against viruses (see chapter 10)

whichever is longest. As a general rule, if you do not see some improvement within 2 days, you are using the wrong drug.

How you administer a drug depends on the drug you use, the disease you're treating, the number of birds involved, their condition, and the length of time the drug must be administered. Drugs are applied in one of four main ways: topically, orally, inhaled, or injected.

Topical, or local, medications are applied directly to the skin, eyes, nose, or other external organs. Examples of topical drugs are antibiotic powders or ointments used to prevent infection of wounds, and liquids applied to an infected eye.

Oral medications are given by mouth. They work either by controlling microbes in the intestine or by being absorbed through the intestine, to be distributed to other parts of the body. Oral drugs take effect slowly, usually in 4 to 12 hours, depending on the drug used, the bird's metabolic rate, and the amount of feed in its crop. Oral drugs are convenient and safe but can be unpredictable in their absorption rates, especially when a bird has diarrhea. Examples of oral medications are pills, feed or water additives, and drenches (liquid medications that are swallowed).

Inhaled medications work against microbes in the respiratory system, or are absorbed through the respiratory system to be carried to other parts of the body. Such a drug may be a liquid solution applied as a drop to the nostril, by means of a fine mist, or as a dust puffed into the air. Specialized equipment is needed to put particles of just the right size and density into the air, making the use of most airborne drugs impractical for small flocks.

Injected medications, which take effect rapidly, are inserted with a needle and syringe into one of three places: beneath the skin, into the muscle, or into the bloodstream.

Giving a Shot

Whenever you administer a drug by injection, use a fresh or sterile needle and syringe. To sterilize a used needle and syringe, separate them, boil them in clean water for 15 minutes, dry them on a clean paper towel, and store them in a clean, dust-free place.

If you use the same needle to inject more than one bird, before refilling the syringe between birds, dip the needle in alcohol (unless you are applying a live-virus vaccine, which the alcohol will kill), or pass the needle through a match flame. Keep extra needles on hand in case the one you're using gets too dull to pierce easily.

Use a 20- or 22-gauge needle, ½ or ¾ inch long. Needles and syringes may be purchased at a farm store, from a veterinarian, or from a supplier of poultry, livestock, or veterinary products.

Liquid Medication

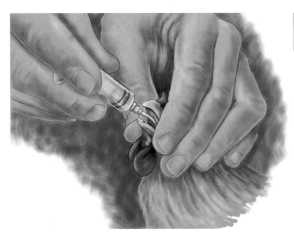

A liquid medication, or drench, may be squirted onto the back of the bird's tongue, taking care not to get any into the windpipe.

Inhaled Medication

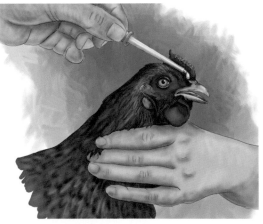

When applying a liquid medication as a drop on the chicken's nostril, watch to make sure the chicken inhales the medication before releasing the bird.

Syringes are marked off in cubic centimeters (cc). Drug dosages are specified either in cc or in cc per pound of weight. To determine how many cc you need, multiply the bird's weight by the number of cc per pound. Sometimes dosages are given in milliliters (mL). Since one mL equals 1.000027 cc, for practical purposes they are the same. Use a syringe large enough to hold the entire dose in one shot.

Subcutaneous injections (SC or SQ) are given directly under the skin, usually at the breast or the nape of the neck where the skin is loose. Pick up a pinch of skin and insert the needle at an angle. If you're injecting chicks, take care not to push the needle all the way through the skin and squirt the drug out the other side (or into your thumb). A subcutaneous injection is easy and safe to administer and lasts a long time, up to 2 days. On the other hand, the drug takes effect slowly because it requires a long time to migrate to the bloodstream for distribution throughout the body.

Intramuscular injections (IM) go into the meaty portion of the breast. They take effect fast — in about an hour — and last about 8 hours, but you must take care not to touch a bone or nerve. A safe bet is to place the shot about an inch above the keel.

Intravenous injections (IV) insert medication directly into the bloodstream, where it takes effect almost immediately. They are the trickiest shots to give and should be used only for drugs designed for IV administration, and only on a bird that's comatose, paralyzed, or otherwise in imminent danger of dying. Intravenous administration of *Clotridium botulinum* antitoxin, for example, might be used on a valuable breeder that's been paralyzed by botulism.

Subcutaneous Injection

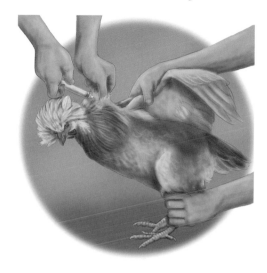

To inject medication under the skin, take a pinch of skin at the back of the bird's neck with one hand and with the other hand insert the needle under the skin.

Intramuscular Injection

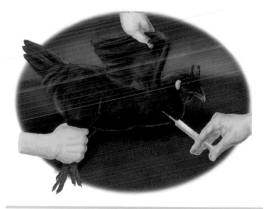

To inject medication into the muscle, insert the needle at a 45-degree angle about an inch above the breastbone.

Intravenous injections are best left to a veterinarian. The procedure is to pull a few feathers from the depression in the upper part of the underside of one wing — to better see the vein — then insert a needle into the main wing vein, or brachial, pointed toward the wing tip (away from the chicken's body), and slowly depress the plunger to release the drug *very* slowly. The position of the needle is the same as for drawing a blood sample, illustrated on page 325.

Feed and Water Additives

When medications are added to feed or water, low birds in the peck order may not spend enough time at the trough to obtain a sufficient dose. Furthermore, there's always the danger that birds won't eat or drink at all, or will eat or drink to excess and overdose.

If a medication must be administered by means of feed or water, adding it to water is preferable for these three reasons:

- Many diseases cause appetite loss but increase thirst.

- Diluting a drug in water is easier than evenly distributing it in feed.

- Compared to feed based, a water-based treatment takes effect more rapidly.

The most effective way to administer a water-soluble treatment is to divide the recommended dosage in half and mix half in the morning and half at night. Since chickens drink the most in the morning and in the evening, dividing the dosage ensures more consistent water consumption and therefore a more consistent distribution of medication. Further, the medicated water is less apt to get dirty, and the medication is less apt to settle out.

Some small-scale flock owners medicate feed or drinking water as a precaution against disease, either routinely or during times of stress. The practice is not only expensive but counterproductive, since it has little or no effect in preventing disease, and can cause resistant strains of microbes to develop so that drugs won't work if a disease does strike.

Commercial growers add low levels of drugs to rations to improve egg production and to stimulate the growth rate and feed-conversion efficiency of broilers. Antibiotics cause a bird's intestinal wall to thin, improving nutrient

INDIVIDUAL VERSUS WHOLE-FLOCK TREATMENTS

Shots, pills, and drenches are suitable for treating individual chickens.

Pro: You can be sure each bird gets an adequate dose.

Con: Treating individual birds is time consuming, and handling each bird increases stress and thus can worsen an ailing bird's condition.

Drugs administered by feed, water, or through the air are suitable where many birds are involved or the drug must be administered over a long period of time.

Pro: Treating the whole flock at once saves time.

Con: You can never be sure each bird gets an adequate dose.

absorption. But the routine nonmedicinal use of antibiotics in food-producing flocks has contributed to antibiotic resistance in pathogens affecting humans as well as those affecting chickens.

Avoiding Drug Residues

When you medicate chickens kept for meat or eggs, take special care to observe any precautions listed on the label. Especially important to human health is the drug's withdrawal time for meat birds or egg-discard time for layers.

When a medication is absorbed, it is first distributed throughout the chicken's body tissue and fluid, then is gradually eliminated through the filtering processes of the kidneys and liver. Different drugs, or the same drug administered in different amounts, are eliminated at different rates. The elimination of a drug that is absorbed by fat can take an especially long time, if ever. Residues remaining in meat and eggs can be harmful to humans in the following ways:

- They may disturb the natural balance of microflora in the intestines and elsewhere.

- They can cause a severe reaction in anyone who is allergic, such as to penicillin or sulfa drugs.

- They can cause microbes to become resistant to medications prescribed by a physician.

- They may adversely interact with a prescription drug being taken by a person who consumes the contaminated meat or eggs.

The withdrawal time on a drug label tells you the drug's elimination rate, or the number of days that must pass between the time you discontinue the drug and the time you butcher the birds for food or eat their eggs. The withdrawal time is the minimum required by law — it doesn't hurt to err on the side of caution and add several extra days.

Few drugs are approved for laying hens. When a drug is stored in fat and released over a period of time, residue can appear in the yolks of eggs laid long after the drug is discontinued. Unofficial guidelines for discarding eggs are as follows:

- When a withdrawal time is given for meat birds, add 10 days for discarding eggs.

- When no withdrawal time is specified, discard eggs for at least 3 weeks, and preferably 8 weeks, after discontinuing drug use.

Nondrug Therapies

Along with an increasing interest in home-grown foods, including chicken meat and eggs, coupled with increasing awareness of the risks of using conventional drugs, a lot of today's chicken keepers are seeking natural means of maintaining healthy flocks. While some natural preparations may be used to treat diseases, they generally require a certain degree of knowledge regarding how to select preparations that work for the situation at hand, and how to use them effectively. Luckily, most nondrug therapies also serve as powerful immunity enhancers, generally resulting in healthier chickens and therefore less need for conventional drugs to treat illnesses.

Vitamin Therapy

Coccidiosis and other intestinal diseases reduce a chicken's ability to absorb fat-soluble vitamins. The affected chicken will benefit from a

A sick or recovering chicken should be isolated in a clean, comfortable cage or small pen, referred to variously as an isolation pen or hospital pen. The chicken should be kept apart from the flock. If it's ill or injured, isolation will prevent other chickens from picking on it, and if it has a contagious disease, it won't spread the disease to others.

The pen should have a low perch or no perch and should be clean and warm, in the 80°F to 85°F (27°C to 29°C) range. Hanging a low-watt lightbulb to one side of the pen will allow the chicken to maintain its own comfort level by moving closer to or away from the heat.

The isolation ward should be away from pesky flies. It should not be drafty, although good ventilation will ensure that the bird doesn't keep breathing the same stale air. It should not be completely dark, although keeping it somewhat darkened will encourage the chicken to remain calm.

Provide clean water and fresh feed. Vinegar added to nonmedicated water at the rate of 1 tablespoon per gallon (15 mL per 4 L) will make the water more appealing to the chicken and encourage the bird to drink. If the chicken is disinclined to eat, entice it with some of its favorite healthful treats.

vitamin supplement, especially containing the fat-soluble vitamins A, E, D_3, and K.

You can boost your flock's ability to fight any disease, and minimize the chance of a secondary infection, by adding a vitamin supplement to their drinking water. A vitamin supplement may also be used to ward off disease in times of stress, such as during a move, before and after a show, during breeding season, or when the weather extremes are particularly unpleasant. Chicks will get a healthy start if you treat them to a vitamin supplement throughout their first 3 weeks of life.

Probiotics and Prebiotics

Useful information for backyard chicken keepers has resulted from the poultry industry's practice of crowding broilers into unsanitary facilities. Such birds are especially susceptible to intestinal diseases, which affect their digestion and therefore their growth rate.

To maintain the intestinal health of broilers, industrial producers have used antimicrobial drugs as so-called "growth promoters."

However, because of increasing concern among consumers over bacterial resistance to antimicrobial drugs, the industry began seeking alternatives in the form of natural probiotic and prebiotic dietary supplements. The basic concept of using probiotics and prebiotics is to encourage competitive exclusion.

COMPETITIVE EXCLUSION

The intestine of a healthy chicken (and also a healthy human) is populated with a huge number of different kinds of bacteria that provide many benefits. Among these benefits are aiding digestion, producing vitamins and other important nutrients, detoxifying harmful compounds, keeping the intestinal tract healthy, and producing antibacterial compounds and enzymes that stimulate the immune system.

The beneficial bacteria also protect the chicken's digestive tract from invasion by pathogenic bacteria through the process of competitive exclusion. By competing with invaders for limited available resources — in the form of nutrients and intestinal attachment sites — the beneficials effectively shut out, or exclude, the invaders. For good measure some beneficials also produce compounds that are toxic to invaders.

Faulty conditions in the digestive tract encourage the beneficials to overpopulate the intestines, causing illness by competing with the chicken for nutrients and by producing an overabundance of unhealthful toxins. If, on the other hand, conditions result in an underpopulation of beneficials, invaders take over and cause intestinal disease, usually indicated by diarrhea. Invading bacteria can also migrate from the digestive tract to cause problems in other parts of the chicken's body; for instance, settling in joints and causing lameness.

Both probiotics and prebiotics are natural components of some foods and of all fermented foods. They may be used to maintain or restore a healthy population of normal intestinal bacteria. As prepared dietary supplements, they may be fed separately or combined together to work synergistically, in which case the supplement is called a synbiotic. Some foods, such as yeast, cultured foods, and certain grains can be both probiotic and prebiotic.

PROBIOTICS

Probiotics are live beneficial bacteria that restore or improve the small intestine's normal population of bacteria. Poultry suppliers offer probiotics formulated specifically for chickens. A chick acquires some beneficials through the egg and gains more from the environment, particularly from properly composting litter. Probiotics are naturally present in certain foods, including root crops, grains, and fermented milk, such as yogurt and kefir.

Probiotics are advantageous in any situation in which naturally acquired beneficials may be in short supply. Chicks that have been shipped, and therefore haven't eaten for their first day or two, benefit from a probiotic in their first meal. Any chicks raised on improper rations or in a poor environment may not develop beneficial bacteria fast enough to ward off pathogenic bacteria. Chickens raised entirely on wire, and therefore lacking opportunities to peck out some of their sustenance from the environment, may not acquire sufficient beneficial bacteria to maintain good health.

The use of antibiotics and other antimicrobials kills both disease-causing and beneficial bacteria alike. Any chicken that is subjected to extreme stress would benefit from a probiotic, as would any chicken that has been treated with an antibiotic. Following drug treatment, a simple way to restore the balance of beneficials is to feed each chicken a heaping tablespoon of plain active-culture yogurt every day for a week.

A varied and well-balanced diet keeps a chicken's population of beneficial intestinal bacteria strong and healthy. Chickens that eat a varied diet or are free to peck in the environment typically do not need a supplemental probiotic. For healthy birds the benefits of feeding a probiotic decrease with age. Overuse of probiotics can, in fact, be detrimental to a chicken's health by unbalancing the intestine's bacterial ecology.

Note, too, that bacteria and protozoa do not inhabit the same ecological niche in a chicken's intestines. Therefore, competitive exclusion

On the label of a bag of prepared chicken ration, probiotics should be listed according to species of live microbes, and prebiotics should be listed as specific ingredients. Here are some typical indications of the inclusion of each:

Probiotics: *Bifidobacterium* (or *B. "something"*), *Lactobaccillus* (or *L. "something"*)

Prebiotics: lactose, inulin, oligosaccharides (fructooligosaccharide [FOS], oligofructose), pectin

Being live cultures, probiotics deteriorate during prolonged storage, while prebiotics — as inert fiber — do not.

resulting from a probiotic does not directly apply to coccidial protozoa. However, any boost to your chickens' immune systems will make them healthier and better able to resist diseases of all kinds, including coccidiosis.

PREBIOTICS

Prebiotics are natural soluble fiber sources that cannot be digested by the chicken, but that stimulate the growth and activity of beneficial bacteria colonizing the large intestine. Prebiotics are quite selective; each specific prebiotic influences only one type, or sometimes a limited number, of beneficials. The most common prebiotics are carbohydrates known as oligosaccharides, a word derived from the Greek words *oligos*, meaning "scanty," and *sakkharon*, meaning "sugar."

Some oligosaccharides are fructooligosaccharides, or FOS (also called oligofructose), and the related fiber inulin. These carbohydrates are derived from fruits and vegetables, such as garlic, Jerusalem artichokes, jicama, dandelion greens, most legumes, and some grains, including barley, oats, and wheat. Chickens cannot digest FOS, but beneficial bacteria can, and most pathogenic bacteria cannot. The beneficial bacteria thus thrive and outcompete the pathogenic bacteria.

Other oligosaccharides are mannanoligosaccharides, or MOS (such as the brand Bio-Mos), derived from yeast. Mannan sugars are one of the main components of yeast cell walls. Unlike FOS, which nourishes beneficials, these prebiotics confuse pathogenic bacteria into attaching to the MOS, rather than to the intestine wall. The chicken, unable to digest MOS, expels it in poop, and the attached pathogens go with it.

Regardless of whether they nourish beneficials or bind and remove invaders, prebiotics can help brooded chicks more rapidly develop a healthy population of beneficials. In chickens of any age, during times of extreme stress prebiotics can help relieve diarrhea, aid digestion, and enhance nutrient absorption. And they are especially useful for helping restore beneficial bacteria following treatment with an antibiotic. As an additional benefit, prebiotics reduce the amount of urates expelled in poop, thus reducing the amount of pungent-smelling ammonia in the henhouse.

The Vinegar Solution

Understanding how to use vinegar to promote chicken health requires first understanding pH. In case you missed, or forgot, this part of chemistry class, here's a quick review.

The acidity or alkalinity of any substance is measured on a pH scale, where low numbers are acidic and high numbers are alkaline (also known as basic). The letters pH stand for "power of hydrogen," so called because the pH scale is logarithmic (in powers of 10) and measures the concentration of hydrogen ions in a water-based solution.

A pH scale typically runs from 0 to 14, with each number 10 times more alkaline than the previous number. Pure water is neutral and has a pH of 7. Working toward lower numbers, a pH of 6 is 10 times more acidic than pure water. Working toward higher numbers, a pH of 8 is 10 times more alkaline than pure water. You can see, then, that a substance with a pH of 1 is strongly acidic, while a substance with a pH of 14 is strongly alkaline.

VINEGAR AND CROP pH

Pathogens thrive in a pH range between 7.5 and 9, and most of them cannot tolerate an acidic environment. Beneficial bacteria (probiotics) prefer a pH range of 5.5 to 7. The pH of a healthy chicken's crop lies between 5 and 6, the ideal range for the beneficial bacteria that produce lactic acid in the crop. The lactic acid keeps the crop at a healthy, slightly acidic pH level. Ingested pathogens therefore have a hard time making it past the unfriendly — to them — crop environment.

A chicken under stress often drinks less than usual, disrupting the activity of beneficial microbes throughout the digestive tract, including the crop. A decrease in the population of beneficial microbes encourages an increase in the population of pathogens.

Vinegar is a natural antimicrobial with a pH range of between 2 and 3. Chickens like the flavor vinegar imparts to their drinking water, which encourages an ill or injured chicken to drink more. Adding a little vinegar to a stressed-out chicken's drinking water both encourages drinking and helps maintain the crop's acidity to discourage alkaline-loving pathogens and encourage the return of acid-loving beneficial microbes.

Only a little vinegar is needed — 1 tablespoon per gallon (15 mL per 4 L), or double the vinegar dose if you have hard (alkaline) water. You want the pH level of the drinking water to be about 4, which you can determine using either a pH meter or pH test strips. Adding

pH in a Chicken's Environment

PH	COMMON SOLUTIONS	CHICKEN'S BODY	MICROBE PREFERENCES
Strongly Acidic			
		Hydrochloric (stomach) acid = 1	
		Proventriculus = 1–3	
	Vinegar = 2–3		
		Gizzard = 3–4	
		Crop, ceca = 5–6	
	Soft water < 6.5	Small intestine = 5.5–6.5	Probiotics = 5.5–7
	Pure water = 7	Saliva = 6.5–7.5	
		Large intestine = 6.5–7.5	
Neutral		Blood = 7.3–7.5	
		Bile = 7.5	
	Hard water > 8.5	Egg = 8	Pathogens = 7.5–9
	Baking soda = 9		
	Ammonia = 11		
	Soapy water = 12		
	Bleach = 13		
Strongly Basic			

too much vinegar can have the opposite of your desired effect by causing chickens to stop drinking.

Besides acidifying the crop, adding vinegar to drinking water has the additional benefit of discouraging the growth of pathogens in the water itself. In a disease outbreak, when healthy and infected chickens drink from the same waterer, vinegar can help slow the spread of disease. Vinegar, used full strength, also makes a good sanitizer for cleaning feeders, drinkers, and other equipment.

VINEGAR AND DIGESTIVE HEALTH

Once vinegar enters a chicken's crop, it has done its job of helping maintain a healthy pH in the crop. When digestive matter from the crop moves down to the chicken's stomach, or proventriculus, it encounters a more powerful acid — hydrochloric acid — which reduces the stomach's pH range to between 1 and 3.

Stress or illness can cause a chicken to lose its appetite, and an empty stomach does not produce acid. As a result, the stomach's pH goes up. The increased pH discourages beneficial bacteria and encourages a proliferation of pathogenic bacteria.

One of the first signs that digestive pH is too high is the appearance of loose droppings. Vinegar in the drinking water encourages chickens to drink more, which in turn attracts them to eat more, which restores digestive pH balance.

Stomach acid not only offers some protection against microbes and parasites but also activates enzymes that are essential for the digestion of protein. Without these enzymes, protein in the chicken's diet would putrefy, making the chicken ill.

As digesting feeds proceed through the system, they get progressively more alkaline, aided by the production of bicarbonate in the pancreas. Bicarbonate is an important part of the ingenious buffering system all animals share, which maintains appropriate pH levels by binding hydrogen ions when the pH tips toward acidity and releasing hydrogen ions when the pH starts to become too alkaline.

The gut's pH is further influenced by bile, which has a pH of about 7.5. By the time digestive matter gets to the small intestine, where alkaline-loving enzymes help move things along, it has a pH range of 5.5 to 6.5. The pH can rise as high as 7.5 by the time digestive wastes leave the chicken as poop.

If you're a gardener, you might be wondering how a chicken's digestive wastes can be alkaline when chicken manure is known to be acidic. It's because droppings contain not only digestive waste but also urates (uric acid), which have an average pH of about 5.6 and therefore reduce poop's total pH. Exactly by how much

THE BEST VINEGAR?

Raw apple cider vinegar is often touted as being superior to pasteurized vinegars because (like yogurt) it contains a live culture. This culture, known as mother of vinegar, consists primarily of acetic acid–producing bacteria, or acetobacter, which need oxygen to survive. By contrast, the crop's lactic acid–producing bacteria require an oxygen-free environment.

Once a chicken swallows raw vinegar containing live acetobacter, the mother of vinegar won't survive long in the crop's anaerobic environment. And any other beneficial nutrients that might be in the mother are in such small amounts as to be inconsequential to the chicken's health.

So for most purposes the type of vinegar you use in a chicken's drinking water is immaterial. To qualify as vinegar a liquid must be at least 4 percent acetic acid. Most household vinegar — whether made from apple cider, distilled vegetables and fruits, or distilled petroleum — contains about 5 percent acetic acid. The pH of white vinegars generally ranges from 2.3 to 2.6, while slightly less acidic cider vinegars range from pH 3 to 3.3.

Every rule has an exception, so here it is: When treating a chicken with a respiratory disease that produces a lot of mucus in the mouth and throat, apple cider vinegar is the way to go. Apple skins contain tannin, the same type of astringent compound found in coffee, tea, and red wine that makes your mouth feel dry. The same property gives a sick chicken relief by helping clear the mucus from its mouth and throat. Add 1 tablespoon apple cider vinegar to each gallon of water (double the dose if you have hard water), and use as the sole source of drinking water until the condition clears up.

depends on the percentage of urates relative to digestive wastes, which in turn depends on many dietary and stress factors and varies throughout the day. Under normal conditions the average pH value of fresh chicken droppings lies somewhere between 6 and 7.

WHEN *NOT* TO USE VINEGAR

A hen suffering from heat stress needs to drink lots of water to cool down. Since chickens like the taste of vinegar, many backyard chicken keepers add vinegar to the drinking water to encourage their hens to drink more and prevent dehydration in hot summer weather.

A hen suffering from heat stress also pants to help keep cool, and rapid breathing increases the loss of carbon dioxide from her body. Carbon dioxide is derived from bicarbonate, which is used by the blood as a pH buffer and is extracted as carbon dioxide by the lungs from the blood. A loss of carbon dioxide therefore results in a loss of blood bicarbonate, increasing the pH level of the hen's blood — a condition called respiratory alkalosis.

Now wouldn't you think that adding vinegar to the drinking water would be a good way to reduce the blood's pH level? Not so! Just as acetic acid has no effect on digestive pH, it also has no effect on blood pH. The blood is self-buffering, using the buffer bicarbonate to maintain a somewhat constant pH.

Further, acidified water reduces the availability of calcium in a hen's diet. And one of the results of respiratory alkalosis is a decrease in blood calcium. Since a hen needs calcium to make eggshells, in hot weather she'll lay fewer eggs with thinner shells. Low blood calcium also interrupts nerve impulses, which results in weak muscles, and the hen will have trouble

pH Levels of a Chicken's Digestive System

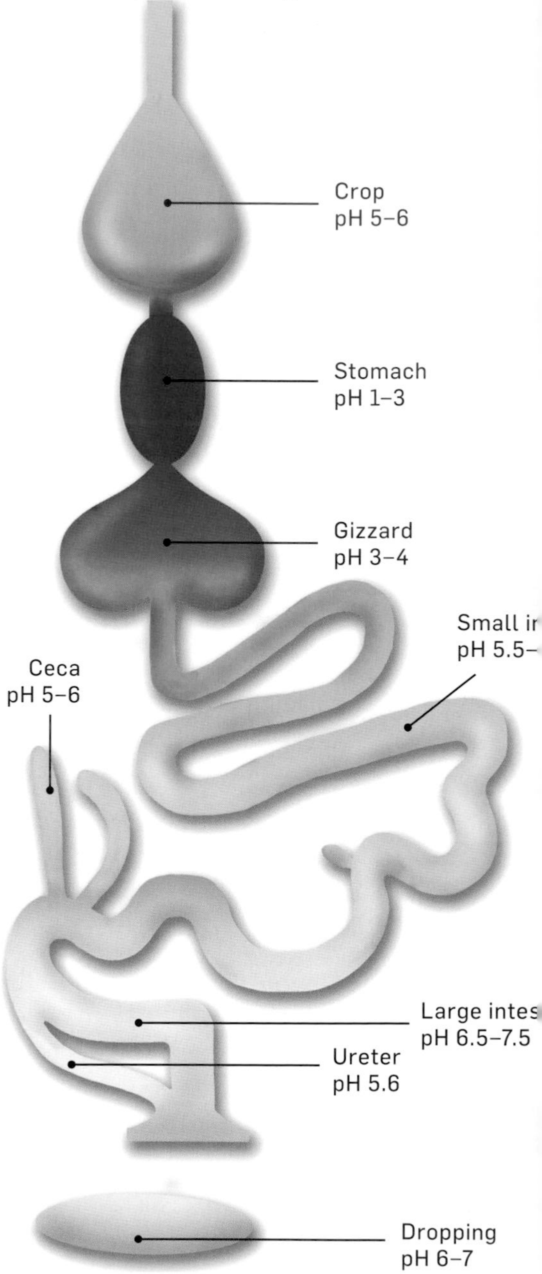

Crop
pH 5–6

Stomach
pH 1–3

Gizzard
pH 3–4

Small in
pH 5.5–

Ceca
pH 5–6

Large intes
pH 6.5–7.5

Ureter
pH 5.6

Dropping
pH 6–7

releasing the eggs she does lay. Since heat stress reduces blood calcium, the last thing you want to do is decrease the availability of dietary calcium by putting vinegar in the drinking water.

So what should you do? Counterintuitively, add sodium bicarbonate (baking soda) to the hen's drinking water. Why? Because when the hen's kidneys detect that the blood is alkaline, the kidneys attempt to decrease the blood's pH by filtering bicarbonate out of the blood and excreting it. Adding ¼ cup sodium bicarbonate per gallon of drinking water will help the hen restore her bicarbonate level; as the blood's buffer, the bicarbonate will do its job to restore blood pH to its proper level. Industrial egg producers know all this, which is why they feed sodium bicarbonate to their hens when hot weather is on the way.

Electrolytes

Also known simply as lytes, electrolytes are natural salts and other minerals — primarily calcium, chloride, magnesium, phosphorus, potassium, and sodium — that are present in the body in small quantities and that help regulate body processes, maintain the body's water balance, and preserve the body's acid/base balance. They are called electrolytes (from the Greek words *electro*, meaning "released," and *lytos*, meaning "dissolvable") because when dissolved in water they split into electrically charged particles (ions) that transmit electrical impulses from nerves to muscles.

Some of these ions have a positive charge, while others have a negative charge. For the body to maintain electrolytic balance, the sum of the positively charged ions must equal the sum of the negatively charged ions. For example, blood and other body fluids contain a high concentration of salt, or sodium chloride. Sodium is the body's major positively charged ion, while chloride is the body's major negatively charged ion, and the two balance each other.

Under ordinary circumstances you don't need to be concerned about your chickens' electrolyte levels, because they are largely determined by feed and water. Maintaining the right balance, therefore, involves providing your flock with proper nutrition and clean drinking water. Dehydration, however — from such things as heat stress, diarrhea, or a worm load — results in a depletion of these minerals from body fluids, upsetting the body's electrolytic balance.

Any time a chicken has loose droppings, or otherwise suffers from dehydration, adding an electrolyte supplement to its drinking water will help restore electrolytic balance, which in turn helps its body replace and retain fluids. That's because one of the many functions of electrolytes is to make sure the water a chicken drinks gets to the body cells that need it.

PH AND ELECTROLYTES

The body's pH balance is intricately related to its electrolyte balance. A pH imbalance can lead to an electrolyte imbalance, and an electrolyte imbalance can lead to a pH imbalance.

Conversely, restoring the electrolyte balance helps restore the body's pH balance, and the other way around.

You can mix up a homemade electrolyte solution from ingredients commonly found in the kitchen, although electrolyte mixtures designed specifically for chickens are available in several brands from most poultry suppliers. Another option is Alltech Acid-Pak 4-Way, which combines electrolytes, organic acidifiers, enzymes, and probiotics all in one solution. Pedialyte works in a pinch and is better for

Electrolyte Caveats

⚠️ *Do not* give electrolytes to a healthy chicken; it can cause an electrolytic imbalance opposite to the desired effect.

Do not consider electrolytes to be a substitute for proper medication if your chickens are suffering from diarrhea caused by coccidiosis or any other disease.

Homemade Electrolyte Solution

INGREDIENT	SOURCE	AMOUNT
Potassium chloride	Salt substitute	½ teaspoon (2 g)
Sodium bicarbonate	Baking soda	1 teaspoon (5 g)
Sodium chloride	Table salt	1 teaspoon (6 g)
Sucrose	Sugar	1 tablespoon (12 g)
Water		1 gallon (4 L)

chickens than Gatorade because it contains less sugar. Offer an electrolyte solution in place of drinking water 4 to 6 hours a day for no more than a week; at other times replace the solution with fresh drinking water.

Garlic Guidelines

Garlic (*Allium sativum*) is well known to have broad-spectrum antimicrobial properties, making it effective against many bacteria, fungi, viruses, and internal parasites, including protozoa. Garlic's principal active ingredient is allicin, the compound responsible for garlic's distinct flavor and pungent odor.

Fresh garlic contains the allicin precursor alliin, which has no odor. Crushing or chopping garlic releases the enzyme alliinase, which acts on alliin to form unstable sulfur-containing organic compounds, allicin being the main one. Interestingly, organic sulfur compounds derived from sources other than garlic include sulfa drugs and penicillin.

Volatile allicin rapidly degrades, meanwhile reacting with garlic's other components to form a variety of additional organic sulfur compounds with varying antimicrobial properties. One of these additional compounds is ajoene, which has antiviral, antifungal, and antiparasitic properties.

SUGAR SOLUTION

A time-honored practice for energizing weak chicks, especially those that have endured being shipped by mail, is to add sugar to their drinking water. When chicks aren't shipped with an electrolyte pack, and you have none on hand, dissolve ¾ cup plain sugar in ½ gallon of fresh water (75 g/L) and offer it as the sole source of drinking water for 1 week. Rinse out the drinker every day, and replace any leftover sugar solution with a fresh batch.

Both allicin and ajoene work by blocking enzymes needed by pathogens for metabolism. At low concentrations they don't inhibit enough enzymes to outright destroy pathogens, but they can reduce the pathogens' virulence. At higher concentrations they can affect enough enzymes to kill pathogens.

Between them allicin and ajoene affect the viability of some two dozen different pathogenic organisms. And — unlike sulfa drugs and penicillin — they do not promote resistance. However — also unlike sulfa drugs and penicillin — garlic does not function as a systemic antibiotic but rather kills on contact. It therefore might be considered to be more of an antiseptic than an antibiotic, although raw garlic should never be applied directly to the skin (for example, to prevent infection of a wound), because it can cause serious blistering.

GARLIC BENEFITS

"If it sounds too good to be true, it probably is" does not entirely apply to garlic, which has so many beneficial properties that researchers haven't yet discovered them all. On a basic level garlic contains oligosaccharides — prebiotics that stimulate the growth of beneficial bacteria in the large intestine, thus stimulating immunity. Small amounts of crushed raw garlic fed to baby chicks twice a week not only help their immune systems develop but also get them used to the flavor so they will be more likely to accept it later in life.

Raw garlic may be used to boost the immune system of a droopy mature chicken by serving as an appetite stimulant. Add crushed garlic to the drinking water at the rate of four cloves per gallon, providing fresh garlic water daily.

Chickens that have been conditioned from a young age to accept the flavor of garlic should have no trouble drinking the water. For chickens that are unfamiliar with garlic, reduce the initial amount until they will drink, then gradually increase the amount up to four cloves per gallon. Meanwhile, should a chicken's condition require antibiotic treatment, garlic will work synergistically with the drug.

Garlic juice spray may be used to control northern fowl mites. For details see Garlic Juice Spray on page 388.

Immersing crushed garlic in oil concentrates ajoenes, making garlic oil effective against fungi, including ringworm. For details see Garlic Oil on page 388.

Garlic powder, added to chicken feed at the rate of 1.5 pounds per 50 pounds (0.6 kg per 20 kg) of ration, has been found to neutralize the odor of manure, but apparently it does not affect the flavor of eggs. Taste testers, in fact, preferred eggs from hens fed garlic, claiming they tasted milder. Researchers speculate that garlic somehow reduces the eggs' sulfur content.

Exactly how garlic works all these miracles, and more, is still pretty much a mystery, largely because of its highly complex chemistry. However, it's fairly clear that allicin and allicin-derived compounds metabolize rather rapidly, working alone or synergistically to exert a variety of beneficial effects on different body systems.

GARLIC CAUTIONS

Different strains of garlic contain varying amounts of alliin; some strains have nearly three times as much as others. Production methods and length of storage also influence alliin content, as does method of preparation — whether used freshly crushed, added to water, made into an extract, or dried by low heat or high heat.

Further, different types of preparations have different antimicrobial properties. And a lot of the research proving garlic's various benefits uses concentrated, refined ("pure") extracts or commercially prepared garlic supplements applied to microbes in a laboratory setting, using test tubes rather than live animals. Additionally, the chemical structures of both allicin and ajoene can, and often are, chemically synthesized to create garlic supplements.

Theoretically, garlic can kill pathogens in the digestive tract, *if* it comes into direct contact with them. In fact, no one has proven that garlic works against any specific disease. Further, although garlic largely targets pathogenic bacteria, to a lesser extent it also affects beneficial bacteria. Based on the possibility that garlic may kill intestinal bacteria, and especially if it is used in combination with an antibiotic drug, follow

GARLIC JUICE SPRAY

To make garlic juice spray, peel cloves from one head of garlic and crush them in a garlic press or whirl them in a food processor. Drain out the juice by pressing the pulp into a mesh strainer over a bowl. To remove small bits of pulp that get through the strainer and might clog your sprayer, strain the juice through a piece of cheesecloth or a paper coffee filter. One head of garlic should yield about ¼ cup of

juice. Combine ¼ cup (about 55 mL) of garlic juice with 2¼ cups (500 mL) of water to make a 10 percent garlic juice spray.

To control northern fowl mites, apply the spray to the affected chicken's vent weekly for 3 weeks, and thereafter as needed to maintain control. If fresh spray irritates the skin around a chicken's vent, age the spray a couple of days before using it.

GARLIC OIL

To make garlic oil, peel garlic cloves and crush them in a garlic press or whirl them in a food processor. Measure the quantity of crushed garlic, and immerse it in four times the amount of oil. For example, if you crush 1 tablespoon (15 g) of garlic, combine it with ¼ cup or 4 tablespoons (56 g) olive oil, peanut oil, or whatever type of oil you normally use in the kitchen. Infuse the garlic in the oil for at least 4 hours.

To treat a chicken with ringworm, wear disposable gloves and either dip your gloved

fingers into the oil or dip a cotton ball into the oil, and apply it directly to the affected areas, taking care not to get any into the chicken's eyes. Apply daily until the ringworm clears up, preparing fresh oil every other day for maximum effectiveness.

Note that garlic oil is not the same as garlic essential oil. Garlic oil uses oil to extract garlic; garlic essential oil is the pure oily component of garlic and, like all essential oils, is potentially toxic.

treatment with a probiotic to ensure an adequate population of beneficial intestinal bacteria.

A much-discussed issue among chicken keepers is that some of garlic's organic sulfur compounds are toxic thiosulfates, which potentially can cause hemolytic anemia, a serious disorder that destroys red blood cells. However, birds are somewhat protected by the fact that their red blood cells have a nucleus — unlike the red blood cells of cats and dogs, both of which are much more sensitive to the toxic effect of thiosulfates. Further, compared to onions, the thiosulphate level in garlic is so minimal as to be barely traceable. When chickens eat small amounts of garlic over a long period of time, their red blood cells regenerate nearly as fast as they are destroyed. Bottom line: a chicken would have to eat an awful lot of garlic all at one time to develop hemolytic anemia. (For signs of thiosulfate toxicity, see Go Easy on Kitchen Scraps on page 307.)

Colloidal Silver

Silver, though rare, is one of the basic elements that make up the earth's crust. Trace amounts of silver are naturally consumed in food and water, and to a lesser extent inhaled from the air. Despite its ubiquity, silver is not an essential nutrient, but neither is it harmful (except when, consumed in excessive quantities, it turns the skin blue). Most silver passes through the body and is excreted within a few days to a few months.

Colloidal silver consists of tiny particles of silver suspended in water. Being a colloidal solution, the particles remain suspended, do not settle out, and cannot be filtered out. Many of the particles are in the form of positively charged silver ions (silver atoms missing an electron). Because they are positively charged,

they repel each other and therefore remain evenly spread throughout the colloidal solution.

Most pathogens have a net negative charge. They therefore attract positively charged silver ions, which then kill the pathogens by binding to and destroying their amino acids (proteins). Although colloidal silver is highly toxic to most bacteria, fungi, protozoa, and some viruses, it is nontoxic to chickens (and humans), making it a safe and natural time-tested antimicrobial.

Online information abounds on where to buy or how to make a colloidal silver generator, which makes sense if you intend to use large amounts and are willing to have your results lab-tested for purity and concentration. Commercially prepared colloidal silver, sold as a dietary supplement or as a homeopathic remedy (which it is not), is relatively expensive, but for most uses a little goes a long way. It is available by the quart or pint, or in smaller quantities with an eyedropper or a fine mister, or as a first-aid salve or gel.

For chickens the best use of colloidal silver is for relief from infections of the eye, skin, or upper respiratory tract. For an eye infection, put a couple of drops into the eye. For a skin infection, apply drops, mist, or salve/gel. For an upper respiratory infection, spray into the chicken's mouth, place a few drops into the mouth for the chicken to swallow, or put a few drops on the chicken's nostrils for the chicken to inhale. Repeat the treatment twice daily until the condition clears up. You should start seeing results within a day or two.

As a broad-spectrum antibiotic, colloidal silver can bind good bacteria as well as harmful bacteria. After treating a chicken internally, follow up with a probiotic to ensure an adequate population of beneficial bacteria in the digestive tract.

Benefits of Biochar

Charcoal is a black, porous, solid form of carbon obtained by heating wood in the absence of air, which keeps it from burning down into ashes. Although some people equate biochar with charcoal, the difference is that biochar is made by burning any kind of organic matter — which in fact could be chicken litter or chicken bones — and is typically used as a soil amendment. Charcoal and biochar are considered to be elemental forms of carbon, in contrast to activated charcoal, which has been treated by heating it in the presence of air to remove noncarbon impurities and increase its porosity; then it's cooled and crushed into a powder to increase its surface area.

For centuries, elemental and activated charcoal have been used to counteract toxins consumed by humans and other animals. In nature, animals have been observed eating bits of natural char in burned-over areas. Charcoal is therefore a normal part of the diet of animals living in a natural environment. Exactly how it is so effective as a detoxifier is not well understood. What is known is that it binds toxins, then is excreted along with the toxins.

Charcoal in all forms is flavorless, inert, nonsoluble, and indigestible and has no nutritional value or medicinal properties. But thanks to its porous nature, it has the ability to soak up toxins and remove them from an animal's system.

When fed to chickens, charcoal has the ability to bind mycotoxins that might be in the feed (see Mycotoxicoses on page 247). It also has the ability to bind pesticides contaminating feed and herbicides in feed ingredients, such as those that result from spraying weed killers on GMO corn and soy crops (see Avoiding GMOs on page 39). Such feed contaminants can adversely affect a chicken's digestive system, not to mention the beneficial microbes living therein.

Charcoal can absorb up to five times its weight in moisture. Fed to a chicken suffering from diarrhea, it not only absorbs the excess moisture to tighten up the droppings but also binds any pathogenic bacteria that might be causing the diarrhea. By removing pathogens, it stimulates the activity of beneficial microbes in the digestive system.

Charcoal also has the ability to deodorize chicken droppings. Here's how it works: The end product of protein metabolism is nitrogen, which the chicken expels from its body as urates (the white cap on top of a brown poop). Bacteria convert urates into ammonia. When chickens eat charcoal, the bacteria convert urates into the odorless salt ammonium, rather than the smelly gas ammonia. As a result, the litter remains drier and doesn't develop a strong ammonia odor, and because the nitrogen isn't gassed off as ammonia, the litter makes better compost for your garden.

Little chicks will readily pick at char, and studies have shown that chicks fed char during their first 4 weeks of life grow better. Hens offered char free choice lay eggs with better shell quality, resulting in fewer eggs cracked in the nest or during collection. Hardwood charcoal is gritty and, when broken into pieces about the size of kitty litter, lodges in the gizzard and enhances digestion.

SOURCES FOR CHAR

Pharmaceutical-grade activated charcoal, typically derived from vegetable matter, is readily available in capsule or powder form. Closely related is elemental charcoal that comes from burning wood. A keyword Internet search will yield an abundance of instructions on how to make biochar. You can also glean charcoal from your fireplace or wood-burning stove. You would, of course, want to use only natural, untreated firewood with no additives and no chemical fire starter.

When the ashes have cooled, screen out the chunks of charred wood, smash them into smaller pieces, and feed them to your chickens free choice in a bowl or hopper separate from their regular ration. You will know the chickens are eating it not only because the char disappears but also because their droppings will become darker and firmer.

Offering char free choice, rather than mixing it into the ration, gives chickens the opportunity to take it or leave it. Too much mixed into the ration can cause chickens to fill up on char, which has no nutritional value, at the expense of needed nutrients. Further, activated charcoal is not fussy about what it binds and can bind essential nutrients as well as toxins.

OMRI AND AAFCO NIX CHARCOAL

Charcoal works so well against both natural and synthetic toxins that it essentially has been banned from commercial livestock feeds. The principle objection is that it might be used by unscrupulous producers to deliberately feed animals contaminated rations, or it might be used to remove, and thus mask the use of, illegal drug residues from food-producing animals. Although charcoal itself is nontoxic, if it is used indiscriminately to mop up toxins and overused drugs, the sheer volume thus passed through livestock can cause the resulting char to become a hazardous substance.

In 2002 the Organic Materials Review Institute (OMRI) issued a report admitting that activated charcoal is considered to be a universal poison antidote. However, the report pointed out, commercially prepared carbon may be obtained from a variety of sources, some of which are not acceptable in organic production. In addition, different brands are activated by a number of different processes, some of which include chemicals that are not acceptable in organic production. Because not all activated charcoal is created equal, OMRI considers activated charcoal in general to be synthetic, and therefore may be used by organic producers only with restrictions: limited to therapeutic purposes and prohibited in routine feeding in the absence of poisoning. Along with expressing concern about the carbon source and method of activation, OMRI's report indicated that if charcoal were approved as a feed supplement, unscrupulous producers might use it to conceal substances that are prohibited in organic production.

In 2012 the Association of American Feed Control Officials (AAFCO) withdrew support of activated charcoal as a feed ingredient. AAFCO is responsible for regulations governing the manufacture, labeling, distribution, and sale of animal feed. By listing activated charcoal in its table of withdrawn ingredients, AAFCO effectively made the commercial use of charcoal powder in animal feeds or supplements illegal. Among the reasons cited are that charcoal has no nutritional value; that the charcoal itself could be contaminated; and that feed manufacturers may be tempted to indiscriminately use charcoal as a binder of toxins and other feed contaminants.

Laxative Flushes

When a chicken suffers from an intestinal disease, poisoning, or botulism, and you have no activated charcoal on hand, you can hasten recovery by flushing the bird's system with a laxative that rapidly removes toxins from the body. Epsom salt (magnesium sulfate) makes the best flush, especially for a chicken that is unable to eat or drink and therefore must be treated individually. Molasses or milk powder, as well as Epsom salt, may be used as a flock-wide flush.

When Epsom salt or milk powder is added to feed, the chickens will drink more than usual. To prevent dehydration, make sure plenty of water is available at all times.

Flushing makes a mess, so be prepared to follow up with a thorough cleaning and fresh litter. If the chickens are on pasture, move them to new ground daily.

Epsom salt flush, individual: 1 teaspoon Epsom salt dissolved in 2 tablespoons of water, gently poured or squirted down the bird's throat twice daily for 2 or 3 days, or until the bird recovers

Epsom salt flush, in feed: 1 pound Epsom salt per 15 pounds feed (1 kg/15 kg) as the sole ration for 1 day

Epsom salt flush, in water: 1 pound Epsom salt per 5 gallons water (0.5 kg/20 L) as the sole source of drinking water for 1 day

Molasses flush: 2 cups molasses per 5 gallons water (250 mL/20 L), offered for no longer than 4 hours; then clean the drinker, and fill with fresh, untreated water

Milk flush, in feed: 1 pound of milk powder per 3 pounds of feed (1 kg/3 kg) as the sole ration for 1 day

Some chicken keepers believe that milk, offered occasionally or continuously, will prevent coccidiosis. Not so. Feeding an excessive amount of lactose to induce diarrhea is a method of controlling an existing outbreak of coccidiosis by flushing out the coccidial protozoa. It works only if scrupulous cleanup prevents the chickens from ingesting the expelled coccidia, thereby avoiding reinfection until the disease runs its course.

Note, too, that the bacterium *Escherichia coli* considers lactose to be prime food. *E. coli* bacteria are normally present in small numbers in every chicken's gut, but during times of stress or illness, these bacteria can proliferate out of control. Feeding milk to chickens at such times also feeds the *E. coli*, giving them extra nutrients (in the form of lactose) that allow them to multiply in excessive numbers.

Herbal Remedies

Herbal medicine uses whole plants and plant extracts to treat disease and maintain health. Herbs have a variety of desirable properties, from containing healthful nutrients that are lacking in pharmacological drugs to the ability to work synergistically with drugs to reduce required dosages. Unlike antibiotics, the active components of herbal compounds are readily absorbed along with other digestive contents and rapidly excreted, with little (if any) risk of accumulated residues.

A problem with herbal therapy, however, is that the effectiveness of different herbs for specific diseases has not been scientifically validated. Accordingly, instructions found online and in print publications describing herbal medicine for backyard chickens suggest that such-and-such herb "is said to" work for a certain disease, or that you "try" such-and-such herb as a treatment — which sounds suspiciously like experimenting at the expense of an ailing chicken.

Another problem with herbs is that their potency varies with cultivar, as well as with growing, harvesting, and storage conditions. Most herbal research involves the use of essential oil, which is a concentrated form of a plant's volatile aromatic compounds. Such an oil is "essential" in the sense that its complex chemistry comprises the plant's essence. Because essential oils are highly concentrated, their misuse can lead to toxicity. Therefore, unless you are a trained herbalist, use only fresh or dried herbs for your backyard chickens.

Although you probably wouldn't want to treat an ailing chicken with unproven herbal remedies, nothing is wrong with taking advantage of the various beneficial properties of herbs to stimulate your chickens' immunity. Herbs may be tied in bunches and hung around the coop, where the chickens can pick what they want. Or they might be grown in the chicken yard, protected by wire cages, so chickens can peck at any leaves they can reach without destroying the whole plants.

Herbs also may be added to feed or drinking water. First dry and crush the herbs (or grind them into a powder). Then either stir the herbs into the chickens' regular ration, or steep them in hot water — as you would make tea — cool the water, strain out the herbs, and add the resulting herbal tea to the chickens' drinking water.

Start with small amounts to make sure your chickens continue eating and drinking as usual. If a particular herb puts them off feed or discourages drinking because they don't like the taste, back off. Some of the most commonly used herbs for chickens are listed in the table on page 394.

Homeopathic Remedies

In contrast to drugs, many of which merely treat symptoms, the intent of homeopathic medicine is to restore health by curing the underlying cause of illness. The word "homeopathy" derives from the Greek words *homoios*, meaning "similar," and *patheia*, meaning "suffering." Accordingly, homeopathic remedies consist of small amounts of natural substances that, in a healthy individual, produce symptoms similar to the condition the treatment is designed to cure. In homeopathic terms, like cures like.

HOMEOPATHIC PRINCIPLES

The principles of homeopathy are pretty simple, although the practice is anything but. Every remedy is associated with countless conditions, and every condition may be treated with countless remedies. The skill is in finding the right remedy, or combination of remedies, for a given situation.

Since its discovery some 200 years ago, homeopathy has focused more on human ailments than on those of animals. Trained homeopathic practitioners use two huge reference volumes, both of which come in several different versions: a *Repertory*, which lists conditions and gives appropriate remedies for each, and a *Materia Medica*, which lists remedies and indicates what conditions they treat.

Here are some examples of common homeopathic remedies: Arnica, derived from a member of the sunflower family, is a treatment for blunt trauma that causes bruising or swelling. Spongia, derived from marine sponges, is used to treat respiratory issues. Symphytum, derived from comfrey, is used to mend broken bones.

Homeopathic remedies are packaged in the form of either a liquid or pills. Since a remedy must be applied to mucous membranes for absorption, liquid drops are easier to use on a chicken, but a pill may be dissolved in a little water and applied as a liquid. A drop is applied either inside the chicken's mouth (to be swallowed) or on a nostril (to be inhaled).

Remedies given to chickens and other animals are based on conditions that appear similar to human illnesses. One of the problems in selecting a correct remedy for an animal is that the animal can't tell you what hurts, so a remedy must be selected based on visible signs.

A chicken poses the additional complications that a bird's body differs in both structure and metabolism from that of a human or other mammal, and birds are susceptible to conditions that don't affect humans.

So the best anyone can do is to take an educated guess as to the correct remedy for the situation and go from there. A trained homeopathic practitioner documents what worked in the past and therefore is quicker to use the correct remedy to treat the same condition again in the future.

Herbs for Chickens

HERB	PROPERTIES	USES
Basil (*Ocimum basilicum*)	Antioxidant, antimicrobial, anti-inflammatory	Improve circulatory health and bone health; reduce stress
Dandelion (*Taraxacum* spp.)	Antioxidant, anti-inflammatory	Improve digestion, kidney health, liver health, and bone health; relieve pain
Dill (*Anethum graveolens*)	Antioxidant, antibacterial, anti-inflammatory	Improve digestion and respiratory health; reduce stress; relieve diarrhea
Lavender (*Lavandula angustifolia*)	Antiseptic, antifungal, anti-inflammatory	Heal wounds and insect bites; improve digestion; reduce stress; relieve pain
Marigold (*Calendula officinalis*)	Antioxidant, antiseptic, antibacterial, anti-inflammatory	Heal wounds and insect bites; improve liver health; relieve diarrhea
Mint (*Mentha* spp.)	Antiseptic, antioxidant	Heal wounds and insect bites; improve digestion; reduce stress
Nasturtium (*Tropaeolum majus*)	Antiseptic, antibacterial, antifungal	Heal wounds; improve digestion; relieve congestion
Oregano (*Origanum vulgare*)	Antioxidant, antimicrobial, anti-inflammatory	Improve respiratory health and digestion
Parsley (*Petroselinum crispum*)	Antioxidant, anti-inflammatory	Improve circulatory health, bone health, nerve health, and digestion
Rosemary (*Rosmarinus officinalis*)	Antiseptic, antioxidant, antibacterial, anti-inflammatory	Heal wounds; improve circulatory health, digestion, and respiratory health; relieve pain
Thyme (*Thymus vulgaris*)	Antioxidant, antibacterial, antifungal	Improve respiratory health and digestion

HOMEOPATHIC RESOURCES

Learning to determine correct remedies takes many years of training and experience. Some simple first-aid remedies are safe to attempt at home, but treating a serious condition should be left to a homeopathic veterinarian. Although using an incorrect remedy on an ailing chicken is neither beneficial nor harmful, if the chicken is seriously ill you could lose valuable time while seeking an appropriate remedy. Veterinarians who are certified by the Academy of Veterinary Homeopathy add the letters CVH (certified veterinary homeopath) or CHom (certified homeopath) following DVM (doctor of veterinary medicine) after their names.

A number of beginner's guides to homeopathy are available, most of which deal with human issues. A good deal of information may be found online by doing a keyword search of "homeopathy for chickens."

Remedies for Health Problems of the Organic Laying Flock is a compendium of homeopathic remedies and other natural treatments for chickens, compiled by Karma E. Glos under a Sustainable Agriculture Research and Education Project grant (SARE project FNE02-415, 2002). It is available online as a free PDF download by doing a keyword search for the title.

Whether or not homeopathic remedies work is a matter of debate. Disbelievers attribute any success to the placebo effect, whereby human patients who believe they will get better do. However, naysayers aren't able to explain the successes homeopathic veterinarians have in dealing with animal issues that have proven difficult or impossible to treat with pharmaceuticals, since an animal has no expectation that any particular treatment will or won't make it better.

Treating Wounds

The most common causes of bleeding wounds are a rooster's treading on a hen while mating; mauling by a dog or other predator; and getting snagged on a protruding nail, stiff wire, or other barnyard hazard. Peck-order fighting may also result in wounds, but they are rarely deep or serious.

Any injury must be treated promptly, or it will attract picking that can quickly become outright cannibalism. As soon as you discover an injured bird, isolate it. If the injury is serious, pull feathers from around the edges so you can more easily assess the damage, and so surrounding feathers won't stick in the wound and hinder healing. Flush away dried blood, broken tissue, feather bits, and other debris with a wound wash.

Aspirin for Pain

A chicken that is suffering pain from inflammation due to an injury, infection, or frostbite can be relieved with aspirin. One way is to open the chicken's beak and pop in a low-dose (baby) aspirin. An easier way is to dissolve the aspirin in the bird's drinking water. The operative word here is "dissolve." Most aspirin tablets do not readily dissolve. If you crush and stir the tablets into water, within a few minutes much of the aspirin will settle to the bottom of the drinker.

For this purpose you need readily soluble, uncoated aspirin (such as the GeriCare brand). The approximate dosage for a chicken is 25 mg per pound (0.5 kg) of body weight per day, which for a 5-pound chicken amounts to approximately one-third of a standard 325 mg aspirin tablet.

To make life simple, dissolve five aspirin tablets in 1 gallon of fresh water and offer it to the ailing chicken as its only source of drinking water. Mix a fresh batch daily for 3 days or until the inflammation subsides and the chicken perks up.

Like other nonsteroidal anti-inflammatory drugs, aspirin increases blood flow through the kidneys and can eventually lead to kidney damage. So although regularly giving aspirin to a chicken with a chronic condition such as articular gout may decrease pain and thus increase mobility, it may also shorten the chicken's life.

Aspirin and Bleeding

⚠ Never give aspirin to a chicken with a visible bleeding injury, or that may have internal bleeding after being mauled. As a blood thinner, aspirin inhibits clotting.

Wound Washes

Antiseptic solutions such as chlorhexidine (Hibiclens), hydrogen peroxide, and povidone iodine are fine for initially flushing a wound, but if the injury is deep enough to require regular flushing, such harsh solutions can damage tissue and inhibit healing. Frequent flushing of a deep wound helps prevent the healing tissue from drying out and reduces the chance of a deep infection by allowing tissue to heal from the inside outward.

Saline wound wash has the same salt concentration as blood. Compared to using plain water, saline wash causes less tissue damage and doesn't sting. It also discourages the growth of bacteria in the wound and is relatively inexpensive, especially if you make your own (see Make a Saline Wound Wash on the next page.) Purchased saline solution goes by many names, including normal saline solution, sodium chloride 0.9 percent solution, and isotonic sodium chloride.

For a really nasty wound, sodium hypochlorite (household bleach) wash has the advantage of killing most bacteria found in open wounds, as well as flushing dead cells away from healing tissue. On the downside, this wash will damage healthy tissue. Take care not to get any in the chicken's eyes, protect healthy tissue surrounding the wound with petroleum jelly (Vaseline), and use bleach solution for no more than 48 hours, then switch to a saline wash. If

---

MAKE A DAKIN'S WOUND WASH

Dakin's Solution comes in full strength, half strength, and quarter strength. This formula makes a half-strength solution. For a weaker, and therefore less irritating, one-quarter-strength solution, use half the amount of bleach.

In a clean pot with a lid, bring 1 quart of water to a boil with the lid on, and continue boiling for 5 minutes. (Instead of boiling the water, you could use distilled water.) Remove the pot from the heat, and stir in 3 tablespoons household bleach (5.25 percent sodium hypochlorite) and ½ teaspoon baking soda.

Pour the solution into a clean jar, seal tightly, label it, and keep it at room temperature in a dark place, or exclude light by tightly wrapping the jar with foil. Unopened, this wash will keep for up to a month. After opening the jar, use the remaining solution within 48 hours, or discard it and prepare a new solution.

In a clean pot with a lid, combine 1½ teaspoons noniodized table salt with 1 quart of water (9 g/L). If your tap water is alkaline (hard water), use distilled water instead. Leaving the lid on, bring the water to a boil, allow it to boil for 5 minutes, then remove the pot from the heat to let the solution cool.

Use the solution as soon as it has cooled to body temperature, or pour it into a clean jar, label it, and store it in the refrigerator. To avoid contamination, use homemade saline wound wash within a week. If the wash gets cloudy, discard it and prepare a new solution.

the bleach solution causes the chicken's skin to become reddened, swollen, or blistered, discontinue it immediately.

Sodium hypochlorite solutions of varying strengths are commercially available under the brand Dakin's, named after one of the men who developed the formula to treat wounded soldiers during World War I, a time when today's antiseptics were not yet available. You can mix your own Dakin's, but it won't keep as well as the commercial brand (see Make a Dakin's Wound Wash on the facing page.) Dakin's is, after all, a bleach solution, so be prepared for it to bleach out your towel and possibly whatever you are wearing when you use the wash.

Flushing Out a Wound

The first thing to do on discovering that a chicken has been injured is to clean out the wound to assess the damage, prevent infection, and promote healing. If the chicken is tame, you might handle it without restraint. If it is not tame, wrap it in a towel to keep it from struggling and causing further injury to itself or you. Either way, you'll need a towel to soak up the wound wash.

Use a 10 mL or 12 mL syringe to apply the wash. You can use either a catheter-tip syringe (which looks like a regular syringe but has an extended tip) or a regular syringe with the needle removed.

A certain amount of pressure is needed to successfully flush out a wound. A syringe allows you to squirt the wash in a steady stream. But too much pressure will drive bacteria and debris deeper into the wound, so press on the plunger just enough to let the flush carry out debris. Pick out stubborn debris with a pair of tweezers.

The more wash you use, the better the wound will be cleaned, up to a point. Flush until you see no more debris, then keep flushing a little longer. The more pathogens that are flushed out the less likely it is that the wound will become infected.

How much wash is needed depends on the size of the wound. As a general rule each 1 inch (25 mm) of laceration can require as many as 15 syringes full of flush for the initial cleaning. Continue to flush a relatively minor wound once a day; flush a draining or contaminated wound twice daily. *Do not* flush a wound that is deep enough to extend into the body cavity.

CALMING A NERVOUS BIRD

A chicken that's not accustomed to being handled, or one that's been traumatized by a predator attack, may struggle enough to make treatment difficult. In such a case you can calm the chicken by putting it into a trance. In this hypnotic state the bird's heart rate and respiration rate are slightly reduced, and the bird temporarily loses its ability to move.

Sometimes turning a chicken onto its back is enough to put it into a trance. A reluctant chicken may be encouraged to relax by gently stroking its throat or running your finger slowly from the wattles down the chest and between the legs. If the chicken still doesn't cooperate, place its head under one of its wings and gently rock the bird back and forth until it relaxes in your hands.

Generally, the flightier the bird, the longer it will remain in a trance, which can last anywhere from 15 seconds to a minute or more. If the bird awakens before you finish treatment, repeat the trance-inducing procedure. When you're done, let the bird revive on its own, give it a gentle nudge, or turn it onto its feet and hold it until it stands on its own.

How to Calm a Nervous Chicken

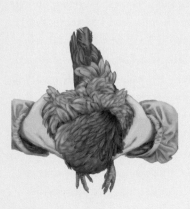

1. Tuck the chicken's head under one wing.

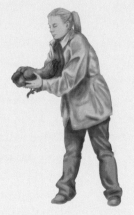

2. Firmly grasp the chicken in both hands.

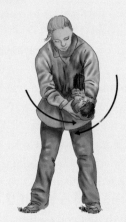

3. Rock it back and forth until you feel it relax.

Wound Flushing

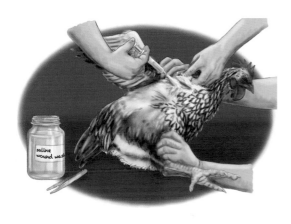

Use a syringe to squirt wash into a wound to clear out bacteria, dead skin, feather bits, and other debris. Use tweezers to remove any stubborn debris that remains visible.

Wound Care

A wound that dries out can lead to cell damage, but a wound that remains moist will heal faster. To a certain extent a chicken will moisten its own wound with oil from its preen gland. You can help it along by coating the wound with a hydrogel (water-based) wound ointment for the first 2 days.

As the wound heals, a lanolin cream or a thick ointment such as Ichthammol will keep the tissue soft and elastic. After 5 days the wound should be well on the way to healing. Leave the wound open, and keep an eye on it to make sure it stays clean.

Since flies spread bacteria on their feet, keep your recovering patient where flies can't get to the wound. Throughout the chicken's recovery, isolate it from other chickens, so they won't peck at the wound, and provide adequate feed and fresh water. A recovering chicken that is disinclined to eat may be encouraged by frequent feeding or stirring of the feed and might be tempted with a variety of the treats it likes best.

Wound Complications

If the injury is on the bird's foot or is quite large, or the chicken picks at it and makes it worse, cover it with a gauze pad and first-aid tape, and fashion a wrap with tape to hold the dressing in place and keep the chicken from picking it off. Exactly how to wrap the tape depends, of course, on the location of the wound. Regularly change the dressing, and examine the wound to make sure it is healing properly and doesn't become infected.

If the wound becomes infected, you'll need to remove the scab so you can treat the underlying infection. An infected wound might drain a murky fluid, develop a yellow scab or a scab that gets larger as time goes by, become increasingly more tender to the touch, become surrounded by increasing redness, or not heal within 2 weeks. Repeatedly coat such a wound with baby oil, or a thick ointment such as Desitin or Ichthammol, for a few days until the scab softens and comes loose. Clean out the infection, and retreat the wound as if it were fresh.

If the wound is really deep, or is the result of an animal bite, you may need an antibiotic to prevent infection. A vet should be able to advise you, but if you can't find a local vet who is knowledgeable about chickens, your next best option is to use a relatively safe broad-spectrum tetracycline antibiotic (as described on page 242), according to directions on the package. The most common bacteria to infect wounds are staphylococci and streptococci.

A wound that's deep enough or wide enough to require stitching is best attended to by a veterinarian or other person experienced with sterile needles, sutures, and numbing medication, and who can determine whether the wound needs a drain tube. However, lots of chicken keepers have successfully stitched up wounds with a sharp sewing needle and thread. A wound that needs stitching is generally one that goes beneath the skin, is too wide to be easily held closed with surgical tape, and occurs in a part of the chicken's body that stretches whenever the bird moves.

Depending on how seriously the chicken is injured, it may go into shock, and the more you handle it, the deeper into shock the bird will sink. To reduce the possibility of shock, work gently on the wound, then let the chicken rest in a quiet, stress-free, warm environment.

What Went Wrong?

If, despite your best efforts, a sick or injured chicken doesn't get better, one or more of the following may be the reason:

- The diagnosis was wrong.

- The organism causing the disease was resistant to the treatment used.

- An inadequate dose of medication was used.

- The medication was administered improperly (reread the label).

- The medication's expiration date has long since passed (try a fresh batch).

- An incompatible combination of medications was used.

- The treatment caused adverse side effects.

- The bird was reinfected (treatment was discontinued too soon).

- An inflammation, abscess, or other condition interfered with treatment.

- The bird had more than one type of infection, and not all of them were treated.

- A biosecurity breach was not corrected (look for ways to improve management).

- The disease was caused by a nutritional deficiency that was not corrected.

- Supportive therapy was inadequate.

- The bird's immune defense was too low (due to the disease, drug use, or poor nutrition).

TREATING SHOCK

Shock is a condition brought on by a sudden drop in blood pressure. It can result from excessive bleeding, a bacterial infection, or severe stress, such as having been chased and caught by a dog and shaken in the dog's mouth. Signs of shock include cold, pale skin; rapid breathing; dilated pupils; weakness; and sometimes prostration and death.

If a bird-oriented vet is close at hand, the chicken *may* recover after emergency veterinary treatment with steroids and fluids. Otherwise, the best you can do is keep the bird warm and calm until it either recovers or — sadly — dies.

CHAPTER 15

Your Chickens and Your Health

Two questions I hear often from first-time chicken owners are: "Will my chickens make me (or my neighbors) sick?" and "Do I have to give up my chickens if I get pregnant?" The important thing to remember is that you can't catch a disease from a chicken that doesn't have the disease in the first place.

As for pregnancy, starting your first flock during pregnancy or while your child is a vulnerable infant is not a great idea. However, if you had chickens for a while before you got pregnant, you likely have developed antibodies against most of the microbes encountered in their environment. Still, you might want to get someone else to handle the nasty cleanup jobs for the duration.

Now, will your chickens make you (or your neighbors) sick? Despite the rumblings of lawmakers and cranky neighbors, chickens do not pose a greater threat to public health than any other domestic animal. Indeed, a 5-year study of chickens submitted to the California Animal Health and Food Safety laboratory in Davis, California, concluded that "backyard chickens do not seem to pose a major risk to public health." Bottom line: the chance of getting some disease from a backyard flock is mighty slim, especially if you endeavor to keep your chickens healthy and you observe a few basic precautions.

Basic Precautions

Disease-causing organisms in a chicken's environment get into a human body in one of three basic ways: by mouth, by inhalation, and through a skin wound. You can therefore protect yourself from most diseases by observing the following commonsense precautions:

- Do not eat or drink (or smoke) while working with your chickens.

- Wash your hands after handling your chickens or working in or around their housing.

- Teach children to keep their hands out of their mouths until they wash their hands after being around chickens.

- Do not wash chicken equipment — including feeders, drinkers, and incubator parts — in the kitchen sink or dishwasher.

- Ventilate the coop well during clean-out, and start by misting the litter to knock down airborne dust.

- Wear a dust mask (N95 respirator) while cleaning the coop.

- Cover any exposed skin scratches or wounds with a protective bandage when working around chickens; clean and disinfect the wound afterward.

- Wear long sleeves and disposable gloves when handling a sick chicken or its body waste.

- After handling a sick chicken or its waste, wash your clothing in a separate batch from other laundry.

- Handle, prepare, and serve homegrown eggs and chicken meat in a sanitary manner.

- Know the signs of disease, especially those that pose a potential threat to humans.

- Do not eat the meat of a chicken that appears to be diseased or was found dead.

- If you suspect you have acquired a disease from your chickens or their environment, seek qualified medical care.

Who's at Risk

Many of the organisms that cause the diseases described in this chapter are fairly common in the human environment, whether or not that environment includes chickens. Ordinarily, those organisms cause no problems to humans. Exceptions are in people with impaired immune systems or low resistance due to systemic therapy (immunosuppressive or antibacterial treatments, for example), pregnancy, obesity, diabetes, or an illness from some disease unrelated to chickens.

The low risk of getting a disease from chickens is no consolation to the few people who do get sick. This chapter, then, is offered in the spirit of helpfulness — physicians tend to overlook or misdiagnose diseases they don't often see. If you visit your doctor about a condition you suspect might be related to your chickens, mention your concern to your doctor.

Although many of the diseases described in this chapter may have sources other than the poultry environment, the focus here is on their relationship to chickens. Diseases that humans can get, directly or indirectly, from chickens may be grouped into four categories: environmental, zoonotic, parasitic, and toxic.

Environmental Diseases

A human can get an infection from some of the same sources that chickens do, the result of environmental exposure rather than interspecies contagion. Most of the diseases a human can get from the poultry environment are mycoses or fungal infections.

Aspergillosis

A fungus that feeds on decaying organic matter, *Aspergillus fumigatus* is quite common in both poultry and human environments. Because chickens have a more delicate respiratory system, this infection affects chickens more often than humans. Either chickens or humans may become infected by inhaling spores from decaying litter.

This disease rarely affects a person with a healthy immune system. In someone with low resistance or compromised immunity, however, it may cause a serious case of pneumonia that can be fatal without prompt medical treatment. In someone with asthma it may cause allergic bronchitis, a respiratory condition characterized by coughing and generally not feeling well, which usually requires prolonged medical treatment.

The aspergillus fungus is so common that it's hard to avoid. Precautions include good coop ventilation to reduce airborne dust, misting litter before cleaning out the coop, and wearing a dust mask during coop clean-out.

Hen Worker's Lung

Technically known as hypersensitivity pneumonitis or allergic alveolitis, hen worker's lung is an allergic reaction to blood protein from feathers, dander, and droppings inhaled in poultry dust. It involves inflammation of the lung's air exchange units, or alveoli. Few people develop this disorder, which usually requires many years of intense exposure, such as a professional poultry worker might experience.

Symptoms may come on suddenly, approximately 6 hours after exposure. They include difficult or painful breathing, cough, fever, chills, and sometimes loss of appetite, nausea, and vomiting. The symptoms, easily mistaken

Some Human Illnesses Potentially Associated with Chickens

HUMAN CONDITION	NATURE OF DISEASE	RISK LEVEL	CHICKEN CONDITION
Environmental			
Aspergillosis	Respiratory infection or allergy	Extremely low	Aspergillosis
Farmer's lung	Respiratory allergy	Low	None
Hen worker's lung	Respiratory allergy	Low	None
Histoplasmosis	Lung infection	Extremely low	None
Pseudomonas	Skin infection	Extremely low	Pseudomonas
Tuberculosis	Lung infection	Extremely low	Avian tuberculosis
Zoonotic			
Bird flu	Flu	Extremely low	Avian influenza
Erysipeloid	Skin infection	Low	Erysipelas
Listeriosis	Eye inflammation	Extremely low	Listeriosis
Ornithosis	Flulike infection	Low	Chlamydiosis
Pinkeye	Eye inflammation	Moderate	Newcastle
Ringworm (tinea)	Skin infection	Low	Ringworm (favus)
Parasitic			
Mites	Skin irritation	Low	Mites
Ticks	Skin irritation	Low	Ticks
Toxoplasmosis	Flulike infection	Sporadic	Toxoplasmosis
Worms	Yuck factor	Extremely low	Worms
Meat-/Egg-Borne Toxins			
Campylobacter	Intestinal infection	Moderate	Campylobacteriosis
Colitis	Intestinal infection	Moderate	Colibacillosis
Salmonella	Intestinal infection	Moderate	Paratyphoid

for flu, may last several hours or up to 2 days, although complete recovery may take weeks.

The allergy sometimes develops gradually, starting with bouts of coughing and breathing difficulties that increase in frequency and severity. The allergy occasionally takes a chronic form, resulting in difficult or painful breathing brought on by physical activity, accompanied by coughing up phlegm, extreme fatigue, and gradual weight loss. Without treatment, the end result may be respiratory failure.

This disease is difficult to diagnose. The primary clue is the relationship of symptoms to exposure; for example, when professional poultry workers feel better on their days off.

Backyard chicken keepers may experience symptoms 4 to 8 hours after exposure, something that can be hard to determine if you visit your coop more than once a day. Frequent attacks reduce the lung's elasticity and eventually cause scar tissue, although an early chest X-ray may appear normal.

An early case of hen worker's lung can usually be cleared up by avoiding the poultry environment. Complete recovery is possible if avoidance occurs before lung tissue becomes scarred. Once the disease becomes chronic — which usually takes 10 to 20 years — even minute quantities of dust can set off a severe respiratory attack; the only recourse is to give up chickens completely.

Whether or not you suffer from hen worker's lung, take the precaution of wearing a good dust mask when you work in the coop, particularly during cleanup. And if necessary, install a fan in the coop to remove floating dust particles from the air.

Farmer's Lung

An allergic reaction similar to hen worker's lung, farmer's lung results from inhaling spores in dust released by moldy grains or moldy straw and other litter. In the medical profession such an allergy is known variously as extrinsic allergic alveolitis, hypersensitivity alveolitis, or hypersensitivity pneumonitis.

It is caused by the spores of heat-tolerant bacteria and molds, including *Micropolyspora faeni, Thermoactinomyces vulgaris,* and *Aspergillus* spp. These microbes typically thrive in grain, straw, and other crops that are harvested in wet weather and that subsequently heat up during storage and eventually crumble to create a dark, dry, spore-laden dust.

Symptoms are nearly identical to those of hen worker's lung, including shortness of breath and generally not feeling well. Diagnosis is difficult, but the allergy should be suspected if shortness of breath and other typical symptoms occur within 4 to 8 hours of handling spoiled feed or litter.

Prolonged breathing of spores can result in permanent lung damage. On the other hand, the condition generally clears up with future avoidance of moldy dust. Prevention includes properly disposing of moldy litter or grain and wearing a face mask with a high-efficiency particulate air (HEPA) filter when working in a dusty area.

Histoplasmosis

Inhaled *Histoplasma capsulatum* fungus spores from old, dry chicken droppings can cause a rare though potentially fatal infectious disease. Histoplasmosis occurs in nitrogen-rich soils mainly in the Ohio and central Mississippi river valleys, where the altitude is low, rainfall is 35 to 50 inches a year, and temperatures remain relatively even.

Histoplasmosis does not infect chickens, thanks to their high body temperature. The fungus therefore does not come from within their bodies into their droppings but rather moves from the soil to colonize droppings, which is why this fungus occurs in aging droppings but not in fresh chicken poop. People become infected by inhaling the fungal spores while cleaning or dismantling an old chicken house, especially one with a dirt floor, or while working in a garden that has been fertilized with contaminated droppings.

Most people who are infected either have no symptoms at all (other than an abnormal chest X-ray that mimics tuberculosis — a doctor who suspects TB will run tests to obtain a positive diagnosis), or may briefly experience minor aches and pains and a dry cough, similar to a mild case of flu. Symptoms generally appear within 3 to 18 days of having inhaled the fungal spores and go away without treatment. Thereafter, the infected person enjoys partial immunity — any future reinfections will be briefer and milder.

Occasionally this infection affects other body parts than the lungs. For instance, it can infect the eyes, permanently impairing vision. In a person who inhales large numbers of spores or who has a weakened immune system, the infection can cause a serious illness similar to tuberculosis. It may also spread from the lungs into the bloodstream, requiring immediate treatment with specific antifungal drugs to prevent a fatal outcome. The patient should tell the doctor about having chickens, in order to be tested. Tests include an antibody test for histoplasmosis, a biopsy of infected tissue, a complete blood count, a chest CT scan, and a urine test for *Histoplasma capsulatum* antigen.

Avoid infection by misting litter to control dust before cleaning out or demolishing an old chicken house. During cleanup, wear a respirator, preferably one equipped with a high efficiency particulate air (HEPA) filter capable of filtering particles as small as 2 microns. Since young children and elderly people generally have weakened immune systems, keep Grandpa and the kids away from the cleanup area until the dust settles.

Pseudomonas

Particularly in humid environments, *Pseudomonas aeruginosa* bacteria are commonly found in soil. In the rare case where chickens become infected, it typically occurs in commercial broilers from contaminated hatchery eggs. Although these bacteria are associated with meat spoilage, they are rarely harmful to humans. However, their presence on the surface of chicken meat serves to protect campylobacter bacteria, which can cause serious food poisoning, as described on page 411.

In an otherwise healthy human, pseudomonas infection is extremely rare. When it does occur, it is most likely to be caused by bacteria from the environment entering an open wound or a deep puncture, typically on the foot. Within 3 days the puncture turns purplish-black toward the center with a reddened area around the outside. A pretty good sign of this infection is wounded tissue that smells sweet, like freshly mown grass, and stains bandages green.

These bacteria are resistant to most antibiotics, so treatment typically requires multiple antibiotics and possibly surgical removal of the infected tissue. However, please note that you are far less likely to get a pseudomonas infection from your chickens' environment than from swimming in a public pool, lounging in a well-used hot tub, or even spending time in a hospital. Still, don't tempt fate by going barefoot (or letting kids go barefoot) while working with your chickens or cleaning their coop.

Tuberculosis

Chickens that are treated as pets and kept well into their old age may eventually develop tuberculosis, which is caused by a different bacterium from the one that normally causes TB in humans. However, in extremely rare cases, avian TB can infect a human — especially one who has been sensitized to human or bovine TB or who suffers from acquired immune deficiency syndrome (AIDS) — and is particularly difficult to treat.

A human gets avian TB by inhaling *Mycobacterium avium* bacteria in dust from dried droppings or contaminated soil, rather than directly from handling infected chickens. However, *M. avium* bacteria are common in the soil worldwide, and even live in the bodies of most humans without causing illness in people with strong immune systems.

Zoonoses

Many diseases are species specific — affecting only a single species, whether it be chickens, humans, or some other animal. Some diseases are zoonoses, a word derived from the Greek words *zoo*, meaning "animal," and *noso*, meaning "disease." As the word implies, zoonotic diseases may be communicated from animals to humans.

A few diseases of chickens are caused by zoonotic organisms — creatures so flexible that they can adapt to the human species. Don't be too quick to suspect you are infected with a zoonosis unless your chickens have been positively diagnosed as having that particular disease. A disease that's rare in chickens is even rarer in humans.

Bird Flu

Every now and then the media go on a bird flu frenzy, stirring up panic about the possibility of a worldwide epidemic. While the potential is real, the threat is by no means imminent. Let's look at the facts related to avian influenza.

Influenza viruses are categorized into three types: A, B, and C. Types B and C infect only people. Type A is subdivided into 144 known subtypes, which can infect a wide range of animals, including chickens and people. With the occasional rare exception, each subtype tends to be host specific, meaning (for instance) that the subtypes affecting chickens may be readily transmitted from one chicken to another, but are not readily transmitted from chickens to humans or other animals.

The type A flu viruses that typically circulate among humans each year are combinations of subtypes H1, H2, and H3 plus N1 and N2 (for an explanation of what this code means, see The Numbers Game, page 275). Two of the most common of these viruses are H1N1 and H3N2.

Other subtypes typically circulate among birds but do not normally affect people. Three subtype groups, however, are capable of infecting both birds and people; they are H5, H7, and H9. Most of these subtypes have low pathogenicity and pose little health threat to humans. Some, however, can be highly pathogenic (see Low-Path and High-Path Flu, page 275).

Most H5 viruses are low-path viruses. The best-known H5 subtype is H5N1, which can be either low path or high path. Highly pathogenic avian influenza subtype H5N1 appears sporadically in other countries and can cause serious pneumonia in humans; about 60 percent of the people who get this flu die. So far, high-path H5N1 has not appeared in the United States.

H7, too, is typically a low-path virus that rarely infects humans. People who handle chickens infected with low-path subtypes H7N2, H7N3, or H7N7 may experience conjunctivitis (pinkeye) or a mild to moderate flulike illness. High-path subtypes H7N3, H7N7, and H7N9, on the other hand, may cause a more serious respiratory illness that can be fatal. High-path H7N9 is nearly as serious to humans as high-path H5N1 but differs in its alarming ability to spread among chickens without causing apparent signs of illness. Like H5N1, H7N9 has so far not made its way to the United States.

All known H9 viruses are low-path viruses that rarely infect humans. Among these, H9N2 sporadically causes mild upper respiratory disease in people, primarily in Asia.

A human gets bird flu through direct contact with infected or dead birds or their droppings, and the illness does not typically spread from one human to another. Bird flu has affected mainly people living in Asia, the Middle East, and Eastern Europe, where large numbers of chickens are crowded together in unhealthful conditions. Even then, only rarely are humans infected, and those who do get sick have had extensive direct contact with sick birds. Chances are slim to none that you can or will get bird flu from your backyard chickens.

Erysipeloid

Erysipeloid is a bacterial infection that invades through a cut or other wound on the hand or arm of a person who handles or slaughters a bird infected with erysipelas. The wound might be caused by the bird itself, such as a toenail slice inflicted by a struggling chicken.

Infection usually appears within a week, starting out as bright red or purplish shiny, itchy skin. The infected area gradually expands, may develop tiny blisters around the edges, and may feel warm and tender or burning and painful.

The infection usually clears up on its own within about 4 weeks. However, recovery is quicker with antibiotic treatment, which also reduces the chance that the infection will spread to internal organs and possibly prove fatal.

This infection is an occupational hazard that is most likely to occur in butchers, kitchen workers, veterinarians, and artificial inseminators — and more often those handling fish, pork, and turkey than chickens. Avoidance is a matter of wearing long sleeves and gloves while handling sick chickens or their droppings.

Listeriosis

Listeriosis is more common in animals other than chickens and is even rarer in humans than in animals. It is, however, life threatening to elderly people and to unborn children infected through their mothers' blood. The disease can infect a human who handles or butchers infected chickens or who eats improperly cooked infected meat.

The most likely result of infection in humans is conjunctivitis (eye inflammation). However, symptoms can range from mild skin irritation to fever and muscle aches, to meningitis (inflammation of the brain covering), to fatal blood poisoning.

Diagnosis requires blood tests. Be sure to tell your doctor you suspect listeriosis, or the lab won't think of looking for *Listeria*. The disease is easily treated with antibiotics.

Ornithosis

Humans can contract ornithosis, a rare form of pneumonia, by inhaling dust from feathers or dried droppings of chickens infected with chlamydiosis, and the disease sometimes spreads from one person to another. It was first recognized in psittacine birds (parrots), hence was called psittacosis or parrot fever. When transmitted to humans from nonpsittacine birds, the same disease is called ornithosis.

Virulent strains appear in cycles, but not every avian outbreak causes human illness. The two most likely poultry-derived sources of chlamydiosis in humans are heavy exposure while dressing birds, more often turkeys than chickens (solution: wet feathers with detergent and water before plucking), and exposure to dusty, crowded facilities (reduce crowding, improve ventilation, and wear a dust mask and gloves during coop clean-out).

The time between exposure and first symptoms ranges between 4 days and 2 weeks. Symptoms include fatigue, loss of appetite, fever, chills, severe headache, dry cough, muscle and chest pain, sweating, and sensitivity to light; sometimes rash, diarrhea, and vomiting. Since chickens can shed *Chlamydophila psittaci* bacteria without showing signs of illness, consult a physician if you experience these symptoms.

Early symptoms may easily be confused with flu or other forms of pneumonia. A telltale sign that it is not the flu is that no one else around you gets sick.

Left untreated, an uncomplicated infection may last a week or so before going away on its own. A complicated infection can be fatal, especially in a pregnant woman or a person over the age of 50, but usually may be successfully treated with a stringent regimen of antibiotics.

Pinkeye

If you vaccinate your chickens against Newcastle disease, chances are that within 1 to 4 days you will suffer from conjunctivitis, an uncomfortable eye inflammation commonly known as pinkeye. Conjunctivitis can also occur in people who butcher chickens infected with Newcastle or, much less likely, who handle infected chickens or their droppings. The virulence of virus in chickens has no bearing on whether or not humans become infected.

Serious complications include fever, seizures, and respiratory distress. The most common symptom is an itchy, bloodshot, watery, sometimes swollen eye (usually only one). No treatment is known. Recovery is spontaneous and complete, usually in 4 days but may take as long as 4 weeks.

Ringworm

Ringworm is not caused by a worm and is not always round, although its signature symptom is a coin-shaped pink patch on the skin. The condition is caused in chickens by *Microsporum gallinae* fungus, which can infect a human who carelessly handles or treats an infected bird. In humans the infection is called tinea, a Latin word meaning "gnawing worm," and is more often caused by one of several fungi that differ from the one that infects chickens.

Besides causing a circular skin infection, tinea can get under a fingernail or toenail, causing the nail to become thick, yellow, and brittle, or on the scalp, creating red pimples and dandrufflike flakes. Symptoms appear within a few days of exposure to the fungus or up to 2 weeks in the case of a scalp infection.

An adult with a strong immune system is not as likely to acquire ringworm from an infected chicken as would a child or a person with diabetes or other immune disorder. Treatment usually is the same as for any superficial fungal infection; for example, an ointment containing the antifungal miconazole (brand name Lotrimin) or any of many other over-the-counter antifungals. Treating a scalp infection requires a prescription shampoo and possibly an oral antifungal medication as well. Avoidance includes wearing disposable gloves when handling or treating a chicken with ringworm and scrubbing your hands with soap and water afterward.

Parasitic Issues

Parasitic diseases are among the most unlikely illnesses a human can get from a chicken. Most of the parasites that thrive on or within chickens aren't much interested in humans.

Mites and Ticks

Mites may crawl onto your body if you handle infested chickens, but they usually won't stay long. Minimize discomfort by taking a shower and washing your clothing.

A tick can also get on you from a chicken. If the tick bites, it could possibility transmit a disease such as tick paralysis (causing loss of appetite, weakness, incoordination, and gradual paralysis) or Rocky Mountain spotted fever (causing severe headache, chills, and muscle pains). You won't get these diseases from the chicken but from the tick.

Remove a tick from yourself the same way you would remove one from a chicken, as described under Tick Removal on page 134. Disinfect the bite with rubbing alcohol. See your doctor if you experience any of the symptoms of a tick-borne disease.

Toxoplasmosis

As more people keep chickens along with cats in their backyards, more people have the potential to become infected with *Toxoplasma gondii* protozoa (described in detail on page 209). Humans can get toxoplasmosis (toxo) in many different ways, most of which do not involve chickens.

The methods that do involve chickens are primarily by eating the raw or undercooked meat of infected chickens and failing to use proper sanitation (including washing hands, cutting boards, and other utensils)

when handling the meat of infected chickens. Although a cat is likely to get toxo by eating infected rodents or wild birds, the cat (like a human) can become infected after being fed the raw or undercooked meat of an infected chicken. Toxo is a potential issue with homegrown and pastured chickens raised for meat but does not occur in industrially produced chickens raised in a controlled environment that excludes cats, wild birds, and rodents.

Most healthy humans — as well as healthy chickens, cats, and other animals — show no signs of being infected. Some humans, however, may have temporary, mild flulike symptoms that include sore throat, headache, muscle pain, low fever, fatigue, diarrhea, and swollen lymph nodes.

The most serious effects occur in people with immunodeficiency disorders and in unborn children whose mothers are infected while pregnant. A woman infected during pregnancy can pass the infection to her unborn child. Luckily, toxo infection during pregnancy is uncommon; an estimated 0.4 percent of pregnant women become infected, and about one-third of them infect their unborn children. Of those, about 10 percent result in serious damage to the baby, which can include blindness, retardation, miscarriage, or stillbirth.

No comprehensive statistics are recorded on how many people have been infected by this parasite, but estimates are that up to 25 percent of the population in the United States has been exposed to toxoplasmosis from all sources (and, it bears repeating, most sources are unrelated to chickens). People who have been infected by this parasite develop antibodies against future infection. The disease is self-limiting, and any symptoms that develop usually go away on their own. The parasite, however, remains in an infected person's body for life and has been implicated in mood disorders.

The easiest way to avoid getting this parasite from homegrown chickens raised for meat is to wash hands, cutting boards, countertops, and utensils after butchering chickens or handling their meat. Cooking the meat to 150°F (66°C) destroys any parasites that might be present.

Worms

You aren't likely to get worms from your chickens, since most worms that prefer poultry do not invade humans. You can, however, accidentally ingest worm eggs if you eat without washing your hands after handling contaminated soil or litter, but you would likely experience few or no symptoms.

A heavily worm-infested hen may occasionally lay an egg with a roundworm inside the shell. As unappetizing as that may be, it will not infect a human, although it is a clear indication that the hen needs to be dewormed.

Meat and Egg Contaminants

One of the reasons people raise their own food-producing chickens, even though doing so costs more than purchasing store-bought meat and eggs, is their concerns about pesticide and herbicide residues, antibiotics, and microbial contaminants in industrially produced poultry products.

Pesticides and herbicides are used on most feed crops that make up chicken rations. Unless you have a source of so-called organic rations, your eggs and chicken meat will contain no fewer residues from pesticides and herbicides

than industrially produced meat, which in any case is extremely low. Residues can also come from treating chickens or their facilities for external parasites using chemicals that enter a chicken's body by inhalation or through the skin. Chemical treatments should therefore be used with care, and cleanliness is far preferable.

Antibiotics at low levels are used industrially to make meat birds reach market weights faster with lower feed costs. Antibiotics are not routinely given to industrial layers but are occasionally used as needed to control disease. You can easily avoid antibiotics in homegrown meat by not making drugs part of your management routine and by observing the withdrawal time for any drug you do use for therapeutic purposes (see Avoiding Drug Residues on page 377).

Pathogenic microbes pose the greatest threat among contaminants in poultry meat or eggs, especially those that are industrially produced, since large-scale production and processing lend themselves to unsanitary practices. Homegrown meat birds, by contrast, are usually killed and cleaned individually, are rinsed under a running faucet (rather than in a vat of rapidly contaminated water), and are refrigerated promptly. Similarly, homegrown eggs are exposed to fewer sources of contamination. Nevertheless, remaining aware of the dangers of contamination is an important step toward avoiding them.

Food-Borne Bacteria

If meat or eggs are held at room temperature for too long, any bacteria present will proliferate. Some multiply more rapidly than others. Since there's no way to tell whether or not bacteria are present, you can't go wrong if you

EGG SANITATION

A freshly laid egg is warm and moist and therefore attracts bacteria and molds that exist in the poultry environment. After leaving a hen's warm body, the egg immediately starts to cool. As its contents contract, a vacuum is created that can draw bacteria and molds through the 6,000-plus pores in the shell, potentially causing egg spoilage and human illness.

Eggs produced in a clean environment, collected often, and promptly placed under refrigeration (after cracked or seriously soiled eggs are discarded) rarely pose a human health problem. Eggs that are slightly soiled with dirt or dried droppings should be dry-cleaned with fine sandpaper. Improperly washing them can do more harm than good.

Eggs produced in a not-so-clean environment and those destined for market may need to be washed. Market eggs are often subjected to temperatures that are higher than desirable (causing bacteria and mold on the shell to multiply) and to repeated warming and cooling during transportation (drawing more microbes through the shell each time).

If you feel the need to wash eggs, use water that is 20°F (11°C) warmer than the eggs are; otherwise vacuum action may draw microorganisms through the shell or tiny cracks may develop in the shell that expose eggs to invasion by bacteria and molds. Wash eggs with detergent (not soap) to remove soil. Rinse them in water of the same temperature as the wash water, adding a sanitizer to reduce the number of microbes on the shell (a sanitizer won't eliminate *all* bacteria and mold). If you wash a large number of eggs, change the wash and rinse solution often, since both can rapidly become contaminated.

Egg sanitizers are available from many poultry suppliers. A chlorine solution (such as 5.25 percent Clorox bleach) will not introduce an off odor or flavor when used at the rate of 1 tablespoon per gallon of water (2 mg/L). Dry eggs thoroughly before placing them in cartons, since wet shells will more readily pick up bacteria. If you are packaging the eggs for sale, check your state's regulations regarding legally acceptable procedures for cleaning them.

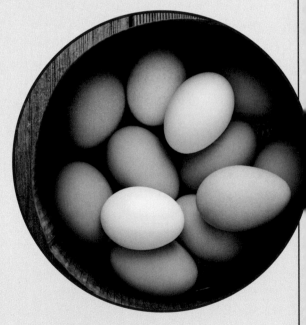

always handle meat and eggs as if they were contaminated.

In a healthy human adult, bacterial food poisoning is typically little more than an annoyance. In a young child, an elderly person, or someone with a compromised immune system, however, bacterial food poisoning can be serious or even fatal. General symptoms are loss of appetite, nausea, vomiting, abdominal cramps, and diarrhea that comes on suddenly. A clue that it is a food-borne problem is when illness strikes a group of people who have shared a meal.

Most cases are resolved with bed rest and plenty of fluids. For many people the most serious consequence is loss of body fluids and electrolytes. Since symptoms resemble the flu, most cases go untreated and end in spontaneous recovery. Unless the illness is complicated by other factors, antibiotics may be of little help and may actually make matters worse. With salmonella, for instance, antibiotic treatment prolongs the period during which the recovered person remains a carrier, and is associated with relapse. Antibiotics also kill the good gut flora that would have helped the patient recover. Unless the person requires hospitalization, the best course of action is to rest and replace lost fluids and electrolytes.

The most common causes of bacterial food poisoning are campylobacter, *E. coli*, and salmonella. Some food-borne bacteria produce toxins that inhibit nutrient absorption, while others are infective — causing disease by invading the intestine wall. Some work both ways.

SALMONELLA

You would have a hard time finding meat, eggs, or any other food that did not harbor one of the 2,500 known strains of salmonella bacteria. *S. Enteriditis* is the version that causes food poisoning outbreaks periodically reported in the news. No one knows exactly how many people experience salmonella poisoning each year, since mild cases are rarely reported. Of the 40,000 annual cases that are reported, only about 5 percent have been traced to chickens.

Poultry disease experts once believed *S. Enteritidis* infected an egg through the shell after the egg was laid and that frequent egg collection and disinfection would minimize contamination. In the 1980s they discovered that salmonella bacteria in hens' ovaries can infect eggs before they are laid. Since then, *S. Enteritidis* bacteria have become more common in both chickens and humans, as well as becoming resistant to antibiotics.

No one can guess how commonly salmonella bacteria occur in eggs from backyard

Food-Borne Illness Quick Check

PATHOGEN	ONSET TIME	SYMPTOMS	DURATION
Campylobacter jejuni	2–5 days	Cramps, diarrhea, headache, fever	3–6 days
Escherichia coli	1–10 days	Cramps, watery or bloody diarrhea, rarely fever	1–12 days
Salmonella spp.	12–74 hours	Cramps, diarrhea, nausea, vomiting, fever	4–7 days
Toxoplasma gondii	7–21 days	Muscle pain, headache, tiredness, fever	2–4 weeks

chickens. According to the Centers for Disease Control and Prevention, only about one in 5,000 to 10,000 industrially produced eggs is contaminated. Despite alarmist press coverage, experts claim your chance of getting salmonellosis from those eggs is only about one in two million. Illness in a healthy person requires eating a large number of bacteria. Further, most cases occur not in homes but in restaurants, schools, hospitals, and other institutions where eggs are mixed in large batches and may not be cooked long enough or may sit on a counter too long, allowing any bacteria present to multiply.

Salmonella bacteria concentrate in the yolk. They may also be present in chicken meat, typically from contamination with fecal matter from the intestines during butchering. Preventing illness is a matter of careful sanitation during butchering, combined with serving chicken meat well done. Thoroughly cooked chicken reaches a temperature well above the 142°F (61°C) necessary to kill salmonella.

Most people who experience salmonella poisoning never know it, believing instead that they have an upset stomach or a mild case of flu. Symptoms begin 12 to 74 hours after eating contaminated food, which tastes and smells normal. Symptoms include nausea, fever, abdominal cramps, and diarrhea. Most infections are relatively mild, and most people recover in a week or less without treatment, as long as they avoid dehydration by drinking lots of fluids.

A serious infection, however, can spread from the intestines to the bloodstream and other body sites, resulting in death, especially among infants, the elderly, anyone with an impaired immune system, a patient undergoing treatment with antibiotics (which remove beneficial bacteria from the intestines, clearing the way for disease-causing bacteria), or an ulcer patient taking antacids (which reduce bacteria-killing stomach acids). Hospitalization is needed if symptoms persist or diarrhea is severe or accompanied by high fever, weakness, or disorientation.

CAMPYLOBACTER

Although it gets less press than salmonellosis, campylobacteriosis is the world's leading food-borne pathogen and the most common cause of diarrheal illness in humans. Of

HANDLING MEAT BIRDS

When butchering your own chickens, select only plump, healthy-looking birds. Avoid rough handling and other forms of stress, which can both increase bacterial contamination and affect the meat's taste and texture. To reduce the possibility of fecal contamination, hold the birds overnight without feed but with continuing access to drinking water.

Once each chicken is plucked and gutted, thoroughly rinse it in clear running water. Rapidly chill the birds in fresh cold water with plenty of ice before packaging them for refrigeration. Allow muscle (meat) to tenderize in the fridge for no less than 1 day and no more than 4 days, by which time it should be either cooked or frozen.

the three species that cause human disease, *Campylobacter jejuni* — the cause of campylobacteriosis in chickens — is identified more than 90 percent of the time, and chicken meat has been identified as the main source of human illness.

Unlike salmonellosis, campylobacteriosis is not transmitted through contaminated eggs. People become ill by handling infected birds (campylobacteriosis is an occupational hazard in poultry processing plants) or by eating undercooked infected chicken meat.

The bacteria produce a toxin that irritates the lining of the intestine, causing abdominal cramps and watery, sometimes bloody diarrhea, occasionally accompanied by a fever ranging from 100°F to 104°F (38°C to 40°C). Usually the illness goes away on its own, but an infant, an elderly person, or someone with compromised immunity may require medical treatment.

No one can say how common these bacteria are in backyard flocks, but they are of growing concern because of their prevalence in industrially produced poultry and their increasing resistance to antibiotics. On the other hand, the stress of rough handling and being transported to a distant processor dramatically increases the presence of campylobacter in the chickens' meat, compared to backyard chickens that are humanely handled at home. At any rate, you can avoid campylobacteriosis by observing basic hygiene precautions and by not eating raw or undercooked chicken meat.

EGG STORAGE

Whether or not your fresh eggs need to be hustled into the refrigerator is a matter of some debate. Because of the possibility of salmonella poisoning, in 1990 the United States Food and Drug Administration decreed that shell eggs are a "potentially hazardous food." Industrially produced eggs therefore must be washed and sanitized, remain under constant refrigeration from farm to consumer, and cooked thoroughly before being eaten.

Although backyard hens can, and occasionally do, get bacterial infections, keepers who take care to maintain a healthful environment are returning to the tradition of not refrigerating homegrown eggs. In 2013 the British-based firm Foodtest Laboratories stored unwashed eggs from healthy hens at room temperature (generally considered to be 68°F/20°C) for 2 weeks, at the end of which the eggs remained bacteria-free. While eggs that have been washed should always be refrigerated, eggs that are clean when collected and remain unwashed to preserve their protective bloom may be kept at room temperature for up to 30 days.

However, consider this: The American Egg Board has determined that eggs age more in 1 day at room temperature than in 1 week in the fridge. So qualitywise, 2-week-old countertop eggs compare to eggs that have been in the fridge for 14 weeks, and 30 days on the counter compares to 7 months in the fridge. Aging eggs may not be laden with bacteria, but they gradually become less appetizing, with runny whites and yolks that break easily.

Don't Swallow the Bug

⚠️ A person can get salmonellosis or campylo-bacteriosis directly from handling an infected chicken by inadvertently swallowing bacteria, as can happen if you eat (or smoke) while working with or around chickens or fail to thoroughly wash your hands afterward. Children are especially susceptible unless they are trained to keep their fingers out of their mouths, avoid kissing chicks and chickens, and always wash hands after visiting the family flock.

ESCHERICHIA COLI

Although it rarely results from eating properly processed homegrown chicken, *Escherichia coli* (*E. coli*) infection is included here because it is of increasing concern to people who work with industrially produced chickens routinely treated with antibiotics, backyarders who persist in using antibiotics to prevent disease in their flocks, and people who eat undercooked contaminated chicken meat. Studies have linked antibiotic treatment of chickens to the emergence of drug-resistant strains of *E. coli* and to an increasing number of difficult-to-treat human infections.

Of the many different types of *E. coli* bacteria existing throughout the environment, most are harmless, some are beneficial, and only a few will make you sick. Among the pathogenic types, some produce a toxin called Shiga (named after the bacteriologist who discovered it). Unlike with many disease-causing bacteria,

ingesting only a tiny amount of *E. coli* can make you sick. Further, the bacteria spread easily from an infected person to others.

People who are at greatest risk for serious infection are children, pregnant women and their newborns, elderly adults, and anyone with a weak immune system. Signs of infection include severe abdominal cramps and diarrhea that may turn bloody within about 24 hours. *E. coli* can also cause a urinary tract infection, respiratory illness, bloodstream infection, kidney failure, and even death. Most infections are mild, however, clearing up on their own within about a week, and remain undiagnosed or unreported.

Avoidance includes thoroughly cooking chicken meat, especially if you are unsure about the sanitation procedures during butchering, and thoroughly washing your hands any time you may have come into contact with infected chickens or their droppings, or potentially contaminated chicken meat.

Quick Guide to
Diseases
and Disorders

THIS CHAPTER IS intended to serve as a quick reference to critical information about the most common diseases and disorders. The entries are organized alphabetically and cross-referenced for easy retrieval. Unless otherwise noted, all cross-references are found within this chapter. The following Sample Entry on page 419 explains the terminology used in describing each disease and disorder.

Reportable/Notifiable Diseases

Certain diseases are such a threat to either the poultry industry or to human health that, by law, your veterinarian or state diagnostic laboratory must report them to your state veterinarian. Some states designate such diseases as "reportable"; others call them "notifiable." Each state has its own regulations as to which diseases are reportable.

The immediate result of the appearance of a reportable disease is quarantine of the affected flock, and often neighboring flocks as well, to keep the disease from spreading. In some cases the affected birds may be treated under strict veterinary supervision. In other cases the infected flock, and sometimes neighboring flocks, will be depopulated — a polite way of saying the entire flock is destroyed. If the chickens were kept for commercial purposes, the owner *may* be reimbursed for the loss.

In addition to diseases that may be reportable in some states, all states must report certain diseases to the Animal and Plant Health Inspection Service (APHIS) in the United States, and to the Canadian Food Inspection Agency (CFIA) in Canada. These agencies, in turn, are required to report to the World Organisation for Animal Health (Office of International Epizootics, or OIE), which maintains its own list of notifiable diseases. The OIE publishes reported outbreaks to alert neighboring countries and maintains a list of poultry diseases at www.oie.int.

The APHIS website shows the current status and date of last occurrence of federally reportable diseases. Data for the previous year may be found at www.aphis.usda.gov. Canada, in addition to OIE-reportable diseases, lists notifiable diseases for which the country has no control or eradication programs. Information may be found at www.inspection.gc.ca under "Terrestrial Animal Health."

Reportable Diseases

GOVERNING BODY	DISEASE	THREAT TO
OIE	Avian influenza	Poultry industry & public health
	Chlamydiosis	Public health
	Chronic respiratory disease	Poultry industry
	Fowl typhoid	Poultry industry
	Infectious bronchitis	Poultry industry
	Infectious bursal disease	Poultry industry
	Infectious synovitis	Poultry industry
	Laryngotracheitis	Poultry industry
	Newcastle disease (neurotropic & viscerotropic)	Poultry industry
	Pullorum disease	Poultry industry
APHIS*	Marek's disease	Poultry industry
	Fowl cholera	Poultry industry
CFIA*	Epidemic tremor	Poultry industry
	Eggdrop syndrome†	Poultry industry
Some states**	Arizonosis	Public health & poultry industry
	Avian tuberculosis	Public health & poultry industry
	Colibacillosis	Public health & poultry industry
	Cryptosporidiosis	Public health & poultry industry
	Fowl pox	Poultry industry
	Paratyphoid	Public health & poultry industry

*Additional to OIE notifiable diseases

**Additional to APHIS notifiable diseases

†To date egg drop syndrome does not occur in the United States or Canada.

Sample Entry

Common Name

Also called: Alternative names, scientific names (for the benefit of specialists and readers who consult technical works), and names no longer in use (for readers who peruse old poultry books). Conditions missing this entry are not commonly known by alternative names.

Prevalence: How common the disease is and where it is likely to occur

System/organ affected: Primary body part or body system the disease affects

Incubation period: Amount of time from exposure to the first sign of infection (this information helps to diagnose the disease based on past contacts and to identify the source of infection once the disease has been diagnosed). For conditions missing this entry, incubation period is not relevant.

Progression: How hard the disease hits a flock, how fast it spreads, and whether it is acute (short term, ending in recovery or death) or chronic (long term). For conditions missing this entry, progression is not relevant.

Signs: Most common signs or combinations of signs; since no two cases are ever exactly alike, not all signs will always appear; age groups are approximations only. (Note: Signs are similar to symptoms, except a sign is what you see, while a symptom is what the chicken feels, which of course we cannot readily ascertain.)

Percentage affected: Proportion of an affected flock likely to be involved

Mortality: Percentage of affected birds likely to die

Postmortem: The most common irregularities found inside a diseased bird's body (for details on conducting a postmortem examination, see chapter 13)

Resembles: Diseases with similar signs and, when practical, how to tell them apart

Diagnosis: A disease can often be identified by some combination of flock history, signs, and postmortem findings; some are so similar to other diseases that laboratory tests are required for a certain diagnosis, and some can only be identified by laboratory tests (for diagnostic guidelines, see chapter 12)

Cause: Primary cause of the disease

Transmission: How the disease spreads

Prevention: Steps for preventing the disease

Treatment: Possible approaches toward dealing with the disease; specific dosages are not included because drugs can vary in potency (always follow manufacturer's directions)

Human health risk: Any potential risk this disease poses for humans (additional information may be found in chapter 15)

⚠️ Entries that include this symbol are reportable in some or all jurisdictions. Please refer to Reportable/Notifiable Diseases on page 417.

Common Abbreviations

AA	avian arizonosis		ILT	infectious laryngotracheitis
AC	avian chlamydiosis		LL	lymphoid leukosis
ADS	acute death sydrome		LP	fowl cholera (chronic) (localized pasteurellosis)
AE	epidemic tremor (avian encephalomyelitis)		LT	laryngotracheitis
AI	avian influenza		MD	Marek's disease
AIS	avian intestinal spirochetosis		MG	chronic respiratory disease (*Mycoplasma gallisepticum*)
AT	avian tuberculosis			
BWD	pullorum (bacillary white diarrhea)		MS	infectious synovitis (*Mycoplasma synoviae*)
CRD	chronic respiratory disease		NE	necrotic enteritis
EL	epididymal lithiasis		NVND	neurotropic velogenic Newcastle disease
END	exotic Newcastle disease		ORT	ornithobacteriosis
FC	fowl cholera (acute)		PD	pullorum disease
FT	fowl typhoid		PPLO	chronic respiratory disease (pleuropneumonia-like organism)
GD	gangrenous dermatitis			
HPAI	high-pathogenicity avian influenza		SDS	sudden death syndrome
IB	infectious bronchitis		TB	tuberculosis
IBD	infectious bursal disease		UE	ulcerative enteritis
IC	infectious coryza		VVND	viscerotropic velogenic Newcastle disease

A

A-avitaminosis. See *Roup (nutritional)*

Acariasis. See *Mites and Ticks, page 126*

Acute Death Syndrome. See *Sudden Death Syndrome*

Acute Gout. See *Gout (visceral)*

Acute Heart Failure. See *Sudden Death Syndrome*

Acute Leukosis. See *Marek's Disease*

Aflatoxicosis
Also called: *Aspergillus toxicosis, aflatoxin mycotoxicosis*
Prevalence: Low levels of aflatoxin are common in feedstuffs
System/organ affected: Systemic
Progression: Acute or chronic
Signs: In incubated eggs from affected hens, early embryo death; defects in hatchlings
In growing birds, huddling, decreased appetite, slow growth, impaired feathering, weakness, incoordination, increased susceptibility to bruising and heat stress, convulsions, sudden death with head drawn back
In hens, pale mucous membranes and shanks, increased susceptibility to infection, reduced egg production, smaller eggs with decreased hatchability
In cocks, weight loss, reduced fertility
Percentage affected: 100% of those consuming contaminated feed
Mortality: High for acute illness, low for chronic illness
Postmortem: None, or large, pale, or yellow soft liver, or (in a chronic case) small, firm liver with swollen gallbladder
Resembles: Fatty liver syndrome, except aflatoxicosis is not related to obesity
Diagnosis: Difficult; signs, feed analysis (often inconclusive), postmortem findings (often absent)
Cause: Four types of poison produced by *Aspergillus flavus, A. parasiticus,* and *Penicillium puberulum* mold in litter, in corn and other grain (especially grain that's insect damaged, drought stressed, or crushed), and in peanut meal

Transmission: Does not spread from bird to bird but can affect all birds that eat the same moldy grain, seeds, or nuts
Prevention: Avoid moldy or insect-ridden feed; store feed in a tight bin in cool, dry place and use within 2 to 3 weeks
Treatment: Birds may recover once contaminated feed has been replaced; although no treatment reverses physical damage caused by toxicity, supportive therapy may improve an affected chicken's overall health: minimize stress; boost dietary energy and protein; offer a vitamin supplement that includes vitamin K to improve blood clotting; including a little oil, such as sunflower or soybean oil, with the ration may be beneficial; a probiotic containing several species of lactobacillus bacteria may be helpful in binding toxins in the gut; a liver support supplement designed for pets may help stimulate liver function
Human health risk: Aflatoxin (a human poison and a carcinogen) is rapidly excreted in the chicken's droppings, resulting in little danger of residue in meat by 3 days after contaminated feed is removed; toxin may continue to deposit in egg yolks up to 10 days after contaminated feed is removed; humans can be poisoned by eating the same moldy grains, seeds, or nuts that poison chickens

Air Sac Disease
Also called: Air sac cold, airsacculitis, air sac infection, air sac syndrome (one form of colibacillosis and/or mycoplasmosis). See *Ruptured Air Sac, page 76*
Prevalence: Common
System/organ affected: Respiratory
Incubation period: 4 to 21 days
Progression: Acute to chronic
Signs: In young birds, 5 to 12 weeks old (most commonly 6 to 9 weeks old): coughing, nasal discharge, breathing difficulty, decreased appetite and rapid weight loss, watery eyes, droopiness, stunted growth or uneven growth among same-age birds
Percentage affected: 100%
Mortality: Up to 30%
Postmortem: Thick mucus in nasal passages and throat; cloudy or beaded air sacs containing cheesy material
Resembles: Chronic respiratory disease, except CRD affects older birds and does not always involve the air sacs

Diagnosis: Flock history, signs, postmortem findings (heavy involvement of air sacs), confirmed by laboratory identification of bacteria
Cause: *Escherichia coli* and/or *Mycoplasma gallisepticum* (sometimes *M. synoviae*) bacteria, often in combination with or following vaccination for chronic respiratory disease, infectious bronchitis, laryngotracheitis, or Newcastle; may also result from environmental stress such as cold temperatures or poor ventilation, or from injury to delicate air sacs
Transmission: Contact with infected or carrier birds; inhaling contaminated dust or respiratory droplets; spreads from breeders to chicks through hatching eggs
Prevention: Avoid dusty litter; provide good ventilation; avoid chilling and other forms of stress; acquire mycoplasma-free birds
Treatment: Keep birds warm and well fed with high-protein rations and a vitamin E supplement; treatment may be effective *if* started early *and* pathogens are identified so ineffective drugs can be avoided; survivors of mycoplasma infection remain carriers
Human health risk: None known

Aleukemic Myeloid Leukosis. See *Typical Diseases Caused by Avian Leukosis Viruses, page 266*

Ammonia Blindness. See *Conjunctivitis (ammonia induced)*

Arizona Infection. See *Arizonosis*

Arizonosis
Also called: AA, Arizona infection, paracolon (one form of salmonellosis)
Prevalence: Rare, appearing mostly in western states (and more often in turkeys than in chickens)
System/organ affected: Intestines
Incubation period: 5 to 7 days
Progression: Acute in chicks, lasting up to 5 weeks, chronic in mature birds
Signs: In chicks 1 to 3 weeks old, droopiness; decreased appetite; increased thirst; huddling near heat; bulging navel; diarrhea with vent pasting; high death rate with sudden deaths; survivors are likely to be stunted
Percentage affected: 100%
Mortality: Variable, usually not more than 50%, starting soon after hatch and peaking at 8 to 10 days

Postmortem: Nonabsorbed yolk sac containing watery fluid or yellow cheesy matter; yellowish, mottled, swollen liver; ceca filled with cheesy matter
Resembles: Paratyphoid (almost identical)
Diagnosis: Testing negative for paratyphoid; laboratory identification of bacteria
Cause: *Salmonella arizonae* bacteria that persists in the environment for months and affects turkey poults more often than chicks
Transmission: Contaminated droppings in soil, litter, feed, or water; contaminated feathers, dust, hatchery fluff; carrier breeders to chicks on the shells of hatching eggs (eggs can explode during incubation, further spreading bacteria); spread by infected eggs and chicks in incubator and brooder; spread on dirty equipment, boots, feet of insects and rodents, droppings of infected birds and reptiles
Prevention: Collect hatching eggs often; hatch only eggs from *S. arizonae*-free breeders; hatch only clean eggs; clean and disinfect incubator and brooder after each hatch; avoid brooder chilling, overheating, parasitism, withholding of water or feed; keep water free of droppings; control reptiles, rodents, cockroaches, beetles, fleas, and flies; *S. arizonae* is easily destroyed by disinfectants
Treatment: None effective; survivors are carriers
Human health risk: Diarrhea may result from failing to wash hands after handling infected chicks; septicemia is possible in immunocompromised individuals

 Arizonosis is a reportable disease in some states.

Arthritis. See *Gout (articular)*

Arthritis (staphylococcic)
Also called: Arthritis/synovitis, staph arthritis (one form of staphylococcosis)
Prevalence: Common
System/organ affected: Joints
Incubation period: 1 to 3 days
Progression: Chronic, developing over the course of weeks, often following septicemic staphylococcosis
Signs: In all ages (most often growing birds 4 to 6 weeks old), ruffled feathers, lethargy, weight loss, lameness, reluctance to move, swollen joints (hot to the touch), resting on hocks and keel with resulting breast blisters
Percentage affected: Usually low

Mortality: Usually low

Postmortem: Joints (especially hock) and surrounding area are inflamed and contain whitish, fleck-filled fluid that becomes cheesy in an advanced infection

Resembles: In young birds, injury to the bones and joints; joint infections (synovitis) caused by other bacteria

In mature birds, septicemic form resembles acute fowl cholera, except cholera has a high death rate

Diagnosis: Signs, laboratory identification of bacteria

Cause: *Staphylococcus aureus* and other staph bacteria commonly found in the poultry environment

Transmission: Not contagious; bacteria enter the body through a wound, as the result of a secondary infection, or through drinking from contaminated puddles

Prevention: Provide a safe, uncrowded environment

Treatment: Staph bacteria are resistant to many antibiotics, but treatment *may* be successful *if* a suitable antibiotic is determined through laboratory sensitivity testing

Human health risk: *S. aureus* strains that infect chickens do not infect humans; however, strains that produce enterotoxins can cause food poisoning (See page 411)

Arthritis/synovitis. See *Arthritis (staphylococcic)*

Articular Hyperuricemia. See *Gout (articular)*

Articular Urate Deposition. See *Gout (articular)*

Ascariasis/Ascaridiasis. See *Large Roundworm, page 168*

Ascites

Also called: Dropsy, pulmonary hypertension syndrome, waterbelly

Prevalence: Common in broilers and aging layers

System/organ affected: Cardiovascular

Incubation period: Not applicable

Progression: Acute or chronic

Signs: In broilers, especially cockerels, 4 to 7 weeks old: swollen abdomen, bluish skin, slow growth, ruffled feathers, bluish comb and feet, reluctance to move; sometimes sudden death

In aging layers, bloated, sagging abdomen; panting without heat stress; sudden death (especially when startled or frightened)

Percentage affected: Up to 25% in intensively raised broilers; up to 15% in pastured broilers; individual aging layers

Mortality: 20 to 30%

Postmortem: Straw-colored liquid or jellylike fluid in abdominal cavity; enlarged heart, especially the right side; dark red muscles; liver may be either swollen, bloody, and mottled or pimpled (early stage) or small, pale, and lumpy (later stage) with a thickened or blistered outer membrane; lungs may appear bloody or pale and gray

Resembles: A hen's bloated abdomen may be mistaken for egg binding, egg peritonitis, cystic ovary, infected uterus, internal laying

Diagnosis: Signs, postmortem findings

Cause: Abnormally high blood pressure to the lungs (see Ascitic Layers, page 111), for a list of contributing factors); in a broiler, it is usually the result of excessively rapid growth; in a layer, it may result from restricted breathing caused by tumors or internal laying

Transmission: Does not spread from bird to bird but may affect birds subject to the same conditions

Prevention: In broilers, restrict feed intake or reduce the energy content during the first 3 weeks to allow heart and lungs to keep up with the amount of oxygen needed for rapid growth; in layers, maintain good ventilation and avoid obesity

Treatment: Carefully removing ascitic fluid (about 1 cup) from a layer using a hypodermic needle will relieve abdominal pressure but will not solve the underlying condition

Human health risk: None known

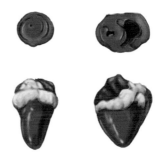

Cross section of a heart from an ascitic chicken (right) compared to the cross section of a normal heart

Asiatic Newcastle Disease. See *Newcastle Disease (velogenic)*

Aspergillosis (acute). See *Brooder Pneumonia*

Aspergillosis (chronic)
Also called: *Aspergillus* infection, bronchomycosis, fungal pneumonia, mycotic pneumonia, pneumonomycosis, pulmonary aspergillosis
Prevalence: Less common than acute aspergillosis (brooder pneumonia); more likely in confined chickens than in those with outdoor access
System/organ affected: Respiratory
Incubation period: Months
Progression: Chronic
Signs: In mature birds, difficulty breathing without making the sounds typical of other respiratory conditions, bluish comb, darkened skin, twisted neck
Percentage affected: Low, usually one at a time
Mortality: Less than 5%; more typical in confined chickens than in outdoor birds and more likely after birds have been handled, especially carried by legs
Postmortem: Mold growing in windpipe; cheesy-looking disks in lungs; fluid-filled abdomen (ascites)
Resembles: Any chronic respiratory condition, except aspergillosis usually does not cause gurgling, rattling, or other typical respiratory sounds
Diagnosis: Flock history, signs, postmortem findings, laboratory culturing of mold spores from respiratory tract
Cause: Spores of *Aspergillus fumigatus* fungus and other molds comonly found in the poultry environment, especially in areas surrounding feeders and waterers (appear blue-green and can easily be seen while growing); infects confined chickens heavily exposed to moldy litter or grain
Transmission: Inhaled mold spores that gradually impair respiration as the maturing chicken needs increasingly more oxygen; does not spread from bird to bird
Prevention: Avoid alternating conditions of wet (when fungi multiply) and dry (when fungi spread through spores blowing in dust); control dust (open windows work better than a fan); remove contaminated litter, especially surrounding feeders and drinkers
Treatment: None effective
Human health risk: Allergic pneumonitis can affect humans who frequently handle moldy litter; the same molds that affect chickens can affect humans with impaired immunity; *see* Aspergillosis, page 253

***Aspergillus* Infection.** See *Aspergillosis (chronic)*

***Aspergillus* Toxicosis.** See *Aflatoxicosis*

Avian Arizonosis. See *Arizonosis*

Avian Borreliosis. See *Spirochetosis*

Avian Chlamydiosis. See *Chlamydiosis*

Avian Cholera. See *Fowl Cholera (acute), Fowl Cholera (chronic)*

Avian Diphtheria. See *Laryngotracheitis (acute)*

Avian Encephalomyelitis. See *Epidemic Tremor*

Avian Flu. See *Avian Influenza (high pathogenicity), Avian Influenza (low pathogenicity)*

Avian Hemorrhagic Septicemia. See *Fowl Cholera (acute)*

Avian Infectious Bronchitis. See *Infectious Bronchitis*

Avian Influenza (high pathogenicity)
Also called: HPAI, avian flu, AI, bird flu, fowl pest, fowl plague, highly virulent avian influenza, hot avian influenza
Prevalence: Sporadic
System/organ affected: Cardiovascular system, nerves, systemic
Incubation period: 14 to 21 days
Progression: Acute, spreads rapidly, runs through flock in 1 to 3 days
Signs: In birds of all ages, sudden death of apparently healthy chickens, soon followed by signs in remaining birds that may include decreased activity, lethargy, loss of interest in feed and water; swollen and darkened head, comb, wattles; swollen, reddened legs; eggs with soft or no shells, rapid drop in laying to near zero; sometimes coughing, sneezing, rales; sometimes bloody discharge from nose and mouth, greenish diarrhea; quivering of the head and neck, neck twisted to one side or bent over the back, inability to stand, death within about 48 hours
Percentage affected: 100%
Mortality: Depending on virulence of the virus and age of the chickens, up to 100%, peaking at about 5 days after first signs appear

Postmortem: None in cases of sudden death; otherwise, large and small reddish-brown spots or blotches (hemorrhages) along the interior of the upper and lower digestive tract, on the ovaries, and over the fat of the abdomen; straw-colored fluid beneath skin of face; swollen blood vessels; loose gizzard lining

Resembles: Fowl cholera (acute), laryngotracheitis, Newcastle (velogenic), heat exhaustion, ornithobacteriosis, water deprivation, acute poisoning

Diagnosis: Signs (sudden high death rate), confirmed by laboratory identification of virus

Cause: Highly contagious strains of type A influenza orthomyxoviruses evolved from mutations of low pathogenic strains

Transmission: Contact with infected birds (either domestic or wild) and their body discharges, especially droppings; spreads on contaminated equipment and the feet of insects, rodents, and humans

Prevention: Not likely to occur in the typical back-yard flock

Treatment: None; infected flocks are quarantined and destroyed, followed by thorough cleaning and disinfecting of the facility

Human health risk: Highly pathogenic bird flu has the potential for seriously infecting humans and other mammals but rarely does

 Highly pathogenic avian influenza is reportable.

Avian Influenza (low pathogenicity)

Also called: LPAI, avian flu, AI, bird flu, low virulence avian influenza

Prevalence: Common

System/organ affected: Primarily respiratory, sometimes digestive, reproductive, and urinary systems

Incubation period: 14 to 21 days

Progression: Spreads rapidly

Signs: None, or ruffled feathers, coughing, sneezing, rattling, rales, watery eyes, nasal discharge, lethargy, loss of interest in water and feed, sometimes diarrhea; hens lay less and tend to become broody more easily

Percentage affected: Usually low unless some other infection is also involved

Mortality: Usually less than 5%, mostly among young chickens

Postmortem: Mucus or cheesy plugs in sinuses, throat, lungs, and air sacs; in hens: egg yolk in abdomen; oviduct shriveled or swollen and fluid filled

Resembles: Aspergillosis, chlamydiosis, chronic respiratory disease, infectious bronchitis, laryngotracheitis, Newcastle disease (lentogenic)

Diagnosis: Difficult, requires laboratory identification of virus

Cause: Several strains of type A influenza orthomyxoviruses that affect a wide variety of bird species but do not survive long in the environment

Transmission: Contagious; ingesting contamination from droppings or inhaling respiratory secretions; contact with infected birds (either domestic or wild) and their body discharges, especially droppings; spreads on contaminated equipment and the feet of insects, rodents, and humans

Prevention: During a local outbreak do not visit flocks or let people visit your flock; consult your vet about the availability of a vaccine against the virus strain responsible for the outbreak

Treatment: None; low-path flu may run through a small flock unnoticed, then die out, leaving the chickens immune to future infection from that particular strain of the virus

Human health risk: Possible, but rare, mild conjunctivitis and/or flulike symptoms

 Low pathogenic avian influenza H5 and H7 strains can evolve into highly pathogenic viruses and therefore are reportable.

Avian Intestinal Spirochetosis. See *Spirochetosis*

Avian Leukosis. See *Lymphatic/Lymphoid Leukosis, Marek's Disease, Osteopetrosis*

Avian Lymphomatosis. See *Marek's Disease*

Avian Malignant Edema. See *Gangrenous Cellulitis/Dermatitis*

Avian Mycoplasmosis. See *Air Sac Disease, Chronic Respiratory Disease, Infectious Synovitis*

Avian Pasteurellosis. See *Fowl Cholera (acute), Fowl Cholera (chronic)*

Avian Pneumoencephalitis. See *Newcastle Disease (velogenic)*

Avian Pox. See *Pox (dry)*

Avian Tuberculosis

Also called: AT, TB, tuberculosis
Prevalence: Common, especially in backyard flocks in midwestern states
System/organ affected: Starts in intestines and migrates to other organs
Incubation period: Weeks to months
Progression: Contagious, slow spreading, usually chronic
Signs: Usually in chickens at least 1 year old that live in contact with soil, dull, ruffled feathers; gradual weight loss despite good appetite; pale, shriveled comb and wattles; lethargy; decrease in laying; shrunken breast muscles with knife-edge (often deformed) keel; sometimes lameness and persistent diarrhea just before death
Percentage affected: Few at a time
Mortality: 100%
Postmortem: Firm, grainy, yellowish to grayish nodules (tubercles) in the intestines, as well as in the liver and spleen, increasing in size and number with the length of time the bird has been infected; abscesses in leg joints of birds that developed lameness
Resembles: Blackhead, except blackhead causes organ spots that are dished rather than knobby; avian leukosis complex (e.g., Marek's disease), except leukosis usually affects younger birds; nodular tapeworm disease, which produces bumps in the intestines but not elsewhere; air-sac mites, which can be detected only as tiny translucent dots moving in air sacs soon after bird dies
Diagnosis: Flock history (bird's age, chronic disease condition), signs (extreme emaciation, continuing deaths in flock), postmortem findings (grainy nodules throughout internal organs), laboratory identification of bacteria (as distinguished from nonpathogenic strains); live birds may be tested with avian tuberculin purified protein derivative (PPD)
Cause: *Mycobacterium avium* bacteria, and sometimes other species of mycobacteria, that survive for 6 months or more in bedding and up to 4 years in soil, the concentration of bacteria depending on how long infected animals have been there and on how crowded they are; affects a wide variety of bird species, as well as calves, pigs, rabbits, sheep, and rodents
Transmission: Picking in soil, feed, or water contaminated by droppings of infected chickens or other infected livestock; picking at an infected live chicken (cannibalism) or the carcass of a dead chicken; spreads on contaminated shoes, equipment, and other mechanical vectors
Prevention: Do not combine chickens from various sources, or young chickens with grown chickens; replace entire layer flock by 18 months of age; control rodents; keep chickens away from pigs and sheep; keep chickens off contaminated ground for at least 4 years
Treatment: None effective
Human health risk: *M. avium* is not the same bacterium that normally causes human TB, although in rare cases it may infect people, as described under Tuberculosis on page 406

 Avian tuberculosis is a reportable disease in some states.

Avian Vibrionic Hepatitis. See
Campylobacteriosis

B

Bacillary White Diarrhea. See *Pullorum*

Big Liver Disease. See *Lymphatic/Lymphoid Leukosis*

Bird Flu. See *Avian Influenza (high pathogenicity)*, *Avian Influenza (low pathogenicity)*

Blackhead

Also called: Histomoniasis, infectious enterohepatitis
Prevalence: Sporadic throughout North America
System/organ affected: Ceca and liver
Incubation period: 7 to 12 days
Progression: Acute or chronic
Signs: In young birds 4 to 6 weeks old, no signs or lethargy; droopy wings; dry, rumpled feathers; pale, shrunken comb and wattles; increased thirst; decreased appetite with accompanying weight loss or stunted growth; bloody droppings; sulfur-yellow cecal discharge; death (rare)
Percentage affected: High
Mortality: Low
Postmortem: Thickened ceca filled with grayish- or greenish-yellow cheesy, foul-smelling, sometimes blood-tinged cores that may range from liquid to solid; liver may be swollen and mottled with circular, dished bull's-eye spots, dark at the center and grayish-white or yellowish-green around the rim

Resembles: Cecal lesions resemble cecal coccidiosis or salmonellosis, and often either disease, or both, also may be present; liver lesions (more likely to occur when coccidiosis is also present) resemble avian tuberculosis, canker, leukosis, and mycosis (*see* Mycoses on page 252) but differ in being depressed and yellowish-green or grayish-white rather than raised and yellowish-gray, although healing lesions may look like those caused by lymphoid leukosis

Diagnosis: Signs, postmortem findings (the combination of cecal lesions and liver lesions); when postmortem findings are insignificant, laboratory identification of protozoa required

Cause: *Histomonas meleagridis* protozoan present wherever poultry occur; free-living forms do not live long but may survive for up to 3 years in cecal worm eggs; histomonads first invade the ceca, then spread to the liver

Transmission: Carried by cecal worms (*Heterakis gallinarum*) and spread to chickens that eat histomonads from the droppings from infected chickens, earthworms containing infective cecal worm eggs, or mechanical vectors such as flies, sowbugs, or grasshoppers, or crickets with histomonads attached

Prevention: Control cecal worms and coccidiosis; prevent damp bedding and muddy yards; range rotation of pastured flocks is ineffective because of the longevity of infectious cecal worm eggs

Treatment: None effective; supplementation with fat-soluble vitamins A, E, D₃, and K helps hasten recovery; recovering birds are carriers

Human health risk: None known

Blue Wing. See *Gangrenous Cellulitis/Dermatitis*

Botulism

Also called: Food poisoning, limberneck, western duck sickness

Prevalence: Sporadic

System/organ affected: Nerves and muscles

Incubation period: High dose of toxin produces signs within hours; low dose may take up to 2 days

Progression: Acute; death can occur within 24 hours

Signs: In birds of all ages, sudden death or progressive limp paralysis of legs, wings, and neck; squatting with outstretched neck and eyes partly closed; mucus accumulation in mouth due to difficulty swallowing; ruffled, loose feathers (raised hackles on cocks) that pull out easily; sometimes trembling; coma and death due to heart and/or respiratory paralysis; healthy, sick, and dead chickens in the same yard

Percentage affected: Depends on how many consume the toxin

Mortality: Usually less than 100%, depending on amount of toxin consumed

Postmortem: None obvious; crop may contain maggots or other suspicious organic matter

Resembles: Spirochetosis and other septicemias, except botulism does not produce internal lesions; limp neck paralysis due to Marek's disease (pseudobotulism form), except in pseudobotulism birds typically recover within 24 hours; castor bean poisoning, which also can cause sudden death

Diagnosis: Signs; elimination of look-alike possibilities; flock history (presence of rotted organic matter, including dead chickens); examination of crop contents for source of toxin; absence of postmortem lesions; sometimes laboratory identification of toxin in blood or tissue

Cause: Consuming powerful toxins in decaying vegetable or animal matter, or maggots feeding on rotting meat, generated by *Clostridium botulinum* bacteria that multiply in warm, moist environments lacking oxygen

Transmission: Not infectious, but a poison resulting from consuming toxins in decaying organic matter, maggots feeding on rotting animal tissue, or beetles (in litter) that harbor *C. botulinum* toxin, or drinking water contaminated with it

Prevention: Do not feed chickens spoiled foods or maggots; burn or deeply bury dead rodents, chickens, or other animal carcasses and rotting, solid vegetables such as cabbages; control flies; acidify soil with ammonium sulfate fertilizer; avoid wet spots in litter; keep birds away from marshy or swampy areas where organic matter rots in water; keep chickens from scratching in compost piles

Treatment: Remove source of poisoning from yard; move affected birds to a cool environment and squirt cool water into crop twice daily; exposed but apparently unaffected birds may be flushed with molasses or Epsom salt (*see* Laxative Flushes, page 392); type C antitoxin, when available, is expensive but can be effective if administered in time

Human health risk: Humans are most commonly poisoned by toxin types A, B, and E; chickens are most commonly poisoned by type C; chickens and humans both may be poisoned by consuming the same contaminated water or spoiled food

Breast Blister
Also called: Keel cyst, keel bursitis, sternal bursitis
Prevalence: Common
System/organ affected: Keel
Progression: Chronic
Signs: In growing or mature cocks, particularly of the heavy breeds, large fluid-filled blister on keel that eventually becomes a callus or thick scar
Percentage affected: Usually no more than 50%
Mortality: None, if not infected
Postmortem: Sternal bursa swollen and filled with yellow creamy or cheesy material (infected) or clear or bloody fluid (not infected), or healed into a thickened scar or callus
Diagnosis: Flock history (breed and sex), signs
Cause: Irritated and inflamed sternal bursa due to pressure from the roost, wire cage floor, or damp or hard-packed bedding; if the reason for resting on the breast bone is a bacterial illness caused by *Mycoplasma synoviae*, *Staphylococcus aureus*, or *Pasteurella*, the blister may be infected with that bacteria
Transmission: Uninfected breast blister is not contagious but is the result of weak legs or poor breast feathering combined with an unsuitable environment; infected breast blister is as contagious as the underlying bacterial disease
Prevention: Do not raise heavy breeds on hardware cloth; do not provide roosts for broilers; for others, provide wide, flat roosts that cushion the breast bone better than narrow, round roosts; keep litter clean, dry, and fluffed
Treatment: Uninfected blisters are usually not treated, since they are rarely noticed before butchering of meat birds; for a breeder cock, open and drain an uninfected blister and treat as a wound (*see* Treating Wounds, page 395); a blister infected with *Mycoplasma synoviae*, *Staphylococcus aureus*, or *Pasteurella* is treated the same as the underlying bacterial illness
Human health risk: None if blister is not infected

Bronchitis. See *Infectious Bronchitis*

Bronchomycosis. See *Aspergillosis (chronic)*

Brooder Pneumonia
Also called: Acute aspergillosis

Prevalence: Common
System/organ affected: Respiratory; eyes (less common)
Incubation period: 2 to 5 days
Progression: Acute
Signs: In hatching eggs, green appearance when candled
In newly hatched chicks, (respiratory form), gasping, rapid breathing, watery discharge from nose and eyes, rapid weight loss, sometimes death
In young chicks, (eye form), swollen eye, usually only one, with an accumulation of yellow cheesy matter
Percentage affected: High
Mortality: Up to 10%
Postmortem: Grayish yellow lungs; white or yellowish cheesy nodules in lungs and air sacs
Resembles: Many respiratory infections caused by bacteria and by other fungi; eye form resembles infectious coryza and nutritional roup
Diagnosis: Difficult; age (less than 2 weeks old), signs, postmortem findings, laboratory culturing of mold spores from respiratory tract
Cause: Spores of *Aspergillus fumigatus* fungus and related molds commonly found in the poultry environment
Transmission: Inhaled spores from mold-contaminated hatching eggs, brooder litter, and chicken coop feed or litter; does not spread from bird to bird
Prevention: Keep nests clean; do not hatch eggs with cracked or poor shells or those found on the floor; sanitize hatching eggs and store them to minimize sweating; clean and disinfect brooder feeders and drinkers daily; avoid stress, moldy litter, moldy feed, dusty brooding conditions; thoroughly clean and disinfect incubator and brooder between hatches
Treatment: None effective
Human health risk: The same molds that affect chicks can affect a human with impaired immunity; *see* Aspergillosis, page 253

Bumblefoot
Also called: Foot burn, foot pad dermatitis, plantar pododermatitis (one form of staphylococcosis)
Prevalence: Common
System/organ affected: Foot pad
Incubation period: 1 to 3 days
Progression: Chronic
Signs: In maturing birds, especially among heavy breeds, lameness; reluctance to walk; inflamed foot

(one or both); hot, hard, swollen abscess on bottom of foot, filled with cheesy/waxy material covered by a dark scab; sores may appear under or between toes and on hocks (from resting on hocks)
Percentage affected: Usually low, except among chickens living in poor conditions
Mortality: Rare; an untreated infection can become septic
Postmortem: Cheesy/waxy material in foot pad; sometimes hock joints filled with grayish-white fluid
Resembles: Fowl cholera (chronic), except cholera typically involves other signs in addition to abscessed foot pad
Diagnosis: Sign (abscess in foot pad)
Cause: *Staphylococcus aureus* bacteria, present wherever there are chickens; dietary deficiency, especially in vitamin B_7 (biotin)
Transmission: Bacteria enters foot through injury caused by scratching in hard or rocky soil, jumping from a high roost onto a hard surface, sharp roosts, splintery bedding, or housing on wire; not contagious
Prevention: Make sure the lowest perch is no higher than 18 inches; round off edges of perches and sand off splinters; provide soft, deep, dry bedding; feed a vitamin supplement (especially vitamin A); do not breed susceptible chickens to avoid producing more of the same
Treatment: Can be difficult to cure; for details *see* page 222
Human health risk: Superficial skin infection (impetigo); wear disposable gloves during treatment, wash hands afterward, take care in disposing of abscess contents and bandages

C

Calcium tetany. See *Hypocalcemia*

Campylobacteriosis
Also called: Avian vibrionic hepatitis, campylobacter hepatitis, infectious hepatitis
Prevalence: More common in industrial flocks than in backyard chickens
System/organ affected: Liver
Incubation period: 1 to 4 days
Progression: Contagious, sometimes acute, usually chronic, spreads slowly (a matter of months)

Signs: Usually none, other than a significant drop in egg laying
Percentage affected: High
Mortality: Gradual, but in an acute outbreak the accumulated death rate can be high
Postmortem: Swollen liver, sometimes green- or brown-stained with characteristic yellow star-shaped patches
Resembles: Any disease causing inflamed liver, including erysipelas, fowl cholera, salmonellosis
Diagnosis: Postmortem findings (stars on liver, when present), laboratory fecal examination to identify bacteria (since campylobacters are sensitive to drying, ask veterinarian or pathologist for a suitable collection container)
Cause: *Campylobacter jejuni* bacteria that commonly dwell in the intestines, survive well in the environment, and resist many disinfectants; often become infective in combination with other conditions such as Marek's disease, pox, or parasites; aggravated by environmental stressors
Transmission: Droppings of infected or carrier birds in feed or water; spread by flies, cockroaches, and rodents; spread on contaminated equipment and soles of shoes
Prevention: None effective; probiotics may help to a limited extent; good management and sanitation; do not combine birds from different sources; keep birds free of internal parasites, coccidia, and other stress-inducing infections; control flies, cockroaches, rodents; isolate weak, unthrifty birds
Treatment: None effective; many chickens naturally develop antibodies that fend off infection; in an acute outbreak, antibiotics may reduce deaths, but survivors remain carriers
Human health risk: Eating undercooked meat of infected birds can cause serious diarrhea; *see* Campylobacter, page 414

Candidiasis. See *Sour Crop*

Canker
Also called: Roup, trichomoniasis
Prevalence: Uncommon, occurring mainly in warm climates or during warm weather
System/organ affected: Upper digestive and respiratory tracts
Incubation period: 3 to 14 days
Progression: Acute or chronic

Signs: Usually in young or growing birds, yellowish-white cheesy patches in the mouth and throat; drooling and repeated swallowing; breathing with the neck extended and mouth open; asymmetric appearance of the face, sometimes with the two halves of the beak failing to meet properly; difficulty eating, with accompanying weight loss or failure to gain; dehydration; pendulous crop; sometimes watery or sticky eyes; sometimes diarrhea; rarely wobbling and other nervous signs

Percentage affected: High

Mortality: Limited, usually within 3 weeks or less, due to inability to swallow and/or breathe

Postmortem: White or yellowish buttons coalescing into cheesy masses in the mouth and throat, possibly spreading down the digestive tract into the proventriculus (but no farther); thickened crop lining

Resembles: Several conditions that cause white or yellow growths in the mouth, including roup (nutritional), pox (wet), and sour crop

Diagnosis: Flock history (contact with pigeons or doves), signs (yellow patches in mouth), confirmed by laboratory identification (*see* Canker on page 214) of trichomonads in mouth scrapings, or droppings

Cause: *Trichomonas gallinae* protozoan parasite that infects pigeons and spreads to other birds through infected saliva or droppings

Transmission: Drinking water or feed contaminated with the saliva or droppings from an infected pigeon or other bird

Prevention: Keep pigeons and doves away from chickens and their feeders and drinkers; keep drinkers clean and sanitized; acidify drinking water with vinegar (1 tablespoon per gallon [15 mL per 4 L], double the vinegar if water is alkaline), making it too acidic for the protozoa to multiply

Treatment: Isolate infected chickens and treat with the nutraceutical Berimax, or treat nonmeat birds with the pharmaceutical metronidazole (Flagyl) or ronidazole (Ronivet), neither of which is legally approved for use with poultry; treat exposed but apparently unaffected birds with acidified copper sulfate (combine 1 pound copper sulfate [powdered bluestone] with 1 cup vinegar and 1 gallon water, mix well, add 1 tablespoon [½ ounce] solution per gallon drinking water for 4 to 7 days, served in a nonmetal drinker); recovered birds remain carriers

Human health risk: None known; not the same as trichomoniasis in humans

Cannibalism. See *Cannibalism, page 294*

Capillariasis. See *Capillary Worm, page 169*

Cardiomyopathy. See *Sudden Death Syndrome*

Cauliflower Gut. See *Necrotic Enteritis*

Cestodiasis. See *Nodular Tapeworm Disease,* also *Tapeworms, page 174*

Chicken Pox. See *Pox (dry)*

Chicken Tick Fever/Paralysis. See *Spirochetosis*

Chlamydiosis

Also called: Avian chlamydiosis, AC, ornithosis, parrot fever, psittacosis

Prevalence: Extremely rare

System/organ affected: Respiratory, digestive, or systemic

Incubation period: Virulent strains about a week; mild strains up to 8 weeks

Progression: Acute or (more commonly) chronic, spreads slowly

Signs: Usually none apparent unless birds are under severe stress; eye discharge and swelling, possible respiratory distress, possible bloody diarrhea, lime-green or yellow urates, weight loss, drop in egg laying

Percentage affected: 100%

Mortality: Low, usually less than 5%, and primarily young birds

Postmortem: Not always obvious; inflamed air sacs; dark, swollen liver with white or yellow spots or pinpoint blood spots; dark, soft, swollen spleen; sometimes enlarged heart; *do not necropsy birds suspected of having chlamydiosis*

Resembles: Aspergillosis, colibacillosis, avian influenza, mycoplasmosis, pasteurellosis (except the liver is not involved)

Diagnosis: History (contact with infected birds), signs (lethargy with no other apparent signs), postmortem findings, laboratory identification of bacteria and/or antigens

Cause: *Chlamydophila psittaci* bacteria that affect many species of bird, but most chickens are resistant; often aggravated by stress and complicated by salmonellosis

Transmission: Contagious; contact with infected birds, infected mucus and droppings, or inhaled dust;

spread by wild birds and infected pet birds, especially those in the parrot family; may be transmitted to chicks through hatching eggs

Prevention: Control wild birds; maintain good sanitation; *C. psittaci* is sensitive to most disinfectants

Treatment: None effective, relapse is likely, survivors may be carriers

Human health risk: High risk of lung infection that, left untreated, is potentially fatal; *see* Ornithosis, page 408

 Chlamydiosis is a reportable disease.

Chondrodystrophy. See *Slipped Tendon*

Chronic Respiratory Disease
Also called: CRD, *Mycoplasma gallisepticum*, MG, PPLO (pleuropneumonia-like organism) infection, stress disease (one form of mycoplasmosis), summer respiratory disease (the same disease in turkeys is called infectious sinusitis)

Prevalence: Common, especially in fall and winter

System/organ affected: Respiratory

Incubation period: 4 to 10 days

Progression: Chronic, spreading slowly and lasting longer in cold weather

Signs: In growing or mature birds, no signs or droopiness, coughing, sneezing, rattling, gurgling, swollen face, nasal discharge without odor, ruffled feathers, weepy or foamy eyes surrounded by donut-shaped swelling, squeaky crow, 20 to 30% drop in laying; sometimes darkened head, decreased appetite, weight loss (prominent breast bone)

Percentage affected: Up to 100%

Mortality: Varies with climate and the existence of secondary infections

Postmortem: Thick mucus in nasal passages and throat; red swollen windpipe; thickened, cloudy air sacs, perhaps containing frothy or yellow cheesy material (may also be found in windpipe and lungs)

Resembles: Any viral respiratory disease (such as infectious bronchitis or Newcastle) with secondary bacterial infection, except CRD is more chronic, spreads more slowly, and usually follows the progression described on page 225

Diagnosis: Blood testing; flock history (time of year, age, potential contact with carriers); signs (respiratory distress, weight loss, drop in laying); postmortem findings (bright yellow cheesy material in windpipe, lungs, and air sacs); laboratory

identification of bacteria (distinguished from nonpathogenic mycoplasmas)

Cause: *Mycoplasma gallisepticum* bacteria, often in combination with other respiratory infections; often follows vaccination for infectious bronchitis or Newcastle; susceptibility increases with stress, cold temperatures, and poor ventilation

Transmission: Contagious; contact with infected or carrier birds and their respiratory discharges; inhaling contaminated dust; spreads from breeders through hatching eggs; spreads on shoes, crates, and other mechanical vectors

Prevention: Purchase only mycoplasma-free stock; keep pigeons away from housing; blood-test breeders; minimize stress caused by sudden weather changes, feed changes, drafts, chilling, crowding, transporting, showing, worming, vaccinating, dust, and ammonia fumes; vaccinate (½ cc subcutaneous) at 6 to 8 weeks of age, repeat in 3 to 4 weeks and every year thereafter; after removing an infected flock, thoroughly clean and disinfect housing and leave empty for a few weeks, as *Mycoplasma gallisepticum* is readily eliminated by sanitizers and sunlight

Treatment: None effective; erythromycin (Gallimycin), a tetracycline, or tylosin (Tylan) will reduce death rate, but survivors remain carriers

Human health risk: None known

 Chronic respiratory disease is a reportable disease.

Cloacitis. See also *Pasting*
Also called: Vent gleet

Prevalence: Fairly common

System/organ affected: Cloaca; can spread internally

Incubation period: Depends on cause

Progression: Usually chronic

Signs: Loose droppings, which may have an offensive odor, sticking to vent feathers

Percentage affected: Usually limited

Mortality: Possible, if infection spreads internally

Postmortem: Distended rectum filled with droppings

Resembles: sticky droppings caused by indigestible feeds (*see* Grain Caution, page 45)

Diagnosis: Signs and flock history

Cause: Stress-induced immune dysfunction commonly resulting in a yeast infection, but may also result in infection by bacteria, fungi, protozoa, or parasites

Transmission: Normally does not spread from bird to bird

Prevention: Avoid stressful situations, nutritional deficiencies, and contamination of feed or water; treat as necessary to control parasites

Treatment: Clean vent feathers, rinse out cloaca with saline-solution wound wash, and disinfect cloaca with an iodine-based antiseptic such as Betadine, repeating as necessary to keep vent clean; get a fecal culture to determine appropriate antimicrobial treatment

Human health risk: None

Clostridial Dermatomyositis. See *Gangrenous Cellulitis/Dermatitis*

Coccidiosis (cecal)

Also called: Cocci, coxy

Prevalence: Common, especially in warm, humid environments

System/organ affected: Cecum

Incubation period: 7-plus days

Progression: Usually acute, spreads rapidly, survivors recover in 10 to 14 days

Signs: In chicks, usually 4½ to 6 weeks of age, but may be earlier or later: droopiness, huddling with ruffled feathers, decreased appetite, pale skin, retarded growth, bloody diarrhea in early stages

Percentage affected: 80 to 100%

Mortality: High

Postmortem: Pale breast muscles, bloated ceca filled with bloody or cheesy material

Resembles: Cecal lesions resemble blackhead, necrotic enteritis, salmonellosis

Diagnosis: Flock history, microscopic identification of coccidia through intestinal scrapings or fecal test (*see* Giving a Fecal Exam, page 187)

Cause: *Eimeria tenella* coccidial protozoa parasites

Transmission: Contact with droppings of infected chickens or pecking the flesh of infected chickens (dead or alive); spreads on used equipment, feet of rodents and wild birds, and so on

Prevention: Can defy good sanitation; breed for resistance; hatch and brood chicks early in the season; introduce local soil into the brooder, and keep litter dry to expose chicks gradually and let them develop resistance; avoid crowded, damp conditions; in warm, damp weather, treat chicks to 16 weeks of age with medicated starter or coccidiostat in drinking water, according to directions on label (excessive use of coccidiostats can be toxic); most mature chickens develop immunity

Treatment: *See* Anticoccidial Drugs, page 205; affected chickens spontaneously recover within a few weeks unless they are reinfected; acidify drinking water with vinegar (1 tablespoon per gallon [15 mL per 4 L], double the vinegar if water is alkaline), making it too acidic for the protozoa to multiply; an antibiotic, in addition, guards against secondary infection; follow treatment with a vitamin supplement (especially A and K); survivors are immune but may never be as productive as uninfected birds

Human health risk: None

Coccidiosis (intestinal). See also *Cryptosporidiosis (intestinal)*

Also called: Cocci, coxy

Prevalence: Common, especially in warm, humid environments

System/organ affected: Intestinal tract

Incubation period: 4 to 5 days

Progression: Usually chronic

Signs: In chicks approximately 3 to 5 weeks of age, but can occur much later, droopiness, huddling with ruffled feathers, loss of interest in water and feed, retarded growth or weight loss, watery, mucusy, or pasty, tan or blood-tinged diarrhea; sometimes emaciation and dehydration

In pullets reaching maturity, thin breast, weak legs, drop in laying; sometimes diarrhea

In yellow-skinned breeds of all ages, pale comb, skin, and shanks

Percentage affected: 80 to 100%

Mortality: Usually low

Postmortem: Varies with *Eimeria* species; *see* Identifying Coccidiosis by Intestinal Lesions, next page

Resembles: Intestinal lesions resemble ulcerative enteritis, salmonellosis, worms, and other enteritic diseases

Diagnosis: Flock history (exposure to large number of oocysts), signs, microscopic identification of coccidia through intestinal scrapings or fecal test (*see* page 187)

Cause: One or more species of coccidial protozoa parasites (*see* Identifying Coccidial Species by Signs, page 200)

Transmission: Contact with droppings of infected chickens or pecking the flesh of infected chickens (dead or alive); spreads on used equipment, feet of rodents and wild birds, and so on

Prevention: Same as for cecal coccidiosis; not all coccidiostats are effective against all coccidial species

Treatment: Same as for cecal coccidiosis; survivors become immune to the coccidial species causing the infection but may never be as productive as uninfected birds

Human health risk: None

Coccidiosis (respiratory). See *Cryptosporidiosis (respiratory)*

Cold. See *Infectious Bronchitis, Infectious Coryza*

Colibacillosis. See also *Air Sac Disease, Egg Peritonitis, Omphalitis*

Also called: Coliform infection, *E. coli* infection

Prevalence: Common

Identifying Coccidiosis by Intestinal Lesions*

	LOCATION	POSTMORTEM FINDING(S)	*EIMERIA* SPECIES
	Duodenum	Roughened lining with white patches or stripes, sometimes overlapping	*E. acervulina* (somewhat easy to identify)
	Duodenum	Tiny bloody spots along duodenum wall	*E. hagani* (hard to identify)
	Duodenum	None distinct; intestine may be filled with sticky fluid	*E. praecox* (hard to identify)
	Duodenum to ceca	Scattered red spots becoming more numerous in the ileum and first part of ceca	*E. mivati* (hard to identify)
	Jejunum, ileum	Large oocysts in reddened, distended, thickened lining dotted with small red or purple blood spots; intestine filled with grayish, pinkish, or orange-brown mucus	*F. maxima*
	Jejunum, ileum, ceca	Small white dots mixed with various-size round red spots; intestine may be filled with bloody sticky fluid; in severe case portions of intestine may thicken and bulge to twice the normal size	*E. necatrix* (easy to identify)
	Ileum	None distinct; intestine may be filled with sticky fluid	*E. mitis* (hard to identify)
	Ileum, ceca, colon, cloaca	Pale, thickened intestine lining that in severe cases peels away, filling intestine with dead tissue and blood	*E. brunetti*
	Ceca	Accumulated clotted blood	*E. tenella* (easy to identify)

*Identification becomes difficult where more than one species is involved.

System/organ affected: Respiratory, intestinal (enteric), or all (septicemia)
Incubation period: Variable
Progression: Severe and acute to mild and chronic, spreads rapidly
Signs: In incubated eggs, dead embryos late in incubation with watery, yellowish-brown yolk sacs, instead of normal thick, yellowish green (omphalitis)
In newly hatched chicks, swollen, inflamed navel, bad odor, death within 6 days of hatching (omphalitis)
In growing birds, lameness, lethargy, ruffled feathers, fever, swollen joints, recovery in about a week or emaciation (infectious synovitis)
In growing or mature birds, labored breathing, coughing, respiratory sounds; diarrhea; or no signs followed by sudden numerous deaths of apparently healthy birds with full crops (acute septicemia)
In mature birds, normal-appearing eye that becomes blind, swollen leg joint filled with golden-colored fluid (infectious synovitis); yellow, watery, or foamy diarrhea (enteritis)
In hens, cessation of laying, upright posture, death within 6 months (egg peritonitis)
Percentage affected: Varies with strain of bacteria and susceptibility of chickens
Mortality: Variable
Postmortem: Varies with location of infection, may include dehydration; greenish liver; swollen liver, spleen, and kidneys with grayish dots; cheesy or fibrous material in air sacs and surrounding heart, liver, and lungs; thick, inflamed intestines filled with mucus and blood; yellowish fluid or yolklike material in body cavity of hens, or distended oviduct filled with whitish curdy or yellowish cheesy material (egg peritonitis); acute septicemia leaves few or no lesions
Resembles: Many other diseases; acute septicemia resembles fowl cholera and fowl typhoid
Diagnosis: Flock history, signs, postmortem findings, laboratory identification of bacteria and its pathogenicity, absence of other pathogens
Cause: Many strains of *Escherichia coli* bacteria commonly found in the poultry environment that infect birds with impaired resistance; often occurs as a secondary infection; signs result from bacterial growth and resulting toxins
Transmission: Ingested droppings of infected birds or mammals in feed or water; spread by wild birds, darkling beetles (*Alphitobius diaperinus*),

and houseflies (*Musca domestica*); transmitted by infected hens to chicks that hatch from infected eggs
Prevention: Good sanitation and ventilation; avoid stress; keep drinking water free of droppings; control rodents; practice good incubator sanitation, and hatch only clean eggs
Treatment: Move affected birds to a clean environment; keep birds warm and well fed with high protein rations and a vitamin E supplement; antibiotic treatment may be effective if started early and *E. coli* strain is positively identified in order to select the most effective drug
Human health risk: Infection or toxic reaction possible from eating contaminated eggs or meat, or by handling infected birds (*see* page 416)

 Colibacillosis is a reportable disease in some states.

Coliform Infection. See *Colibacillosis*

Congenital Loco. See *Stargazing, page 97*

Conjunctivitis (ammonia induced)
Also called: Ammonia blindness, keratoconjunctivitis
Prevalence: Common in flocks raised on deep litter, especially in winter where chickens remain indoors and ventilation is poor
System/organ affected: Eyes
Progression: Acute
Signs: In all ages, rubbing eyes against wings, reluctance to move, loss of interest in eating, avoiding sunlight, one or both eyes cloudy, blindness, death from inability to find feed and water
Percentage affected: 80 to 100%
Mortality: Variable
Postmortem: None significant
Resembles: Any upper respiratory disease, roup (nutritional), any septicemic infection, eye worm
Diagnosis: History (detection of ammonia fumes), signs (eye and eyelid damage), absence of pathogenic cause
Cause: Ammonia fumes from accumulated droppings causing inflammation of the mucous membranes covering the front of the eye and lining the inside of the eyelids
Transmission: Common cause; does not spread from bird to bird
Prevention: Reduce crowding; improve ventilation; avoid damp litter; freshen or replace litter if ammonia fumes are detected; add diatomaceous earth (DE)

and/or absorbent clay (bentonite or montmorillonite) to litter to reduce moisture and neutralize ammonia
Treatment: Improving ventilation and refreshing litter in early stages can lead to recovery of damaged eyes within 2 months but will not reverse blindness
Human health risk: Squinting in ammonia fumes is no less unpleasant for humans than for chickens

Contagious Catarrh. See *Infectious Coryza*

Coryza. See *Infectious Coryza*

Crazy Chick Disease. See *Encephalomalacia, Stargazing, page 97*

Crop Binding
Also called: Crop impaction
Prevalence: Rare
System/organ affected: Crop
Signs: In mature birds, distended crop that feels hard when pressed between fingers; failure to poop; emaciation
Percentage affected: Usually limited to one or a few birds
Mortality: Possible, due to impaired digestion
Postmortem: Crop filled solid with feed and roughage, sometimes sores in lining
Resembles: Pendulous crop, except in crop impaction the crop feels round and hard; sour crop, except in crop impaction a bird initially appears otherwise healthy
Diagnosis: Signs; withhold feed overnight to determine if crop fails to empty by morning
Cause: Overeating, usually due to extreme hunger because feed has been withheld or appropriate feed is unavailable; foraging on long, tough, fibrous matter; tumor or other condition that prevents crop from emptying
Transmission: Does not spread from bird to bird
Prevention: Provide proper rations and plenty of clean, fresh water; if feed is withheld prior to worming, feed a moistened ration 1 hour after worming; mow often enough to keep pasture plants tender and succulent
Treatment: Disinfect skin, slit through skin with very sharp blade, pull skin aside and slit through crop, clean out crop, isolate bird and keep wound clean until it heals (best done by a veterinarian)
Human health risk: None

Crop Impaction. See *Crop Binding*

Crop Mycosis. See *Sour Crop*

Crud. See *Necrotic Enteritis*

Cryptosporidiosis (intestinal)
Also called: Coccidiosis, crypto
Prevalence: Fairly common in confined young chickens; otherwise prevalence is unknown
System/organ affected: Digestive system, cloacal bursa, urinary tract
Incubation period: 3 days
Progression: Acute (lasting 2 to 3 weeks) or chronic
Signs: None or paleness in yellow-skin breeds, ruffled feathers, weight loss, diarrhea, unthriftiness
Percentage affected: Unknown
Mortality: Rare
Postmortem: None obvious; detached intestinal lining (*C. baileyi*); swollen ileum (*C. meleagridis*); numerous oocysts attached to proventriculus lining (*C. galli*), identified by microscopic examination
Resembles: Any mild intestinal disease
Diagnosis: Identification of oocysts through fecal examination or tissue scrapings
Cause: *Cryptosporidium baileyi, C. galli,* and *C. meleagridis* protozoa
Transmission: Ingested oocysts from droppings of infected birds
Prevention: None known other than meticulous sanitation
Treatment: None known; survivors are immune
Human health risk: None known, except possibly in an immunosuppressed person

 Cryptosporidiosis is a reportable disease in some states.

Cryptosporidiosis (respiratory)
Also called: Crypto, respiratory coccidiosis
Prevalence: Not common
System/organ affected: Respiratory (windpipe, lungs, air sacs)
Incubation period: 7 days
Progression: Acute (lasting 2 to 3 weeks) or chronic
Signs: In birds 4 to 17 weeks old, coughing, sneezing, swollen sinuses, swollen eyelids, nasal and eye discharge, respiratory sounds, extending neck to breath, sitting with weight on keel, reluctance to move
Percentage affected: Up to 25%
Mortality: Can be high; survivors recover in 2 to 3 weeks

Postmortem: Loss of cilia in windpipe; swollen airways filled with clear, foamy, white or gray fluid or thick, white, cheesy material
Resembles: Any respiratory infection
Diagnosis: Laboratory identification of oocysts through tissue scrapings
Cause: *Cryptosporidium baileyi* protozoa, often in conjunction with *Escherichia coli* bacteria as a secondary infection
Transmission: Inhaled oocysts from respiratory discharges of infected birds
Prevention: None known, other than meticulous sanitation
Treatment: None known; reduce mortality with supportive therapy (*see* Crypto Control, page 212) and treatment of concurrent infection(s); survivors are immune
Human health risk: None known, except possibly in an immunosuppressed person

Curled-Toe Paralysis

Prevalence: Uncommon
System/organ affected: Sciatic nerve, legs
Progression: Chronic
Signs: In chicks 3 to 4 weeks old, slow growth, weakness, and emaciation despite eating well; diarrhea, resting on hocks, reluctance to move, dry skin, toes curled under foot (making a "fist"), inability to stand, paralysis, death
Percentage affected: Variable
Mortality: Variable
Postmortem: Swollen sciatic nerve
Resembles: Crooked toes, except crooked toes occur at the time of hatch and do not affect a chick's ability to walk (*see* Curled Toes versus Crooked Toes on page 121); any condition resulting in leg paralysis, except in no other condition do the toes curl into the foot
Diagnosis: Flock history (age), signs
Cause: Vitamin B_2 (riboflavin) deficiency
Transmission: Nutritional, does not spread from bird to bird, although several chicks may be affected if fed the same deficient diet
Prevention: Feed breeder flock ration and starter ration with adequate vitamin B_2 (riboflavin)
Treatment: For a quick fix, supplement rations with ground raw liver; a water-soluble vitamin supplement may be helpful if started early but won't correct existing permanent damage
Human health risk: None

Cutaneous Pox. See *Pox (dry)*

Cystic Right Oviduct

Prevalence: Common, especially in older hens
System/organ affected: Right oviduct
Signs: In hens, usually none; an extremely large cyst can fill the abdomen and eventually lead to death
Percentage affected: Individual birds
Mortality: Uncommon
Postmortem: Right oviduct expands to a diameter ranging from a fraction of an inch to 6 inches or more and is filled with clear fluid
Resembles: Signs of an extremely large cyst resemble ascites, infected uterus, internal laying, egg peritonitis; postmortem signs resemble ascites
Diagnosis: Postmortem finding (single fluid-filled balloonlike sac)
Cause: Incomplete regression of the normally nonfunctional right oviduct; could be triggered by an illness such as infectious bronchitis
Transmission: Does not spread from bird to bird
Prevention: None known
Treatment: If a cystic right oviduct is diagnosed before it grows massive enough to cause internal damage, the fluid might be drained by a veterinarian
Human health risk: None

D

Deep Pectoral Myopathy. See *Green Muscle Disease*

Dermatitis, Gangrenous/Necrotic. See *Gangrenous Cellulitis/Dermatitis*

Dermatitis, Vesicular. See *Ergotism*

Dermatomycosis. See *Ringworm*

Dermatophytosis. See *Ringworm*

Diphtheritic Pox. See *Pox (wet)*

Drop Crop. See *Pendulous Crop*

Dropsy. See *Ascites*

Dry Pox. See *Pox (dry)*

E

E. coli infection. See *Colibacillosis*

Egg Binding. See *page 92*

Egg Peritonitis
Also called: Salpingitis, salpingoperitonitis (one form of colibacillosis)
Prevalence: Common
System/organ affected: Oviduct
Incubation period: 5 to 7 days
Progression: Usually chronic
Signs: In hens, particularly obese hens and heavy layers: decreased (or no) egg production, occasional deaths (usually in early morning)
Percentage affected: Variable
Mortality: Sporadic
Postmortem: Inflamed oviduct containing bad-smelling, cheesy cooked-yolk-like matter, which may include eggshells, membranes, and/or whole eggs and may spill into abdomen
Resembles: Egg binding, which may accompany egg peritonitis; yolk peritonitis (free yolks in abdomen), except yolk peritonitis is not an infection and does not cause inflammation; peritonitis due to other types of infection, especially fowl cholera or salmonellosis
Diagnosis: Postmortem findings, laboratory identification of bacteria
Cause: Pathogenic *Escherichia coli* bacteria migrating from cloaca up into the oviduct, sometimes following a viral infection such as infectious bronchitis or a bacterial infection such as mycoplasmosis; more common in heavy layers because of their looser muscle separating the vagina and cloaca
Transmission: Fecal contamination
Prevention: Freshen drinking water often (or use nipple drinkers) to minimize contamination by droppings; eliminate rodents (their droppings can spread coliform bacteria); encourage competitive exclusion (*see* Competitive Exclusion on page 378); maintain a healthful environment that includes good ventilation and litter management
Treatment: None effective
Human health risk: None, if hands are washed after handling infected birds and their meat is not eaten

Emphysema. See *Ruptured Air Sac*

Encephalomalacia
Also called: Crazy chick disease
Prevalence: Rare
System/organ affected: Central nervous system (brain)
Incubation period: Depends on degree of dietary deficiency and for how long
Progression: Acute
Signs: In chicks 1 to 8 weeks (most commonly 2 to 4 weeks) old, loss of coordination, spasms in which the head is pulled down between the legs or the neck bends over the back and sometimes twists to one side, loss of balance and falling over, outstretched legs with rapid muscle spasms that stretch and flex the toes, partial paralysis, prostration, death
Percentage affected: Up to 100%
Mortality: 100%
Postmortem: Clearly visible fluid accumulation and blood spots on the brain; in an advanced case the brain may be spotted with yellowish-green dead tissue
Resembles: Epidemic tremor (encephalomyelitis), except chicks with encephalomalacia don't rest or walk on their hocks; neurotropic velogenic Newcastle disease, except chicks with Newcastle have respiratory issues; Vitamin B_1 (thiamin) deficiency, except vitamin E–deficient chicks continue to eat while vitamin B_1–deficient chicks stop eating. Unlike other paralytic conditions, encephalomalacia does not completely paralyze the wings and legs
Diagnosis: Signs, postmortem findings, ration evaluation
Cause: Insufficient vitamin E in diet; ration lacks sufficient antioxidants; diet high in rancid fat
Transmission: A nutritional issue, does not spread from bird to bird
Prevention: Use only fresh feed, fortified with vitamin E and other antioxidants; store feed in cool, dry place, use within 2 weeks of purchase; use vitamin supplements before their expiration date; supplement breeder flock diet with vitamin E
Treatment: Effective only if begun before brain is seriously damaged; for chicks: ½ teaspoon vitamin AD&E powder per gallon of water until signs disappear; for growing birds: ¼ cc AD&E injected into breast (intramuscular) in addition to vitamin powder in drinking water
Human health risk: None

Encephalomyelitis. See *Epidemic Tremor*

Endemic Fowl Cholera. See *Fowl Cholera (chronic)*

Endemic Newcastle. See *Newcastle Disease (lentogenic)*

Enlarged Hock Disease. See *Infectious Synovitis*

Enteritis. See *Colibacillosis, Necrotic Enteritis, Ulcerative Enteritis*

Enterococcal infection. See *Omphalitis*

Enterohepatitis. See *Blackhead*

Enterotoxemia. See *Necrotic Enteritis*

Enzootic Fowl Cholera. See *Fowl Cholera (chronic)*

Epidemic Tremor
Also called: Avian encephalomyelitis, AE, New England disease
Prevalence: Sporadic
System/organ affected: Nervous system
Incubation period: Egg transmitted, 1 to 7 days; otherwise 10 to 17 days
Progression: Rapid, runs its course in 2 to 3 weeks
Signs: In 1- to 3-week-old chicks, dull eyes followed by incoordination, resting or walking on hocks, falling over with outstretched wing, and trembling of the head, neck, wings, and legs; weak peeping; paralysis; death due to inability to eat or to being trampled by other chicks; survivors of acute infection remain unthrifty and may eventually develop cataracts and blindness
In mature hens (signs easily go unnoticed), up to 20% drop in laying for 2 weeks; late embryo deaths in incubated eggs; poor livability of hatchlings
Percentage affected: Up to 60%
Mortality: *In chicks:* 25% average; can be as high as 90%
In mature birds: none
Postmortem: Subtle pale (tan or white) areas may occur in the gizzard muscle of chicks; otherwise none obvious
Resembles: Encephalomalacia (vitamin E deficiency), except encephalomalacia usually affects slightly older chicks; Marek's disease, except Marek's usually affects much older birds and causes damage that is readily visible during postmortem; Newcastle, except

Newcastle can appear at any age; aspergillosis and other brain inflammations caused by bacteria, fungi, or mycoplasmas; salt or pesticide poisoning
Diagnosis: History (age of birds), signs (trembling of head and neck), postmortem (lack of obvious damage), confirmed by laboratory identification of virus (from brain tissue) or antibodies
Cause: Picornavirus that survives well in the environment
Transmission: Ingesting virus from droppings of infected birds, which shed virus for 2 weeks or more; infected breeders infect offspring by shedding virus in eggs; can be spread by turkeys, pheasants, pigeons, quail; spreads on contaminated equipment and shoes of humans
Prevention: Vaccinate pullets at least 4 weeks before they start laying; hatch eggs only from disease-free or immune hens (those having been vaccinated or having survived infection, as determined by blood testing)
Treatment: None; survivors become immune and are not carriers, but chicks may not mature into good layers or breeders
Human health risk: None known

 Epidemic tremor is a reportable disease in Canada.

Epididymal Lithiasis
Also called: EL, premature low fertility syndrome
Prevalence: Common
System/organ affected: Male reproduction (epididymis)
Progression: Chronic
Signs: Low fertility or infertility of cocks past the age of 2 years
Percentage affected: About 50% among backyard chickens (approaching 100% among industrial strains)
Mortality: None
Postmortem: Calculi (stones) in the epididymis region; atrophy of the testicles
Resembles: Any condition causing reduced fertility
Diagnosis: Postmortem findings
Cause: Unknown; theories include infection, hormone imbalance, and genetic predisposition
Transmission: Unknown
Prevention: None known
Treatment: None known
Human health risk: None

Ergotism

Also called: Gangrenous form: sod disease, vesicular dermatitis

Prevalence: Rare

System/organ affected: *Convulsive* — central nervous system
Gangrenous — extremities (comb, beak, toes, etc.)

Progression: Acute (convulsive) or chronic (gangrenous)

Signs: *Convulsive* — incoordination, trembling, neck twisting, inability to stand, convulsions, and death
Gangrenous — slow growth or reduced egg production; abnormal feathering; diarrhea; decay of comb, wattles, and beak; sometimes blisters on the shanks and tops of toes

Percentage affected: Depends on how much contaminated feed was consumed and for how long

Mortality: Depends on how much contaminated feed was consumed and for how long

Postmortem: Sometimes enlarged heart (gangrenous form); otherwise inconclusive

Resembles: Other mycotoxicoses (*see* Mycotoxicoses on page 247)
Convulsive form—any disease affecting the central nervous system
Gangrenous form—gangrenous dermatitis (in which staphylococcal or clostridial bacteria are present)

Diagnosis: Signs, feed or forage analysis, absence of other causative agents

Cause: Toxic alkaloids produced by *Claviceps purpurea* and related molds in rye, wheat, barley, and other cereal grains, as well as in the seed of wild grasses

Transmission: Consuming contaminated grain or grass seed, particularly rye, as well as consuming pelleted rations containing contaminated grain or weed seeds; does not spread from bird to bird

Prevention: Do not feed grains or other rations from questionable sources; keep chickens away from ergot-contaminated cropland or weed fields

Treatment: Replace contaminated feed; increase dietary protein and carbohydrates; offer a vitamin supplement

Human health risk: Humans may be poisoned by eating that same contaminated grain that poisons chickens

Erysipelas

Also called: Erysipelothrix infection, red skin

Prevalence: Sporadic and rare, occurring most often in maturing birds at the start of cold, damp weather

System/organ affected: Entire body (septicemic)

Incubation period: Uncertain

Progression: Acute, sometimes followed by chronic infection

Signs: Sudden death or a brief period of lethargy, decreased appetite, sometimes greenish-yellow diarrhea, sometimes purplish or reddish blotches on skin, death or recovery within 24 hours
In cocks, reduced fertility
In hens, dramatic drop in egg production

Percentage affected: Up to 50%

Mortality: Up to 100%

Postmortem: No significant postmortem signs other than skin blotches; small blood spots in nearly any tissue or organ, especially breast muscle; inflamed intestines filled with thick mucus; possibly swollen liver and spleen

Resembles: Any disease causing acute septicemia, including chlamydiosis, colibacillosis, fowl cholera (except cholera does not cause swollen spleen), Newcastle, salmonellosis, streptococcosis; several noninfectious conditions, including poisoning, predation, or being trampled by other chickens

Diagnosis: Difficult because of lack of specific signs and lesions, and because bacteria are hard to isolate for identification; flock history (chickens ranged on land that once held infected turkeys, pigs, or sheep), signs (sudden deaths among apparently healthy birds), postmortem findings (blood-spotted breast muscle and blotchy skin), laboratory identification of bacteria

Cause: *Erysipelothrix rhusiopathiae* bacteria that affects turkeys more often than chickens

Transmission: Bacteria from droppings of infected chickens (or turkeys, pigs, or sheep) enter through wounds caused by fighting, cannibalism, poorly designed equipment, or procedures such as dubbing, cropping, or spur trimming; bacteria ingested while picking infected live birds (cannibalism) or dead ones; consuming meal from infected fish; spread by red mites (*Dermanyssus gallinae*); may be triggered by stress due to crowding, dampness, bad weather, poor sanitation, ration change, vaccination

Prevention: In erysipelas-prone areas, keep chickens away from pasture occupied by turkeys, pigs, or sheep during the previous 5 weeks; avoid crowding; control rodents

Treatment: Rapid-acting penicillins may be effective if started early; survivors are resistant to future infection but remain carriers; since this disease poses a human health risk, the best course is to eliminate the infected flock and start over on fresh ground

Human health risk: Handling infected chickens may result in a painful infection that can be fatal without medical attention; see Erysipeloid, page 408

Erysipelothrix Infection. See *Erysipelas*

Erythroid Leukosis. See *Typical Diseases Caused by Avian Leukosis Viruses, page 266*

Escherichia coli Infections. See *Air Sac Disease, Egg Peritonitis, Colibacillosis, Omphalitis*

Exotic Newcastle Disease. See *Newcastle Disease (velogenic)*

Exudative Diathesis

Prevalence: Rare

System/organ affected: Skin and muscle tissue

Signs: In chicks, failure to grow well, ruffled feathers, visible greenish-blue fluid accumulation under breast and leg skin, weepy skin between legs and under wings, chicks have trouble walking and stand with legs unusually far apart, paralysis, death

Percentage affected: 100% of chicks eating same faulty ration

Mortality: 100%

Postmortem: Yellow or bluish-green gelatinous fluid under skin; degenerated skeletal muscle

Resembles: Gangrenous dermatitis, for which exudative diathesis may be a precursor

Diagnosis: Signs, postmortem findings, ration evaluation

Cause: Diet deficient in both vitamin E and selenium

Transmission: Nutritional problem, does not spread from bird to bird

Prevention: Use only fresh feed fortified with vitamin E and selenium; store feed in cool dry place and use within 2 weeks of purchase; do not feed rancid polyunsaturated fats such as cod liver oil and soybean oil

Treatment: Vitamin E and selenium supplement in feed or orally (300 IU per bird); replace stale ration or reformulate home-mixed feed

Human health risk: None

F

False Botulism. See *Marek's Disease*

Fatty Liver Disease/Syndrome

Also called: Hemorrhagic fatty liver syndrome, hemorrhagic liver syndrome

Prevalence: Common in overweight hens

System/organ affected: Liver

Progression: Chronic

Signs: In hens, particularly in warm weather: sudden death of an apparently healthy hen, or a sudden drop in laying; obesity (25 to 35% above normal); swollen, pale combs and wattles

Percentage affected: Variable

Mortality: Up to 5%, usually in older hens

Postmortem: Large, bloody liver (sometimes yellow and mushy), excess body fat (sometimes pink), blood clots in the body cavity

Resembles: Campylobacteriosis, except a fatty liver lacks the characteristic star-shaped patches; sudden death syndrome, which involves the heart rather than the liver; aflatoxicosis and hypocalcemia, but neither is related to obesity

Diagnosis: Postmortem findings, signs, flock history

Cause: Obesity resulting from a high-energy feed combined with inactivity; without excess body fat, liver damage may have been caused by mold toxins in feed; death is due to liver rupture

Transmission: Does not spread from bird to bird but can affect all hens subjected to the same conditions

Prevention: Avoid obesity resulting from high-energy feeds (consisting mostly of grains) combined with insufficient space for normal activity; avoid moldy feeds

Treatment: None effective

Human health risk: None

Favus. See *Ringworm*

Flip-Over Disease/Flips. See *Sudden Death Syndrome*

Floppy Broiler Syndrome. See *Marek's Disease*

Food Poisoning. See *Botulism*

Foot Burn. See *Bumblefoot*

Foot Pad Dermatitis. See *Bumblefoot*

Fowl Cholera (acute)

Also called: Avian cholera, avian hemorrhagic septicemia, avian pasteurellosis, FC
Prevalence: Sporadic
System/organ affected: Entire body (septicemic)
Incubation period: 3 to 9 days
Progression: Acute, contagious, spreads rapidly, kills quickly
Signs: In growing chickens, usually 4 months or older, sudden death (typically laying hens found dead in nests) or lethargy, ruffled feathers, decreased appetite and weight loss, increased thirst, increased respiratory rate and rattling sounds when breathing, lameness, mucus discharge from mouth (drooling); white, watery diarrhea later becoming thicker and greenish yellow; death, with bluish comb and wattles, within hours of first signs; chickens that survive longer may either eventually die from emaciation and dehydration or develop chronic cholera
Percentage affected: High
Mortality: 10 to 50%
Postmortem: Engorged blood vessels; flecks of blood on heart, mucous membranes, abdominal lining, and fatty tissue; swollen, grayish liver (looks cooked) with small grayish-white spots (resembles cornmeal); swollen spleen; fluid in abdomen; bruised-appearing tissue lining body cavity; bloody mucus in intestines
In hens: inflamed ovary, bloody immature yolks; yolk in abdominal cavity
Resembles: Poisoning, chlamydiosis, listeriosis, ornithobacterosis, salmonellosis (especially fowl typhoid), staphylococcic arthritis (except arthritis has a much lower death rate), septicemic colibacillosis, and some types of coccidiosis produce similar signs and nearly identical lesions
Diagnosis: Signs (especially sudden death of apparently healthy mature chickens), history (of cholera on or near premises), laboratory identification of bacteria
Cause: *Pasteurella multocida* bacteria that affect a variety of birds and increase in virulence as disease spreads; *P. multocida* survives for 1 month in droppings and 3 months in moist soil but is easily destroyed by sunlight, disinfectants, drying, heat
Transmission: Contagious bacteria enter through the mouth or respiratory system; spreads in mucus (contaminating feed and water and spread on soiled equipment and shoes) from the nose, mouth, or eyes of recovered carriers and chickens with chronic fowl cholera; picking at the carcass of an infected dead chicken; may be spread by pets, rodents, and wild birds
Prevention: Provide clean, safe drinking water; avoid excessive stress; acquire only cholera-free chickens; avoid acquiring growing or mature birds, which may be carriers; do not mix birds of different ages from different sources; keep wild birds, rodents, and other animals away from chickens; responsibly dispose of dead chickens; keep new chickens off old, contaminated pasture for at least 3 months; a bacterin (vaccine) is available for immunizing healthy chickens where fowl cholera has been a problem in the past
Treatment: None effective; disease recurs when medication is discontinued and survivors are carriers; isolate and dispose of infected flock, thoroughly disinfect and dry housing, leave it vacant at least 3 months before introducing new birds
Human health risk: Upper respiratory tract infection (which can in turn infect chickens through mucus discharged from the human's mouth or nose) is possible in people working where large numbers of chickens have died in poorly ventilated housing.

 Fowl cholera is a reportable disease.

Fowl Cholera (chronic)

Also called: Avian cholera, avian pasteurellosis, endemic fowl cholera, enzootic fowl cholera, localized pasteurellosis, LP, mild fowl cholera, roup
Prevalence: Common
System/organ affected: Respiratory, wattles, joints
Incubation period: Weeks to months
Progression: Chronic and slow spreading
Signs: In mature chickens, no signs of upper respiratory distress; cheesy nasal discharge; abscessed wattles (which may rupture and scar over); swollen head and face; inflammation of membranes associated with the eyes; lameness or swelling of leg joints, wing joints, foot pads; sometimes neck twists sideways
In hens, slight decrease in laying, smaller eggs with increased blood spotting
In cocks, loss of typical aggressive behavior and reduced crowing
Percentage affected: Low
Mortality: Low
Postmortem: Yellow cheesy material filling sinuses, along keel, and surrounding joints; cheesy material

in inner ear and skull of birds with twisted neck; wrinkled, bloody, and/or off-color immature yolks

Resembles: Infectious coryza, except coryza is more typically associated with a foul odor; Newcastle, except Newcastle involves other nervous signs besides twisted neck

Diagnosis: Signs, postmortem findings, laboratory identification of bacterial strain

Cause: *Pasteurella multocida* bacteria lingering after an acute cholera infection or of a less virulent strain

Transmission: Bacteria enter through respiratory system or skin wounds; spread in mucus directly from infected chickens or carriers and on contaminated equipment, feed, water; may develop in survivors of acute fowl cholera

Prevention: Avoid combining chickens of different ages or from different sources; isolate infected chickens; remove flock from infected facilities, clean throughly, and leave empty for at least a month; a bacterin (vaccine) is available for immunizing healthy chickens where fowl cholera has been a problem in the past

Treatment: Sulfa drugs are effective, although recovered chickens remain carriers

Human health risk: None known

Fowl Diphtheria. See *Pox (wet)*

Fowl Paralysis. See *Marek's Disease*

Fowl Pest. See *Avian Influenza (high pathogenicity)*

Fowl Plague. See *Avian Influenza (high pathogenicity)*

Fowl Pox. See *Pox (dry)*

Fowl Spirochetosis. See *Spirochetosis*

Fowl Tick Fever/Paralysis. See *Spirochetosis*

Fowl Typhoid

Also called: FT (one kind of salmonellosis)
Prevalence: Sporadic but rare in USA and Canada
System/organ affected: Intestines or septicemic
Incubation period: 4 to 5 days
Progression: Usually acute (running course within a week), can be chronic (lasting up to 5 weeks)
Signs: Usually in growing birds 12 weeks or older, decreased appetite, increased thirst, droopiness, ruffled feathers, huddling near heat, pale comb and wattles, yellow-green diarrhea that sticks to vent feathers, sporadic deaths

Percentage affected: Varies widely
Mortality: Usually less than 30%
Postmortem: Dark, swollen, bronze metallic-looking liver; swollen, mottled spleen; swollen gallbladder; pinpoint hemorrhages in muscles and fat; smelly, slimy, inflamed duodenum; thin, watery blood

Resembles: Paratyphoid and pullorum, except fowl typhoid usually affects growing birds

Diagnosis: Flock history, signs, postmortem findings, laboratory identification of bacteria

Cause: *Salmonella* Gallinarum bacteria that can survive for 6 months or more in litter and soil but are sensitive to sunlight and disinfectants

Transmission: Usually from carrier breeders to chicks through hatching eggs, but also can be spread by contaminated droppings in litter or clinging to equipment, shoes, flies, feet of animals and wild birds

Prevention: Purchase certified typhoid-free chickens; blood-test birds and eliminate carriers; hatch eggs only from disease-free breeders; clean and disinfect regularly; control flies, rodents, animals, and wild birds; keep chickens away from contaminated ponds and other surface water; rotate range-fed chickens

Treatment: None effective; survivors are carriers

Human health risk: Low; not the same disease as typhoid fever in humans

 Fowl typhoid is a reportable disease.

Fungal Pneumonia. See *Aspergillosis (chronic)*

Fusariotoxicosis

Also called: Trichothecene mycotoxicosis, fusariotoxin mycotoxicosis
Prevalence: Sporadic in cool climates
System/organ affected: Mucous membranes and skin, bone marrow
Incubation period: Minutes to hours
Progression: Acute
Signs: Usually in growing birds, refusal to eat, slow growth, unusual wing positions, abnormal feathering with broken feather shafts, lack of reflexes, lethargy, paleness, bloody diarrhea, sores at corners of mouth and on skin, burnlike irritation inside mouth and on tongue, crusty accumulation along edges of beak, reduced resistance to respiratory diseases

In hens, lethargy, sitting around, bluish comb and wattles, sudden drastic drop in egg production, thin shells, reduced hatchability of eggs

Percentage affected: High

Mortality: Low

Postmortem: Sores along upper digestive tract, reddening throughout digestive tract, swollen gizzard lining, mottled liver, swollen gallbladder, shriveled spleen, bloody internal organs, pale bone marrow

In hens: shriveled ovary and oviduct

Resembles: Roup (nutritional), sour crop, any caustic substance that causes mouth blisters or burning when ingested

Diagnosis: Signs (refusal to eat, blisters in mouth and throat), postmortem findings

Cause: Consumed trichothecene toxins produced by *Fusarium sporotrichioides* and related molds in corn, oats, wheat, barley, rice, rye, sorghum, and safflower seed grown under cold, damp conditions; inhaled or skin contact with trichothecene toxins in bedding

Transmission: Contaminated feed or litter; does not spread from bird to bird

Prevention: Avoid grains or litter from questionable sources

Treatment: Toxin is rapidly excreted, so chickens generally recover after contaminated feed is replaced; chicks recover more quickly when given supplements of vitamins C and E

Human health risk: Serious diarrhea from eating some contaminated grains that poison chickens

G

Gangrenous Cellulitis/Dermatitis

Also called: Avian malignant edema, blue wing, clostridial dermatomyositis, GD, gas edema disease, necrotic dermatitis, wing rot

Prevalence: Sporadic, more likely to occur in warm seasons

System/organ affected: Skin

Incubation period: 3 to 6 days

Progression: Acute; runs its course within 2 weeks

Signs: Usually in intensively raised chickens 4 to 16 weeks old, sudden deaths (sometimes with small, moist sores between toes) or birds may become prostrate; feathers look dirty and fall out easily; skin easily rubs off and pops or crackles when touched (from gas underneath); wattles become swollen and weepy; reddish-black patches of dead, featherless skin on wing tips, breast, abdomen, or thighs; death within 24 hours, and body decomposes rapidly, turning green within 1 or 2 hours

Percentage affected: Low

Mortality: Up to 60%

Postmortem: Gas and bloody, gelatinous fluid beneath bad-smelling skin; gray or tan breast and thigh muscles that look cooked; usually shriveled cloacal bursa; sometimes swollen liver, spleen, kidneys, or bloody lungs

Resembles: Any skin infection caused by contact with wet or improperly managed litter; nutritional deficiencies that leave skin unprotected because of slow feathering; exudative diathesis (which may be a predisposing factor)

Diagnosis: Flock history, signs, postmortem findings, laboratory identification of bacteria

Cause: *Clostridium septicum*, *C. perfringens*, or *Staphylococcus aureus* alone or in combination, usually in immunosuppressed birds following severe coccidiosis or a viral infection, especially infectious bursal disease; a selenium–vitamin E deficiency may encourage infection

Transmission: Bacteria enter individual birds through wounds caused by fighting, cannibalism, treading during mating, or poorly designed housing equipment

Prevention: Bedding sanitation and proper nutrition, including avoiding rancid rations; ventilation to prevent excessive humidity in housing; good management to avoid bruises, injuries, and cannibalism; avoiding indiscriminate use of antibiotics

Treatment: Antibiotic selection requires laboratory identification of bacteria; vitamin-electrolyte supplement hastens recovery

Human health risk: None; as a precaution, wash hands well after handling infected chicks

Gapes. See *Gapeworm, page 171*

Gas Edema Disease. See *Gangrenous Cellulitis/Dermatitis*

Gout (articular)

Also called: Articular hyperuricemia, articular urate deposition

Prevalence: Sporadic

System/organ affected: Usually joints

Incubation period: Not applicable

Progression: Usually chronic

Signs: Primarily in cocks age 4 months or older, swollen foot joints with pasty white urate deposits easily seen through the skin; lameness and unwillingness to walk; blisters and sores on feet; in a severe case, comb and wattles may also be involved
Percentage affected: Usually individual birds
Mortality: None
Postmortem: White tissue surrounding joints, white semifluid deposits within joints and possibly in comb, wattles, and windpipe
Resembles: Bumblefoot, except bumblefoot results in a single sore at the bottom of the foot and usually affects only one foot; an extreme case of scaly leg mite, except in scaly leg the foot swelling and deformity results from deposits under individual scales rather than under the skin
Diagnosis: Signs, postmortem findings
Cause: Arthritis as a result of abnormal accumulation of urates in the body following kidney damage caused by hereditary susceptibility or excessive protein in diet
Transmission: Genetic, or nutritionally related
Prevention: None known, other than appropriate diet
Treatment: Decrease dietary protein, and encourage the bird to drink more, which won't cure articular gout but will help keep it from getting worse; aspirin (as described on page 395) may be used to relieve inflammation and pain
Human health risk: None

Gout (visceral)

Also called: Acute gout, visceral hyperuricemia, visceral urate deposition
Prevalence: Common
System/organ affected: Kidneys and other organs
Incubation period: Not applicable
Progression: Usually acute
Signs: In chicks, flockwide deaths soon after hatch In growing or mature birds, sudden deaths or lethargy, increased thirst, decreased appetite, emaciation, darkened head and shanks, white pasty droppings, dull feathers, cessation of laying, sometimes swollen feet
Percentage affected: Up to 100%
Mortality: Gradual, up to 100%
Postmortem: Dry, shrunken breast muscles; both kidneys shriveled or one shriveled and one pale and swollen; chalky white deposits coating the kidneys, heart, liver, and sometimes joints
Resembles: Any inflammation causing kidneys to dysfunction; articular gout, when foot swelling is involved

Diagnosis: Signs, postmortem findings (white chalklike deposits coating various organs)
Cause: Kidney failure caused by an inability to excrete urates for a variety of reasons that include water deprivation, kidney damage from disease (especially infectious bronchitis or intestinal cryptosporidiosis), excessive use of antibiotics (especially gentamicin or sulfa drugs), moldy feed, excessive dietary protein, excess calcium (3% or more), excess sodium bicarbonate, calcium-to-phosphorus imbalance, vitamin A deficiency, blockage of the ureters by kidney stones or tumors
Transmission: Does not spread from bird to bird, although the condition may appear flockwide in birds subjected to the same debilitating conditions
Prevention: Provide plenty of pure drinking water, cool in summer and warm in winter; feed age-appropriate balanced rations; avoid excessively high protein rations
Treatment: None known
Human health risk: None

Gray Eye. See *Marek's Disease*

Green Muscle Disease

Also called: Deep pectoral myopathy
Prevalence: Common among heavy-breast broilers
System/organ affected: Breast (chicken tender)
Incubation period: Not applicable
Progression: Acute or chronic
Signs: None
Percentage affected: Variable
Mortality: None
Postmortem: Depending on how long before slaughter the injury occurred, one or both breast tenders may be swollen and pale, or bloody looking, or dry and yellowish or greenish
Resembles: No other condition
Diagnosis: Postmorten findings
Cause: Excessive wing flapping caused by fright or other stress
Transmission: Does not spread from bird to bird but may affect all broilers subjected to the same stressful conditions
Prevention: Avoid conditions that encourage wing flapping
Treatment: None
Human health risk: None

Gumboro disease. See *Infectious Bursal Disease*

H

Heart Attack. See *Sudden Death Syndrome*

Hemangioendothelioma. See *Typical Diseases Caused by Avian Leukosis Viruses, page 266*

Hemophilus Infection. See *Infectious Coryza*

Hemorrhagic (Fatty) Liver Syndrome. See *Fatty Liver Disease/Syndrome*

Hepatitis. See *Campylobacteriosis*

Histomoniasis. See *Blackhead*

Hock Disease. See *Slipped Tendon*

Hot Avian Influenza. See *Avian Influenza (high pathogenicity)*

Hypocalcemia
Also called: Calcium tetany
Prevalence: Sporadic
System/organ affected: Blood
Progression: Acute
Signs: In pullets or hens, egg binding, muscle weakness, paralysis, death early in the day, often while laying an egg; back feathers may be missing from excessive treading
Percentage affected: Variable
Mortality: Highest in pullets starting to lay and in hens during hot weather
Postmortem: Developing egg in oviduct (often in uterus), sometimes little or no medullary bone
Resembles: Fatty liver syndrome (postmortem signs differ)
Diagnosis: Difficult; flock history, signs, postmortem findings
Cause: Low blood calcium
Transmission: Metabolic, does not spread from hen to hen, although several hens in a flock may be affected by the same underlying cause (such as inadequate diet or heat stress)
Prevention: Avoid feeding layer ration to pullets before they start to lay; offer large-particle calcium supplement (oyster shell or limestone granules); avoid heat stress and dehydration
Treatment: For muscle weakness, sprinkle large-particle calcium on top of ration alternately for 3 days, stop 3 days, repeating for 2 to 3 weeks until signs disappear; for paralyzed hen, intravenous calcium administered by a veterinarian
Human health risk: None

Hypovitaminosis-A. See *Roup (nutritional)*

I

Infectious Bronchitis
Also called: Avian infectious bronchitis, IB, cold
Prevalence: Common
System/organ affected: Primarily respiratory, can infect kidneys, digestive tract, or oviduct
Incubation period: 18 to 36 hours
Progression: Acute; starts suddenly, spreads rapidly, runs through flock in about 2 weeks (a respiratory distress that lasts longer likely has some other cause)
Signs: In chicks up to 6 weeks of age, gasping, coughing, sneezing, rattling, watery eyes, nasal discharge, huddling near heat, decreased appetite, slow growth, sometimes swollen sinuses
In growing and mature chickens, similar to signs in chicks, although respiratory sounds may not be obvious except when birds roost at night; sometimes pasty white diarrhea
In hens, temporary drop in laying by up to 50%, with the few eggs laid being smaller, with shells that are thin (and therefore pale, in brown-egg layers), soft, misshapen, rough, or ridged and whites that are watery; laying resumes in about 6 weeks but at a lower rate than before infection, and recovered hens are subject to reproductive disorders, including oviduct impaction and internal laying
Percentage affected: 100%
Mortality: Up to 30% in chicks under 3 weeks of age, depending on virulence of the virus, but can be up to 90%, especially in cold weather or in the presence of a secondary bacterial infection; uncommon in birds older than 5 weeks
Postmortem: *In chicks:* yellowish cheesy material in windpipe, lungs, and air sacs
In growing and mature birds: swollen, pale kidneys; urate crystals clogging ureters; fluid yolk or whole eggs in abdominal cavity of hens
Resembles: Laryngotracheitis, except laryngo spreads less rapidly and is more severe; Newcastle, except Newcastle is more severe, results in a greater drop in egg production, and often includes nervous signs;

low pathogenic avian influenza; infectious coryza, except coryza often has a foul odor and produces facial swelling (bronchitis rarely does); roup (nutritional), except roup does not affect egg whites or shells

Diagnosis: Difficult; signs (rapid onset of respiratory distress), postmortem findings, laboratory identification of virus, absence of other respiratory pathogens

Cause: Several strains of coronavirus that infect only chickens, do not survive more than about a week in the environment, and are easily destroyed by disinfectants and sunlight

Transmission: The most contagious poultry disease; spreads by contact with infected birds or their respiratory discharges; spreads on contaminated equipment; not transmitted to embryos in incubated eggs, but an infected hen can shed virus on eggshells

Prevention: Avoid mixing chickens of different ages or from different sources; a vaccine is available but is effective only against virus strains found locally, and can permanently reduce a hen's laying rate

Treatment: Provide electrolytes in drinking water (*see* Electrolytes on page 385); keep birds warm and well fed; avoid crowding; as necessary, treat for secondary bacterial infection; where white pasty diarrhea occurs, acidify drinking water with vinegar (1 tablespoon per gallon [15 mL per 4 L], double vinegar dose if water is alkaline) for 5 to 7 days; survivors may continue shedding the virus periodically

Human health risk: None known; a different virus causes bronchitis in humans

Infectious Bursal Disease

Also called: Gumboro disease, IBD
Prevalence: Common, primarily in large flocks
System/organ affected: Lymph tissue, especially cloacal bursa
Incubation period: 2 to 3 days
Progression: Highly contagious, acute, appears suddenly, spreads rapidly, runs through a flock in 1 to 2 weeks
Signs: <u>In young birds 3 to 6 weeks old</u>, none; or lethargy, huddling, ruffled feathers, vent picking (bird picks at own vent), diarrhea (sometimes blood tinged) with watery urates staining vent feathers and making litter sticky, decreased appetite, wobbly gait, slight trembling, dehydration, prostration, death
Percentage affected: Nearly 100%
Mortality: 0 to 20% (more if the strain is highly virulent), peaking in about a week

Postmortem: None significant, or swollen, fluid-filled (sometimes bloody) cloacal bursa; dark, shriveled muscles (especially breast and thighs) flecked with blood; mucus-filled intestine; swollen spleen peppered with gray dots; pale kidneys swollen with urates

Resembles: Coccidiosis, except cocci does not cause bloody flecks in muscles or swelling of cloacal bursa; pale, urate-clogged kidneys resemble infectious bronchitis, except infectious bursal disease does not produce respiratory signs

Diagnosis: Flock history (young birds), signs (sudden illness throughout flock, white or watery diarrhea, birds picking own vents, deaths peaking within a week, rapid recovery of survivors), postmortem findings (appearance of cloacal bursa, blood spots in breast and thigh muscles), laboratory identification of virus or antigens (infected cloacal bursa may be frozen and taken to a pathology lab for inspection)

Cause: Birnavirus that reduces the immunity of young chickens, making them highly susceptible to other infections

Transmission: Highly contagious; survives in feed, water, and droppings for weeks and in housing for at least 4 months after removal of infected birds; spread from infected birds through their droppings in contaminated litter and dust in air and on equipment, feed, shoes, insects, rodents, and wild birds; may be spread by darkling beetle, or lesser mealworm (*Alphitobius diaperinus*) found in litter; not spread by breeders through hatching eggs; survivors are not carriers

Prevention: Once present, this virus defies good management and is difficult to eradicate; where this virus is present, early exposure of chicks reduces signs of illness, and as mature breeders they pass maternal antibodies to future generations; vaccinated breeders also pass paternal immunity to their offspring; vaccinate only where this disease is prevalent

Treatment: None effective; keep birds warm and well ventilated and provide plenty of drinking water with supplemental multivitamin; an antibiotic may be needed to control secondary bacterial infection; recovered chickens are more susceptible to other diseases and may not develop immune response to vaccines, especially Marek's

Human health risk: None known

Infectious Catarrh. See *Infectious Coryza*

Infectious Coryza

Also called: Cold, contagious catarrh, hemophilus infection, infectious catarrh, IC, roup

Prevalence: Common, particularly in fall and winter in the temperate climates of California and the southeastern United States

System/organ affected: Respiratory

Incubation period: 1 to 3 days

Progression: Can be acute and spread rapidly, running its course in about 3 weeks, or chronic and spread slowly, running its course in about 3 months

Signs: Typically in growing and mature birds (but can affect chicks as young as 3 weeks), foul-smelling discharge from nose that may become crusty or cheesy; swollen face, eyes, and sinuses (swollen wattles in cocks); labored or noisy breathing and sneezing; watery eyes with eyelids stuck together; drop in feed and water consumption; drop in egg production; sometimes diarrhea

Percentage affected: High when acute, low when chronic

Mortality: Usually no more than 20% but can be as high as 50%

Postmortem: Thick, grayish fluid, or yellowish solid material in nasal passages and upper respiratory tract

Resembles: Chronic respiratory disease, fowl cholera, laryngotracheitis, Newcastle, roup (nutritional), bronchitis, avian influenza, except none of these produces coryza's characteristic fetid odor

Diagnosis: Flock history, signs (facial swelling, characteristic odor), postmortem (lesions confined to upper respiratory tract); definitive diagnosis only by laboratory identification of bacteria (as distinct from nonpathogenic *Haemophilus* bacteria)

Cause: *Haemophilus paragallinarum* bacteria that do not survive long in the environment and are easily destroyed by disinfectants

Transmission: Contagious; contact with infected or carrier birds and their nasal or respiratory discharges in dust, drinking water, or feed; all chickens in a flock where coryza has occurred should be considered carriers whether or not they exhibited any signs of illness

Prevention: Avoid combining birds from different flocks; vaccinate, but only if the disease has been positively identified; vaccinated breeders pass temporary immunity to chicks hatched from their eggs; remove an infected flock, disinfect, and leave housing vacant for at least 3 weeks before bringing in new birds

Treatment: Antibiotics (the most effective of which should not be used for laying hens) may be used to treat the signs but will not eliminate the disease, which can be accomplished only by removing and destroying the affected flock and cleaning the premises

Human health risk: None known

Infectious Enterohepatitis. See *Blackhead*

Infectious Hepatitis. See *Campylobacteriosis*

Infectious Laryngotracheitis. See
Laryngotracheitis (acute), Laryngotracheitis (mild)

Infectious Synovitis

Also called: Enlarged hock disease, *Mycoplasma synoviae* infection, MS, silent air sac disease, synovitis (one form of mycoplasmosis)

Prevalence: Uncommon except in large commercial layer flocks during cold, damp weather

System/organ affected: Joints, sometimes upper respiratory tract

Incubation period: 11 to 21 days

Progression: Spreads rapidly and is usually acute with slow recovery in young birds; chronic in older birds (survivors of systemic [acute] infection become chronic)

Signs: In chicks, 4 to 12 weeks old, no signs or slow growth; lameness; pale, shrunken comb; ruffled feathers; hunkering around feeders and drinkers; emaciation; sometimes hot, swollen hocks, shanks, and foot pads; resting on hocks; breast blisters filled with yellowish creamy material; greenish diarrhea capped with large amounts of urates just before death In growing and mature chickens, no signs or respiratory sounds, sneezing, head shaking, eye and nasal discharge, facial swelling

Percentage affected: Usually 100%, but only 15 to 20% may show signs

Mortality: Usually less than 10% (most deaths are result of secondary infection)

Postmortem: Yellowish or grayish fluid (acute) or thick orange-yellow cheesy matter (chronic) in joints, keel, and foot pad; if septicemic, kidneys become swollen, pale, and mottled and liver is swollen and greenish; in respiratory form, air sacs are filled with thin, cheesy matter

Resembles: Staphylococcic, except infectious synovitis more often involves wing joints and breast blisters; respiratory form is indistinguishable from chronic respiratory disease

Diagnosis: Blood test, flock history, postmortem findings, laboratory identification of bacteria (distinguish from other mycoplasmas)

Cause: *Mycoplasma synoviae* bacteria

Transmission: Inhaling bacteria from infected or carrier birds; spread by breeders through hatching eggs

Prevention: Do not combine birds from different sources; acquire only MS-free stock; hatch eggs only from MS-free breeders; blood-test and remove positive reactors; vaccinate where infection is prevalent (expensive)

Treatment: None effective; slow recovery may result from injection with tylosin, erythromycin, spectinomycin, or chlortectracycline, although survivors remain carriers

Human health risk: None known

 Infectious synovitis is a reportable disease.

K

Keel Bursitis. See *Breast Blister*

Keel Cyst. See *Breast Blister*

Keratoconjunctivitis. See *Conjunctivitis (ammonia induced)*

Kidney Stones
Also called: Urinary calculi, urolithiasis
Prevalence: Common
System/organ affected: Kidneys
Incubation period: Not applicable
Progression: Chronic
Signs: <u>Usually in laying pullets and hens</u>, lethargy, weight loss, dehydration, pale comb, reduced laying, or sudden death
Percentage affected: High
Mortality: Gradual, usually up to 50%
Postmortem: Swollen ureters containing irregular white stones; atrophy of some or all six kidney lobes, with remaining lobes swollen and pale; possible signs of gout (visceral); possible atrophy of breast and leg muscles
Resembles: Any disease causing kidney degeneration
Diagnosis: Postmortem findings

Cause: Urates obstructing one or both ureters as a result of excess dietary calcium (3% or more) or protein (30% or more), insufficient phosphorus or vitamin A, moldy feed, kidney inflammation following disease (especially infectious bronchitis)
Transmission: Does not spread from bird to bird, although the condition may appear flockwide in hens subjected to the same debilitating conditions
Prevention: Vinegar in the drinking water may prevent stone formation
Treatment: Vinegar in the drinking water may help dissolve stones
Human health risk: None

L

Laryngotracheitis (acute)
Also called: Avian diphtheria, infectious laryngotracheitis, ILT, laryngo, LT, trach (trake)
Prevalence: Sporadic
System/organ affected: Upper respiratory tract
Incubation period: 6 to 12 days
Progression: Acute, spreads slowly, runs through flock in 2 to 6 weeks; most birds die or recover within about a week
Signs: <u>Usually in mature birds</u>, red, swollen, watery eyes with crusty dried discharge clinging to areas surrounding the eyes; nasal discharge; swollen sinuses; coughing and making gurgling, wheezing, or cawing sounds; breathing with mouth open, gasping with neck extended upward during inhale, dropping head to breast during exhale; sneezing while shaking head to dislodge plugs in the windpipe; coughing up bloody mucus that sticks to the face or feathers; drop in laying, and eggs have thinner shells
Percentage affected: 90 to 100%
Mortality: Usually 10 to 20%, but can be as high as 70%; least in young birds during warm weather, greatest in layers during winter
Postmortem: Swollen windpipe clogged with frothy or bloody mucus or a yellowish cheesy plug; pinpoint blood spots along inside of windpipe
Resembles: Avian influenza (high path); pox (wet), except in laryngo the cheesy masses on the throat rub off easily; infectious bronchitis, except laryngo spreads less rapidly and is more severe; Newcastle, except laryngo does not cause nervous signs;

gapeworm, except in laryngo birds die more quickly with no worms in throat
Diagnosis: Flock history, signs (swollen eyelids, coughing up blood, high death rate), postmortem findings, confirmed by laboratory identification of virus
Cause: A herpesvirus that affects primarily chickens and pheasants and does not live long off the bird
Transmission: Highly contagious; inhaled virus (or virus entering the eyes) from infected or carrier birds or contaminated litter; can be spread on equipment or the feet of rodents and dogs, and on the shoes of humans
Prevention: Avoid introducing mature chickens into a mature flock; vaccinate *if* you exhibit your chickens, laryngo is common in your area, you regularly bring in new mature birds, or you visit chicken keepers from laryngo-prevalent areas (*see* Laryngo Vaccination, page 272); do not combine vaccinated or recovered birds with others
Treatment: None effective; use a cotton swab to remove windpipe plugs from gasping birds; vaccinate to keep the disease from spreading; survivors may remain carriers that can infect other chickens and become reinfected themselves when under stress; the only sure way to rid the premises of this virus is to remove the infected chickens, disinfect housing, and leave it empty for 2 months
Human health risk: None known

 Laryngotracheitis is a reportable disease.

Laryngotracheitis (mild)
Also called: Infectious laryngotracheitis, ILT, laryngo, LI, trach (trake)
Prevalence: Common
System/organ affected: Upper respiratory tract
Incubation period: 6 to 12 days
Progression: Spreads slowly, most birds in a flock recover within 2 to 6 weeks
Signs: In young birds, (under 14 weeks of age), coughing, sneezing, difficulty breathing, discharge drying around nostrils, lethargy, failure to grow at a normal rate
In mature birds, watery, sticky, inflamed eyes; swollen sinuses; nasal discharge; coughing; slight drop in laying
Percentage affected: 5%
Mortality: Usually none in young birds, up to 2% in mature chickens

Postmortem: Windpipe is rough and reddened, contains sticky or yellowish mucus, or is dotted with pinpoint red spots (hemorrhages)
Resembles: Aspergillosis, avian influenza (low path), infectious coryza; swallowed feed-sack string wrapped around tongue, except string affects only one bird at a time, and you can usually locate the string
Diagnosis: Signs (swollen, watery eyes), postmortem findings (pinpoint hemorrhages in the windpipe), confirmed by laboratory identification of the virus
Cause: A herpesvirus that affects primarily chickens and pheasants and does not live long off the birds
Transmission: Highly contagious; virus is inhaled, or virus enters the eyes, from infected or carrier birds or contaminated litter; may be spread on equipment or the feet of rodents and dogs, and on the shoes of humans
Prevention: Vaccinate *if* you exhibit your chickens, laryngo is common in your area, you regularly bring in new mature birds, or you visit chicken keepers from laryngo-prevalent areas (*see* Laryngo Vaccination, page 272); do not combine vaccinated or recovered birds with others
Treatment: None effective
Human health risk: None known

Leukemic Myeloid Leukosis. See *Typical Diseases Caused by Avian Leukosis Viruses, page 266*

Leukosis. See *Lymphatic/Lymphoid Leukosis, Osteopetrosis*

Limberneck. See *Botulism*

Listeriosis
Also called: Septicemic listeriosis
Prevalence: Rare, sporadic in temperate areas
System/organ affected: Brain (encephalitic) or entire body (septicemic)
Incubation period: 2 to 8 weeks
Progression: Usually acute in older chickens, chronic in young ones
Signs: In young birds, lethargy, lack of coordination, head arching over the back (encephalitic form); diarrhea, loss of appetite, gradual weight loss, death (septicemic form)
In mature birds, none or sudden death (septicemic)
Percentage affected: Low
Mortality: Usually low but can reach 40%
Postmortem: *Encephalitic form:* none obvious

Septicemic form: swollen spleen; patchy gray spots on liver, which may be swollen and greenish; pale, inflamed heart; inflamed oviduct

Resembles: *Encephalitic form:* encephalomalacia, epidemic tremor, exotic Newcastle
Septicemic form: any septicemic infection including avian influenza, fowl cholera, fowl typhoid, pseudomonas

Diagnosis: Signs (deaths without obvious signs of illness); identifying bacteria, which can be tricky, especially in the encephalitic form (must be distinguished from listeria species that do not cause disease)

Cause: Noncontagious *Listeria monocytogenes* bacteria commonly found in soil and the intestines of birds and other animals, especially ruminants, but to which chickens tend to be resistant

Transmission: Inhaling or ingesting bacteria from the environment, typically near a meat-producing cattle, sheep, or goat operation; contamination of an open wound; may be triggered by damp, humid, or wet conditions; not transmitted through hatching eggs

Prevention: Identify and eliminate the source of infection

Treatment: None effective

Human health risk: A potentially fatal infection can result from handling infected or carrier birds, or eating the meat of an infected chicken (*see* Listeriosis, page 408)

Lymphatic/Lymphoid Leukosis

Also called: Avian leukosis, big liver disease, LL, visceral lymphoma (one disease in the leukosis/sarcoma group; *see also* Osteopetrosis)

Prevalence: Common

System/organ affected: Liver and other organs

Incubation period: 3 to 16 weeks

Progression: Usually chronic; can be acute in individual chickens

Signs: Typically in birds reaching maturity, sudden death or progressive emaciation and weakness, pale and shriveled (sometimes purplish) comb, vent feathers spotted with white (urates) or green (bile); sometimes blood blisters bursting on the skin; sometimes swollen kidney, cloacal bursa, liver, or nodular tumors may be felt through the bird's skin; sometimes a tumor in the eye socket results in bleeding and blindness; green diarrhea is a sign of impeding death
In hens, few signs other than reduced egg production, poor egg quality, swollen abdomen, loose droppings

Percentage affected: Sporadic

Mortality: Up to 20% (rapidly following obvious signs)

Postmortem: In birds at least 4 months old: swollen liver; large and numerous soft, smooth, shiny white or gray tumors in liver, spleen, and cloacal bursa; sometimes swollen grayish crumbly or gritty liver, swollen joints, tumors in kidneys, lungs, heart, bone marrow, and testes or ovary

Resembles: Marek's disease (*see* Lymphoid Leukosis vs. Marek's Disease, page 264), avian tuberculosis, blackhead, fatty liver

Diagnosis: Flock history (birds' age), signs (progression and mortality), postmortem findings (swollen liver, tumorous cloacal bursa, lack of nerve involvement), elimination of other causes

Cause: A group of retroviruses that primarily infect chickens, do not live long off a bird's body, and are sensitive to most disinfectants

Transmission: Ingestion of droppings from infected birds; spread by blood-sucking insects; may be transmitted from infected breeders through hatching eggs (not all chicks are infected via the egg, but those that are spread disease to noninfected chicks at hatch)

Prevention: Acquire chickens from leukosis-free sources; breed for resistance; identify and eliminate breeders that produce infected chicks (requires testing for reactors); thoroughly clean and disinfect incubator and brooder between hatches; do not combine chickens of different ages or from different sources

Treatment: None; survivors may be carriers

Human health risk: None known

M

Marble Bone. See *Osteopetrosis*

Marek's Disease

Also called: Acute leukosis, avian lymphomatosis, fowl paralysis, MD, neural leukosis, neuritis, neurolymphomatosis, range paralysis, visceral leukosis
Eye form: gray eye, ocular lymphomatosis
Transient paralysis: false botulism, floppy broiler syndrome, pseudobotulism

Prevalence: Common

System/organ affected: Nerves, organs (liver, lungs, and others), eye, or skin; *see* Forms of Marek's Disease, page 262

Incubation period: 2 weeks

Progression: Acute in young chickens, chronic in older birds

Signs (*see also* Forms of Marek's Disease, page 262): In chicks 2 to 3 weeks old, transient paralysis followed by twisted neck on recovery from paralysis; or sudden death

In chicks 4 to 8 weeks old, lethargy, paralysis, deaths affecting up to 80% of flock

In growing birds 3 to 7 months, growing thin while eating well (most common form), paralysis in wing(s) or leg(s), classically one leg pointing forward and the other back under the body, greenish diarrhea, death

In maturing birds 6 to 9 months old, swollen feather follicles or firm white bumps (tumors) on skin that scab over with a brown crust (skin form); reddened, bloody-looking shanks; stilted gait or lack of coordination, pale skin, wing or leg paralysis (nerve form); sometimes swollen comb and wattles; sometimes rapid weight loss, gaping or gasping, transient paralysis of a leg or wing lasting 1 to 2 days (pseudobotulism form), dehydration, emaciation, coma; death as result of inability to get to food and water or being trampled by other chickens

In mature birds (vaccinated or not), significant weight loss, weakness, death from massive internal tumors

In birds 10 to 18 weeks old with reddish-gray eyes (gray eye, involves optic nerve), cloudy-grayish, dilated, irregular pupil, distorted or blinded eye, emaciation, diarrhea, death

In all ages, sudden death of apparently healthy birds

Percentage affected: Up to 100% in unvaccinated flock (although not all chickens show signs), up to 5% in vaccinated flocks

Mortality: An acute epidemic can result in 80 to 100%, varying with virulence of the virus and resistance of the breed

Postmortem: In cases of sudden death, massive internal tumors; otherwise, swollen nerves with nodules (usually on one side; compare same nerve on opposite side of body); tumors in the testes or ovary (ovary takes on a cauliflower appearance); pale heart; solidified lungs; extremely swollen and spotted liver, spleen, or kidneys

Resembles: Primarily lymphoid leukosis (*see* Lymphoid Leukosis vs. Marek's Disease, page

264); any respiratory disease when Marek's affects the lungs; lameness and wasting in mature birds resembles avian tuberculosis; general signs resemble spirochetosis, except the latter does not produce tumors; transient paralysis (pseudobotulism) resembles botulism, except in pseudobotulism birds typically recover quickly; paralysis may resemble any joint infection or injury, epidemic tremor (except Marek's typically affects older birds), or Newcastle (except Newcastle does not involve tumors)

Diagnosis: Difficult; flock history (birds not yet mature), signs (especially asymmetric paralysis or discolored iris and irregular pupil), postmortem findings (tumors in nerve tract; asymmetric nerve enlargement; two or more organs affected); identification of virus or antibodies; elimination of other causes

Cause: Herpesviruses that replicate in the feather follicles, are inhaled in shed dander, and survive for a year or more in chicken house dust

Transmission: Contagious; inhaling contaminated dust or dander from infected birds; not spread through hatching eggs or on their shells

Prevention: Brood chicks away from mature birds until they develop natural resistance by 5 months of age; breed for resistance (some chickens carry resistance factor B21, detected through blood testing); keep turkeys with chickens or put a little turkey poop in the chick brooder (turkeys carry a related though harmless virus that keeps Marek's virus from causing tumors); vaccinate newly hatched chicks (does not prevent Marek's disease but does prevent tumors and paralysis if done prior to exposure to the virus)

Treatment: None; survivors remain carriers

Human health risk: None known from the virus, but handling vaccine may make your eyes itch for a few days

 Marek's disease is reportable.

Mesogenic Newcastle Disease. See *Newcastle Disease (mesogenic)*

Moniliasis. See *Sour Crop*

Mushy Chick Disease. See *Omphalitis*

Mycoplasma gallisepticum. See *Chronic Respiratory Disease*

Mycoplasma synoviae Infection. See *Infectious Synovitis*

Mycoplasmosis. See *Air Sac Disease, Chronic Respiratory Disease, Infectious Synovitis*

Mycotic Pneumomia. See *Aspergillosis (chronic)*

Mycotoxicosis. See *Aflatoxicosis, Ergotism, Fusariotoxicosis, Ochratoxicosis*

Myeloid Leukosis. See *Typical Diseases Caused by Avian Leukosis Viruses, page 266*

N

Navel Ill/Infection. See *Omphalitis*

Necrotic Dermatitis. See *Gangrenous Cellulitis/ Dermatitis*

Necrotic Enteritis
Also called: Cauliflower gut, crud, enterotoxemia, NE, rot gut
Prevalence: Rare
System/organ affected: Intestines
Incubation period: 3 to 10 days
Progression: Acute; appears suddenly, progresses rapidly, runs through flock in about 2 weeks
Signs: In intensively raised, rapidly growing chickens, 2 to 5 weeks old, sudden death without signs, or lethargy, decreased appetite, ruffled feathers, reluctance to move; dark, smelly diarrhea; emaciation; death within hours
Percentage affected: High
Mortality: Usually up to 10% but sometimes as high as 30%
Postmortem: Cauliflower-like yellow or green membrane lining small intestine filled with gas or smelly brown fluid
Resembles: Coccidiosis, which is usually less severe; ulcerative enteritis, except necrotic enteritis rarely affects the ceca or liver
Diagnosis: Flock history, signs, postmortem findings
Cause: *Clostridium perfringens* bacteria and their toxins, sometimes following change in feed; often found in conjunction with worms, coccidiosis, and occasionally salmonellosis (all of which increase susceptibility)

Transmission: Droppings from infected birds and spores in built-up litter, dust, or feed; does not spread directly from one bird to another, except if healthy chickens cannibalize diseased birds
Prevention: Good sanitation management to prevent worms, coccidiosis, and other intestinal infections that reduce immunity; avoid overcrowding; make feed change gradually; use probiotics to promote competitive exclusion
Treatment: Bacitracin, neomycin, and tetracyclines are effective treatments, combined with amprolium to control coccidia; a vitamin supplement following treatment hastens recovery
Human health risk: None, if hands are washed after handling infected birds and their meat isn't eaten

Neural Leukosis. See *Marek's Disease*

Neuritis. See *Marek's Disease*

Neurolymphomatosis. See *Marek's Disease*

Neurotropic Velogenic Newcastle Disease. See *Newcastle Disease (velogenic)*

Newcastle Disease (lentogenic)
Also called: Domestic/endemic/low virulence/mild Newcastle disease
Prevalence: Common
System/organ affected: Respiratory system; intestines (asymptomatic-enteric lentogenic ND)
Incubation period: 2 to 15 days
Progression: Spreads rapidly, running through flock within about a week
Signs: In growing birds, coughing, sneezing, gasping, rales
Asymptomatic-enteric lentogenic ND: no signs to mild diarrhea
Percentage affected: Up to 100%
Mortality: Rare
Postmortem: None significant
Resembles: Any mild respiratory disease
Diagnosis: Signs, confirmed by laboratory identification of virus
Cause: Low-virulent strains of paramyxovirus that affect many bird species, do not cause serious illness in chickens, and are used in vaccines to protect chickens in countries where strains of higher virulence are prevalent
Transmission: Inhaling or ingesting the virus shed in body excretions of infected birds

Prevention: Avoid chickens and other birds of unknown health status

Treatment: None; keep chickens warm and well fed; watch for secondary bacterial infections, particularly air sac disease and chronic respiratory disease; survivors are immune to reinfection but will continue to shed the virus for a short period after recovery

Human health risk: Temporary eye infection may, but rarely does, result from handling or butchering infected birds

Newcastle Disease (mesogenic)

Also called: Virulent Newcastle disease
Prevalence: Rare in USA and Canada
System/organ affected: Respiratory system, sometimes nerves
Incubation period: 2 to 15 days
Progression: Starts suddenly, spreads rapidly, runs through flock in about 5 days
Signs: <u>In all ages</u>, nasal discharge, gurgling from mucus in windpipe, cloudy eyes
<u>In growing</u> birds, gasping, coughing, sneezing, rales; sometimes followed within 14 days by nervous disorders (drooping wing, draggy leg; neck twisted to one side, or bent over the back or between the legs)
<u>In mature birds</u>, wheezing; hens temporarily lay fewer eggs with soft, rough, or deformed shells
Percentage affected: Up to 100%
Mortality: Usually less than 10%, primarily among birds with nervous signs
Postmortem: None significant; sometimes mucus in windpipe and thickened air sacs containing yellowish cheesy material
Resembles: Coryza, infectious bronchitis, and other respiratory diseases, except Newcastle may include nervous signs; pox (wet)
Diagnosis: Signs (combination of nervous and respiratory signs), confirmed by laboratory identification of virus
Cause: Highly contagious paramyxovirus that affects many bird species but does not survive long in the environment
Transmission: Inhaling or ingesting the virus shed in body excretions of infected birds
Prevention: Avoid contact with illegally imported pet birds and fighting cocks; do not visit flocks or let others visit your flock if an outbreak occurs in your area
Treatment: None; infected flocks are quarantined and destroyed, followed by thorough cleaning and disinfecting of the facility

Human health risk: Temporary eye infection, and occasionally fever and other flulike symptoms, may result from handling infected birds

 Mesogenic Newcastle disease is reportable.

Newcastle Disease (velogenic)

Also called: Avian pneumoencephalitis, virulent Newcastle disease, pseudo poultry plague
Nerve form: neurotropic velogenic Newcastle disease, NVND
Gut form: Asiatic Newcastle disease, exotic Newcastle disease, END, viscerotropic velogenic Newcastle disease, VVND
Prevalence: Rare in USA and Canada
System/organ affected: *Neurotropic strains:* respiratory system and nerves
Viscerotropic strains: digestive tract and brain
Incubation period: 2 to 6 days
Progression: Acute, spreads rapidly, runs through flock in 3 to 4 days, lasts 3 to 4 weeks
Signs: <u>Both virus strains, in mature birds</u>, rapid drop in laying followed by deaths starting within 24 hours; survivors may be permanently paralyzed (droopy wings, twisted neck, jerky or wobbly movement); hens may lay fewer, smaller eggs with rough misshapen shells, soft bloody yolks, and watery whites
<u>Neurotropic strains</u>, rapid or difficult breathing and progressive weakness soon followed by signs of nerve damage (spasms, neck bent over the back or twisted to one side, circling, partial or complete paralysis)
<u>Viscerotropic strains</u>, sudden, high rate of death without signs, or severe lethargy; swollen head, especially around eyes, with dark circles around eyes (similar to a black eye) and sticky straw-colored fluid dripping from eyes and nostrils; watery, white or greenish and dark (bloody) diarrhea
Percentage affected: Up to 100%
Mortality: Usually 50% in mature birds, 90% in young ones
Postmortem: In acute deaths, no apparent signs; otherwise, bloody intestines and cloaca (viscerotropic); egg yolk in abdominal cavity of hens
Resembles: Variable signs mimic any serious disease infecting the intestines, nerves, respiratory system or causing septicemia, especially aspergillosis, fowl cholera (acute), infectious bronchitis, laryngotracheitis, pox (wet), highly pathogenic avian influenza; also acute poisoning (rapid sudden deaths)

Diagnosis: Flock history (human handler's contact with smuggled pet birds or fighting cocks), signs (rapid onset, sudden deaths), postmortem findings, laboratory identification of virus (especially to distinguish from acute fowl cholera and highly pathogenic avian influenza)

Cause: Several strains of paramyxovirus that survive for up to 30 days in infected droppings, broken eggs, feathers, and drinking water

Transmission: Highly contagious; spreads by contact with infected birds and their body discharges; spreads in feed and water and on the feet of rodents and humans

Prevention: Avoid contact with illegally imported pet birds and fighting cocks; do not visit flocks or let others visit your flock if an outbreak occurs in your area

Treatment: None; infected flocks are quarantined and destroyed, followed by thorough cleaning and disinfecting of the facility

Human health risk: Temporary eye infection, and occasionally fever and other flulike symptoms, may result from handling infected birds

 Velogenic Newcastle disease is reportable.

Nodular Tapeworm Disease

Also called: Nodular disease
Prevalence: Unknown
System/organ affected: Small intestine
Incubation period: 2 to 3 weeks
Signs: In growing chickens, stunted growth
In mature chickens, decreased laying; a heavy infestation can cause emaciation, weakness, paleness, yellow slimy diarrhea, and (rarely) death
Percentage affected: High, if all chickens snack on infective ants
Mortality: Rare
Postmortem: Large tapeworms in small intestine, with a swelling or lump (which may be as large in diameter as ¼ inch [6 mm]) at the site of each head attachment; intestine may be swollen and filled with yellow or bloody mucus
Resembles: Tuberculosis, except that in TB, tumors are found elsewhere in addition to the small intestine and do not involve tapeworms
Diagnosis: Postmortem findings
Cause: *Raillietina echinobothrida*, also known as nodular tapeworm

Transmission: Nodular tapeworms have an indirect life cycle involving ants (see Life Cycles on page 166)
Prevention: None effective; control ants
Treatment: Any dewormer that is effective against tapeworm (see Off-Label Benzimidazoles on page 183)
Human health risk: None

Nutritional Roup. See *Roup (nutritional)*

O

Ochratoxicosis

Also called: Ochratoxin mycotoxicosis
Prevalence: Sporadic
System/organ affected: Kidney
Progression: Gradual and cumulative
Signs: In growing birds, lethargy, diarrhea, dehydration, increased thirst, reduced body temperature, huddling, excessive urates, rapid weight loss, death
In hens, depressed appetite, yellow diarrhea, decreased laying, thin-shelled eggs containing blood or meat spots, poor hatchability
Percentage affected: Depends on age of birds and amount of toxin ingested
Mortality: Usually low, depending on amount of toxin ingested
Postmortem: Hard, swollen, white to pale-tan kidneys, sometimes with white pinpoint urate crystals; sometimes swollen, spotted, yellow liver; mucus-filled intestine
Resembles: Visceral gout (of which ochratoxicosis is one of many potential causes)
Diagnosis: Signs, postmortem findings, feed analysis
Cause: Ochratoxins produced by *Aspergillus* spp. and *Penicillium* spp. in barley, corn, sorghum, and wheat and in pelleted feed made with contaminated grain
Transmission: Consuming contaminated feed; does not spread from bird to bird
Prevention: Avoid moldy or insect-ridden feed; store feed in a tight bin in cool, dry place, and use within 2 to 3 weeks
Treatment: Replace contaminated feed; young birds recover more rapidly when given supplements of vitamins C and E; a probiotic containing several species of lactobacillus bacteria may be marginally beneficial in binding toxins in the gut

Human health risk: Since ochratoxin is rapidly excreted in droppings, danger of residual toxin in meat or eggs is minimal by 4 days after contaminated feed is replaced

Ocular Leukosis. See *Typical Diseases Caused by Avian Leukosis Viruses, page 266*

Ocular Lymphomatosis. See *Marek's Disease*

Omphalitis
Also called: Mushy chick disease, navel ill/infection, yolk sac infection (one form of colibacillosis)
Prevalence: Common
System/organ affected: Navel infection, may become systemic
Incubation period: 8 to 24 hours (present at time of hatch)
Progression: Acute; can last a week before death
Signs: Dead embryos late in incubation; newly hatched chicks feel wet; in chicks up to 4 weeks of age, drooping head, puffed-up down, huddling near heat, lack of uniformity in size, lack of interest in eating or drinking, distended abdomen with unabsorbed yolk sac; unhealed, reddened, swollen, and wet, mushy, or scabby navel; sometimes diarrhea; deaths starting within 24 hours of hatch and peaking at about a week
Percentage affected: Usually low unless incubator sanitation is grim
Mortality: Variable, starting just prior to hatch and continuing for about 2 weeks; may increase as hatching season progresses if sanitation is ignored
Postmortem: Incompletely healed navel, fluid under skin, bluish abdomen, unabsorbed yolk in abdomen (sometimes yellowish-green and watery or yellowish-brown and cheeselike, often bad smelling)
Diagnosis: Signs, postmortem findings, presence of mixed bacteria or absence of a single specific responsible pathogen (other than a coliform)
Cause: *Escherichia coli* infecting the yolk sac of incubated eggs, in combination with *Staphylococcus aureus, Enterococcus faecalis* (formerly *Streptococcus faecalis*), and other bacteria
Transmission: Bacteria deposited in egg by infected hen; contaminated droppings penetrating shells of eggs collected for hatching; high incubation humidity preventing navels from closing properly; poor incubator sanitation, allowing pathogens to accumulate

Prevention: Hatch only clean, uncracked eggs; control incubator humidity; thoroughly clean and disinfect incubator and brooder between hatches
Treatment: None effective; in a nonsepticemic infection, the chick may survive if the navel is cleaned with povidone iodine (brand name Betadine) two or three times a day until it heals; if newly purchased chicks experience a high death rate, notify seller and/or hatchery
Human health risk: None, if hands are washed after handling infected chicks

Ornithobacteriosis
Also called: ORT
Prevalence: Emerging
System/organ affected: Respiratory, joints
Incubation period: 24 to 48 hours
Progression: Acute and highly contagious
Signs: Most commonly in broilers 3 to 4 weeks of age, sudden death (sometimes with neurological signs such as tremors, weakness, paralysis) or mild respiratory distress, nasal discharge, sneezing, coughing, swollen sinuses, loss of appetite and retarded growth, lethargy; may be followed by severe respiratory distress, labored breathing, possible diarrhea, prostration, and death; signs may disappear after about a week, only to reappear in the future
In layers 6 to 12 months old, mild respiratory signs, loss of appetite, decreased laying, small or misshaped eggs with soft shells
In older chickens, joint swelling and lameness, muscle weakness, paralysis
Percentage affected: Variable to high
Mortality: Usually 10% or less, but varies depending on severity of environmental stress factors
Postmortem: Sudden death: brain infection; respiratory: foamy, white yogurtlike material in abdominal air sacs; joint infection: foul-smelling slimy material surrounding joints
Resembles: Sudden death resembles fowl cholera, except ORT infects the brain; respiratory signs and postmortem findings resemble many other respiratory infections, particularly coryza, except coryza produces foul-smelling nasal discharge, and fowl cholera, except cholera generally affects older chickens; joint infection resembles similar infections caused by *E. coli, Staphylococci,* and *Streptococci*
Diagnosis: Laboratory identification of bacteria or antibodies

Cause: *Ornithobacterium rhinotracheale* bacteria that affect a wide range of poultry, as well as wild birds, triggered by some other bacterial or viral pathogen (although *O. rhinotracheale* is known to be a primary pathogen) and primarily affecting chickens that are under significant environmental stress from poor living conditions
Transmission: Inhaled, ingested in drinking water, or passed to chicks via hatching eggs
Prevention: Avoid such environmental stressors as overcrowding, poor sanitation, inadequate ventilation, and ammonia fumes; remove infected flock, thoroughly clean and disinfect housing before introducing new chickens; do not hatch eggs from infected breeders; a vaccine is available for use in broiler breeder flocks to confer immunity to offspring while the broilers reach the age of harvest
Treatment: None effective, as the bacteria rapidly become resistant
Human health risk: None known

Ornithosis. See *Chlamydiosis*

Osteopetrosis
Also called: Marble bone, thick leg disease (one disease in the lymphoid/sarcoma group; *see also* Lymphatic/Lymphoid Leukosis)
Prevalence: Sporadic
System/organ affected: Bones
Incubation period: 30 days
Progression: Usually chronic
Signs: <u>In young or mature birds (more often male than female)</u>, thickened (sometimes unusually warm) leg bones, puffy-looking shanks, lameness or stilted gait, faulty body conformation, stunted growth
Percentage affected: Low
Mortality: Up to 10%
Postmortem: Thickened, deformed bones
Resembles: Osteoporosis, except in osteoporosis the bones twist but do not thicken
Diagnosis: Flock history, signs, postmortem findings, laboratory identification of virus
Cause: Retrovirus, related to and may occur in combination with lymphoid leukosis
Transmission: Contact with infected birds; spread by infected breeders through hatching eggs or by infected chicks to noninfected chicks through droppings; mechanically by blood-sucking parasites
Prevention: Acquire chickens from leukosis-free sources; breed for resistance; identify and eliminate breeders that produce infected chicks (requires testing for reactors); thoroughly clean and disinfect incubator and brooder between hatches; do not combine chickens of different ages or from different sources
Treatment: None; survivors may be carriers
Human health risk: None known

Osteoporosis
Prevalence: Common in high-producing, small-bodied commercial-strain hens and older backyard hens
System/organ affected: Bones
Progression: Chronic
Signs: <u>Usually in older hens, often in summer,</u> weakness, squatting, inability to stand (will eat and drink if feed and water are within reach), thin-shell eggs with low hatchability followed by cessation of laying, paralysis, death (usually lying on one side)
Percentage affected: Variable
Mortality: Variable
Postmortem: Deformed or collapsed rib cage; soft, thin, or brittle bones that break easily; little or no medullary bone
Resembles: Marek's disease and other paralytic conditions
Diagnosis: Flock history (strain, sex, age), signs, postmortem findings
Cause: Diet low in calcium, phosphorus, or vitamin D; disturbance in the metabolism of dietary minerals, particularly calcium, causing hen to draw calcium from her structural bones; *see* Hypocalcemia, page *445*
Transmission: Metabolic, does not spread from hen to hen, although more than one hen may be affected if of the same strain or subjected to the same diet
Prevention: Feed a properly balanced layer or breeder ration supplemented with large-particle oyster shell or limestone granules; encourage hens to spend time outdoors
Treatment: Per immobile hen, 1 g calcium carbonate gelatin capsule daily for 1 week
Human health risk: None

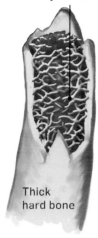

Dense medullary bone

Thick hard bone

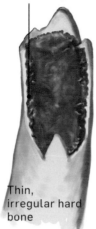

Little (or no) medullary bone

Thin, irregular hard bone

Normal bone   Sign of osteoporosis

P

Paracolon. See *Arizonosis*

Paratyphoid

Also called: PT (one kind of salmonellosis)
Prevalence: Common
System/organ affected: Intestines or septicemic
Incubation period: 4 to 5 days
Progression: Acute, lasting up to 5 weeks, or chronic
Signs: In incubated embryos, numerous dead in shell, pipped or unpipped
In chicks 1 to 3 weeks old, lethargy; decreased appetite; increased thirst; dehydration; "chirping" sounds of distress; huddling near heat with feathers ruffled, eyes closed, head down, wings drooping; sometimes swollen joints, swelling or blindness in one or both eyes, watery diarrhea with vent pasting
In mature chickens (*Salmonella* Enteritidis), no signs (carriers) or reduced egg production; diarrhea; purplish head, comb, wattles (septicemic form); up to 10% death rate
Percentage affected: High
Mortality: Usually up to 20%, peaking at 1 to 2 weeks of age

Postmortem: *In chicks:* none recognizable or unabsorbed yolk sac; dehydration; swollen liver, may be yellowish with red streaks or white dots; creamy or yellowish cheesy cores in ceca
In mature birds: none recognizable or inflamed intestine
Resembles: Arizonosis (nearly identical); any septicemia; synovitis when joints are swollen
Diagnosis: Flock history (birds' age), signs, postmortem findings, laboratory identification of bacteria
Cause: Several different *Salmonella* bacteria, most commonly *S.* Typhimurium, but may also be caused by *S.* Enteritidis, which can affect humans
Transmission: Primarily by carriers; spreads in contaminated soil or litter (persists for up to 7 months); contaminated droppings (persists for up to 28 months); contaminated feathers, dust, hatchery fluff (persists for up to 5 years); feed containing contaminated animal by-products (not including pellets and crumbles) or feed and water contaminated with droppings; spreads from infected breeders to chicks on the shells of hatching eggs or in the case of *S. enterica enterica* is deposited by an infected hen inside the shell of a developing egg (eggs may explode during incubation, further spreading contamination); spreads on dirty equipment, feet of rodents and humans; can be spread by pets, wild birds, rodents, and reptiles
Prevention: Difficult because of bacteria's wide range of animal hosts; collect hatching eggs often; hatch only eggs from paratyphoid-free breeders; do not combine eggs in incubator or chicks in brooder from different sources; replace nesting litter often; clean and disinfect incubator and brooder after each hatch; avoid brooder chilling, overheating, parasitism, withholding of water or feed; keep drinking water free of droppings; control rodents, reptiles, wild birds, cockroaches, beetles, fleas, and flies; avoid mixing chickens of various age groups
Treatment: None effective; survivors may be carriers
Human health risk: Mild to serious illness from eating raw or undercooked contaminated meat or eggs; *see* Salmonella, page 413

 Paratyphoid is a reportable disease in some states.

Parrot Fever. See *Chlamydiosis*

Pasteurellosis. See *Fowl Cholera (acute), Fowl Cholera (chronic)*

Pasting. See also *Cloacitis*
Also called: Pasted vent, paste up, pasty butt, sticky bottom
Prevalence: Common
System/organ affected: Vent
Progression: Usually appears suddenly soon after hatch
Signs: <u>In chicks up to 10 days old</u>, droopiness, vent covered with sticky droppings that harden, sealing the vent shut and eventually causing death
Percentage affected: Usually individuals, rarely an entire brood
Mortality: Possible, if vent becomes sealed shut
Postmortem: Distended rectum filled with droppings
Resembles: Arizonosis and paratyphoid, except pasting usually involves fewer chicks at a time and they otherwise appear healthy
Diagnosis: Signs
Cause: Loose droppings resulting from stress conditions such as chilling or overheating; drinking too-cold water or water with too much sugar or other additives, after being shipped or being left in an incubator long enough to become dehydrated; poor-quality feed, especially containing too much soybean meal
Transmission: Metabolic; does not spread from bird to bird
Prevention: Brood chicks at the ideal temperature for their numbers and age; provide quality starter ration and clean, warm water
Treatment: Moisten and carefully pick away adhering poop, then dab a little hydrogen wound ointment or petroleum jelly (Vaseline) on the vent
Human health risk: None

Pasty Butt. See *Pasting*

Pediculosis. See *Lice, page 142*

Pendulous Crop
Also called: Drop crop
Prevalence: Rare
System/organ affected: Crop
Signs: <u>In mature birds</u>, distended baglike crop, filled with feed and water, that feels squishy when pressed with the fingers; emaciation

Percentage affected: Usually limited to one or a few birds
Mortality: Possible, as result of impaired digestion
Postmortem: Crop filled with feed, water, and sometimes bedding
Resembles: Crop impaction, except in pendulous crop the crop is larger, hangs lower, and feels squishy; sour crop, except in pendulous crop a bird may appear otherwise healthy (pendulous crop may develop into sour crop because of fungal invasion of accumulated crop contents)
Diagnosis: Signs
Cause: Crop loses muscle tone and is unable to empty for unknown reasons; possibilities include eating or drinking too much at once, eating bedding when appropriate rations are unavailable, injury, genetic predisposition, age-related loss of muscle tone
Transmission: Does not spread from bird to bird
Prevention: Maintain a regular feeding schedule, and ensure that palatable drinking water is available at all times
Treatment: None effective
Human health risk: None

Perosis. See *Slipped Tendon*

Plantar Pododermatitis. See *Bumblefoot*

Pleuropneumonia-like Organism Infection. See *Chronic Respiratory Disease*

Pneumoencephalitis. See *Newcastle Disease (velogenic)*

Pneumomycosis. See *Aspergillosis (chronic)*

Pox (dry)
Also called: Avian pox, chicken pox (has nothing to do with human chicken pox), cutaneous pox, fowl pox, sore head (sometimes mistakenly called canker)
Prevalence: Common
System/organ affected: Skin
Incubation period: 4 to 10 days
Progression: Spreads slowly (except where mosquitoes are a problem); lasts up to 4 weeks in individual birds and takes up to 10 weeks to run through a flock
Signs: <u>In birds of all ages, except newly hatched chicks</u>, small, white pimplelike bumps thickening into yellowish wart- or blisterlike swellings on

comb and wattles that grow larger, crust over, and eventually slough off, leaving scabs singly, in clusters, or clumping together before the scabs fall off, sometimes leaving smooth scars; sometimes scabs spread to eyelids, featherless areas of the head and neck, vent, feet, or legs; retarded growth or weight loss (sores around eyes inhibit feeding); drop in egg production

Percentage affected: Low to 100%, depending on virulence of virus strain

Mortality: Rare

Postmortem: *See* Signs, above

Resembles: Comb wound scabs caused by fighting, except wounds do not spread

Diagnosis: Signs (scabs on featherless parts of several chickens), confirmed by laboratory identification of virus

Cause: Poxvirus that affects a wide variety of birds and survives for many months on scabs, dander, and feathers from infected birds

Transmission: Through skin wounds caused by insect bites, dubbing, fighting, cannibalism, or other injury; spreads by means of feathers and scabs from infected birds in which the virus can survive for a long while

Prevention: Control flies, mites, and mosquitoes; vaccinate where pox is prevalent (*see* Pox Vaccination, page 266)

Treatment: *See* Pox Treatment, page 268

Human health risk: None known; chicken pox in humans is caused by a different virus that has nothing to do with chickens

 Fowl pox is a reportable disease in some states.

Pox (wet)

Also called: Diphtheritic pox, fowl diphtheria

Prevalence: Worldwide, but less common than dry pox

System/organ affected: Upper respiratory

Incubation period: 4 to 10 days

Progression: Spreads slowly; lasts up to 2 weeks in individual birds and takes up to 10 weeks to run through a flock

Signs: In birds of all ages, but more commonly mature chickens, raised white or yellow patches in mouth (particularly in the corners of the beak and along the tongue), nose, and throat (and sometimes around the eyes), growing larger until they join into a yellow cheesy mass; sometimes swollen sinuses; sometimes rales or wheezing, nasal or eye discharge; death as result of suffocation from blocked airway or starvation because of inability to swallow or to see well enough to find food

Percentage affected: Low to 100%, depending on virulence of virus strain and measures taken to control spreading

Mortality: Up to 60% in unvaccinated chickens

Postmortem: Yellowish or brownish cheesy masses in mouth, upper throat, windpipe, and sometimes eyes, anchored by cheeselike roots

Resembles: Canker, coryza, laryngotracheitis, sour crop

Diagnosis: Difficult, because signs are similar to several other respiratory diseases; positive diagnosis requires laboratory identification of virus

Cause: Poxvirus invading the upper respiratory tract

Transmission: Inhaling the virus or drinking from the same waterer as infected birds

Prevention: Control dry pox, which can evolve into wet pox; vaccinate where pox is prevalent (*see* Pox Vaccination, page 266)

Treatment: *See* Pox Treatment, page 268

Human health risk: None known; not related to diphtheria in humans

Premature Low Fertility Syndrome. See *Epididymal Lithiasis*

Pseudobotulism. See *Marek's Disease*

Pseudomonas

Also called: Septicemic pseudomonas

Prevalence: Rare

System/organ affected: Respiratory, systemic

Incubation period: 1 to 3 days

Progression: Acute to chronic

Signs: In embryos or newly hatched chicks, death In growing birds, difficulty breathing, loss of appetite, lameness, lack of coordination, swollen head and wattles, swollen hock joints and foot pads, diarrhea; death may occur within 1 to 3 days

Percentage affected: Up to 10%

Mortality: Usually low but can be up to 90%

Postmortem: Swollen, spotty liver, spleen, kidneys; watery fluid under the skin; characteristic fruity odor

Resembles: Septicemic colibacillosis, except colibacillosis does not emit a fruitlike odor

Diagnosis: Odor, laboratory identification of bacteria

Cause: *Pseudomonas aeruginosa* bacteria commonly found in chicken droppings, soil, water, and humid environments

Transmission: Droppings of infected birds in feed, water, litter; infects chicks via hatching eggs (one of the many bacteria causing omphalitis); infects young chickens with reduced resistance as a result of other bacterial or viral diseases

Prevention: Good incubator and brooder sanitation; avoid extreme stress

Treatment: None effective

Human health risk: Infection of healthy humans is rare (*see* Pseudomonas, page 406)

Pseudo Poultry Plague. See *Newcastle Disease (velogenic)*

Psittacosis. See *Chlamydiosis*

Pullorum

Also called: Bacillary white diarrhea, BWD, pullorum disease, PD, white diarrhea (one kind of salmonellosis)

Prevalence: Sporadic but rare in USA and Canada

System/organ affected: Intestines or septicemic

Incubation period: 4 to 5 days

Progression: Acute, lasting 1 to 2 weeks, or chronic

Signs: In chicks up to 3 weeks old, sudden death or droopiness; decreased appetite; huddling near heat; swollen, blistered hock joints; white (sometimes green-stained) pasty diarrhea; sometimes gasping, shrill peeping, or chirping while trying to expel droppings; stunted survivors

In mature birds, no signs or decreased appetite, increased thirst; lethargy; sometimes pale, shriveled comb, green diarrhea, drop in egg production

Percentage affected: Up to 100%, varies with age

Mortality: Up to 90% in chicks, beginning at about 5 days of age and peaking at 2 weeks of age (100% if infected chicks are shipped, chilled, or kept in unsanitary conditions)

Postmortem: *In chicks:* none recognizable or unabsorbed yolk sac; cheesy material in ceca; swollen liver, heart, kidneys, and spleen; small (pinpoint to pea size) grayish-white spots or nodules on organs
In mature birds: small round spots on liver; shriveled ovary with brownish or greenish misshapen yolks in hens; shriveled testes in cocks

Resembles: Many other diseases produce similar signs or lesions; nearly identical to fowl typhoid; white diarrhea may be caused by simple chilling

Diagnosis: Difficult; history (birds' age), signs (pattern of deaths), laboratory identification of bacteria

Cause: *Salmonella* Pullorum bacteria; survives for at least a year in unclean housing but is easily destroyed by cleaning, disinfection, drying, and sunlight

Transmission: From infected hens to chicks through hatching eggs; from chick to chick in incubator or brooder; from breathing feces-contaminated dust, eating contaminated feed, or contact with contaminated litter or equipment

Prevention: Purchase certified pullorum-free stock; hatch eggs only from pullorum-free breeders; do not mix certified pullorum-free stock with other birds; control flies, rodents, and wild birds; blood-test birds (home kits are available), and eliminate carriers until two tests, no less than 21 days apart, are negative (some states require blood-testing of all exhibition birds)

Treatment: None effective; infection settles in the ovaries of survivors, which remain carriers for life

Human health risk: Low

 Pullorum is a reportable disease.

Pulmonary Aspergillosis.
See *Aspergillosis (chronic)*

Pulmonary Hypertension Syndrome.
See *Ascites*

Q

Quail Disease. See *Ulcerative Enteritis*

R

Range Paralysis. See *Marek's Disease*

Red Skin. See *Erysipelas*

Respiratory Coccidiosis. See *Cryptosporidiosis (respiratory)*

Respiratory Cryptosporidiosis. See *Cryptosporidiosis (respiratory)*

Ringworm

Also called: Dermatomycosis, dermatophytosis, favus, white comb
Prevalence: Sporadic
System/organ affected: Skin
Incubation period: 1 to 2 weeks in predisposed birds
Progression: Chronic
Signs: The appearance of a white powder clinging to the comb (rarely on shanks) that thickens to form a dry, scaly, wrinkled crust that smells moldy; sometimes spreads to other skin areas, creating a honeycomb appearance where feathers are lost; possibly leading to lethargy, weakness, emaciation, and death
Percentage affected: Depends on each bird's degree of resistance
Mortality: Rare
Postmortem: Scaly skin, feather loss, depressions ("favus cups") surrounding feather follicles
Resembles: Nothing
Diagnosis: Signs, confirmed by laboratory examination of skin scraping
Cause: *Microsporum gallinae* fungus
Transmission: Contact with infected birds or sloughed-off scales
Prevention: Allow chickens plenty of outdoor time in the sunshine; avoid introducing an infected chicken into the flock
Treatment: Isolate the chicken, peel off crusts if necessary, and apply a miconazole antifungal ointment (such as Lotrimin), or garlic oil (*see* Garlic Oil, page 388) daily until signs disappear
Human health risk: Can, but rarely does, cause ringworm in humans

Rot Gut. See *Necrotic Enteritis*

Roup. See *Canker, Infectious Coryza, Fowl Cholera (chronic)*

Roup (nutritional)

Also called: A-avitaminosis, hypovitaminosis-A
Prevalence: Most likely in chickens confined indoors and fed stale or improperly formulated rations
System/organ affected: Mucous membranes
Progression: Chronic
Signs: In chicks 1 to 7 weeks old, droopiness, pale combs, and failure to grow followed by sore swollen eyelids, sticky or cheesy discharge from eyes and nostrils, swollen sinuses, difficulty breathing, death from organ failure

In hens, runny eyes and nose, eyelids stuck together, ruffled feathers, whitish-yellow mouth sores making swallowing difficult, weakness, emaciation, increased interval between egg clutches, increased blood spots in eggs, decreased hatchability of eggs
In chickens of any age, inability to accurately peck because of poor eyesight
Percentage affected: High
Mortality: Up to 100%
Postmortem: Dry, dull respiratory lining
Resembles: Any respiratory infection; upper respiratory blisters resemble fowl pox
Diagnosis: Signs, postmortem findings, ration evaluation
Cause: Vitamin A deficiency as a result of coccidiosis, internal parasites, or other conditions that interfere with nutrient absorption; dietary vitamin A deficiency for 2 to 5 months; chicks hatched from deficient breeders
Transmission: Does not spread from bird to bird but will affect all chickens subjected to the same conditions
Prevention: Use only fresh feed (buy small quantities so it won't go stale), allow birds to free-range, or feed sources of vitamin A such as new yellow (not white) corn and alfalfa meal; fortify starter ration, or feed chicks a vitamin supplement
Treatment: Mix fresh cod liver oil into feed at the rate of 2 tablespoons per 5 pounds (2.25 kg)
Human health risk: None

Ruptured Air Sac

Also called: Subcutaneous emphysema, windpuff
Prevalence: Rare
System/organ affected: Respiratory (a form of air sac disease)
Progression: May be acute or chronic
Signs: Bird appears to grow large and round without associated weight gain, or an air bubble under the skin may appear at the front of the neck, under a wing, or elsewhere on the chicken's body
Percentage affected: Individual birds
Mortality: Possible if air sac is torn
Postmortem: Accumulation of air beneath the skin
Resembles: No other disease
Diagnosis: Signs, postmortem findings
Cause: Ruptured air sac caused by a defect in the respiratory tract or injury from rough handling, caponizing, crash landing while flying, heavy coughing caused by respiratory infection

Transmission: Does not spread from bird to bird
Prevention: None known
Treatment: May heal on its own; an extreme air pocket may be deflated by puncturing skin with a large hypodermic needle or other sharp instrument (best done by a veterinarian)
Human health risk: None

S

Salmonellosis. See *Arizonosis, Fowl Typhoid, Paratyphoid, Pullorum*

Salpingitis. See *Egg Peritonitis*

Salpingoperitonitis. See *Egg Peritonitis*

Silent Air Sac Disease. See *Infectious Synovitis*

Slipped Tendon
Also called: Chondrodystrophy, hock disease, perosis
Prevalence: Uncommon
System/organ affected: Hock
Signs: In chicks 6 weeks old or less, swollen, flat hock joint, hopping on one leg with the other leg extended diagonally backward; death as a result of inability to reach food and water
Percentage affected: 3 to 5%
Mortality: Low
Postmortem: Achilles tendon out of hock joint
Resembles: Splayed legs, except splaying usually occurs at or shortly after hatch and often involves both legs, while slipped tendon rarely does (*see* Slipped Tendon versus Splayed Leg on page 120)
Diagnosis: History (birds' age), signs, postmortem findings, ration evaluation
Cause: Deficiency in choline, vitamin B_7 (biotin) and other B vitamins, or manganese
Transmission: Related to nutrition; does not spread from bird to bird
Prevention: Add a vitamin supplement to the drinking water of chicks; feed chicks a balanced ration; provide breeders with adequate nutrition
Treatment: Early treatment with a vitamin supplement will minimize future damage but can't reverse deformity after tendons slip
Human health risk: None

Sod Disease. See *Ergotism*

Sore Head. See *Pox (dry)*

Sour Crop
Also called: Candidiasis, crop mycosis, moniliasis, thrush
Prevalence: Common
System/organ affected: Upper digestive tract
Progression: Chronic
Signs: In birds less than 3 weeks old, often none
In growing birds, lethargy, rough feathers, distended crop, sour odor in chicken's mouth, loss of appetite, slow growth or weight loss, greenish-yellow diarrhea
In older birds, none, or pendulous crop, increased appetite, inflamed vent crusted with white droppings, reduced egg production, ulcerlike patches in the mouth
Percentage affected: High in birds exposed to the same conditions
Mortality: Low to none
Postmortem: Grayish-white, rough, circular thickenings that join to create a Turkish-towel appearance in mouth, esophagus, and crop lining, sometimes in the stomach, rarely in the intestine; sometimes cheesy patches that peel off easily
Resembles: Canker, capillary worms, pox (wet), roup (nutritional) trichothecene toxicity (fusariotoxicosis) or ingestion of other caustic substances
Diagnosis: Flock history (age of birds, previous outbreak of another disease, use of coccidiostats or antibiotics), signs (unthrifty birds), postmortem findings, laboratory identification of yeast
Cause: *Candida albicans* yeast commonly living in the digestive tract of chickens that proliferate out of control when normal flora are disrupted by another disease, parasites, or overuse of antimicrobials; sometimes found in combination with another disease (especially coccidiosis or chlamydiosis)
Transmission: Fecal contamination of feed, drinking water, or ground where chickens peck; does not spread from bird to bird
Prevention: Avoid prolonged or inappropriate use of antibiotics or other drugs; discard feed that has gotten wet and started to ferment; clean and sanitize drinkers frequently; add vinegar to drinking water at the rate of 1 tablespoon per gallon (15 mL per 4 L) — double in alkaline water; sour crop in brooded chicks resulting from shell contamination of hatching eggs may be prevented by disinfecting shells with an iodine solution prior to incubation
Treatment: *See* Sour Crop Treatment, page 25)

Human health risk: The same yeast that infects chickens can cause mouth and genital infection in humans

Spirochetosis
Also called: Avian borreliosis, avian intestinal spirochetosis, AIS, chicken tick fever, chicken tick paralysis, fowl spirochetosis, fowl tick fever, fowl tick paralysis
Prevalence: Rare but sporadic in free-range flocks in the U.S. South and Southwest
System/organ affected: Septicemic
Incubation period: 3 to 12 days
Progression: Acute, spreads slowly
Signs: In birds of all ages, sudden death without signs of illness or drowsy and lethargic, ruffled feathers, purplish comb and wattles, huddling and shivering, greenish diarrhea with large amounts of white urates, increased thirst, decreased appetite, rapid weight loss, leg weakness, resting on hocks with eyes closed, lack of coordination, lying on side with head on ground, convulsions, progressive limp paralysis; death or recovery within about a week; recovering chickens may be temporarily weak or paralyzed in one or both wings or legs
In hens, fewer and smaller eggs; egg production of survivors drops dramatically; shells stained with diarrhea
Percentage affected: 1 to 2% in a flock with immunity from constant exposure to ticks; up to 100% in susceptible birds mingled with immune birds
Mortality: Usually less than 75% but can be as high as 100%
Postmortem: None or swollen, mottled spleen; greenish mucus in intestines; sometimes swollen liver with pinpoint bloody or gray spots; swollen, pale kidneys with urate-packed ureters
Resembles: Avian influenza or Newcastle, except spirochetosis does not cause respiratory signs and bloody intestines; botulism, except botulism does not produce internal lesions; Marek's disease, except spirochetosis does not produce tumors; fowl cholera, fowl typhoid, and septicemic colibacillosis, except *Salmonella*, *Pasteurella*, or *E. coli* bacteria are absent in spirochetosis
Diagnosis: Presence of fowl ticks (*Argas* spp.) on chickens; signs; postmortem findings; identification of *Borrelia* spirochetes or antigens in the blood
Cause: *Borrelia anserina* bacteria that affect many birds; can survive for up to 2 months in droppings but are sensitive to many disinfectants

Transmission: Eating or being bitten by an infective fowl tick; spread from infected chickens by lice, mites, mosquitoes, and other bloodsuckers; spread through contact with moist droppings, blood, tissue, and mucus of infected birds, contaminated feed or water, and cannibalism (including picking at dead birds); can be spread by wild ducks and geese
Prevention: Control ticks and other blood-sucking insects; do not combine tick-infested chickens with susceptible birds; discourage wild ducks and geese from your chicken yard
Treatment: Most antibiotics, including penicillin derivatives, streptomycins, tetracyclines, and tylosin are effective, but use only under supervision, as treating chickens with large numbers of spirochetes in their blood can result in more deaths than no treatment; survivors become immune and are not carriers
Human health risk: Some strains of spirochetes that affect chickens can also infect humans

Staph Arthritis. See *Arthritis (staphylococcic)*

Staph Infection. See *Staphylococcosis*

Staphylococcic Septicemia. See *Staphylococcosis*

Staphylococcosis. See also *Arthritis (staphylococcic)*, *Breast Blister*, *Bumblefoot*, *Omphalitis*
Also called: Staph infection
Prevalence: Common
System/organ affected: Usually bones and joints (staphylococcic arthritis); also skin (breast blister, bumblefoot), navel or yolk sac (omphalitis); can be septicemic
Incubation period: 1 to 3 days
Progression: 1 week if acute (septicemic); up to 5 weeks if chronic (local infection)
Signs: Septicemia: lethargy; loss of appetite; reluctance to move; foul-smelling diarrhea
Percentage affected: Usually low
Mortality: Usually low
Postmortem: Acute septicemia: yellow fluid in swollen joints; watery digestive contents in intestines; dark, swollen liver
Resembles: Septicemic form resembles acute fowl cholera, except cholera has a high death rate
Diagnosis: Laboratory identification of *Staphylococcus* spp. as the primary cause, which is difficult when other bacteria contribute to the infection

Cause: *Staphylococcus aureus* and other species of staph bacteria
Transmission: Opportunistic infection by normal bacteria living in soil and on skin and mucous membranes; septicemia may occur after drinking water from a stagnant puddle; not contagious
Prevention: Provide proper nutrition and a sound environment; do not breed chronically infected chickens
Treatment: Can be difficult, as *S. aureus* resists most antibiotics; erythromycin and spectinomycin can be effective against strains that have not become resistant (as determined by antibiotic sensitivity test)
Human health risk: *S. aureus* strains that infect chickens do not infect humans; however, strains that produce enterotoxins can cause food poisoning (*see* Food-Borne Bacteria, page 411)

Stargazing. See *Stargazing, page 97, and Neck Twisting, page 338*

Sternal Bursitis. See *Breast Blister*

Sticky Bottom. See *Pasting*

Streptococcosis
Also called: Streptococcal infection
Prevalence: Worldwide but not common
System/organ affected: Entire body (septicemic)
Incubation period: 5 to 21 days
Progression: Acute (septicemic) or chronic
Signs: In mature birds, lethargy, weight loss; sometimes lameness, head tremors, yellow diarrhea, blood from mouth staining feathers around mouth and head, pale combs and wattles, eventual or sudden death
In hens, drop in laying
Percentage affected: Up to 50%
Mortality: Up to 50%
Postmortem: Swollen spleen, liver, and kidney; light-colored or dark-red patchy areas on liver
Resembles: Any septicemic bacterial disease, including staphylococcosis, colibacillosis, pasteurellosis, erysipelas
Diagnosis: Signs and laboratory identification of bacteria
Cause: *Streptococcus zooepidemicus* bacteria that normally live in a chicken's intestines; infection is considered secondary, since it occurs only if resistance is reduced by some other disease

Transmission: Inhalation, ingestion, skin wounds; bacteria are extremely susceptible to drying and so do not spread on equipment
Prevention: Avoid extreme stress; maintain good sanitation
Treatment: *S. zooepidemicus* resists many antibiotics; amoxycillin *may* be effective *if* started early *and* its suitability is determined through laboratory sensitivity testing
Human health risk: Rare but potentially serious infection in humans and other mammals

Stress Disease. See *Chronic Respiratory Disease*

Subcutaneous Emphysema. See *Ruptured Air Sac*

Sudden Death Syndrome
Also called: SDS, acute death syndrome, ADS, acute heart failure, cardiomyopathy, flip-over disease, flips, heart attack
Prevalence: Common
System/organ affected: Heart and lungs
Progression: Acute
Signs: In apparently healthy broilers, primarily cockerels, peaking at 2 to 3 weeks of age, convulsions consisting of loss of balance, gasping or squawking, violent wing beating and leg pumping, flipping onto back and dying within 1 minute of first signs
In laying hens, dead in the nest
Percentage affected: Up to 4%
Mortality: 100%
Postmortem: Bloody, enlarged heart; bloody lungs; large, pale, crumbly liver; small, empty gallbladder; pale kidneys; feed-filled crop, gizzard, and intestine; sometimes blood in body cavity; in hens: egg in shell gland
Resembles: Ascites, except an ascitic chicken doesn't die on its back; fatty liver syndrome, which involves the liver rather than the heart
Diagnosis: Signs (flipping onto back), postmortem findings (good condition, full digestive tract, bloody lungs, no indication of other diseases)
Cause: Acute heart failure; in broilers it is most likely a combination of genetics (irregular heartbeat), nutritional factors (excess carbohydrates), and environmental stress (crowding); in layers it may be caused by low dietary calcium, potassium, phosphorus, or vitamin D_3

Transmission: Can affect a large number of genetically related birds in the same flock but does not spread from bird to bird
Prevention: In broilers: avoid crowding, discourage rapid growth up to 3 weeks of age, avoid startling birds with loud noises and other disturbances; in layers: provide a balanced diet, prevent obesity
Treatment: None
Human health risk: None

Summer Respiratory Disease. See *Chronic Respiratory Disease*

Synovitis. See *Arthritis (staphylococcic), Infectious Synovitis*

T

Thick Leg Disease. See *Osteopetrosis*

Thrush. See *Sour Crop*

Toxoplasmosis
Also called: Toxo, toxoplasma
Prevalence: Sporadic
System/organ affected: Muscles, central nervous system, eyes, heart, other organs
Incubation period: Uncertain; approximately 1 to 3 weeks
Progression: Usually acute in young birds, chronic in older birds
Signs: In birds under 8 weeks of age, decreased appetite, emaciation, pale comb, white diarrhea, lack of coordination, head twisted back or to one side, muscle spasms (especially jerking of head and neck), paralysis, blindness; eventual or sudden death In mature birds, usually no signs, although acute infection can develop in birds that are otherwise stressed
Percentage affected: Up to 100%
Mortality: Usually none but can be high in acute cases
Postmortem: Cystic muscles; inflamed sciatic nerve; inflamed brain
Resembles: Marek's disease, Newcastle, or any infection involving the nerves
Diagnosis: Antibody detection via blood testing
Cause: *Toxoplasma gondii* protozoan parasite that survives in damp soil for up to 18 months

Transmission: Cats are the primary source; transmitted to chickens that pick in the infected droppings of house cats or related animals, contaminated soil, or infected animals, including other chickens (dead or live); inhale dusty air; eat earthworms, flies, or cockroaches in an area contaminated with oocysts; eat feed on which flies or cockroaches have deposited infective oocysts from their feet
Prevention: Keep cats and kitty litter away from chickens; control rodents, wild birds, flies, cockroaches, and dung beetles
Treatment: None effective
Human health risk: Eating raw or undercooked meat of infected chickens will cause infection in humans; *see* Toxoplasmosis, page 410

Trach (Trake). See *Laryngotracheitis (acute), Laryngotracheitis (mild)*

Trichomoniasis. See *Canker*

Trichothecene Mycotoxicosis. See *Fusariotoxicosis*

Tuberculosis. See *Avian Tuberculosis*

Typhoid. See *Fowl Typhoid*

U

Ulcerative Enteritis
Also called: Quail disease, UE
Prevalence: Not common in otherwise healthy chickens
System/organ affected: Intestine and ceca
Incubation period: 3 to 6 days
Progression: Acute or chronic, runs its course in 2 to 3 weeks
Signs: Usually in layer pullets 4 to 12 weeks old (commonly 5 to 7 weeks), sudden death with no signs, or lethargy, dull and ruffled feathers, droopy wings, hunched-up posture with head pulled in and eyes closed, diarrhea, extreme emaciation, recovery or death within 2 to 3 weeks
Percentage affected: High
Mortality: Usually less than 10%, peaking within a week

Postmortem: Yellowish buttonlike bull's-eye dots (ulcerations) throughout the intestinal tract, concentrating in the lower intestine, ceca, and upper colon; raised patchy tan or yellow areas on liver; sometimes swollen, mottled spleen; shriveled breast muscle in chronic cases

Resembles: Coccidiosis, except UE alone does not cause bloody droppings (although chickens may be infected with both coccidiosis and UE); necrotic enteritis, except NE rarely involves the liver; blackhead, except blackhead results in dished rather than raised liver lesions

Diagnosis: Signs, postmortem findings (buttons in intestine, colorful patchy liver)

Cause: *Clostridium colinum* bacteria that affect game birds more often than chickens, persist under varying conditions (hot, cold, dry, humid), and resist disinfection; often occurs in combination with coccidiosis, mycoplasmosis, or parasites (internal or external); often follows infectious bursal disease

Transmission: Highly contagious; spreads in droppings of infected or carrier birds picked from litter, feed, or water; spread by flies

Prevention: Raise chickens away from quail and other game birds; avoid crowding; manage chickens to prevent coccidiosis, internal and external parasites, and viral diseases (which reduce resistance); do not combine birds of different ages or from different sources if carriers are suspected; remove and replace all litter between flocks

Treatment: Bacitracin and streptomycin are both effective, although medicated chickens may be susceptible to reinfection; natural survivors are resistant, treated survivors remain susceptible, all survivors may be carriers

Human health risk: None known

Urinary Calculi. See *Kidney Stones*

Urolithiasis. See *Kidney Stones*

V

Velogenic Newcastle. See *Newcastle Disease (velogenic)*

Vent Gleet. See *Cloacitis*

Vesicular Dermatitis. See *Ergotism*

Vibrionic Hepatitis. See *Campylobacteriosis*

Visceral Hyperuricemia. See *Gout (visceral)*

Visceral Leukosis. See *Marek's Disease*

Visceral Lymphoma. See *Lymphatic/Lymphoid Leukosis*

Visceral Urate Deposition. See *Gout (visceral)*

Viscerotropic Velogenic Newcastle Disease. See *Newcastle Disease (velogenic)*

W

Waterbelly. See *Ascites*

Western Duck Sickness. See *Botulism*

Wet Pox. See *Pox (wet)*

White Comb. See *Ringworm*

White Diarrhea. See *Pullorum*

Windpuff. See *Ruptured Air Sac*

Wing Rot. See *Gangrenous Cellulitis/Dermatitis*

Y

Yolk Sac Infection. See *Colibacillosis, Omphalitis*

Glossary

abscess. A swollen area filled with puslike fluid

acariasis. Infestation with mites

active ingredient. The component of a drug or pesticide that is responsible for its effect

acute. Having a severe and swift development, often measured in hours and ending in death or recovery; opposite of chronic

agricultural lime. Calcium carbonate, used to condition chicken coop litter, although it also facilitates the generation and release of harmful ammonia fumes

airsacculitis. Any inflammation of the air sacs

alternate host. Intermediate host

amino acids. The basic constituents of proteins

amino acids, essential. Amino acids that must be furnished through diet

amino acids, nonessential. Amino acids that are synthesized within the body

anemia. Deficiency of the blood in quantity or quality because of blood loss or disease, characterized by weakness and pale skin

anthelmintic. Also called vermifuge; any dewormer

antibacterial. An antibiotic

antibiotic. Any drug that kills or inhibits the growth of bacteria

antibody. A blood protein that attacks a specific antigen, causing an immune response to infection or vaccination

antigen. Any foreign substance that excites the immune system into developing antibodies

antimicrobial. Any drug that destroys or inhibits the growth of microorganisms

antinutrient. Any natural compound in a feedstuff that interferes with the absorption of nutrients

antioxidants. Organic chemicals of plant origin that destroy free radicals and reduce, prevent, or help repair the damage they do

antiseptic. Anything that destroys or inhibits microorganisms that cause disease, decomposition, or fermentation

antiserum. A blood serum containing antibodies against a specific antigen, injected to treat or protect against a specific disease (plural: antisera)

antitoxin. An antibody that neutralizes a bacterial toxin

arthritis. Any inflammation of a joint and surrounding tissue

ascariasis. Infestation with roundworms

ascaridiasis. Infestation with roundworms

ascites. An accumulation of fluid in the body cavity

atrophy. To shrivel up or waste away

attenuated. Describes a virus made less infectious for use in a vaccine that will not produce disease

avian. Pertaining to birds

bacteria. One-cell microscopic organisms with plantlike characteristics (singular: bacterium)

bactericide. An antibiotic that kills bacteria outright

bacterin. A vaccine derived from bacteria, rather than from viruses

bacteriostat. An antibiotic that inhibits or prevents bacteria from multiplying

basal metabolism. The amount of energy (fuel) needed to keep a chicken alive and healthy but not engaged in activity, growth, or egg production

benign tumor. Abnormal tissue growth that develops and remains where it started

binary fission. Multiplying by splitting in two

biological pest control. The control of a pest population through the use of its natural enemies, such as predators, parasites, or pathogens

biosecurity. Collective disease-prevention management practices

blood poisoning. A bacterial infection or toxin that circulates in the blood; also called septicemia

blowout. Uterine tissue that remains protruding outside a hen's vent after an egg is laid; commonly called prolapse

booster. Any vaccination following the first in a series

brachial. The main vein of the wing

breeder ration. A feed designed to optimize the hatchability of eggs and the health of the resulting chicks

broad spectrum. Description of a drug that affects a wide variety of pathogens

bumblefoot. An infected abscess in the foot pad

bursa. A fluid-filled sac that cushions a pressure point to reduce friction between body tissues

bursa of Fabricius. The cloacal bursa

bursitis. Inflammation of a bursa

cancer. A malignant growth or tumor

cankers. Ulcerous sores, usually on the face or in the mouth

cannibalism. Pecking or eating the flesh of one's own species

capillariasis. Infected with capillary worms

capillary. Any of the fine blood vessels branching out from the larger arteries and veins

capsid. The protective protein coat of a virus

carbohydrates. Plant- or animal-derived feedstuffs that provide a source of energy

carrier. An outwardly healthy individual that is capable of transmitting disease-causing organisms to other individuals

cecum. A blind pouch at the juncture of the small and large intestine (plural: ceca)

CEO vaccine. Chicken embryo origin vaccine, dangerous for use in backyard chickens

cervical. Pertaining to the neck

cestode. A tapeworm

cestodiasis. Infestation by tapeworms

cholecystitis. Any inflammation of the gall bladder

chondrodystrophy. Shortening of the leg's long bones

chronic. Developing gradually and having a long duration measured in days, months, or even years and being difficult to treat; opposite of acute

cilia. Short, tiny hairlike structures that vibrate to keep the trachea clear of debris

cloaca. The chamber at the lower end of the digestive tract where the digestive, reproductive, and urinary tracts come together

cloacal bursa. A grape-shaped organ above the cloaca that primarily controls antibody production and immunity in chicks

cloacal drinking. A reflexive action in which a young chicken's cloaca samples the environment in order to develop antibodies against existing pathogens

cloacitis. Any inflammation of the cloaca

clubbed down. Chick down that fails to emerge from the sheaths, most commonly around neck and vent

coccidia. Microscopic single-cell protozoa that have a life cycle involving both sexual and asexual reproduction, become infective in the asexually produced sporozoite stage, and multiply in the intestinal tract

coccidiasis. A coccidial infection that produces no detectable signs

coccidiosis. Infection with coccidial protozoa

coccidiostat. A chemical added at low levels to feed or water to prevent coccidiosis

cockerel. A male chicken under 1 year of age

coliform bacteria. *Escherichia coli* and other members of a large group of bacteria that inhabit the intestinal tracts of warm-blooded animals and that may cause disease

colitis. Any inflammation of the large intestine

competitive exclusion. The dominance of one species over another when both compete for the same resources, as occurs when beneficial gut flora keep out harmful organisms

congenital. Existing at birth but not necessarily genetic

conjunctiva. Mucous membrane covering the eyeball and inner surface of the eyelid

conjunctivitis. Any inflammation of the conjunctiva; also called pinkeye

contagious. Readily transmitted from one individual or flock to another

core temperature. The temperature of internal organs; also called deep body temperature

critical high temperature. The air temperature at which a chicken starts suffering heat stress

critical low temperature. The air temperature at which a chicken starts suffering cold stress

crop. An expandable pouch at the base of a chicken's neck where feed accumulates and is softened by digestive juices before moving into the chicken's stomach

crumble. A complete ration, usually intended for chicks, consisting of crushed pellets

cull. To permanently remove an undesirable chicken from its flock

culture. The propagation in a laboratory of microorganisms or body tissue from a diseased bird to determine the cause of disease; also the sample so propagated

cutaneous. Affecting the skin

cyanosis. A bluish discoloration of the skin resulting from low blood oxygen

cyst. An abnormal membranous sac structure containing fluid or semisolid material

dander. Sloughed-off skin and feather cells

debeaked. Having had the tip of the beak amputated (to prevent cannibalism)

definitive host. Natural host

dehydration. The loss of a large amount of body fluids (a loss of more than 12 percent results in death)

depopulate. Dispose of an entire flock, typically by euthanasia

dermatitis. Any inflammation of the skin

detergent. A surfactant that improves the cleaning action of water, helps water penetrate and soften organic matter, and is mildly germicidal

developer. A ration formulated to optimize the growth of pullets

diagnosis. The identification of the nature and cause of a disease by examining external and internal signs

diarrhea. Droppings with the fecal portion too loose to retain its shape

diathesis. A tendency to suffer from a particular medical condition, such as exudative diathesis, in which seeping (exuding) fluid accumulates under a chicken's skin

differential diagnosis. A preliminary list of possible causes of a disease

digestion. The process by which feed is converted into a form that can be absorbed into the body from the digestive tract

diluent. A liquid used to reconstitute and dilute a vaccine

diphtheric. Affecting mucous membranes

direct life cycle. A life cycle that does not involve an intermediate host

disease. An abnormality of any body function resulting from infection and recognized by identifiable signs

disinfect. To inactivate or kill microbes on housing and equipment, but not on a chicken's body

disorder. An abnormality of body functions that may or may not be the consequence of a disease

diverticulum. A finger-shaped blind pouch

drench. A fluid drug administered by mouth; also to orally administer a fluid medication

dropping. A combination of feces and urates

dropsy. Ascites

dub. To surgically remove the comb

edema. An excessive accumulation of low-protein fluid in swollen or damaged tissues

egg discard time. The number of days that must pass after discontinuing drug use before eggs are considered safe for human consumption

electrolyte. Natural salts and other minerals present in small quantities in the body to help regulate body processes, maintain water balance, and preserve the acid/base balance

emaciation. Abnormal thinness

embryo. A unhatched chick developing within an incubated egg

embryonate. To develop an embryo inside a parasitic worm egg

encephalitis. Any inflammation of the brain

endospore. A bacterium in a dormant state protected within a tough triple-layer wall

energy. The amount of power produced when feed is metabolized

enteric disease. Any illness that causes inflammation of the intestines

enteritis. Any inflammation of the intestines

enterotoxin. A poison affecting the intestines, such as the cause of food poisoning

envelope. An outer layer that protects the capsid of some viruses

enzyme. A complex protein produced by living cells that serves as a catalyst for some aspect of cell metabolism, such as the digestion of food or the metabolism of energy

esophagus. The flexible tube that carries feed from the mouth to the crop and from there to the stomach

eversion. Condition of being turned inside out

extra-label. Description of a veterinarian-prescribed medication that is not approved by the FDA for treating chickens

exudate. Any fluid secretion associated with inflammation

fecal. Pertaining to feces

fecal-oral transmission. The spreading of an infection through ingesting contaminated poop

feces. The solid brownish or grayish portion of a poop consisting of digestive waste

finisher. A ration formulated to fatten meat birds prior to harvest

fluke. A leaf-shape trematode parasite

flush. To cleanse a body part by causing large quantities of water to pass over or through it

fomite. Any inanimate object on which pathogens may be transported from one place to another

free radicals. Unstable molecules that damage body cells and contribute to the development of disease

fungus. Any of a diverse group of plantlike organisms — including mushrooms, molds, mildews, and yeasts — that lack chlorophyll, live on dead or decaying organic matter, and reproduce through spores (plural: fungi)

gangrene. A potentially life-threatening condition in which body tissue dies because of infection (wet gangrene, as in gangrenous dermatitis) or a lack of blood flow to the affected part (dry gangrene, as in frostbite)

gaping. Opening the mouth wide while stretching the neck to get a good gulp of air; the chicken version of a yawn

gasping. Short, rapid inhaling caused by the inability to take a deep breath

genes. Parts of chromosomes that carry hereditary factors

genetic. Pertaining to genes or heredity

genetically engineered. Genetically modified

genetically modified. Describes a living thing into which genetic material from an unrelated organism has been unnaturally inserted; also called genetically engineered or transgenic

germs. Common collective name for disease-causing microbes

GMO. A genetically modified organism

going light. Growing thin while eating ravenously; synonym for anemia

gram-negative bacteria. Bacteria that have a thin wall surrounded by an outer membrane and that turn pink or red when stained

gram-positive bacteria. Bacteria that have a thick wall with no outer membrane and that turn blue or purple when stained

grit. Small, hard objects that accumulate in the gizzard to help grind up feeds

grit, inert. A hard form of grit that is not readily ground up in the gizzard

grit, mineral. A substance that serves as a source of both calcium and grit; also called calcium grit

gross. Easily seen with the naked eye

gross lesion. Any readily observable change in the color, size, shape, or structure of tissues or organs

grower. A ration formulated to optimize the growth of young chickens

gurgling. An intermittent, low-pitched bubbling respiratory sound at the beginning of inspiration and sometimes during expiration

hardware disease. Piercing of the gizzard by a sharp object that has been swallowed. Also called traumatic ventriculitis

helminth. A parasitic worm

helminthiasis. Infestation with parasitic worms

hemorrhage. The escape of blood from a ruptured blood vessel, especially resulting in heavy or uncontrolled bleeding

hepatitis. Any inflammation of the liver

horizontal transmission. The spread of a disease from one chicken to another by means other than from an infected breeder to offspring through eggs that hatch

hormone. A natural substance produced in the body that circulates in blood and other body fluids to control the activity of certain cells or organs

host. A bird (or other animal) on or in which a parasite or an infectious agent lives

hydrated lime. Calcium hydroxide, used to destroy pathogens in buried organic matter. Also called slaked lime, builder's lime, or mason's lime

hypervitaminosis. Any vitamin overload resulting in toxicity

immune. Resistant to a particular infection or toxin, thanks to the presence of specific antibodies or sensitized white blood cells. Also called resistant

immunity. The ability to resist a particular infection or toxin by means of antibodies or sensitized white blood cells. Also called resistance

immunity, active. Long-term resistance to a disease conferred by antibodies produced as a result of having had the disease or having been vaccinated against it

immunity, passive. Short-term resistance to a disease conferred by antibodies introduced from an outside source, such as maternal antibodies or injection with antiserum or antitoxin

immunoglobulin. A protein in the serum and cells of the immune system that has the same function as an antibody

immunosuppression. A partial or complete immobilization of the immune response

impaction. Any blockage of a body passage or cavity

incubation period. The time interval between exposure to a pathogen and the appearance of the first sign of disease; also, the time it takes for a bird's egg to hatch

indirect life cycle. A life cycle that involves an intermediate host

inert/inactive ingredients. Components of a compound that enhance the effectiveness of the active ingredient

infection. Invasion of body tissue by a pathogen that causes disease by developing or multiplying

infectious. Capable of invading and multiplying in the living tissue of another organism, causing disease

infertility. The inability to reproduce

inflammation. A swelling, often reddened, hot, and painful, occurring as a reaction to an injury or infection

ingest. To eat

inoculate. To introduce an infective agent or antigen to stimulate

resistance or produce disease for study

intermediate host. An animal in which a parasite lives during an immature stage in its life cycle. Also called an alternate host

intramuscular (IM). Administered into muscle tissue

intranasal. Administered into the nose

intraocular. Administered into the eye

intravenous (IV). Administered into a vein

-itis. A suffix indicating inflammation (e.g., sinusitis means inflammation of the sinus cavities)

keel. The breastbone or sternum

laceration. A jagged wound

lentogenic. Mildly virulent

lesion. Any change in the size, shape, color, or structure of body tissue or an internal organ as a result of damage caused by injury or disease

leukocytes. White blood cells

leukosis. An excess of leukocytes, or white blood cells

lime. See: agricultural lime; hydrated lime; quicklime

limiting. Description of an environmental variable, such as a nutrient, the presence or absence of which restricts growth, reproduction, and overall health

local infection. An infection confined to a limited area of the body

lymph. A watery fluid containing white blood cells that bathes the body's tissues and returns to the blood via the lymphatic system

lymphatic system. The part of the immune system consisting of a network through which lymph drains from body tissues into the blood

malabsorption. Poor intestinal absorption of nutrients

malignant tumor. Abnormal tissue growth that worsens, spreads, or recurs; also called cancer

maternal antibodies. Antibodies that protect newly hatched chicks by means of parental immunity

mesogenic. Moderately virulent

metabolism. All the physical and chemical processes that produce and maintain a living body

microbe. A microorganism, especially one that causes disease

microflora. Beneficial microorganisms living in the gut of a healthy chicken

microorganism. A microscopic organism, especially a bacterium, virus, or fungus

microscopic. Too small to be seen by the naked eye

minerals. Soluble nutrients derived from the weathering of chemical elements in the earth's crust and needed in small amounts for good growth and reproduction

mite. A small, spiderlike creature with a single-segmented body, exterior skeleton, and four pairs of jointed legs

mold. A type of fungus growing as a colony of slender tubular branches with a fuzzy appearance

molt. The natural periodic shedding and renewal of feathers

molt, hard. A rapid shedding combined with slow renewal of feathers

mortality. Percentage killed by a disease

mucous membranes. Tissues lining the body cavity and the tubular passages of the digestive and respiratory systems and that secrete mucus. Also called mucosa

mucus. A slimy substance produced by mucous membranes as a protective lubricant coating

mutate. To undergo a change in genetic character

mycosis. Any infection caused by members of the fungus family

mycotoxicosis. Any illness caused by a mycotoxin

mycotoxin. Any poison generated by the mold members of the fungus family

myocarditis. Any inflammation of the heart

myopathy. Any disease of the muscles

myositis. Any inflammation of the muscles

narrow spectrum. Description of a drug that affects a limited variety of pathogens

natural host. Also called definitive host or primary host; an animal in which a parasitic worm matures and reproduces sexually

natural immunization. Development of antibodies through exposure to viruses naturally occurring in the environment

necropsy. A postmortem examination (equivalent to a human autopsy)

necrotic. Pertaining to dead tissue

nematode. A roundworm

neoplasm. A tumor

neural. Pertaining to nerves

neuritis. Any inflammation of the peripheral nerves

neurotoxin. A poison that affects the nervous system

noninfectious. Describes an illness resulting from things other than an invading organism (such as nutritional issues, poisons, injury, or stress)

notifiable. Designation for diseases that are such a threat to the poultry industry or to human health that they must, by law, be reported to a state or federal veterinarian; also called reportable

nutraceutical. A food that provides health benefits, including the prevention and treatment of disease

nutrient. Any consumed substance that provides nourishment needed for growth and the maintenance of life

ocular. Pertaining to the eye

off-label. Description of a medication or other product used for poultry that is not specifically approved by the FDA

omphalitis. Any inflammation of the navel

oocyst. A tough membrane, or cyst, containing the fertile egg of a parasitic protozoa

opisthotonos. Muscle spasms in which the back arches and the head and tail are pulled over the back

opportunistic. Description of a pathogen that is noninfectious to a healthy individual but causes infection in an individual with weakened immunity

oral syringe. A syringe without a needle attached, used for washing out eyes or wounds

organism. Any living individual

osteopetrosis. A disorder in which the bones become hard and dense

osteoporosis. A disorder in which the bones become thin and weak

oviduct. The hen's 2-foot-long, multicompartmented passageway in which an egg develops

parasite. A living organism that invades the body of another organism, relying on its host for survival without returning benefit

parental immunity. Egg-transmitted antibodies acquired by a chick against diseases to which the mother hen is immune

pasting. Loose droppings sticking to the vent of a chick

pathogen. Any disease-causing organism

pathogen, primary. A pathogen that is capable of infecting an individual with a healthy immune system

pathogenic. Capable of causing disease

pathogenicity. Degree of ability to cause disease

pathologist. A veterinarian who specializes in diagnosing diseases primarily as a consultant

pathology. The science of studying the nature of diseases and their causes and consequences

pediculosis. Infestation with lice

pellets. A complete ration consisting of ingredients ground, mixed, and compressed

perosis. A metabolic condition in which the legs' long bones are shorter than normal; also called slipped tendon

persistence. Enduring effectiveness

pH. A number indicating the acidity or alkalinity of a solution; 7 is neutral, above 7 is alkaline, below 7 is acidic

pickout. Fatal vent damage due to cannibalism

pneumonia. Any inflammation of the lungs

post. To conduct a postmortem examination

postmortem. Pertaining to or occurring after death

prebiotic. A nutritional supplement that provides nutrients for the intestine's beneficial microbial population

predator-prey transmission. The spreading of an infection through eating a contaminated animal; regarding parasites it implies an indirect life cycle

predispose. To make susceptible (to disease)

prevalence. Measure of disease frequency

primary host. Natural host

primary pathogen. An organism that can infect a chicken with a healthy immune system

probiotic. A live microbial supplement that improves the intestine's beneficial microbial balance

progeny testing. Evaluating parents based on the health of their offspring

prolapse. The natural process by which a hen's vagina temporarily turns inside out to deposit an egg in the nest; failure of the tissue to retract is a potentially life-threatening condition

protein. A plant- or animal-derived feedstuff used by the body to build cells, tissues, and organs

protein, complete. A protein source, often of animal origin, that furnishes a balance of all the essential amino acids; also called high-quality protein

protein, ideal. The optimum combination of amino acids for a specific stage in life

protein, incomplete. A protein source of plant origin that is low in one or more of the essential amino acids

protozoa. One-cell microscopic organisms with animal-like characteristics (singular: protozoan)

proventriculus. The chicken's stomach

pullet. A female chicken under 1 year of age

quicklime. Calcium oxide, not to be confused with hydrated lime (calcium hydroxide) or agricultural lime (calcium carbonate)

rales. A brief, intermittent clicking or rattling sound caused when air is forced through respiratory passages narrowed by fluid or mucus

ration. The combination of all feed consumed

ration, complete. A feed that is supposed to furnish all the nutrients a chicken needs

reportable. Designation for diseases that are such a threat to the poultry industry or to human health that they must, by law, be reported to a state or federal veterinarian; also called notifiable

reservoir of infection. Any animate or inanimate object on which an infectious agent survives or multiplies and from which it can be transmitted to a susceptible host

residual effect. The amount of time a substance remains active after being applied or administered

resistance. The ability to resist a particular infection or toxin by means of antibodies or sensitized white blood cells; also called immunity

respiration rate. The number of breaths per minute

roup. A respiratory disease specific to poultry

salpingitis. Any inflammation of the oviduct

sanitize. To reduce pathogenic microbes to a level considered to be safe

sarcoma. A type of malignant tumor

secretion. A substance produced and released by a cell, gland, or organ

self-limiting. Description of a disease that runs its course and ultimately resolves itself without treatment

septicemia. A systemic infection that invades the body through the bloodstream; also called blood poisoning

serum. The clear, pale yellow, protein-rich liquid that separates out when blood clots (plural: sera)

shedding. The release of pathogens from an infected body

sign. A readily observable indication of illness

sinus. One of the four cavities in the dense portion of a skull bone that connect the nasal cavities, and through which air enters and mucus drains

sinusitis. Any inflammation of the sinus cavities

species specific. Associated with or affecting a single species

spirochetes. Bacteria in the order Spirochaetales that have a spiral shape and wiggle like a worm when viewed through a microscope

spleen. A round, purplish abdominal organ near the stomach that filters blood as part of the immune system

spore. A reproductive cell produced by fungi, and some bacteria and protozoa, capable of developing into a new individual without being fertilized by another reproductive cell

sporocyst. A tough membrane, or cyst, enclosing sporozoites within an oocyst

sporozoite. The infective stage of a parasitic protozoa

sporulate. The asexual development of sporozoites within an oocyst

spp. Abbreviation for *Species pluralis*, a Latin phrase meaning multiple species (as in *Salmonella* spp.)

stargazing. Backward arching of the head and neck, with the beak pointing skyward

starter. A ration formulated for baby chicks

stem cell. Any cell capable of producing an unlimited number of like cells with the potential to develop into many other kinds of cells with differing functions

sterile. Thoroughly clean

sternum. The breastbone or keel

stress. Any unfavorable condition that causes physical or mental disruption, thus creating anxiety and reducing resistance to disease

subcutaneous. Directly beneath the skin

superficial mycosis. A fungal infection of the skin or feather follicles, as opposed to an infection within the body

susceptibility. The inability to resist a particular infection or toxin

symptom. A subjective indication of disease as experienced by the affected individual

syndrome. A group of signs that typically occur together and appear as a specific, but poorly defined, disease

synergism. The phenomenon whereby two substances together have a greater total effect that the sum of their individual effects

synergist. An additive used to increase the potency of a compound's active ingredient

synovitus. Any inflammation of the membranes lining joints

syringe. A tube with a plunger used to release liquid in a thin stream (such as for flushing out wounds) or fitted with a hollow needle for injecting drugs or withdrawing blood or other fluids

systemic. Affecting the entire body

take. A reaction that indicates successful vaccination

TCO vaccine. Tissue culture origin vaccine, safe for use in backyard chickens

thermoregulation. The ability to maintain core temperature within certain limits despite changes in air temperature

topical. Applied directly to an external body part

torticollis. Twisting of the neck; also called twisted neck or wryneck

toxin. A poison produced by or derived from microorganisms

toxoid. A toxin that has been treated to reduce its toxic effect for use as a vaccine to confer active immunity

trachea. The windpipe

transgenic. Genetically modified

transovarian transmission. Transfer of an infection from a hen to her chicks through the eggs they hatch from; also called vertical transmission

trauma. A distressing situation; also a physical injury

traumatic ventriculitis. The piercing of the gizzard from the inside by a sharp object that has been swallowed; also called hardware disease

trematode. A parasitic flatworm known as a fluke

trickle infection. Gradual exposure to a pathogen, resulting in immunity

tumor. A mass of tissue that abnormally develops and grows, usually without inflammation, which may be either benign or malignant

twisted neck. A condition in which the head turns to one side or to some other abnormal position; also called wryneck; technically, torticollis

ulcer. An open sore that fails to heal

unthrifty. Eating well while growing thin and/or laying poorly

urates. Uric acid (salts found in urine), the off-white, cream-colored, or yellowish cap on poop — the chicken version of urine

urolith. A kidney stone

vaccine. A biological preparation derived from disease-causing organisms and used to produce immunity against those same organisms

vector. An organism, typically a biting or bloodsucking insect or tick, that spreads a disease or parasite

vehicle. Any object or living thing that mechanically transports disease organisms or parasites from one place to another

velogenic. Highly virulent

vent. The outside opening of the cloaca

ventriculus. The gizzard

vermifuge. Also called anthelmintic; any dewormer

vertebrae. The small bones collectively forming the backbone (singular: vertebra)

vertebrate. Any animal, including a chicken or a human, that has a backbone

vertical transmission. Transfer of an infection from a hen to her chicks through the eggs they hatch from; also called transovarian transmission

VetRx. An old-time natural veterinary remedy used to relieve respiratory signs; its corn oil base makes it also effective as a treatment against leg mites

virulent. The degree of infectiveness of a pathogen as indicated by the severity or harmfulness of disease it produces

virus. A microscopic parasitic entity able to multiply only inside the living cell of another being, and consisting of a genome, protein coat, and sometimes an outer envelope

viscera. The soft internal organs within the main body cavity

visceral. Pertaining to the viscera

vitamins. A variety of nutrients that are essential in small amounts to regulate metabolism

vitamins, fat-soluble. Vitamins that are stored in body fat and used as needed

vitamins, water-soluble. Vitamins that are not stored by the body, but are used as immediately needed and the remainder excreted in droppings

water. An essential nutrient required by all body functions

waterbelly. Ascites

withdrawal period. The number of days that must pass after discontinuing drug use before the chicken's meat is considered safe for human consumption. Also called withdrawl time

wryneck. A condition in which the head turns to one side or to some other abnormal position; technically, torticollis

zoonosis. A disease transmissible from a chicken (or other animal) to a human (plural: zoonoses)

Index

Page numbers in *italics* indicate drawings and photographs. Page numbers in **bold** indicate tables and charts.

A

Acariasis, 126. *See also* Mites
Acquired immunity, 28–29, *29*
Active immunity, 28, *29*
Active ingredients, 126
Aerosol vaccination, 285
Aflatoxicosis, 248–249, **248**, *249*, 421
Agrobacterium tumefaciens, 41
Air flow, 11–13, 109
Air sac disease (airsacculitis), 76, **220**, 328, 421–422
Air-sac mite, **127**, 130
Air sacs, 73–74, *74*, **75**, 76–77, 359
Ajoene, 386–387
Albendazole, 183, **184–185**
Aleukemic myeloid leukosis, **266–267**
Algae biofilm, 303–304
Alkaloids, 216, 310
Alkalosis, 116–117
Allergies, 180, 245, 403–404
Allicin, 386–387
Alltech Acid-Pak 4-Way, 386
Alternative remedies. *See* Natural remedies
Amanita mushrooms, *307*
American Association of Feed Control Officials (AAFCO), 391
Amino acids, 45, 46–50
Aminocyclitols, 243
Aminoglycosides, **239**, 243, **244**
Ammonia, 15, 75–76, 96, 311, 399
Amprolium, 206, **206**, **207**
Amputation, 300–302
Anemia, 100, 357
Animal and Plant Health Inspection Service (APHIS), 418, **418**
Anthelmintics, 179, 181, 373. *See also* Dewormers

Antibacterial agents, 238. *See also* Antibiotics
Antibiotics. *See also* Specific antibiotics
  aminoglycosides, **239**, 243, **244**
  bacitracin, 182, **239**, 242, **244**
  botulism and, 231
  for canker, 216
  caveats for use of, 244–245
  colloidal silver, 389
  commonly used for bacterial infections, **245**
  erythromycin, **239**, 243–244, **244**, **245**
  fowl cholera and, 232
  gram staining and, 240
  hygromycin and, 182
  overview of, 238–241, **239**
  penicillins, **239**, 242, **244**
  relative effectiveness of, **244**
  salmonellae and, 228
  sour crop and, 255
  spectinomycin, **239**, 243, **244**
  spectrum ranges of, 239
  sulfa drugs, 206, **207**, 241
  tetracyclines, **239**, 241, 242–243, **244**
  tylosin, 243–244, **244**, **245**
Antibodies, 28, 64, 65, 67
Anticoccidials, 204–207, **206**, **207**
Antigens, 28, 64
Antinutrients, 45, 46, 310
Antioxidants, 38, 45, 50, 57. *See also* Specific antioxidants
Antiprotozoals, 204–207, **206**, **207**, 373
Antiseptic solutions, 396
Antiviral agents, 277. *See also* Vaccines
Apple cider vinegar, 383
Apteria, 62, *63*
Aragonite, 55, **55**

Arizonosis, **220**, 227, 422
Arthritis, **220**, 223, 422–423
Articular gout, 443–444
Ascites, 110–112, *112*, 328, 423, *423*
Aspergillosis, *254*, **254**, 403, 424
Aspirin, 395–396
Atlas of Avian Diseases (Cornell), 363
Atrophy, 62, 357
Attachment, 259, *259*
Autonomic nervous system, 67, 95
Avian influenza
  in humans, **404**, 407–408
  NPIP certification and, 8
  overview of, **260**, 274–276, **275**, 424–425
Avian leukosis viruses (ALV), 42, 263–264, **266–267**
Avian tuberculosis, **220**, 235–236, 426

B

Bacillus thuringiensis (Bt), 39–41
Bacitracin, 182, **239**, 242, **244**
Bacteria, 217–219, *219*, 240, **240**. *See also* Specific bacteria
Bacterial diseases. *See also* Antibiotics; Clostridial diseases; Colibacillosis; Salmonellosis; Staphylococcosis; Zoonoses
  antibiotics commonly used for, **244**, **245**
  avian tuberculosis, **220**, 235–236, 426
  campylobacteriosis, **220**, 236–237, **404**, **413**, 414–415, 429
  chlamydiosis, **220**, 237, 430–431

of neurologic disorders, 337–
338, **337**, **339**
of respiratory disorders,
329–330, **330**
signs of health and illness,
327–329, **327**
syndromes and, 328
of untimely death, 349,
350–351
Diarrhea, 324, 333
Diatomaceous earth (DE), 15,
137, 155–156, 186–187
Diet, 60, **60**. *See also* Nutrition
Differential diagnosis, 329, 353,
354
Digestive system
crop binding and, 79
diagnosis of disorders, 331–
333, **331**, *333*, **333**, **334**,
335, 336, **336**
enteric diseases and, 84, **84**
hardware disease and, 80
intestines, 81, **81**, 84
liver, 80, 81
low calcium and, 118
necropsy and, 361
overview of, 78, 82, *83*
pendulous crop and, 79–80
pH levels of, *384*
stomachs, 80
vinegar and, 382–383, *384*
Direct contact, 5, 6
Direct life cycle, 166, *166*, 167,
168
Dirt, 9, 30
Discharge chamber, 85, *85*
Discoloration, conditions causing, 346, **347–348**
Disease-resistant chickens, 42
Disinfection, 16–19, 311
Disposal of dead birds, 370
Diverticula, 70
DL-methionine, 115
DNA viruses, 258, **258**
Drenches, 181
Drinkers, 10, 36–37, *36*, 109
Drinking water. *See* Water
Droppings. *See* Feces; Poop
Droppings boards and pits, 9, *10*

Drug interactions, 180
Drugs. *See* Medications
Drying, disinfection and, 21
Duodenum, 81, 82, *83*
Dust bathing, 158–159, *159*

E

Ears, 98–99
Egg binding, 92–93, **92**, 232
Egg eating, **295**, 297
Egg peritonitis, 220, 437
Eggs
binding and, 92–93, **92**
calcium and, 116–117
causes of decline in production of, 315–321, **322**, 343,
343–345
causes of odd, 320
contamination of, 404, 411–
416, **413**
development of, 89–90, *90*
dewormers and, 180
diagnosis and, 343, **343–345**
heat stress and, 107
medullary bone and, 70
passive immunity and, 28
as protein supplement, 48
reproductive disorders and,
91–94
salmonellosis and, 226
sanitation and, 412
storage of, 415
toxins in, 306
vertical disease transmission
and, 5
withdrawal period and, 180–
181, 245, 377
Eggshells, 55
Eimeria spp., 197–201, **200**
Electrolytes, 116, 385–386, **386**
Emasculatomes, 357
Encephalomalacia, 52, 119, *119*,
437
Endospores, 229
Energy, 43–45, 67, 102. *See also*
Metabolism
Enlist Weed Control System, 41
Enteritis, overview of, 84, **84**

Enterococcosis, **220**, 238
Enveloped viruses, 258, **258**
Environment. *See* Day length;
Housing; Temperature
Epidemic tremor, **260**, 276–277,
277, 438
Epididymal lithiasis, 89, 328, 438
Epididymis, *87*
Epsom salts, 58, 190, 255, 392
Ergotism, **248**, 249–250, 439
Erysipelas, **220**, 237, 439–440
Erysipeloid, **404**, 408
Erythrocytes, 100
Erythroid leukosis, 266–267
Erythromycin, **239**, 243–244,
244, 245
Escherichia coli infections, **220**,
231–232, *232*, 413, 416
Esophagus, 78, 359
Essential amino acids, 46
European chick fleas, 137
Euthanasia, 356–357
Evaporation, 106–107
Exotic Newcastle disease, 273
Exploratory behavior, 26
Extension Toxicology Network
(EXTONET), 148
Extra-label use, 181, 241
Exudative diathesis, 52, 440
Eyedrop vaccination, 283
Eyes, 50, 96–97, 98, **262**, 340,
341–342
Eye worm, 170–171, **194**

F

Fabricius, Hieronymus, 65
Farmer's lung, **404**, 405
Fat, 47, 108, 360
Fatty liver syndrome, 80, 112,
328, 440
Feather mite, **127**, 130, **160**
Feather picking, 295–296, **295**
Feathers, 48, 62, *63*, 108, *251*,
296
Feather tracts, 62, *63*
Fecal chamber, 84, *85*
Fecal exams, 187–192, *189*,
193–195

Pendulous crop, 79–80, 458
Penetration, 259, *259*
Penicillins, **239**, 242, **244**
Penis, 87, *87*
Peritonitis, 94, **220**, 232, 437
Permethrin, 152
Pesticides, 126, 311. *See also*
 Insecticides
Petroleum jelly, **160–161**
Peyer's patches, 66
pH, 19, 381–385, *382, 384. See*
 also Vinegar
Phenols, 11, 18–19
Phosphorus, 54–55, **55**, 116
Pickout, 93
Piling, 311–312
Pillbugs, 177–178
Pinkeye, **404**, 409
Pink tissue, 199, 332
Piperazine, 180, 181, **184–185**
Piperonyl butoxide (PBO), 154
Plants, 164, **308–309**, 392–393,
 394
Pneumatic bones, 70, *71*
Poisoning. *See also* Botulism;
 Mycotoxicoses
 chicks and, 311
 coccidiostats and, 206
 insecticides and, 152
 plants and, **308–309**
 preventing, 305–311,
  308–309
 rodents and, 293–294
Polysporin, 242
Polyunsaturated fats, 47
Poop, 332–334, *333*, **334**, **335**,
 336, **336**. *See also* Digestive
 system; Feces
Postmortem examinations
 disposal of dead birds and,
  370
 do-it-yourself, 355–363
 overview of, 353
 pathology laboratories and,
  352–354
 potential findings of,
  364–369
Potatoes, **308–309**, 310
Poultry bugs, 136

PoultrySulfa, 206, **207**
Povidone iodine, 396
Prebiotics, 378–380, 387
Predator-prey transmission, 166
Preen glands, 64
Primary pathogens, 2, 247, 253
Probiotics, 378–380, 382
Progeny testing, 28, 31–32
Prolapse, 93, *94*
Protein, 33, 47–50, **48**
Protozoal diseases. *See also*
 Coccidiosis
 blackhead disease, **197**, 212–
  214, *213*, 426–427
 canker, **197**, 214–216, *214*,
  215, **215**, 429–430
 cryptosporidiosis, **197**, 211–
  212, 435–436
 overview of, 196, **197**
 toxoplasmosis, **197**, 209–211,
  210, **404**, 410–411, **413**,
  465
Proventriculus, 80
Pseudobotulism, **262**
Pseudomonas infections, **220**,
 238, **404**, 406, 459–460
Pterylae, 62, *63*
Pubic bones, 315
Pullorum, 8, **220**, 227, 228, 460
Pyrethrins, 137, 153–154,
 160–161
Pyrethroids, 150–152, **160–161**
Pyrethrum, 153, 154
Pyridoxine, **54**

Q

Quarantine, 22
Quats, 19
Quicklime, 370
Quinoa, 46

R

Radiant space heaters, 109
Range confinement, 8
Rations. *See* Diet; Feeds
Rats, 288–289, **288**, *289*, 291
Recombinant vaccine, 272

Red blood cells, 100
Red Cell supplement, 100
Red mite, 126–128, **127**, **160**
Redworm, 48
Reflex behavior, 25–26
Remedies for Health Problems
 of the Organic Laying Flock
 (Glos), 395
Replication, 259, *259*
Reportable diseases, 258, 417–
 418, **418**
Reproductive system (female),
 89–95, *90*, 362
Reproductive system (male),
 87–89, *87*, 362
Reservoirs of infection, 2–3
Resistance
 antibiotics and, 244–245
 Bacillus thuringiensis (Bt)
  and, 39–41
 breeding for, 30–32
 to dewormers, 179
 to insecticides, 148
 to sulfa drugs, 241
 to tetracyclines, 242
 vaccines and, 277
Respiration rate, **64**
Respiratory alkalosis, *384*
Respiratory heat transfer, 106
Respiratory mite, **127**, 130
Respiratory system
 air flow and, 74, *75*
 airsacculitis and, 76
 air sacs, 73–74, *74*, **75**, 76–77
 body temperature and, 106
 conditions affecting, 77, 78,
  78
 defenses of, 75–76
 diagnosis of disorders, 329–
  330, **330**
 dust bathing and, 158–159
 overview of, 73, *76*
 pneumatic bones and, 70
 ruptured air sacs and, 76–77,
  77
 voice box and, 73
Resting the coop, 20
Rest patterns, 26
Riboflavin, **54**, 121

Other Storey Books by Gail Damerow

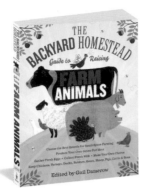

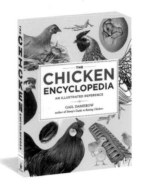

Now you can raise chickens, goats, sheep, cows, pigs, honeybees, and more, in your own backyard! With expert advice on everything from housing to feeding and health care, learn how to keep happy, productive animals on as little as one-tenth of an acre.

From albumen to zygote, the terminology of everything chicken is demystified in this illustrated, A-to-Z reference. With breeds, common chicken conditions and behaviors, and much more, here are all the answers to any chicken quandary.

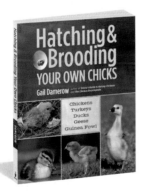

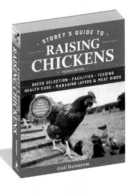

A definitive guide to hatching healthy baby chickens, ducklings, goslings, turkey poults, and guinea keets, this has information on everything from selecting breeds, having the proper incubator and setup, sanitary conditions, embryo development, and much more.

This ultimate guide has all the information you need to raise happy, healthy chickens, from selecting breeds and building coops to hatching chicks, incubation, sanitation, complete health care, safety from predators, and much more.

Join the conversation. Share your experience with this book, learn more about Storey Publishing's authors, and read original essays and book excerpts at storey.com. Look for our books wherever quality books are sold or call 800-441-5700.